Handbook on Mental Health Administration

Michael J. Austin
William E. Hershey
General Editors

Handbook on Mental Health Administration

Jossey-Bass Publishers

San Francisco • Washington • London • 1982

HANDBOOK ON MENTAL HEALTH ADMINISTRATION
by Michael J. Austin and William E. Hershey, General Editors

Copyright © 1982 by: Jossey-Bass Inc., Publishers
433 California Street
San Francisco, California 94104
&

Jossey-Bass Limited
28 Banner Street
London EC1Y 8QE

Library of Congress Cataloging in Publication Data
Main entry under title:

Handbook on mental health administration.

Includes bibliographies and indexes.
1. Mental health services—Administration.
I. Austin, Michael J. II. Hershey, William E.
RA790.5.H29   1982   362.2'1'068   82-48058
ISBN 0-87589-544-1

Manufactured in the United States of America

The paper in this book meets the guidelines for
permanence and durability of the Committee on
Production Guidelines for Book Longevity of the
Council on Library Resources.

JACKET DESIGN BY WILLI BAUM

FIRST EDITION

Code 8226

The Jossey-Bass
Social and Behavioral Science Series

❦ Preface ❧

Many administrators in community and institutional mental health programs have not had the opportunity to acquire management training. More often than not, practitioners have been promoted within agencies to management positions without either a solid background in managerial knowledge and skills or a clear understanding of their new roles and responsibilities. As more and more clinicians assume administrative responsibilities and as staff training funds are cut as a result of overall agency belt tightening, the mental health field will increasingly need practical, agency-related, managerial resources. Unfortunately, the recent literature has focused almost exclusively on *top* management and has not taken into account the information needed by middle managers to effectively administer and supervise programs and staff.

Handbook on Mental Health Administration is designed to fill the need for current and comprehensive coverage of both general administration and specific service delivery problems. It discusses clinical and policy issues related to supervisory management, the managerial skills necessary for program and service management, and ways to manage service delivery to clients with different mental health needs. Written by experienced mental health practitioners, administrators, and educators, it combines practical wisdom with relevant social and behavioral science theory and knowledge. Each chapter was specially commissioned for this volume.

Conceived as a working administrative resource, the handbook will benefit mental health professionals with varying degrees of managerial experience, responsibility, and interest in program administration. Experienced middle managers as well as higher-level administrators can refresh their knowledge or gain new insights by selecting chapters on specific issues or ones suited to the problems at hand. Recently appointed managers can read the chapters consecutively for a solid understanding of management issues and effective mental health administration—as can clinicians who are considering the transition to administrative roles. Students in mental health, health services administration, and public administration programs can gain an overview of what program management and staff supervision involves. In short, the handbook provides both a knowledge base and a skill repertoire for administering a variety of mental health programs.

The introduction puts the various issues of management practice into perspective, pointing out the special difficulties clinicians face when they make the transition to managerial roles. Part One begins with a discussion of how administrators and clinical staff members view one another and then reviews current treatment methodologies and delineates medications management. Part Two presents societal perspectives on the administration of mental health programs and discusses mental health public policy and law, minority group perspectives, and the changing role of women in the management of mental health services.

Part Three covers a range of key program management functions and skill areas, including general planning; analysis of mental health organizations; management of interdisciplinary teams; staff-meeting management; management as problem solving; work with governing boards; management of volunteers; labor-management relations; human resource planning; financial management; use of management information systems; program evaluation; quality assurance; and community needs assessment.

Part Four deals with the management of a wide range of specialized mental health services and related human service programs—residential mental health facilities; community support programs; services for the mentally ill offender; alcohol and drug abuser services; occupational therapy services; services for the developmentally disabled; mental health services for women, for the aged, and for children; preventive mental health services; and rural mental health services.

Acknowledgments

This book became a reality with the assistance, in part, of the National Institute of Mental Health, Division of Manpower and Training, Social Work Education Training Branch. With the support of the University of Washington School of Social Work, a special post-master's degree management certificate program in mental health administration was begun in 1979. The material in all the chapters was developed to further the education of middle-management personnel in mental health programs in the Pacific Northwest. The success of this program is the result of collaboration between an advisory committee of experienced mental health administrators, a group of talented certificate program participants, a dedicated project support staff, and the able program leadership of an experienced mental health administrator, who left the directorship of the Seattle Crisis Clinic to manage the mental health administration and planning project.

Many people were involved in the development of this handbook. We wish to express our appreciation to Scott Briar, dean of the University of Washington School of Social Work, for his encouragement and support. The field test of the chapters was greatly facilitated by Elissa Dyson, Sally Graves, Gail Nyman-York, and the special typing talents of Joan Hiltner and Cindy Della Monica. Comments and feedback on each chapter were gained from members of an advisory committee and the participants of the management certificate program. The advisory committee was composed of experienced mental health administrators, and we gratefully acknowledge the assistance of Jack Bartleson, Donald Berg, Al Casale, Robert Cherniack, Joann Costello, Betty Docekal, Jack Ellis, Carl Gaddis, John Lavalle, Barbara Mauer, Paul Peterson, Helen Schwedenberg, Donald Seidemann, Patricia Steele, Florence Stier, Calvin Takagi, and Johan Verhulst. Participants in the management certificate program provided detailed feedback on each chapter; we wish to thank Scott Bond, Martha Calabretta, Maureen A. Conroyd, Jeannette Dezsofi, Mary Jane Dunlap, Fred Edward, Jr., Lisa Giles, Ann Harvey, Martin Hemmann, Harriet Kirk, Nellbyrt Landstad, Robert Lenigan, Roland Lindstrom, Sharon Nations, Cynthia Neuffer, Kenneth Pearce, John Powers, Roberta Rohr, Theresa Rubin, Carol Simmons, Melvin Warn, W. Brent Winderbaum, Miriam Wise, and Arnold Wrede.

We also wish to acknowledge the valuable assistance of the Jossey-Bass staff. We hope that the handbook provides the relevant knowledge and skills needed by busy program managers seeking to deliver quality mental health services to people in need.

Seattle, Washington   Michael J. Austin
July 1982   William E. Hershey

ଓ Contents ଓ

   Perspectives of clinical staff members should be taken
   into account by the mental health program manager who
   wants to increase job satisfaction, improve organizational
   communications, and enhance staff supervision.

   A review of the basic mental health treatment methodologies of crisis intervention, the psychotherapies, advocacy,
   and consultation can help managers maintain a clear
   focus on the goals of community mental health programming and the implications of treatment orientations
   for staffing programs.

Part Two: Social Issues Affecting Administration and Planning

Part Three: Key Management Roles and Functions

Part Four: Managing Special Services

Community support programs require managerial skill
in helping consumers secure government benefits, providing crisis stabilization support and medical services,
and implementing a case management system.

The administrative and clinical tasks involved in serving
the mentally ill offender include developing services for a
wide range of client needs and staff roles related to deinstitutionalization and improving coordination between
the mental health and criminal justice systems.

Current knowledge about mood-changing drugs, their effects, and their implications both for staff and for agency
relations with other community agencies is critical.

Mental health managers should not overlook the potential of occupational therapy services, including evaluation and treatment, in meeting the needs of the mentally
ill.

How legislation defines developmental disabilities, ways
to meet the psychosocial needs of the developmentally
disabled, current service provisions and gaps, and future
directions for mental health services are all issues that
need to be addressed by mental health managers serving
the developmentally disabled.

Assessing the mental health needs of women and exploring new approaches for planning and delivering nonsexist mental health services can help program managers
move beyond traditional ideas about women in society.

> Program managers serving the aged should be aware of the mental health needs of older persons, relevant treatment approaches for them, community network considerations, and the importance of upgrading staff capabilities in geriatric mental health services.

> Analyzing the critical administrative issues of service costs, staff training, program coordination, and service accountability can better enable program managers to understand and meet the mental health needs of children.

> Prevention and promotion in mental health services begins with the positive attitude of administrators and staff and can evolve through a continuum of services that takes into account target populations, methods of treatment, and worker roles.

> Delivery of mental health services in rural areas requires the development of generalist skills among staff, outreach services, and personal relationships that respect local customs.

❦ The Authors ❦

Michael J. Austin is professor and director, Center for Social Welfare Research, the School of Social Work, University of Washington. He also is chairperson of the Community and Organizational Services Track, which prepares graduate social work students for careers in planning, policy, and administration.

Austin was awarded the B.A. degree in political science and the M.S.W. degree from the University of California at Berkeley in 1964 and 1966, respectively; he was awarded the M.S. degree in public health and the Ph.D. degree in social work from the University of Pittsburgh in 1969 and 1970, respectively.

Austin served as director of the Mental Health Administration and Planning Project at the University of Washington, which facilitated the development of this handbook. At the National Institute of Mental Health, he was regional mental health services consultant in Denver, as well as grants review consultant to the Center of State Mental Health Manpower Planning. Recently, he was consultant to the Division of Mental Health, Washington State Department of Social and Health Services, and to the King County Mental Health Division on the management of involuntary treatment services.

Austin is author and/or coauthor of several books, including *Administration for the Human Services* (with W. H. Ehlers, 1976); *Delivering Human Services* (1977); *Professionals and Paraprofessionals* (1978); *Management Simula-*

tions for Mental Health and Human Services Administration (1978); and *Supervisory Management for the Human Services* (1981). He has contributed articles to *Administration in Mental Health* and is a member of both the American College of Mental Health Administration and the National Association of Social Workers.

WILLIAM E. HERSHEY is associate faculty in the School of Social Work, University of Washington. He also directs the Certificate of Management Program sponsored by the Office of Continuing Education in the School of Social Work, which prepares clinicians with post-master's degrees for careers in middle management.

Hershey has a broad background in the management of mental health services. He served as coordinator and curriculum specialist of the Mental Health Administration and Planning Project and wrote a number of the modules that are included as chapters in this handbook. He was planning budget director for the United Way of Pierce County, Washington, and executive director of the Seattle Crisis Clinic. He has served as management consultant to the Division of Mental Health, Washington State Department of Social and Health Services, and to the United Way of King County, Washington. Hershey is also a volunteer trainer for the Kellogg–United Way Governing Boards training project in the Pacific Northwest. He is a member of the American Association of Suicidology and of the National Association for Social Workers.

Hershey was awarded the B.A. degree in history from Gettysburg College in 1955, the M.Div. degree from Lutheran Theological Seminary in 1960, the M.A. degree in history from the University of Pennsylvania in 1965, and the M.S.W. degree from the University of Washington in 1973.

Linda Bellerby, research associate, Regional Research Institute for Human Services, Management Information System Project, Portland State University

John R. Brinkley, lecturer, Department of Psychiatry and Behavioral Sciences, School of Medicine, University of Washington; attending psychiatrist, Harborview Community Mental Health Center

Maureen A. Conroyd, coordinator, Family and Child Services, Eastside Mental Health Center, Seattle

Gary B. Cox, research associate professor, Department of Psychiatry and Behavioral Sciences, School of Medicine, University of Washington

Jill Crowell, management consultant, Division of Mental Health, Washington State Department of Social and Health Services, Olympia

Linda Dreyer, assistant professor, Regional Research Institute for Human Services, School of Social Work, Portland State University

Ellen Russell Dunbar, professor, School of Social Work, Eastern Washington University

Stephanie J. FallCreek, research associate, School of Social Work, University of Washington

Robert T. Fraser, research assistant professor, Epilepsy Center, Department of Neurological Surgery, University of Washington

Barbara J. Friesen, doctoral candidate, School of Social Work, University of Washington

Joseph S. Gallegos, assistant professor, School of Social Work, University of Washington

Naomi Gottlieb, professor and associate dean, School of Social Work, University of Washington

Mary Davis Hall, assistant professor, Graduate School of Public Affairs, University of Washington

Sylvia Harlock, hospital planner, Puget Sound Health Systems Agency, Seattle

Nancy R. Hooyman, associate professor, School of Social Work, University of Washington

Benson Jaffee, professor, School of Social Work, University of Washington

Nancy Koroloff, assistant professor, Regional Research Institute for Human Services, School of Social Work, Portland State University

Jean Marie Kruzich, assistant professor, School of Social Welfare, University of Wisconsin, Milwaukee

Bernadette I. D. Lalonde, research associate, School of Social Work, University of Washington

LeNora B. Mundt, former associate professor, School of Social Work, University of Washington; now in private practice

Kermit B. Nash, professor, School of Social Work, and director, University Hospital Department of Social Services, University of Washington

Anne Strode Nelson, program consultant, Division of Mental Health, Washington State Department of Social and Health Services, Olympia

Rino J. Patti, professor, School of Social Work, University of Washington

Peter J. Pecora, doctoral candidate, School of Social Work, University of Washington

Nancy Peterfreund, health planning specialist, Seattle-King County Department of Public Health, Seattle

Herman B. Resnick, professor, School of Social Work, University of Washington

Mary Richardson, instructor, Department of Health Services Administration, School of Public Health, and administrator, Clinical Training Unit, Child Development and Mental Retardation Center, University of Washington

Roger A. Roffman, associate professor, School of Social Work, University of Washington

Theresa Aragón Valdez, director, City of Seattle Department of Human Services

Richard A. Weatherley, associate professor, School of Social Work, University of Washington

❦ Handbook ❦
on Mental Health
Administration

᭰ Introduction ᭰

Issues in Management Practice

Michael J. Austin
William E. Hershey

The management of community mental health programs has become a complex job for mental health practitioners, irrespective of their previous clinical training experiences. Clinicians are assuming middle-management positions as coordinators of outpatient, day treatment, and consultation services or as directors of inpatient, children's, or community support services. These positions demand a working knowledge of a wide range of community mental health programs, a recognition of the transition from clinical to middle-management roles and functions, and the acquisition of mental health management knowledge and skills. This introductory chapter addresses these three demands.

We begin with a description of twelve types of community mental health services reflected in federal legislation, although we cannot be certain that these major service components will continue to serve as the foundation for community mental health programming in the future. New directions emerging from our nation's capital appear to be changing the face of the mental health map in this country. Most notably, the Mental Health Systems Act of 1980, which sought to provide community services related to the chronically mentally ill, unserved and underserved populations, and the prevention of mental illness, appears to have died for lack of federal funding authorization. The new political philosophy de-emphasizes federal directions and guidelines and encourages decision making at the state level through the use of block grants. How states will determine funding allocations for mental health services is not clear. Some may follow the principles underlying the Mental Health Systems Act of 1980. Others may further reduce their support of community mental health programs. Still others may proceed on the basis of "business as usual," thereby continuing their current approach to funding mental health services. In some states, the increasing demands of state hospitals—brought about, in part, by new state involuntary treatment laws—may result in the increased allocation of state funds to support state hospitals.

In any event, the role and structure of community mental health services are likely to change in the decade ahead. At present, however, twelve basic community mental health services are in various stages of implementation and consolidation in communities across the country.

Community Mental Health Services

Inpatient Services. Under Public Law (PL) 94–63, federally funded community mental health programs are required to provide inpatient services, which may include milieu therapy, psychotherapy, chemotherapy, recreational therapy, occupational therapy, and medical treatment when needed, as well as diagnostic assessment and evaluation for the courts and for community physicians. Full-time or part-time psychiatrists admit patients directly to hospitals and supervise their treatment, attempting to link a patient's hospital stay and follow-up to outpatient services by involving mental health center staff and the patient's physician before, during, and after hospitalization.

Inpatient programs usually provide short-term intensive services: 80 to 90 percent of all patients who receive inpatient care are released within two to six weeks. Transfer at this point is to another service in the community mental health system, to a local physician, or to a nursing home or state mental hospital for long-term care. Persons who need twenty-four-hour care include potentially suicidal clients, persons suffering deep depression and unable to function, acute schizophrenics requiring close supervision because of disordered behavior, violently acting-out youths, and elderly persons who are extremely confused and unable to manage themselves.

Because of the traditional shortage of local inpatient beds and/or stringent admissions criteria, community mental health programs needing to hospitalize clients must be prepared to use whatever resource is available and appropriate for the client. For example, a network of informal relationships among community hospitals may be used to facilitate emergency admissions. Across the country, members of health planning councils, hospital associations, and mental health agencies are developing plans for the coordinated delivery of inpatient care services.

In recent years, the number of adults and children involuntarily committed to inpatient care facilities has increased greatly, far surpassing the capacity of local psychiatric units to care for them. As a result, increasing numbers of clients are referred to state hospitals. In addition, some states utilize special long-term care facilities to treat chronically mentally ill adults who have had one or more hospital admissions for psychiatric treatment. If the trend toward more hospitalizations increases because of changes in involuntary treatment statutes, there will be heavy demands on the inpatient portion of the community mental health system. Administrators will need to seek improvements in the whole system so that relief of pressure at one point in the system will not cause difficulties in other areas. A well-defined, well-designed, and well-implemented continuum of care is needed for mentally ill adults.

Further, there seems to be a growing recognition that the widespread state hospital deinstitutionalization of the 1960s has not been altogether successful because of the lack of funds to support community mental health services, and, as a result, the chronically ill person is shuttled between uncoordinated, inadequate services before the inevitable readmission. The comprehensiveness of treatment demanded by the chronically ill person, the difficulty in managing such treatment on an outpatient basis, and the huge expense of the admission-readmission cycle all suggest a possible role for long-term hospitalization. It appears that the optimism of the 1960s, which resulted in predictions that state hospitals would completely disappear, has yielded to more rational and more realistic views of long-term care.

Outpatient Services. Outpatient community mental health services—which include the evaluation, diagnosis, and treatment of psychiatric problems, along with referral to other resources as needed—are designed to help clients continue functioning in their daily lives. Outpatients usually receive one hour or more per week of either individual or group therapy, with the choice of treatment approach left to the clinician. In some programs, a variety of therapeutic approaches is represented among members of the staff, with easy referral to a therapist with the special competencies best suited to meet a particular client's needs. Other outpatient programs develop a primary treatment approach, such as a medical model with heavy emphasis on medications or a behavioral model with emphasis on learning new coping behavior. A typical outpatient caseload would range from twelve to twenty-four clients seen for short-term treatment of up to three months, with a portion of the caseload seen in group therapy sessions. One approach to screening and assigning outpatients is the use of the Global Assessment Scale to assess the degree of severity of mental illness and the client's capacity to function. Using a hundred-point scale, expectations of behavioral functioning are attached to each level of the scale—for example, "21–30" reflects an inability to function in almost all areas and usually indicates that the client is seriously disturbed (see Table 1).

In addition to contracting with local mental health centers for basic outpatient services, counties may also contract with various nonprofit agencies for specific outpatient services. Such outpatient contracts might include drop-in centers providing activity therapy, emotional support groups, training programs for seriously disturbed adults, culturally sensitive services oriented to the needs of Hispanic, Asian, and American Indian populations, services oriented to the needs of sexual minorities, or vocationally oriented outpatient services that include work evaluation and adjustment services with related job sampling, job placement, and sheltered workshops.

Table 1. Global Assessment Scale.

No Dysfunction

100   No symptoms; superior functioning in a wide range of activities; life's problems
       never seem to get out of hand; is sought out by others because of his or her warmth
91   and integrity.

90   Transient symptoms may occur, but good functioning in all areas; interested and
       involved in a wide range of activities; socially effective; generally satisfied with
81   life; everyday worries that only occasionally get out of hand.

Mild Dysfunction

80   Minimal symptoms may be present, but no more than slight impairment in func-
       tioning; varying degree of everyday worries and problems that sometimes get out
71   of hand.

70   Some mild symptoms (for example, depressive mood and mild insomnia); or
       some difficulty in several areas of functioning, but generally functions pretty
       well—has some meaningful interpersonal relationships, and most untrained
61   people would not consider him or her ill.

60   Moderate symptoms; or generally functioning with some difficulty (for example,
       few friends and flat affect, depressed mood and pathological self-doubt, euphoric
51   mood and pressure of speech, moderately severe antisocial behavior).

Priority Group (Called Seriously Disabled)

Moderate Dysfunction

50   Any serious symptoms or impairment in functioning that most clinicians would
       think obviously require treatment or attention (for example, suicidal preoccupa-
       tion or gesture, severe obsessional rituals, frequent anxiety attacks, serious anti-
41   social behavior, compulsive drinking).

40   Major impairment in several areas, such as work, family relations, judgment,
       thinking or mood (for example, depressed woman avoids friends, neglects family,
       unable to do housework); or some impairment in reality testing or communica-
       tion (for example, speech is at times obscure, illogical or irrelevant); or single
31   serious suicide attempt.

Severe Dysfunction

30   Unable to function in almost all areas (for example, stays in bed all day); or be-
       havior is considerably influenced by either delusions or hallucinations; or serious
       impairment in communication (for example, sometimes incoherent or unrespon-
21   sive) or judgment (for example, acts grossly inappropriately).

20   Needs some supervision to prevent hurting self or others or to maintain minimal
       personal hygiene (for example, repeated suicide attempts, frequently violent,
       manic excitement, smears feces); or gross impairment in communication (for ex-
11   ample, largely incoherent or mute).

Profound Dysfunction

10   Needs constant supervision for several days to prevent hurting self or others; or
       makes no attempt to maintain minimal personal hygiene.
1

Source: Spitzer, Gibbon, and Endicott (1977).

A number of problems affect the delivery of outpatient services. Persons who are not severely disturbed and not eligible for Medicaid, but who still need service, experience long waiting periods and mounting charges for services. Programs that are understaffed may have to rely on prescribing medications in the absence of trained personnel. Yet another problem in the delivery of outpatient services is that procedures for the transfer of clients from inpatient to outpatient services are often not systematized, with the result that local mental health agencies frequently do not know that a client has been released to their catchment area, and physicians sometimes release clients without adequate follow-up procedures.

Partial Hospitalization. Partial hospitalization services are designed to provide treatment alternatives to hospitalization and to supplement outpatient services. Whether in day, night, evening, or weekend treatment services, the client is treated in a therapeutic environment that allows him or her to maintain family and community ties. Also known as *day treatment,* partial hospitalization can include such services as intake/evaluation, individual and group therapy, activities therapy, family/marital therapy, and medications management and can provide the most intensive therapy short of total hospital care.

While clients are frequently transferred to day treatment from outpatient services, more often they enter the program after hospitalization. The term *milieu therapy* usually characterizes the day treatment activity program, which can be located inside or outside a mental health agency. The typical program schedule varies from three mornings or afternoons per week to a full-day session one or more times per week. Most programs include periodic medications review; group therapy sessions; recreational activities such as volleyball, swimming, picnics, and field trips; vocational activities such as job assessment and training, cooking, sewing, and sheltered workshops; and the possibility of simply being in a safe environment for developing friendships and enhancing one's self-concept.

Within most day treatment programs, there are structured activities related to life-skills training, job training, and job placement. Some day treatment programs are organized into clubs in which client-members manage club newspapers, snack shops, or thrift stores, thereby learning daily living and work skills. This approach encourages clients to assume as much independence as possible while they are in treatment and provides an intermediate step back to regular daily life for those becoming increasingly functional.

Groups are sometimes divided into levels of functioning. When persons become more independent or more functionally capable, they are transferred to the advanced group and eventually moved out of the program either to outpatient service, a vocational training program, or some other community support program. Most day treatment programs build on client strengths by helping those persons who are improving as well as those who are coping with a chronic condition. Since this positive reinforcement, or "overnurturing," provides incentives to improve, some clients may stay in the program for a year or longer.

Emergency Services. Emergency community mental health services must be available twenty-four hours a day, seven days per week. Programs consist of twenty-four-hour walk-in service, telephone service, and/or outreach and referral service with a mental health professional available at all times (PL 94–63).

In addition to hospital discharge planning, crisis counseling, and case management, emergency services include crisis outreach programs, which are designed to serve as alternatives to hospitalization and which respond to crisis calls by sending staff out into the community for assessment, crisis resolution, and referral to appropriate community agencies. Crisis outreach programs can fill critical gaps in service to severely disturbed individuals by providing case management, liaison between state and local hospitals, and support to clients' family members. Emergency service staff can serve as dispatchers for crisis outreach, directing some clients to a hospital emergency room, calling for police support when needed, or referring nonemergency clients to community mental health centers' crisis units. When emergency service staff assume case management functions, especially in the case of involuntary commitment, assessments for seventy-two-hour detentions can be initiated immediately; clients need see only one professional, thereby eliminating referral delays; and emergency staff can act as advocates for clients to gain access to counseling or evaluation for psychiatric hospitalization.

Consultation and Education. The consultation and educational services of a community mental health agency are usually available to a wide range of individuals and organizations, including health professionals, schools, courts, state and local law enforcement and correctional agencies, members of the clergy, public welfare agencies, and health services delivery agencies. They often include activities designed to develop effective mental health programs within the agency's catchment area, promote the coordination of mental health services in the community, and inform residents about the nature of mental health problems and available services (PL 94–63).

Educational programs often take the form of classes or conferences—on subjects ranging from weight control to family life education—which have none of the stigma so often associated with mental health programs. And in recent years, some local community mental health center directors have begun to develop low-key lobbying programs to inform state legislators and citizens in their districts about the need for services and financing.

Mental health education requires careful planning and precise tailoring to meet specific needs. For example, a rural area with a high concentration of senior citizens requires different mental health education programs than does a suburban metropolitan area with a large population of children. Similarly, materials focusing on family relations, divorce, or death might be more valuable to clergy than to police, who in turn might find background on juvenile delinquency or suicide more appropriate to their work. Mental health consultation to community agencies and professionals involves a systematic dissemination of mental health information through problem solving within a voluntary consulting relationship. The consulting service might involve the schools, clergy, law enforcement agents, or physicians.

Children's Services. Specialized community mental health services for children often include a full range of diagnostic, treatment, liaison, and follow-up services (PL 94–63). In addition to outpatient services, children's mental health services may include psychiatric beds in general hospitals, residential facilities for children, psychiatric halfway houses, and specialized foster homes. As with services to adults, children's mental health services are part of a network of community services including schools, courts, vocational rehabilitation agencies, and developmental disability agencies.

Geriatric Mental Health Services. Mental health services for the elderly often involve specialized programs, including a full range of diagnostic, treatment, liaison, and follow-up services (PL 94–63) for those living alone as well as for those living in long-term care facilities, such as nursing homes, congregate care facilities (CCFs), and intermediate care facilities (ICFs). The residential care staff in these facilities often need training in psychosocial treatment and in outreach techniques for communicating with the mentally ill geriatric patient and coordinating relevant services with agencies in the community.

Mental health agencies often provide consultation and educational services to nursing homes and other congregate care facilities, services that usually involve coordinated service planning with residents and residential care staff. These service plans include referrals to specific mental health agencies or other community support agencies that can provide supplemental counseling and activities programs. One difficulty involved in sustaining this approach to decentralized service delivery is the frequent absence of physician services, services that are required if a program is to qualify for reimbursement by Medicaid funds.

In-home care to homebound elderly persons needing mental health services may include evaluation and diagnosis; development of a treatment plan; medication management and evaluation; individual, marital, and family therapy; and case management. One of the advantages of a home care program is that services can be linked with the broad range of resources in the health care system.

As with services to children, there is conflict regarding responsibility for elderly clients. Elderly persons are served by state agencies operating under authorization of the Older Americans Act or by those under authorization of the Community Mental Health Centers Act. Although agreements have been reached and exchanged at the state level, it is still up to local community mental health agencies to coordinate services.

Screening Services. Mental health screening services to courts and other public agencies relate primarily to referral to a state facility for inpatient treatment and are designed to link individuals with the least restrictive treatment setting. The Global Assessment Scale noted in Table 1 is frequently used as an assessment tool in the screening process (PL 94–63).

Community mental health agencies continue to serve as the primary entry point for access to state hospitals, despite problems of inadequate staffing of screening services, transporting of clients, frequently poor communication between agencies and state hospitals, and recent involuntary-treatment legislation requiring state hospitals to admit difficult cases. Often a substantial number of individuals are referred by private physicians, therapists, or family members who may not be aware of community resources. Sharing information on available community mental health resources with these independnt referral agents can improve the screening and discharge-planning process.

Discharge and Follow-up Services. Arrangements must be made for the client's return to the community—and thus an appropriate planning process for discharge, transportation, and follow-up is needed (PL 94–63). A discharge and post-hospital plan usually involves identifying community support programs to help maintain the patient's mental health and coping capacity in the community. A copy of the plan is given to the client and additional copies are sent to the local community mental health agencies that receive referrals of discharged persons. For clients initially served by crisis outreach units, emergency service staff may provide extended follow-up and counseling. Follow-up can also include case management services, provided through community support programs that offer liaison and coordination with both state and community hospitals for discharge planning of clients.

Based on the recognition that mental health treatment is only one of many services needed in order for a client to remain in his or her local community, community support programs are designed to reduce the frequency and severity of behavior leading to hospitalization and to improve the functional level of severely disturbed clients. Such programs may include inpatient care at hospitals, prevocational activities, activity therapies, and home-delivered services, as well as assistance in satisfying routine needs for food, clothing, recreational activities, and supportive personal relationships. In addition, a case manager assigned to the client provides liaison with hospitals, appropriate assessment of the client's needs for community services, coordinating and brokering of community services, and advocacy services to resolve any organizational barriers to effective service delivery. The case manager monitors the client's use of community services and coordinates such services as housing, financial support, medications, and crisis counseling.

Transitional Care Services. Transitional mental health services are needed for mentally ill clients who have been discharged from a mental health facility or who require a treatment alternative to inpatient care. Such services are usually oriented to seriously disturbed clients who are at risk of hospitalization or who have the potential to move to a less restrictive living or treatment setting. The goal of most transitional care services is to maintain severely disturbed individuals in the community in the least restrictive setting possible (PL 94–63).

Transitional care services provide day treatment, outpatient services, consultation with facility staff, assistance with in-facility activities programs, in-facility counseling, and related case management services for individuals living in private residences and in intermediate care, congregate care, and residential care facilities. Rehabilitation services are also provided through vocational training projects. Transitional care services can be developed for special groups such as the elderly, handicapped, minorities, and low-income individuals. Another important goal for delivering transitional care services is the integration of mental health services with the other social and health services necessary to maintain mentally ill clients in the community.

Transitional programs may also include outpatient services to clients in alternative living situations, such as group houses, boarding homes, or foster homes. These living arrangements are designed to help clients deal with stress, develop coping skills, learn to negotiate employment systems, and manage the general problems of community living. For example, a fifty-bed, single-occupancy living facility can provide twenty-four-hour emotional support and supervision by employees familiar to the client-residents. The facility manager and assistant should have immediate access to case managers and psychiatric backup. Other housing arrangements include leased apartment units for clients and adult foster care.

Alcoholism and Alcohol Abuse Services. Alcoholism and alcohol abuse services are closely related to community mental health services and seek to prevent, treat, and rehabilitate alcohol abusers (PL 94–63). Many communities have a separate administrative, planning, and service delivery system for alcoholism services, frequently related to special state legislation. Alcoholism is usually defined as an illness characterized by habitual lack of self-control in the use of alcoholic beverages to the extent that the user's health is substantially impaired or endangered or his or her social and economic functioning is substantially disrupted. A comprehensive and coordinated alcoholism program usually includes informational and referral services, alcohol information schools, and outreach programs for elderly and indigent persons.

Emergency treatment services are typically provided by emergency police patrols, local hospitals, and detoxification centers. A police patrol is generally responsible for picking up persons incapacitated by alcohol and delivering them to the local hospital receiving room for medical screening and emergency services. Medically controlled withdrawal from alcohol is usually accomplished at a detoxification center.

Clients often begin at designated public facilities or hospitals, where inpatient treatment is provided, and then move to recovery houses, which are both supportive communities and providers of outpatient services. Long-term treatment is usually provided at private residential treatment facilities.

Outpatient services are frequently delivered by the community alcoholism centers, of which Alcoholics Anonymous (AA) is perhaps the most notable example. Although AA is usually not affiliated with any agency, referrals to AA are regarded as a key component in the continuum of care. Many of the outpatient alcoholism counselors are ex-alcoholics, who bring a special commitment to service programs.

Alcoholism services may also be offered through a day treatment program at a community mental health agency, where a treatment philosophy can be developed to serve persons who want to overcome problems related to alcohol and drug abuse within the context of a therapeutic community. Daily contact with such a treatment program—which may involve group, individual, and family counseling, substance information and antabuse groups, art therapy, recreation therapy, physical exercise, monitoring of sobriety, and the support of the treatment community—can help the patient maintain a substance-free life. In the initial stages of treatment, the program can provide external controls and supports to help establish abstinence through daily monitoring of antabuse, educational and informational classes, and emphasis on changing one's life-style. The focus may then shift to addressing individual problems through supportive outpatient services.

Drug Addiction and Drug Abuse Services. Drug abuse services include the prevention, treatment, and rehabilitation of drug addicts, drug abusers, and persons with drug dependency problems (PL 94–63). A typical drug abuse service includes emergency telephone services and informational and referral services that address the special needs of minorities, youth, and the elderly. Most mental health agencies include at least one drug abuse specialist who handles intake services and referrals to appropriate drug treatment services in the community.

Drug treatment services usually include residential treatment centers or therapeutic communities that provide around-the-clock supervision, living accommodations, counseling, and recreational opportunities. The goal of all such therapeutic communities is client abstinence and withdrawal from illegal behaviors and drug use, but the intensity of supervision and therapy differs from center to center, ranging from the unsupervised sign-in/sign-out approach to a high degree of control, with continual observation of, and reaction to, client behavior. In some centers, methadone is used as a substitute for other narcotic-type drugs, and methadone maintenance is provided in conjunction with counseling and rehabilitation services.

The provision of drug abuse services is largely accomplished today outside of community mental health agencies. In the future, with the rising abuse of prescription drugs, more attention to drug abuse problems will be required.

Service Directions for the Future

One of the most comprehensive catalogues of identified mental service needs is found in the report of the President's Commission on Mental Health (1978). Despite progress in the treatment of the mentally ill, the commission reported, many persons still receive inadequate care, including persons with chronic mental illness, children, adolescents, older Americans, social and ethnic minorities, the urban poor, and migrant and seasonal farm workers. The commission noted that a basic premise of the movement toward community-based services was that care would be provided in halfway houses, family and group homes, foster care settings, and community mental health settings. However, the commission found that the transition from state hospital to community was not effectively achieved in most cases, and that people with chronic mental disabilities who had been released from hospitals did not receive the basic necessities of food, shelter, financial assistance, and support services.

The commission also noted the inconsistencies that exist between what we know should be done and what we do—we know that services should be tailored to the needs of people in different communities and circumstances, but we do not provide the choices that make this possible, especially since the bulk of funds still go to nursing homes and state mental hospitals. With these inconsistencies in mind, the President's Commission on Mental Health (1978) made the following recommendations:

1. A major effort should be developed in the area of personal and community supports that will recognize and strengthen the natural networks to which people belong and on which they depend and that will improve the links between community support networks and formal mental health services.

2. A more responsive community services system should be established by developing new alliances between the public and private sectors and between federal, state, and local governments, and by setting a national priority for meeting the needs of people with chronic mental illness through a new federal grant program for community mental health services. Priorities in this new array of services would also include specialized services for children, adolescents, the elderly, and racial and ethnic minorities.

3. A more comprehensive and coordinated public and private strategy for financing mental health services should be provided by modifying public and private health insurance programs to expand benefits, including coverage for emergency, outpatient, and inpatient care; partial hospitalization; and twenty-four-hour residential treatment for youth—as well as by guaranteeing freedom of choice of services. Such changes would mean amending the federal Medicaid legislation to give provider status to community mental health agencies.

4. Mental health specialists should be encouraged to work in areas and settings where severe shortages exist; the number of qualified minority personnel in mental health professions, as well as the number of mental health personnel trained to deal with the special problems of children, adolescents, and the elderly, should be increased.

5. The legal rights of consumers must be assured by establishing advocacy systems for the representation of mentally disturbed individuals and by encouraging states to review their laws covering civil commitment, guardianship, the right to treatment in least restrictive settings, the right to refuse treatment, and the right to due process. In addition, mentally disturbed persons in detention or correctional institutions should have access to appropriate mental health services.

Although these recommendations clearly outline the priority issues and needs of the future, the political response to these priorities remains to be seen. Federal, state, as well as private resources will all be needed to address the mental health problems of the future.

In addition, training needs for future mental health administrators and clinicians are definitely changing. The mental health system will require more sophisticated administrators with broad skills in management and planning and clinicians who are trained in a combination of therapeutic and community relations skills as community organizers. The growth of increasingly complex organizational structures and the pressure for accountability in the expenditure of public funds require of the administrator a familiarity with more sophisticated management information systems. Future funding for community mental health programs is also a major problem for administrators, who frequently find themselves seeking to implement mandated programs without adequate funding or constantly juggling financial resources as public mental health policies change.

In addition to funding dilemmas, administrators face growing community interest in the planning of mental health services. Advocates for the mentally ill are becoming increasingly vocal in demanding a change in the allocation of mental health dollars. Clients' rights, clients' access to treatment plans, and clients' choice of treatment are affecting service delivery patterns.

The future of mental health services, like the future of so many other social programs today, is linked to economic and political circumstances. A creative response to community mental health needs will require a recognition of the role of the private sector, as well as other social service providers, and the assistance of local mental health advocates. Mental health program goals will need to emphasize reduced dependency on the mental health care system through the use of community support programs, consultation and educational services to the private sector, and the recruitment of new care givers and constituency groups to help address the complex mental health needs of each community. Clinicians must identify and confront these major issues as they make the transition to the role of mental health program manager.

Transition from Clinician to Program Manager

The clinician's transition from providing treatment services to managing a mental health program is both challenging and frustrating. The challenge of acquiring a new position and searching for new skills is frequently offset by the frustration that emerges from feelings of self-doubt and isolation. New program managers may often wonder: Why did I take the promotion to become the coordinator of outpatient services? Why do my former colleagues treat me differently now that I supervise the day treatment program? Why do I feel caught in the middle between my clinical staff and top agency management? How do I use the skills acquired in helping clients in my new job of helping staff? These and other questions reflect the common concerns of clinicians recently promoted to program managers. Some of these questions can be answered by assessing the individual and interpersonal roles assumed by clinicians and managers.

When contrasting the predispositions of clinicians and managers, several interesting observations can be made (Patti and Austin, 1977). First, differences in temperament are apparent. Clinicians emphasize the expressive aspects of empathy, compassion, altruism, and sharing within the context of clinician-client relations. Program managers, on the other hand, emphasize the instrumental aspects of organizing, manipulating, investigating, and integrating. However, the expressive attributes of the clinician are needed by the program manager to work effectively with staff inside and outside the agency, and the instrumental attributes of the program manager are needed by the clinician to effectively serve a wide range of client needs.

Second, there are notable differences in intellectual interests and job rewards. Clinicians tend to be interested in the psychology, cultural anthropology, and philosophy of human survival, whereas program managers tend to be more interested in the sociology, political science, and economics of human survival. Again, these differences are not always clearly apparent, and there is obvious overlap in the intellectual interests of clinicians and managers. In relation to job rewards, the clinician views rewards in terms of client treatment success and his or her own personal growth through self-actualization, whereas the program manager views rewards in terms of program credibility and funding and pride in building an organization.

In addition to differences in temperament, intellectual interests, and job rewards, differences also exist in the realm of interpersonal relations. Five major areas of discontinuity between the clinician's perspective and the program manager's perspective are as follows (Patti and Austin, 1977):

- *Orientation to Authority.* The authority of clinicians derives largely from their knowledge and expertise in the areas of therapy or rehabilitation. The exercise of that authority is contingent on both client and collegial recognition of expertise. In contrast, although program managers may seek to establish authority with clinical staff on the basis of knowledge and skill and to elicit worker behavior on the basis of consensus, they must also be prepared to press for compliance and cooperation on the basis of their position's authority.
- *Modes of Decision Making.* Mental health practitioners are trained to treat each client relationship as an entity in itself, with its own needs and requirements. It is the practitioner's professional responsibility to provide those services that will maximize benefits in any given case. Program managers, on the other hand, can seldom afford to think in terms of optimal solutions for each worker, unit, or department for which they are responsible. Rather, they must consider the best possible alternatives available under circumstances that nearly always involve scarce resources. The managerial culture recognizes this decision mode—in contrast to clinical optimizing decision mode—as both necessary and ethical.
- *Orientation to Relationships.* Open communication, rapport, trust, and caring are essential ingredients in the clinician-client relationship. The relationship between program managers and clinical staff, however, is likely to be more functionally specific and instrumental, since the program manager must be concerned with maximizing the contribution of staff to the organization. Guardedness and restraint are also likely to characterize this relationship, because program managers are responsible for evaluating staff performance and for ensuring equity in relationships with all clinical staff.

- *Orientation to Effectiveness.* Although clinicians are increasingly being
trained to specify treatment goals and objectives in terms of measurable,
observable outcomes, many subtle and more difficult-to-measure process
phenomena—for example, the extent to which the client understands himself
or herself, the client's recognition of the need for help, or the client's acquisition of skills that contribute to improved personal relationships or problem-
solving capacities—are equally important in the clinical culture. Increasingly,
however, program managers are called on to provide evidence that services
contribute to the attainment of tangible, publicly valued changes in the life
circumstances of clients, such as improved academic performance, job retention, and reduced recidivism. Program managers tend to be more oriented to
program impact expressed in terms that are valued and understood by influential publics than to the process phenomena valued by clinicians.
- *Collegial Relationships.* It is commonly believed that the environment of
mental health agencies provides clinicians with support, counsel, and opportunities for exchanging ideas and advice on methods and techniques and sharing information on case experiences. A good agency is thought to be one where
both expressive and instrumental needs are met, where group membership and
involvement are important corollaries of clinical effectiveness and professional
growth. Program managers, however, are often preoccupied with program
turf, competition for resources, and the selection and retention of personnel,
and they consequently are reluctant to share information and ideas openly.

With these predispositions and interpersonal factors in mind, it is useful to
identify some of the generic supervisory management knowledge and skills a
clinician needs to make the transition to program manager. Such relevant knowledge and skills are of two kinds: analytical knowledge and skill related to thinking
and conceptualizing one's managerial practice, and interactional knowledge and
skill related to individual and group relations and the process of involving staff in
program management activities. The following components of the generic approach to supervisory management can be found in more detail in *Supervisory
Management for the Human Services* (Austin, 1981).

- *Interpreting Supervisory Practice.* Program managers experience considerable
doubt and confusion about the most meaningful way to carry out their supervisory role. In order to appreciate the value of supervision, it is necessary to
gain some understanding of the organizational context of supervisory management and of the middle-management bind that stretches program managers
between the needs of clinicians and the needs of top management. In addition,
program managers who have been clinicians need to recognize the importance
of their abilities to conceptualize and articulate the nature of mental health
work and technology in order to assist subordinates.
- *Developing Supervisory Leadership.* Assuming positions of leadership can be
both exhilarating and frightening. Clinicians who look to program managers
for leadership obviously shape the type of leadership provided. How program

managers acquire or demonstrate the qualities of effective leadership is still open to question and continuing research. However, it is possible to describe a process for developing, managing, and testing supervisory leadership in mental health agencies.

- *Analyzing Mental Health Work.* The knowledge and skills related to analyzing the nature of mental health work are useful in creating job specificity and mutual agreement about work expectations between program managers and clinicians. Without such common understandings of job tasks and the standards of mental health service delivery, the program manager and clinician will continue to pass each other like ships in the night, since no formal or informal contract of understanding will exist, and, therefore, excessive amounts of time may be spent on clarifying expectations.

- *Guiding the Case Management Process.* This process involves developing and monitoring client service objectives. Program managers provide case, process, and program consultation to clinicians and also coordinate the work of clinicians according to the service objectives developed for the overall service program.

- *Managing by Objectives.* Building on job analysis and case management skills, a program manager continuously seeks to link the efforts of clinicians in the program to the prevailing goals and objectives of the agency. This process requires translating agency goals and objectives into viable clinician activities—which is commonly known as managing by objectives.

- *Deploying Staff.* Program managers frequently experience difficulties in delegating work and deploying staff in such a way as to maximize their full potential. Clinicians often display considerable skill in recognizing the dynamics of client behavior; program managers need the same level of skill in recognizing and utilizing differences among staff. This is not always a matter of the direct transference of good clinical skills, however. Although effective interpersonal relations are common to both sets of skills, the problems and situations related to task group management, management of "troubled" clinicians, and grievance handling provide challenges that are very different from the challenges of clinician-client interactions.

- *Monitoring Clinician Performance.* Program managers often experience considerable anxiety in conducting periodic clinician evaluations. Therefore, it is important to learn to conduct periodic career development conferences and to use job performance appraisal tools in assessing clinician work performance.

- *Assessing and Educating Staff.* The results of monitoring clinician performance serve as the basic ingredients for assessing and educating staff. The program manager assumes four major roles: the educational planner, who helps to orient, update, and upgrade staff; the tutor, who shares professional and personal philosophy, ethics, and beliefs about change; the facilitator, who seeks to match learning styles of clinicians with teaching styles of program managers, as reflected in individual and group conferences; and the trainer, who confronts negative clinician attitudes toward learning, translates poorly performed clinician tasks into learning objectives, participates in the selection of appropriate training and learning resources, and assists clinicians with their career-planning process.

- *Managing Time and Stress.* How well administrators manage the issues of time and stress affects the degree of personal pressure and staff burnout they experience as well as the amount of demand for organizational change from inside and outside the agency. Time management involves periodic assessment of personal and professional goals and objectives; stress management involves assessing sources of stress and managing distorted overreactions to stressful situations by modifying ideas, attitudes, and philosophies.

The self-evaluating program manager is continuously appraising several functions of a middle manager—those of consideration, facilitation, and participation. Consideration (social support) includes creating a climate of approval, developing personal relationships, providing fair treatment, and enforcing rules equitably. *Facilitation* (technical support) includes providing adequate help and assistance to clinical staff and demonstrating competence as a technically proficient program manager. *Participation* involves promoting worker autonomy and job enrichment and not supervising too closely.

Conclusion

As program managers work in complex mental health systems, they need skills in handling the transition from clinical work to managerial work as well as the skills of administration. They need a clear understanding of the broad array of services available to clients and a sense of vision of what programs will be required in the future. This chapter highlighted services that comprise the essential ingredients of a comprehensive community mental health agency: inpatient, outpatient, partial hospitalization, emergency, consultation and education, geriatric, children's, screening, discharge and follow-up, transitional care, alcohol abuse, and drug abuse.

Acquiring management skills adequate to supervise staff and to plan, develop, maintain, and evaluate programs represents a major challenge. Knowledge of the wide range of mental health services available for treatment purposes will give managers latitude in selecting treatment methodologies, choosing appropriate program modalities, and coordinating their own mental health programs with others in the service system.

References

Austin, M. J. *Supervisory Management for the Human Services.* Englewood Cliffs, N.J.: Prentice-Hall, 1981.

Bloom, B. L. *Community Mental Health, A General Introduction.* Monterey, Calif.: Brooks/Cole, 1977.

Mechanic, D. *Mental Health and Social Policy.* Englewood Cliffs, N.J.: Prentice-Hall, 1980.

Patti, R. J., and Austin, M. J. "Socializing the Direct Service Practitioner in the Ways of Supervisory Management." *Administration in Social Work,* 1977, *1*(3), 266–280.

President's Commission on Mental Health. *Report of the President's Commission on Mental Health.* Vol. 1. Washington, D.C.: U.S. Government Printing Office, 1978.

Public Law 94–63. 1975 Amendments to The Community Mental Health Centers Act of 1963.

Spitzer, R. L., Gibbon, M., and Endicott, J. "Global Assessment Scale." In W. A. Hargreaves, C. C. Attkisson, and J. E. Sorenson (Eds.), *Resource Materials for Community Mental Health Program Evaluation.* Washington, D.C.: U.S. Government Printing Office, 1977.

ৡ 1 ৡ

Understanding
Clinical Staff's Views
of Administration

Jill Crowell

Clinical staff represent a valuable agency resource, and managers who can move comfortably into and out of clinical staff territory should contribute to improved communications based on understanding of staff perspectives. Jill Crowell reviews staff perceptions of administrative processes and suggests strategies for increasing job satisfaction, improving organizational communications, and enhancing supervision. The respective roles of the administrative staff and the clinical staff are described as a means of clarifying channels of communication. Clinical staff perspectives on accountability, the nature of power, organizational decision making, and job satisfaction are also discussed.

Administrators often wonder how they are perceived by the clinical staff or are perplexed over the seeming incompatibilities between clinical and administrative mind sets. Research findings suggest that these concerns are well founded. For example:

1. A 1969 study of mental health center staff revealed that agency administration and administrators were the most frequently mentioned sources of job dissatisfaction. This finding was consistent across the major mental health professions of social work, psychology, and psychiatry (Glasscote and Gudeman, 1969).

2. The technical incompetence of supervisors was the most frequently mentioned source of job dissatisfaction in a study of beginning social workers (Miller, 1970).

3. Four of the six major complaints of social workers who had resigned from a large department of social welfare were directly related to the quality and nature of first-line supervision (Kermish and Kushin, 1969).

4. Olmstead and Christensen (1973) studied 1,600 workers in thirty-one social welfare and rehabilitation agencies and reported that high scores on supervision were accompanied by greater job satisfaction, better individual performance, less absenteeism, better agency performance, and higher agency competence.

5. Aiken, Smits, and Lollar (1972) found that among 360 counselors in state rehabilitation agencies, the interaction between supervisor and counselor was considered the most important aspect of employment.

6. In their seminal work *The Motivation to Work,* Herzberg, Snyderman, and Mausner (1959) reported that job satisfaction was primarily related to job environment, of which supervision and administration were primary components.

These findings may lead to the conclusion that there is simply no way of pleasing the clinical staff. But we have taken a more optimistic viewpoint. First, these findings suggest that program administration is an important function and that clinicians expect, want, and need competent administration to carry out their work effectively. This interpretation contradicts the common myth that clinicians view administrators as a necessary evil, something to be tolerated and, when possible, ignored. Second, findings suggest that clinicians are able to differentiate between competent and incompetent administrators and between administrative behaviors that either enhance or hinder their own performance in the delivery of services to clients. Therefore, administrators can continue to learn by monitoring and assessing clinical perspectives.

It would be misleading for administrators to assume that, simply because they are former clinicians, they now maintain both a clinical and an administrative perspective. It is important to remember how quickly we forget, and how the further removed from the situation we become, the less we are able to recall in detail and intensity the feelings associated with past experiences.

The goal of this chapter is not to reinforce the common stereotype of clinicians who complain about administration, but rather to stress the importance of clinician perspectives on the administration of a mental health center organization. In some cases, staff grievances are well founded—many organizations *are* poorly managed. One explanation is that, historically, administrators have assumed their new roles with minimal or no specific training in fiscal or program planning, budgeting, grant writing, evaluation, personnel, organizational behavior, or planned change. Today, although more administrative personnel are seeking additional training, specific management training and experience are still not universally required for administrative positions. In addition, there are few, if any, guidelines or standards for monitoring and assuring effective management practices. If clinicians are known to complain, it is not without some justification.

It is also important to remember that clinicians too have had little training as organizational change agents and often lack conceptual frameworks either for understanding organizational behavior or for bringing about change themselves. In many instances, administrators inadvertently encourage staff complaints, either because the administrators themselves lack the necessary skills to encourage or facilitate organizational problem solving by clinical staff, or because they resist staff-initiated change.

It is not our intention to portray clinical staff and administrative staff as two homogeneous groups; in fact, no one clinician or administrator is exactly like another. With this consideration in mind, let us identify the different roles played by administrators and clinicians in delivering mental health services.

The Roles of Administrators

The term *administrator* is used in a general sense to refer to those persons who hold supervisory, program management, or agency director roles and does not include secretarial and other support staff. In the 1970s, administrative tasks became considerably less clinical in nature and more specifically directed toward program management and efficiency. For example, local, state, and federal accountability and reporting requirements, the lobbying of consumer and advocate groups, and the governance of citizen and coordinating boards led to an influx of management technologies borrowed from the business community, such as planning, programming, and budgeting systems (PPBS), management by objectives (MBO), and management information systems (MIS). Problem-oriented record keeping, utilization reviews, and program evaluation found their way into the mental health field as administrators scrambled to compete for increasingly scarce resources. As clinical and administrative roles become more keenly differentiated, administrators must be alert to the impact of such changes on the effective management of professional clinical staff.

The Roles of Clinicians

The term *clinician* refers to the broad range of professionals who deliver mental health services. Most clinical staff members are persons who have acquired professional training in one of the core mental health disciplines (psychology, social work, psychiatry, and psychiatric nursing) or in a related field (for example, guidance and counseling, rehabilitation therapy, occupational therapy). Since clinical staff perspectives on mental health administration are partly functions of clinical training, ideological orientation, and the organizational environment, it is important to identify the characteristics of a typical mental health agency staff.

Mental health agency staffs are typically multidisciplinary, professional, and autonomous. Although the multidisciplinary nature of such staffs offers potential for service innovativeness and healthy collegial exchange, it has also created territorial, status, and power conflicts, particularly among the professions of social work, psychology, and psychiatry. Historically, mental health administrative roles were predominantly held by psychiatrists. Today, however, most community mental health agencies are administered by psychologists or social workers. Since there is considerable overlap in the technical skills of the various mental health professions, roles, responsibilities, and status are no longer differentiated simply on the basis of professional training.

Clinicians derive their power from their specialized knowledge and expertise, power which is reinforced by clients who often view them as all-knowing and all-powerful. Many mental health organizations have essentially provided a context for the conduct of private practice, and the interests of practitioners have in many cases directly shaped program policies and priorities. Only in recent years have practitioners been expected to participate as members of a larger system whose program policies and agency goals are influenced by an array of forces often external to the organization, such as consumer groups, coordinating boards, and legislative action.

Like other professionals, mental health professionals derive satisfaction largely from internalized standards of excellence reinforced by their professional identities. The conventional concept of hierarchical authority poses problems for mental health professionals, not only because of their sense of power and their perception of themselves as professionals but also because of their democratic ideals, which place great value on fairness and equality.

The autonomy of mental health professionals is derived largely from the confidential nature of their clinical contacts and the varied, nonroutine, and ill-defined nature of their work. Clinicians have been largely responsible for defining their practice and judging achievement. More recently, mental health centers are relying on utilization and case reviews to monitor service quality and performance standards. Administrators, however, must still rely heavily on their own confidence in their staff and on the personnel practices of the agency to assure effective implementation of the agency's purposes and objectives.

The multidisciplinary, professional, and autonomous nature of the mental health agency staff may at once challenge, inspire, frustrate, and anger the mental health administrator. Even administrators who have risen from the clinical ranks will no doubt gain a new perspective on mental health professionals as their own tasks and functions take on an administrative focus. Whittington (1975) describes the new administrator's response to the challenge in terms of these stages. First, personnel problems are considered an annoyance and much staff behavior is seen as an effort to frustrate the administrator's aspirations and block his or her legitimate exercise of authority. In the second stage, the administrator begins to see staff with a clinical eye and brings his or her therapeutic skills to bear on personnel problems. Finally, the administrator comes to view professionals within a broader systems perspective that acknowledges the interplay of leadership style and personal and professional characteristics, as well as the nature of organizational and environmental characteristics.

Clinician Perspectives on Administrative Processes

Clinical staff perspectives are neither right nor wrong; they are simply often different from those of administrators. Different clinicians may hold different views of a single administrator or administrative behavior. Further, since administrative tasks and roles change as mental health programs evolve through developmental stages of program design, implementation, and stabilization, clinical staff perspectives may reflect program development, with one set of administrative behaviors appreciated at one point but unappreciated at another. With these considerations in mind, the following sections discuss clinician perspectives on several administrative processes.

Accountability

We begin with the issue of accountability because of its current significance to the management and survival of mental health programs. The accountability era brought with it management information systems, program evaluation, problem-oriented recordkeeping, management and service audits, externally imposed priorities, fee-for-service funding systems, coordination among community services, and broad legislative and community involvement—all requiring clinicians to increase their output and to define, count, and evaluate services delivered. Many clinicians view such detailed documentation as bureaucratic red tape that only detracts from the quality of the service they provide. However, clinician resistance sometimes prods administrators to make concerted efforts to streamline their data reporting and collection procedures. For example, new forms can be designed to replace existing agency paperwork or to serve multiple purposes, and paperwork can often be handled more efficiently and more reliably by support service staff. Further, administrators can arrange for staff members to become informed about funding, policy, and legislative matters that dictate accountability practices and can make visible their own use of data for agency self-evaluation and internal management purposes. Often, systematically collected data about clients, services, and staff activity are not seen to be in the domain of the clinical staff, when in fact many clinicians use them skillfully to manage, monitor, and evaluate client progress and their own performance.

Implementing and maintaining accountability procedures can be a trying, disruptive, and, at the same time, exciting and challenging process in mental health organizations, and clinician resistance is often the result of the clinical staff being denied active involvement in that process. To mitigate the resistance and ultimately produce a more reasonable and useful product, staff members should be encouraged, even drafted, to participate in the design and implementation of new accountability practices.

The Nature of Power

In our society, the concept of power more often than not carries with it a negative connotation and is readily associated with authority, force, dominance, inequity, injustice, and undemocratic process; "to want power, or to have power, is somehow indecent" (Friesen, 1980). Levinson and Klerman (1972) write that mental health administrators need to learn more about power, but note that mental health professionals view power much as the Victorians viewed sex—as something vulgar, which an upstanding professional would not stoop to engage in.

Power struggles are played out daily in the life of every organization. To deny the existence, or even the "power," of power is to miss opportunities for effecting desired change, mobilizing resources and action, and improving the quality and character of the workplace. The term *power,* as we use it here, refers to a person's ability to obtain and use whatever he or she needs to get a job done or achieve desired goals (Kanter, 1977). This meaning implies mastery or autonomy, rather than dominance or control over others.

Feelings of powerlessness have numerous manifestations: nonparticipation or nonattendance at staff meetings, competitiveness with coworkers or supervisors, noncompliance with agency procedures, and hostile or passive-aggressive behavior. The feelings of incompetence or low self-esteem that frequently accompany powerlessness tend to block initiative, assertiveness, creativity, and innovativeness. The successful manager will find ways to exercise what McCluskey (1976) has termed "liberating power," the power to assist others in taking risks and discovering undeveloped talents.

Although there are many kinds of power—based on one's knowledge, expertise, information, position, authority, ability to reward or punish, and affiliation—we will discuss three sources of power: information, extraordinary activities, and social affiliations.

Information. Persons with information are necessarily valued and given attention. Since energetic and forward-looking staff members are not infrequently viewed as a threat to those above them in the hierarchy, administrators may maintain their own sense of power by deliberately withholding information from clinicians or by excluding them from important planning or problem-solving meetings. Since clinicians must rely on supervisors or program managers to channel information both up and down the hierarchy, they are frequently irritated by supervisors who present staff ideas at management meetings as if they were their own. Recognition and credit, therefore, do not flow to those to whom they are rightly due, and staff members must find other than formal channels to obtain recognition for their contributions; often, they simply learn not to contribute.

Administrators can help their own cause by keeping staff informed about broader agency issues. Through their contacts with a host of service agencies in the community, clinicians hear and see much that would be of interest to administrators; but, if they have not been given a framework for processing or acting on their observations, they are unnecessarily hampered in their role as information gatherers.

Extraordinary Activity. Persons have power also by virtue of their involvement in new or innovative projects. Neither persons nor organizations get credit for doing the mandatory or expected (Kanter, 1977). Risk takers and innovators are rewarded not only by those who observe them but also by the excitement and tension that accompany innovation. Administrators are frequently better able than clinicians to volunteer for new positions or initiate organizational change because they are generally better informed of impending policy changes or deficiencies in the organization. Staff resentment at not being informed is a normal response to opportunities taken by administrators before clinicians are aware that they exist.

Social Affiliations. Power often comes through one's social connections or through the informal network of an organization. Influential social contacts may give administrators the opportunity to get inside information, to bypass the hierarchy, or to shortcircuit cumbersome procedures and cut red tape. A staff person's familiarity with administrators is visible not only to clinical peers but also to other administrators who have the power to recognize and reward the work of others. Formal results are frequently the by-products of informal network exchanges. The ability to get things done or to achieve desired ends is enhanced, then, by virtue of one's acquaintances, and staff members who do not have such social contacts may feel unappreciated, unrecognized, and unfairly treated in the allocation of resources, promotions, and job opportunities.

Power by virtue of information, extraordinary activities, and social affiliations can be made available to a broader range of staff through what we referred to earlier as the administrator's exercise of liberating power. The exercise of liberating power assists clinical staff members in achieving satisfaction by providing them with opportunities to be creative, to be challenged, and to strive for new goals, and it benefits administrators through increased staff accomplishments. However, the exercise of liberating power demands thought and risk-taking on the part of administrators and is often more time-consuming than reliance on a comfortable or dependable *modus operandi*. It requires administrators to learn more about the skills, aspirations, and potentials of a wide range of staff members, not just those who have visibility, and to assign new tasks to persons not comfortable, confident, or powerful enough to volunteer. Exercising liberating power means sharing information, delegating responsibility, recognizing the accomplishments of staff, and providing opportunities for staff to participate in new organizational ventures.

Organizational Decision Making and Organizational Change

Organizational decision making and organizational change are processes which go hand in hand in the life of an organization. It is important to reflect on how the concerns and perspectives of clinical staff relate to both processes. To have lived and worked in the mental health field during the last two decades has meant witnessing and participating in an ongoing and dynamic process of change. Compare the small, self-contained outpatient clinic of the 1950s and early 1960s with today's mental health bureaucracies—staffs of up to two and three hundred, treatment programs that include day treatment (for children, adults, and the elderly), inpatient facilities, outpatient programs, drug and alcohol services, involuntary treatment services, crisis intervention teams and crisis phone programs, sexual abuse and sexual- and criminal-offender programs, emergency foster-home services, consultation services, educational and training services, and, more recently, community support-system activities—which in and of themselves represent new philosophies, new treatment modalities, and new concepts for the delivery of services to clients.

Decisions and directives for change in mental health organizations reflect state and federal legislation, regulations and requirements of state and county mental health programs, court decisions, accrediting agency and financial grant guidelines, the reports of special-purpose study committees, the views of dissatisfied citizenry, the input of innovative and creative practitioners and administrators, and the pressures of cultural change. As participants in complex mental health systems, professionals can no longer rely only on their past training but must participate, grow, make decisions, and change in response to a myriad of mental health constituencies. How decisions are made and how changes come about are as important as the decisions and changes themselves.

Decision Making. Participatory decision making is consistent with the professional and personal values of most mental health professionals and is often, in theory, the decision-making preference professed by mental health administrators. Participatory decision making implies that staff members have a voice and a vote in management decisions that affect their work. In practice, however, and in spite of good intentions by administrators to involve them, clinicians frequently view organizational decision making as democratic in theory but, in reality, the domain of a few. Staff feedback is frequently sought only after decisions have been made. Feedback sought in advance is often ignored or, when incorporated, is not given adequate recognition.

Participatory decision making is unquestionably more frustrating for the administrator than autocratic processes. Not only do multiple and sometimes uninformed perspectives need to be considered and processed, but the process itself may involve heated disputes, lengthy and painful deliberations, unanticipated delays, and the exercise of tolerance and patience. Although some administrators are intolerant of the process in their own agencies, they would protest if they were excluded from important decisions affecting their own work—whether by boards, state and county agencies, or legislatures. The returns on participatory decision making manifest themselves in (1) greater cohesiveness of staff members among themselves and with the organization, (2) a staff with broad organizational, rather than narrow departmental, views, (3) decreased hostility, conflict, and cut-throat competition within the organization, and (4) a work climate that promotes initiative, risk taking, and involvement (Argyris, 1955).

Not all decision making need be participatory in nature. Clinicians would resist the tedious processing of every minute decision. The use of authority should not be avoided, but it should be handled with wisdom and discretion. When an authoritarian model is appropriate, however, the successful administrator will keep staff informed about problems, solutions, progress, and future plans to facilitate a cohesive movement toward the realization of agency goals.

Organizational Change. Although mental health organizations undergo many changes, implementing change remains an enormous source of frustration to administration and staff alike. Curiously, administrators often fail to learn from past experiences, leading predictably to more frustrations. In mental health organizations, all changes, regardless of their nature or magnitude, should be considered problems of human relations. Administrators should be cautious not to underestimate the impact of proposed changes on staff even when change has been initiated by staff or has involved staff participation. Johns (1973) makes several observations, paraphrased below, that are easily and disastrously forgotten by would-be implementers of change:

1. Change regarded as trivial by administrators may be anything but trivial to those persons directly affected by the change.
2. Change promotes conflict if only because worker autonomy is threatened by an increase in the flow of orders.
3. Change is resisted if it threatens existing or anticipated levels of need satisfaction.
4. When people are told to change, they tend to become stubborn, hostile, or defensive.
5. Changes that reduce opportunities for social interaction are particularly vulnerable to resistance.

Easily forgotten too is that resistance to change has its positive aspects. It may help (1) pinpoint sources of low morale and motivation in the organization, (2) identify communication weaknesses—for example, inadequate or understated explanations of the reasons for change, and (3) force those initiating the change to reexamine their arguments and give more thought to human relations in the future (Johns, 1973).

Bringing about change successfully will continue to be a major administrative function. Since change comes about primarily through changes in staff behavior, strategies for change must include staff involvement at all levels of the change process.

Job Satisfaction

When we consider the accumulated staff knowledge and expertise in the field of human behavior and motivation, it is bewildering to consider how infrequently it is applied to the work environment of mental health organizations. Mental health workers are experts on communication, possess the analytical skills to understand the family as a social system, engage others in problem solving, mobilize resources, and bring about change. Yet mental health organizations are frequently characterized by low staff morale.

Although we believe that job satisfaction is a legitimate and important aspect of every administrator's job, it seems particularly important in mental health organizations, where staff members are highly vulnerable to the syndrome of burnout. Unfortunately for both administrators and staff, administrators are frequently ill-equipped to handle issues of staff morale and often fall into the trap of a patronizing approach to burned-out staff. Boredom, anger, frustration, and feelings of being unproductive and misunderstood can lead clinicians to take longer coffee breaks, forget to take vacations or take them at the wrong time, look for or think about other jobs, withdraw or become submissive, or become cynical about clients or about the whole mental health system. Job dissatisfaction also affects both work efficiency and the quality of services delivered to clients. Three potential sources of clinical staff job dissatisfaction are (1) organizational communication, (2) the physical environment of the organization, and (3) benefits and opportunities.

Organizational Communication. Communication is infinitely more than a two-way process of sending and receiving information. Within an organization, it is the social process through which meaning is conveyed, energy is generated, power and authority are exercised, support and feedback are given, instructions are provided, conflict is resolved, and loyalty and a sense of mission are inculcated. As such, communication is the very essence of an organization. Without communication, there is no organization.

Communications problems are less characteristic of small organizations, where problems can be explored and decisions made and shared simply by word of mouth. As administrative levels in the organization increase, memoranda, reports, and meetings often substitute for spontaneous one-to-one communications. As distance between administrators and staff increases, contacts among staff members become more formal and reserved in nature (coworkers may remain relative strangers), rivalry and factionalism develop among units, procedures become more formal and routinized, and staff members lack a sense of control, feel alienated and unimportant, and function largely as receivers of information. These circumstances contribute to low staff morale, reduced commitment to the purposes of the organization, less role consensus, and decreased performance quality and effectiveness. It is no small task for administrators to prevent the disturbing but often inevitable effects of organizational growth. Particularly today, when mental health centers change and grow so rapidly, the effects of the change process on organizational communication often escape the administrator's awareness and understanding. Administrative efforts to promote a healthy climate for free and open communication can take many forms:

1. Model and promote tolerance for diversity, conflict, and expression of grievances.
2. Model and promote constructive approaches to conflict resolution.
3. Encourage and facilitate unit or program interdependency and team approaches to tasks that cut across programs and professions.
4. Minimize the "height" of the organizational hierarchy—"flat" hierarchies tend to promote communication and improve staff morale.
5. Delegate authority and responsibility to all levels of the hierarchy, particularly in those areas that directly affect job performance.
6. Provide opportunities, incentives, and rewards for participation in organizational planning and decision making.
7. Establish predictable and effective formal channels for sharing information across all levels and programs—memos and reports should flow in all directions, not just from the top down.
8. Clarify and promote understanding of organizational goals, ethics, and ideology.
9. Clarify staff roles and responsibilities.

Physical Environment. A second potential source of job dissatisfaction is the physical environment of the organization. Consider some typical comments of clients:

"As a client, my first impression of that dreary building gave
me a very uneasy feeling."

"The office was small and very crowded. It was difficult for
my wife and me to move around."

"The room was cold and empty, and it seemed like they
couldn't afford anything else. If they changed it, maybe the staff
would like it better. Maybe they could change the color and make it
more homelike with lamps and pictures."

How curious that mental health organizations often fail to make use of
readily available information on the effects of color, lighting, furniture arrangement, and the use of space, when it is widely recognized that staff and clients are
influenced by their physical environment. Clinicians are still crowded three or
four to an office, sharing dilapidated furniture and other office amenities and
using dull, dirty conference rooms, while the director has a large, well-furnished
private office.

The physical environment includes not only furnishings and surroundings
that make our environment pleasant and uplifting, but also those that promote
efficiency and convenience.

1. Mailboxes, secretarial stations, records rooms, and bulletin boards can be
    functionally located to facilitate prompt retrieval of messages, to discourage
    hoarding of client records in private offices, and to promote informal com-
    munication and gatherings. Or, as in many offices, their locations can serve
    to keep staff physically fit but inefficient.
2. How offices are arranged in relation to others should be a serious considera-
    tion in both designing and assigning office space. Although it is useful to
    have staff members in the same program unit within close proximity to one
    another, consideration should also be given to how office arrangements en-
    hance and expedite interunit communication and cooperation.
3. Clinical staff members like private offices, primarily to exert control over the
    environment in which they see clients. Private offices give them a sense of
    privacy, a sense of control, and a sense of status and recognition.

Opportunities and Benefits. Clinicians receive the most gratification from
work with clients (Glasscote and Gudeman, 1969). Not surprisingly, they also
enjoy professional exchanges with their work associates and opportunities for
learning new treatment approaches. Since there are a few opportunities for clinicians to move up in the organization if they wish to remain in direct services,
growth within clinical practice is an important component of job satisfaction.
Growth opportunities take the form not only of financially supported training,
workshops, and conferences, but also of quality in-service training, varied job
assignments through job rotations and lateral promotions, supervisory and staff
training assignments, and agency-supported clinical supervision from a respected
professional of their choice.

Job benefits are also important to clinical staff. Many clinical staff members, particularly those in their late twenties and early thirties, leave mental health positions because of characteristically low salaries, even though they may find their work satisfying and rewarding. Many mental health centers do not have career ladders or pay scales that adequately recognize and reward tenure. Although most administrators would claim that salaries are constrained by limited resources, it is important for them to remember that job benefits can also take the form of flexible hours, longer paid vacations, mental health days, broad health insurance coverage, paid and unpaid sabbaticals, and pay based on services provided rather than hours spent in the office. Administrators should also recognize that some agencies are able to offer their clinical staff comparatively high salaries, which may reflect administrative practices that effectively generate income and efficiently manage the agency's resources.

To heighten administrators' awareness of morale issues, we have identified three potential sources of staff dissatisfaction: organizational communication, physical environment, and staff benefits and opportunities. In the following sections, emphasis is given to the clinical staff's perceptions of supervisors, agency directors, and boards of directors.

Clinician Relationships with Administrators

Clinician Relationships with Program Managers

Clinical staff members expect program managers to provide leadership, to keep them informed about important program management and agency administrative issues, to represent them to top-level administration and other program units, to protect them from excessive administrative detail, to facilitate conflict resolution, to carry out personnel policies fairly, to be technically competent and therefore serve as a resource on clinical matters, and to facilitate fruitful program meetings that are both instructive and enjoyable to attend. These expectations are not unrealistic, since they typically characterize a program manager's job description. Yet inadequate or incompetent supervision and program management is a primary source of job dissatisfaction among clinicians. Listed below are several clinician perspectives on supervisory program managers:

1. Technically incompetent supervisors (that is, those with inadequate knowledge and expertise) are viewed with resentment and intolerance by clinicians, who invest considerable energy in working around them and in wondering what it would take to have them removed.
2. Boring, nonproductive, or conflict-ridden staff meetings are seen largely as a reflection of an incompetent program manager.
3. Although clinicians value the human relations skills of program managers, they prefer competence over niceness. Nice managers who are otherwise incompetent or who lack upward power often provide obstacles to getting things done and are a source of embarrassment to the staff.

4. Insecure managers are often seen as withholding information from staff and
    preventing upward mobility or visibility of their staff members by excluding
    them from important planning activities or other situations that would ex-
    pose them to more powerful persons within the organization.
5. Managers who align themselves strongly with administration and neglect
    their responsibilities to champion staff concerns find little cooperation from
    clinical staff. Misuse of authority, arrogance, and involvement in staff con-
    flicts are seen as untrustworthy, insincere, and irresponsible behavior.

    Program supervisors are vital to the success of a mental health organiza-
tion. They, more than top-level administrators, are responsible for inspiring,
mobilizing, and coordinating the efforts of a multidisciplinary staff. To the extent
that managers are unable to enlist the support of staff, programs will suffer.
Persons to fill such managerial roles should therefore be selected and groomed
with a great deal of forethought and care.

Clinician Relationships with Agency Directors

    In contrast to supervisors, agency directors—particularly in moderate-to-
large-size agencies—usually have very little direct contact with clinical staff. Clinical staff perceptions of directors are, therefore, of a different nature. In a recent
study of mental health staff, Glasscote and Gudeman (1969) found that the most
frequently mentioned source of dissatisfaction was agency administration. There
are no easy explanations for this finding nor, for that matter, any easy solutions to
problems seemingly inherent in the clinician-agency director relationship.
    Directors have been described as puppets with hundreds of people pulling
the strings. Most string pullers, however, are unaware of both the number and the
nature of the other string pullers, and relate to the director from their own parochial perspectives. This applies not just to clinicians but to board members,
legislators, state and county agency directors, funding sources, community representatives, and so on. Mental health administrators are not often or freely praised.
Their inability to be all things to all people leads them to adopt adaptive and
coping mechanisms that are sometimes interpreted as isolationist, uncaring, cold,
and calculating. In a sense, they learn not to care so intensely, to take things less
personally, and to keep in perspective all the criticisms and unrealistic expectations that unsympathetically fall their way. Successful and effective administrators can, however, be differentiated from those who are less skillful, and a growing
body of literature and training opportunities in mental health administration
attests to the fact that mental health programs can be more effectively managed.
Clinician perceptions of agency directors comprise one type of information that
directors can use to examine their impact on the organization. A number of
commonly held perceptions are identified below:

1. The concept of the "invisible" director derives mainly from large organiza-
    tions, where the director seldom attends program or unit meetings and is

frequently out of the building or tied up in closed-door meetings, and where leadership roles of the director are preempted by other administrative tasks.

2. Clinicians sometimes see themselves as concerned with clients and directors as concerned with dollars—a micro versus macro perspective on mental health.

3. Directors are seen to show preference for those who are socially or professionally similar to themselves, reproducing themselves in kind through their management selection process.

4. There is a tendency for clinicians to respect administrators who have paid their dues as competent mental health practitioners.

5. Directors do not readily give personal recognition to staff members for their contributions to the organization.

6. Directors seldom share information from the board of directors.

7. Administrative style is less important to staff than being kept informed about organizational problems, future directions, proposed changes, and so on (Whittington, 1975).

Although directors seldom have substantial contact with clinical staff, their influence is often felt in ways they would perhaps find surprising. Administrators, by virtue of their position in the organization, frequently are ascribed more power, more knowledge, and more expertise than they experience themselves to have. Also, because clinicians usually know very little about the director, transference and projective processes are likely to influence their perceptions of directors, as well as vice versa. Consequently, the relationship between clinician and director is often superficial and based on inaccurate or incomplete information.

Clinician Relationships with Boards of Directors

If we were to ask clinicians for their impressions of board members, most would be unable to identify board members by name or to identify what it is they do, how often, or with whom. Perhaps the most distinguishing feature of board-clinician relationships is that they are characterized by distance. Since clinical staff members seldom interact with board members and are seldom privy to the processes that lead to their decisions, clinicians often assume they are indifferent to or uninformed regarding clinical matters, preoccupied with unit costs, and overly concerned with administrative issues.

Board members have also been known to be unsympathetic to salary matters where the clinical staff is concerned, inferring from their own volunteer status that staff members should be willing to work for low salaries and put in the necessary overtime for the cause of mental health. Board members often do not understand the roles and functions of the clinical staff, and, similarly, clinicians do not understand the power and authority which board members exercise. Although in some agencies clinicians complain about the lack of representation on the board, in other agencies the board is so remote to them that little thought is given to lack of staff involvement in board activities.

It has been said that there are two kinds of boards—those that are effective and those that are ineffective. Effective boards take their responsibilities seriously and are active in setting priorities, policies, standards, and guidelines. Ineffective boards are token in nature, rubber-stamping the view of agency directors. In one sense, the ineffective board may be more acceptable to clinicians since it is the least intrusive. However, as boards take on more governing responsibilities, the potential for greater board-clinician conflict increases, and administrators need to develop effective means for channeling information between board members and clinical staff members.

A Comparison of Administrative and Clinical Roles

Thus far, we have presented how clinicians perceive several administrative functions—accountability, the exercise of power, organizational decision making/organizational change, and job satisfaction—as well as how they view program managers, agency directors, and agency boards of directors. In this section, we suggest some ways in which administrators can help clinicians better understand administrative roles and the administrative process.

Administrators who at one time made the transition from clinical to administrative roles can well testify to their own lack of socialization to assume administrative behaviors, attitudes, and perceptual screens (Patti and Austin, 1977). We should not be surprised, therefore, to find that most clinicians possess inadequate or distorted role information about administrative functions. One explanation for inadequate role socialization lies in the apparent lack of overlap in administrative and clinical roles. Typical roles are contrasted in Table 1.

Because most administrators come from clinical backgrounds, clinicians and administrators have a relatively common base for understanding clinical roles. The administrative roles in Table 1, however, may not be well understood by clinicians or, in fact, by administrators who themselves think of their tasks as those of planning, organizing, coordinating, and controlling.

The interpersonal roles—figurehead, leader, and liaison—arise directly from administrators' formal authority. The figurehead role is largely ceremonial in nature—for example, greeting touring visitors, giving public awards, taking important constituents to lunch. The leadership role relates to administrators' responsibilities for hiring and training staff, motivating and encouraging employees, and reconciling individual staff member needs with the goals of the organization. In the liaison role, administrators make contacts with persons outside the vertical chain of command: peers, state and county officials, and other constituent representatives.

Administrators' informational roles—monitor, disseminator, spokesperson—emerge from their interpersonal contacts both with subordinates and with the network of contacts outside the vertical chain of command. As monitors, administrators perpetually scan the environment for information, not infrequently receiving unsolicited information (often in the form of gossip, hearsay, and speculation) from a network of personal contacts. In the disseminator role,

Table 1. Comparison of Administrative and Clinical Roles.

	Administrative Roles*	Clinical Roles
Interpersonal	Figurehead	Team member
	Leader	Intake worker
	Liaison	Case conference participant
		Crisis counselor
		Treatment implementor
Informational	Monitor	Trainer/educator
	Disseminator	Program or case consultant to
	Spokesperson	other agencies
		Agency information sensor
		Program developer
		Outreach specialist
		Client advocate and broker
Decisional Roles	Entrepreneur	Diagnostician
	Disturbance handler	Treatment planner
	Resource mobilizer	Treatment evaluator and follow-
	Resource allocator	up specialist
	Negotiator	
	Program evaluator	

*Administrative roles and categories are adapted from Mintzberg (1975).

administrators pass privileged information directly to subordinates who would otherwise not have access to it. As spokespersons, administrators send information to persons outside their units, often in the form of speeches and reports to persons or groups who influence program funding and direction.

Administrators' decisional roles emerge both from formal authority and from the accumulation of information. As entrepreneurs, administrators seek to improve their own programs or units. As disturbance handlers, they respond to pressure or constraints imposed from the environment, over which they frequently exert little influence. Administrators also have decisional responsibilities for mobilizing and allocating program resources and authorizing program decisions before they are implemented. As negotiators, administrators handle grievances, bargain for territory and staff, and influence agency priorities. Finally, in the evaluator role, administrators have responsibilities for assessing the operation and effectiveness of their units.

With little experiential understanding of these administrative roles, clinicians are easily influenced by popular beliefs and misconceptions about human services administration, including the belief that formal organizations and those who run them have little commitment to the quality of human services, the belief that administrators must compromise their values and ethics in order to survive, the belief that good management is a function of personality rather than acquired knowledge and skill, and the belief that administrators are more concerned with things and abstractions than with people (Patti and Austin, 1977). Such beliefs contribute to a lack of appreciation on the part of clinicians for the concerns and actions of administrators.

It is our contention that better understanding of administration by clinical staff will not only enhance communication but also facilitate more cooperative and productive working relationships and ultimately increase agency effectiveness. In addition, the exposure of clinicians to administrative behaviors, attitudes, and perceptual screens can greatly facilitate the transition to administrative roles. In what ways can we bridge the gap between clinical and administrative worlds? What degree of fusion between the two worlds is both feasible and appropriate? Although it is not our intent to address these questions here, a mental health administrator's ongoing process of self-assessment must include an examination of his or her relationships with clinical staff members, perhaps by asking questions like the following:

1. What information do I disseminate in my organization? How important is it that clinicians get the information that I have? Do I keep too much information to myself because dissemination is time-consuming or inconvenient? How can I get more information to others so that they can be more responsible decision makers and participants in the organization?

2. How do I gather information? Can I make greater use of the clinical staff to obtain the information I need? Can the clinical staff do some of the scanning for me?

3. What pace of change am I asking my organization to tolerate? Do we sufficiently analyze the impact of proposed changes on both the day-to-day functioning and the future of the organization? To what extent do I involve clinicians in program planning and other important changes that influence their work performance?

4. How do clinicians react to my administrative style? Am I sufficiently sensitive to the powerful influence my actions have on them? Do I fully understand their reactions to my actions? Do I find an appropriate balance between encouragement and pressure? Do I stifle their initiative?

5. Do I use different modes of communication appropriately? Do I know how to make the most of written communication? Do I rely excessively on memos or excessively on face-to-face communication? Do I spend enough time touring the organization to observe activity firsthand? Am I too detached from the heart of the organization's activities, seeing things only abstractly?

6. Do clinical staff members feel like cogs in a machine, or do they feel that their efforts will be recognized and mean something to the organization? How do I assess staff motivation, conviction, and morale? Do I have an effective program for staff development and advancement?

7. Do I focus on what the organization can become, rather than on what it has been? How do I bring new blood into the organization? How do I combat vested interests and procedures that no longer serve the organization's interests? Do I rely upon jurisdictional boundaries, or do I view the internal structure as fluid and flexible in response to changing interests and needs? Am I open to criticism?

In many respects, the clinical staff has been an untapped resource for administrators. Insight into clinical staff perspectives on administration and inclusion of clinical staff members in what is typically considered administrative territory offer promise and direction for improving the administration of mental health organizations. This chapter should serve as one point of departure for understanding and improving administrative practices and the administrator-clinician relationship.

References

Aiken, W. J., Smits, S., and Lollar, D. J. "Leadership Behavior and Job Satisfaction in State Rehabilitation Agencies." *Personnel Psychology*, 1972, *25*, 65–73.

Argyris, C. "Organizational Leadership and Participative Management." *Journal of Business*, 1955, *28* (1), 1–7.

Friesen, B. "Power and the Middle Manager." Unpublished paper, School of Social Work, University of Washington, 1980.

Glasscote, R. M., and Gudeman, J. E. *The Staff of the Mental Health Center.* Washington, D.C.: Joint Information Service, 1969.

Herzberg, F., Snyderman, B., and Mausner, B. *The Motivation to Work.* (2nd ed.) New York: Wiley, 1959.

Johns, E. A. *The Sociology of Organizational Change.* New York: Pergamon Press, 1973.

Kanter, R. M. *Men and Women of the Corporation.* New York: Basic Books, 1977.

Kermish, I., and Kushin, F. "Why High Turnover? Social Work Staff Losses in a County Welfare Agency." *Public Welfare*, 1969, *27*, 134–137.

Levinson, D. J., and Klerman, G. L. "The Clinician-Executive: Some Problematic Issues for the Psychiatrist in Mental Health Organizations." *Administration in Mental Health*, Winter 1972, pp. 53–67.

McCluskey, J. E. "Beyond the Carrot and the Stick: Liberating Power Without Control." In W. G. Bennis and others (Eds.), *The Planning of Change.* (3rd ed.) New York: Holt, Rinehart and Winston, 1976, 383–403.

Miller, S. O. "Components of Job Satisfaction for Beginning Social Workers." Kalamazoo: School of Social Work, Western Michigan University, 1970 (mimeograph).

Mintzberg, H. "The Manager's Job: Folklore and Fact." *Harvard Business Review*, 1975, *8*, 49–61.

Olmstead, J. A., and Christensen, H. E. *Effects of Agency Work Contexts: An Intensive Field Study.* Washington, D.C.: U.S. Department of Health, Education, and Welfare, 1973.

Patti, R., and Austin, M. "Socializing the Direct Service Practitioner in the Ways of Supervisory Management." *Administration in Social Work*, 1977, *1* (3), 267–280.

Whittington, H. G. "People Make Programs: Personnel Management." In S. Feldman (Ed.), *The Administration of Mental Health Services.* Springfield, Ill.: Thomas, 1975.

❧ 2 ❦

Mental Health
Treatment Methods

LeNora B. Mundt

Information about the broad array of treatment methodologies used by mental health practitioners is important for (1) managers who have come up through the clinical ranks and now experience some distancing from treatment issues; (2) those who had limited clinical experience and need a breadth of understanding; (3) managers who need to balance different treatment orientations within a program in order to guarantee a mix of perspectives; (4) those who need to see the importance of individual, group, and community intervention approaches; and (5) those who seek to relate relevant treatment orientations to the stages of program development. This chapter examines four treatment methodologies—crisis intervention; the psychotherapies, including cognitive, behavioral, and affective therapies; advocacy; and consultation—from the perspective of the whole person and the multidimensional aspects of human functioning. Since the community mental health movement is based on treating individuals within the context of normal everyday living, treatment methods are also examined with regard to the attention given to an individual family, neighborhood, and community.

Based on the ethics of his or her profession, a clinician's first priority is the treatment of the client, whereas the administrator's first priority and ethical responsibility is to the effective and efficient management of the financial and staff resources of the organization. So long as these two priorities are understood and shared within the organization, harmony prevails. The absence of such mutual respect and collaboration leads to mistrust and misunderstanding. The intent of this chapter is to help mental health managers identify the treatment responsibilities of the clinician in the context of the skills, knowledge, values, and goals required in delivering mental health services. With this information, administrators can do their jobs more effectively and aid in the prevention of conflict within mental health systems.

Historical Perspective

Many factors influence the manner in which methodologies develop and are practiced in the treatment and prevention of mental illness. Medical advancements, myths about mental illness, societal attitudes and beliefs, theories of causation, prevention and treatment, and costs for care of public charges have all been known to influence the planning of mental health programs and the treatments chosen in the prevention and reduction of mental illness.

Perhaps the most significant influence on treatment methodologies has been the theories of causation of mental illness. Over the centuries, priests, physicians, social scientists, and politicians have postulated various explanations. Hippocrates theorized that "madness" was related to the mixing of different types of bile. Others believed that mentally ill people were possessed by the devil. Mental illness has been described as an irritation of the brain, a behavior disorder due to reactions to psychological and biological stress, a hereditary phenomenon caused by brain degeneration, a nervous system disorder, and a process of the unconscious.

These various explanations of causation have affected how society in general has perceived and cured mentally ill persons. For example, when mental illness was viewed as a sign of witchcraft or possession by the devil, the mentally ill person was "cured" by being burned at the stake. Later, when illness was believed to be inherited, families would hide ill members and, instead of treating them, would aid in their demise. When thought to be an organic disease of the brain, mental illness was treated with lobotomies and electroshock. With Freud's theory of the unconscious came treatment by hypnosis and psychoanalysis. Later still, the emphasis on cultural causes brought about efforts to reform ghettos, child-rearing practices, and the community mental health movement. More recently, schizophrenia has been treated by developing and improving communication patterns within families, and current studies of blood chemistry are underway to help effect chemical change in the brain processes of schizophrenics by dialysis.

Some explanations of mental illness are based on research data, whereas others are based on belief systems, and mental health professionals need to discriminate between fact and fantasy when planning mental health programs. Obviously, the program of choice would be the program that has been planned and developed according to the findings of systematic research. Unfortunately, however—perhaps because of incomplete research or inadequate evaluation of treatment methodologies—little program planning is done in this way. For example, inappropriate program planning can result in therapists with general degrees and broad experience being assigned to a set caseload without extensive examination of treatment methodology or client background. Such an approach is neither cost effective nor treatment efficient.

In setting up a mental health program or in selecting a treatment of choice for a particular illness, mental health clinicians must address themselves to several important issues. First, they must understand the theory and its underlying assumptions, addressing themselves to questions like the following: According to the theory, how do people change in their thinking, feeling, and behaviors? Is this assumption appropriate to the specific program or client in question? To what extent does the social environment influence the process of change?

Second, they must consider population variables. For one reason or another—for example, discrimination against certain population groups by the mental health care system, increased visibility of certain populations, disproportionate stresses on certain groups of people—certain population groups receive more mental health treatment than others. The President's Commission on Mental Health (1978) revealed that more women than men are treated for schizophrenia and depression and receive prescriptions for tranquilizers, more black people than members of any other group are institutionalized for mental illness, and more married women than single or divorced women report mental disturbance. These factors influence the diagnosis rendered, the treatment type and length, and the sexual and racial composition of the mental health staff.

With these issues and this historical perspective in mind, we will describe the major treatment methods used today by identifying the underlying assumptions of each theory, describing the treatment process, and specifying the research and evaluation components of the treatment. Methodological bias to certain population groups will be noted, and case examples will be used to demonstrate the use of the therapy. The therapies presented—the psychotherapies, crisis intervention, advocacy, and consultation—include those directed toward the correction of illness as well as those aimed at prevention, and the client of a mental health agency may experience one (or more) of these intervention therapies in the course of treatment.

The Psychotherapies

Psychotherapy, a broad term encompassing a multitude of treatment techniques and procedures carried on by a number of different professions, may be defined as a form of treatment for problems of an emotional, behavioral, physiological, or environmental nature in which a client is assisted—by a trained person using suggestion, counseling, or psychoanalysis—in removing, modifying, or retarding existing symptoms or disturbed patterns of behavior and in promoting positive personality growth and development. Since body, mind, and environment are so thoroughly intermeshed, psychotherapy must take into account all the important dimensions of human functioning—thought, emotion, behavior, and interaction with the environment.

The Assessment Process

In the diagnostic phase of treatment, the clinician uses his or her knowledge of the person's symptoms and of the physical, emotional, social, and environmental context of the person's problem to formulate an assessment. Knowing how the person deals with life and change will aid in selecting an intervention that does not seem strange, frightening, or alien. Tailoring intervention to a person's coping style should result in more client involvement in the treatment process.

An assessment formulation includes five main areas: the unit to be treated, the dynamics of the problem or illness, factors maintaining the illness or problem, the treatment plan, and the method of evaluation. The treatment plan outlines a step-by-step process for correcting the illness, specifying the methodology to be used.

The unit of treatment includes the person who is manifesting the mental illness or disturbance and may also include other significant persons, most often family members, who are influencing or affected by the illness. For instance, if the interactions of several members of the family were helping to maintain the illness, treatment might involve changing the behaviors, thoughts, or feelings of the whole family with conjoint family therapy. As an example, we cite the following case study:

> Tommy, age eight, presented problems of crying, fighting, bed-wetting, fire-setting, and running away from home. The parents disagreed on discipline and on expectations of Tommy's behavior. The father, who was feeling depressed and had been hospitalized one year before for depression, was unemployed. The mother was anxious and threatened to leave the family unless things changed. Each family member was under stress, and there was a threat of family disruption.

Although Tommy's behavior was the presenting problem, the data indicate that many more factors were involved, each interacting to perpetuate a "family illness." In order to facilitate congruency in communication, discipline, and positive supports for behavior change, the family as a whole is taken as the unit of treatment. The family can be seen by an individual therapist or by cotherapists in consultation with a psychiatrist for possible medication and evaluation. Since the father may need rehospitalization if the stress within the family is not corrected, treatment is aimed not only at alleviating Tommy's dysfunction, but also at preventing the recurrence of the father's illness.

Determining the unit of treatment and collaborating with other mental health professionals are important activities in delivering mental health services. This approach to service delivery requires a staff with multiple skills in treatment and physical facilities to accommodate the treatment of several people at one time, and may well require the capacity and resources to make home visits, consult with school personnel, and seek medical consultation.

Also significant in assessment formulation is an understanding of the dynamics of the problem or illness, which involves more than just a cursory examination of the symptoms. Such an understanding must include a prioritizing of the problems to determine their interrelatedness and how the solution of one problem affects the others. In the above example, it would be important to know how the father's depression may or may not be affecting Tommy's symptoms, the mother's anxiety, and the family's motivation to receive help. Each problem is maintained through certain behaviors, thoughts, and/or feelings of each family member within the context of their living situation (for example, financial resources, extended family/friend relationships, and neighborhood conditions). It is important to gather data related to the problem: the onset, intensity, frequency, duration, and context. Tommy's bedwetting may be preceded by the onset of father's depressive symptoms or by the parents' disagreement about discipline. Such thoughtful examination of each dynamic within the case situation clarifies the interrelationship of the problems presented and may facilitate the client's understanding of the connections between events and encourage participation in the treatment plan.

The assessment process should conclude with specification of a treatment procedure including the goals or outcomes expected from implementation of the treatment and the rationale for its use, as well as a plan for evaluating the treatment's effectiveness.

Treatment Planning and Monitoring

The goal of therapy is change—to make maladaptive thoughts, behaviors, feelings, and/or environments more functional. As mentioned earlier, these dimensions of human functioning are interrelated: a change in one dimension causes change in the others. The majority of methodologies focus change on only one dimension at a time and assume the change will generalize to others. For example, there are studies (McFall and Marston, 1971) that indicate that changed behavior, by affecting the way in which a person interacts with other people and the environment, may generate more positive responses to that person, thus enhancing his or her self-perception (thoughts) and self-esteem (feelings) and enabling him or her to manage the environment more effectively. With this assumption in mind, the mental health professional should (1) assess which dimension is likely to engage the client most quickly in the change process, (2) select ways to monitor whether the change affects the other dimensions of functioning, and (3) determine whether the change remains in effect over a period of time.

The person seeking help desires relief from stress as soon as possible, and usually presents priorities as to what is most desirable to change. A proper assessment will provide guidelines as to which symptoms can be affected most quickly and will provide information about how that person made and responded to changes in the past. Some persons are very rational in their approach to life and problem solving; others need to feel comfortable or safe before risking change. Still others are action-focused and try behavior change first. If the therapist uses these data to select a methodology that seems familiar and makes sense to the client, the probability of the client's engaging and remaining in treatment will be higher.

Monitoring change involves knowledge of all dimensions of the person in which the symptoms of illness are operational. For example, if a person changes behavior by becoming less claustrophobic, does his or her thinking about the phobia also change and is anxiety reduced? Further, does the change in behavior indicate a solution to life circumstances, such as being able to ride in an elevator or maintain a job? For example:

May, a thirty-two-year-old mother of two preschool children, became immobilized when leaving her house, experiencing increased heart rate, sweating, thought confusion, and feelings of loss of control. These symptoms were interfering with activities with her husband and her children and threatened her with the loss of her job. The symptoms had first appeared within a week after an automobile accident six months earlier, and the severity had increased during the past month. Her history revealed that her mother had died in an auto accident when she was twelve years old, resulting in her being placed in foster care and separated from the rest of her family. May had always been an active, social person and was involved in many school, church, and job-related activities. She did not understand her feelings and wanted only that the symptoms go away.

The phobia that May was experiencing was affecting her behavior, her thoughts, her feelings, and her relationships with her husband, her children, and her employer. Since her focus for change was on the removal of the behavior, the most relevant methodology was a behavioral one; in this case, desensitization. When she was able to leave the house for gradually increased periods of time, she was then able to examine and gain insight into the irrational thoughts that presented themselves at such times and to change the thoughts to more rational ones. As she experienced success, her feelings about her ability to control her life increased and her relationships with her husband and children improved.

The clinician can develop a treatment plan that addresses the interrelatedness of the symptoms of the phobia and monitors the change of behavior in all areas of the client's life in which the symptoms created problems. If the selected method, desensitization, is not achieving the expected goal, another method must be implemented. Evaluating the progress of treatment is vital.

The probability of change remaining stable is higher if all dimensions of the person's functioning have changed. In the case cited, May not only changed her behavior but also dealt with her irrational thoughts, understood her desire to be in control of her life, and changed her relationship with her environment. Unless all four of these areas—behavior, thought, feeling, and environment—had changed, the probability of the return of the phobia would have been higher. With change in all areas comes a process of integration that ensures stabilization.

Since it is imperative that methods of treatment consider the whole person and situation, it is often necessary to use more than one method in the treatment planning. The sequencing of the therapeutic methods depends on the dynamics found in the assessment—for example, if the symptoms require beginning with a behavioral approach, then cognitive or affective methods may be used sequentially; if the personality of the client requires that the clinician begin with an affective method, then a cognitive or behavioral method may follow. The environment or milieu of the person is always a factor, and in some instances may be the first to require intervention, as in the case of foster care for children who need different parenting before behaviors, thinking, or attitudes can change.

In the sections that follow, four major types of psychotherapy—cognitive, behavioral, affective, and environmental—will be discussed, and each description will include the theory underlying the therapy, the process of treatment, and a critique of the method.

Cognitive Therapies

Cognitive therapies seek to change, modify, or strengthen the thought processes in ways that are more functional for the person. Some of the basic assumptions in cognitive therapy are that people are born with a potential to be rational as well as irrational; that people's tendencies toward irrational thinking, self-damaging habituations, wishful thinking, and intolerance are frequently exacerbated by their culture and family group; that humans tend to perceive, think, emote, and behave simultaneously; and that introspection, insight, reality testing, and learning are basic cognitive processes. Proponents of cognitive therapies believe that the major treatment procedure is to identify the irrational belief systems or thoughts which lead to dysfunctional behavior and then correct those thoughts to more readily correspond to the reality of the individual's life. This process then brings about change in the individual's behavior patterns and feelings.

Types of cognitive therapy include rational-emotive therapy (Ellis and Grieger, 1977), cognitive therapy (Beck and others, 1979), cognitive-behavioral therapy (Mahoney, 1977), cognitive behavior modification (Meichenbaum, 1977), and Adlerian therapy (Corsini, 1979). Other therapies that include the prominence of thought change are psychoanalysis, transactional analysis, and person-centered therapy.

Most clinicians do not deal with unconscious motivations and processes but with the thoughts that a person is able to verbalize, based on the assumption that human beings strive to avoid unpleasant experience and devise ways to explain traumatic life experiences. The lifestyle of the individual can perpetuate and extend irrational thoughts and misconceptions that may lead to feelings of distrust, inferiority, self-deprecation, depression, and anxiety and to phobias and other neuroses. Since one of the premises is that reactions, motivations, and overt behavior are guided by thinking, the clinician helps increase the client's awareness of maladaptive ideas that interfere with the ability to cope with life experiences and produce inappropriate, excessive, and painful emotional reactions. The clinician must understand the client and his or her environment and circumstances well enough to locate the activating stimulus that gives rise to the maladaptive thought, recognize the thought that this stimulus provokes, and identify the maladaptive behavior in which the client then engages.

Verbal probing on the part of the clinician helps to increase client self-awareness by clarifying the distortions, self-injunctions, and self-reproaches that lead to distress or disability. Awareness of the sequence of the thoughts often helps to reveal the rules that produce these faulty self-signals. For example, an activating stimulus might be the sight of a couple walking down the street holding hands, which begins a sequence of thought processes like the following: They are happy; they have each other; I am alone; I am unhappy; I have no one that loves me; I am not worth loving; I must have something wrong with me; I am no good.

This may lead to morbid ideation, suicidal thoughts, or other self-destructive behaviors.

Together, the clinician and the client examine each of these thoughts to evaluate their validity and the assumptions on which they are based. If the thought is an irrational one, therapist and client substitute a rational thought that is true to the client's life situation. If the thought is accurate—for example, "I am alone," therapist and client find ways not to be alone and also probe the meaning of aloneness for the client. The client must work at realistic life situations and not substitute unrealistic thoughts, even though positive. This process might involve the client in some reality testing—for example, talking with friends or applying for a job—to reaffirm the existence of worthwhile qualities.

Besides the thought-substitution and reality-testing techniques, some cognitive therapists use role-reversal exercises, humor, task assignment, and reflective procedures, which focus constantly on the recognition and correction of maladaptive or irrational thoughts. A system for practicing outside the therapeutic session is formulated and integrated into the client's lifestyle in order to keep the client aware of his or her thoughts and thought substituting. The mode of therapy can be either individual, family, or group. The advantage of group process or family therapy is the reinforcement the person receives from group or family members for thought substitution and reality checking, whereas reflection and self-monitoring can best be handled in individual therapy.

Other therapies that deal primarily with the cognitive dimension but hold a more extensive explanation as to rationale than the purely cognitive therapies are psychoanalysis, transactional analysis, Adlerian psychotherapy, and person-centered therapy. These treatment methods are based on Freudian, neo-Freudian, or ego psychology and have some major theoretical differences from other cognitive therapies—for example, the concepts of the unconscious (id, ego, and super-ego) underlie the formulation of the treatment methodology—but the techniques used are not dissimilar. Psychoanalysis deals with conscious and unconscious thought processes and the symbolic meanings of thoughts and leads to a rational understanding of the behavior, symptom, or illness. Transactional analysis, with its division of the personality into adult, parent, and child, focuses on the cognitive understanding of how these parts of the person operate together to cause dysfunction. In person-centered therapy, "the theoretical base . . . is a belief in the exquisite rationality of human growth under optimal conditions. . . . The task of the therapist is to facilitate the client's awareness of and trust in his own actualizing process" (Corsini, 1979, pp. 180–181).

Limited outcome studies indicate that cognitive therapies are effective in the treatment of depression, phobias, and some neuroses. The studies do not, however, control for racial, class, or sexual differences. Clients most likely to benefit from these methods are those whose orientation to life is cognitive and rational, who have enough intelligence to recall and verbalize thought processes, and who are motivated to look for reasonable substitutions or explanations for their "rules." Proponents claim that cognitive therapies work well with most people and that changes in cognitive functioning generalize to behavior, feelings, and environmental functioning.

Behavioral Therapies

The behavioral therapies aim at changing the person's behavior—with the expectation that feelings and thoughts will change as a result—and focus on observable changes. Techniques are primarily action-focused, with the client interacting with the therapist and others in the environment, and include behavior modification, task-centered casework, assertion training, play therapy, parent effectiveness training, and reality therapy.

The psychotherapies draw their primary theoretical assumptions from social learning theory. Behavioral intervention does not rest so much on theory as on the relationships between behavior and environment observed in a wide range of animal species, behaviors, and situations (Gambrill, 1977). Basic assumptions include: (1) People have become what they are through learning processes, or, more correctly, through the interaction of the environment with their genetic endowment; (2) Problems are learned and can be unlearned; (3) Deficits occur when there has been inadequate learning, but these deficits can be corrected through provision of necessary learning experiences; (4) Past events are not to be used as an excuse for behaving in an irresponsible manner.

Certain practice principles are developed from these assumptions. Emphasis is placed on current controlling conditions and on the relationship between behavior and the current antecedent and consequent events. Diagnostic labeling is deemphasized, and attention is paid to observable, countable responses and the measurement of effects. Reality therapy emphasizes the need to accept and be accountable for one's behaviors and their consequences. Task-centered casework emphasizes the need to focus on current behaviors, rather than on their historical roots. All the behavioral therapies utilize a corrective behavioral experience and see change as occurring within a brief period of time.

As described earlier, behavioral therapies require careful assessments that focus on the antecedents, contingencies, and consequences of events and behaviors. Careful attention is paid to specific behaviors that the client has identified as maladaptive, and treatment is based upon the assumption that all behaviors, thoughts, and feelings occur in response to external or internal stimulation. Although the behavior therapist focuses on the correction of one behavior, the interrelatedness of other problems or behaviors is noted.

Techniques involve an active, directive role in the analysis of behaviors as well as in the therapy process. Modeling, task assignment, self-monitoring, role playing, systematic desensitization, relaxation exercises, flooding, assertion training, and token economy represent but a few of the techniques and procedures used in behavioral therapies. Although behavioral therapies originally were devised for individuals, they are commonly applied to groups and families. As with other therapies, the unit of treatment is determined on the basis of who is included within the problem definition. In addition, since it focuses on observable, measurable dysfunction, behavioral therapy lends itself to more reliable assessment of results than do some other forms of therapy. The techniques are replicable, and tangible rewards increase client motivation to continue change.

Behavioral therapy has been developed specifically for the treatment of maladaptive behavior; it requires cooperation of the client, must be tailored to the unique behavior patterns of each client, and must follow the client's specific desire to alter behavior. The use of behavioral therapy with psychotic patients was never a goal of its originators, although some advocates of implosion therapy have claimed to benefit schizophrenics. Once psychotic symptoms are in remission or controlled by medication, the use of some behavioral therapy techniques, particularly those of assertion training, may be indicated. The client's intelligence level does not seem to be highly correlated with successful behavioral therapy treatment, although it generally requires the client to be capable of carrying out instructions between sessions. Since most behavioral therapies are action-oriented and directive in technique, problems may arise with clients whose strong need for interpersonal control makes them resist instruction. Also, clients requiring long-term supportive care may have difficulty with *only* this kind of intervention (Corsini, 1979; DiLoreto, 1971; Beck and others, 1979).

Affective Therapies

The aim of the affective therapist is to effect change in the expression of feelings and emotions. Although cognitive and behavioral therapies talk about feelings and their change, such therapies do not direct their specific techniques to the identification, quality, or handling of feelings. Feelings are considered a by-product, important but not central to therapy. Affective therapies are based on the assumption that, with a change in feelings, the person's behavior and thinking will change. The clinician is interested in facilitating emotional growth that will enhance the quality of life for the client.

Of all the therapies, this type of therapy deals with the most unknown, immeasurable qualities; it is a therapy of experiencing life. Defining specific terminologies is difficult and believed unimportant. The affective therapies do, however, pay attention to the environment, behavior, and thoughts and claim that these components make up, with feelings, the gestalt of human functioning.

Gestalt therapy, experiential therapy, psychodrama, encounter groups, guided group interaction, primal scream, and bioenergetics are some of the therapies which focus on affective change. Rather than having an organized theoretical foundation, these therapies are based on a philosophy that is similar in many respects to existentialism and humanism. For example, gestalt therapy is defined by Simkin (1979) as a noninterpretive, ahistorical, existentially based system of psychotherapy that focuses on the immediate, present awareness of one's experience and rejects cognitive explanations or interpretations of causes or purposes.

The affective therapies direct the client to internal feelings and an awareness of self in relationship to others and the environment. Homeostasis and self-actualization are basic concepts. The primary techniques involve verbal and experiential interchange with the therapist in which clients are asked to report their subjective reality—what they are aware of at the moment, including thoughts, sensory-motor impressions, and feelings. In order to do this, the client is guided to examine support systems—breathing, bodily tensions, physical comfort or discomfort—and connections between body and emotions. Techniques allowing feedback from others help the person to differentiate self from others, to remain in the here and now, to confront any falsity of expression, and to remain authentic. Psychodrama allows the client to reenact past, present, or future events considered to be unfinished business en route to getting to the present. Old issues are dealt with in terms of how they affect current feelings. Having a conversation with a remembered adversary, for example, may elicit feelings needing expression.

The treatment process of affective therapies requires a commitment of time and effort. The time involved ranges from several months to a year or more. The most widely used mode is the group, although some clinicians work individually or with families. Most affective therapists do not believe in an assessment or diagnostic phase but start with what the client defines as the problem. The verbal and experiential exercises are spontaneous and depend on what the person brings to each session. Treatment is terminated when the client determines that desired solutions have been achieved. The clinician encourages the client to experiment with new behaviors and to share, cognitively and emotionally, the nature of his or her experience.

Although few clinicians use a purely affective methodology, many of the techniques are used in general practice to develop emotional expression and awareness (Barnwell, 1968; Moreno and Enneis, 1950; Simkin, 1979; Perls, 1969; Zinker, 1977). The techniques focus on the importance of relationships in deepening emotional awareness, legitimizing expression of repressed emotions, and accepting unpopular emotions like anger, jealousy, fear, and envy. Clients report that when suppressed emotions are expressed anxiety is decreased, thus freeing them to engage in more productive behavior. The emphasis on focusing on the here and now, recognizing and handling emotional exchanges, and realizing the value of being authentic, open, and genuine with emotions contributes a new and needed dimension to psychotherapy and tends to even the distribution of power between clinician and client in the therapeutic encounter.

Environmental (Milieu) Therapies

Direct intervention in the client's environment is referred to as milieu therapy, environmental manipulation, or environmental support. It is not usually perceived as being a psychotherapy or as requiring great skill and is often overlooked or discounted as a viable methodology. It is, however, an important form of therapy designed to change or modify the client's environment and thereby effect change in thoughts, feelings, and behaviors. Supportive group therapy, recreational therapy, vocational and social skills training, self-care training, behavioral therapies, affective therapies, and cognitive therapies represent but a few of the specific techniques utilized in milieu therapy. The latter three techniques may be introduced into the milieu process by a therapeutic team or used in individual sessions.

As in other therapies, the assessment process includes a careful examination of the problem to be corrected and the personality factors to be affected. If the data indicate that the problem or behavior could best be changed by direct change of the environment, this methodology would be the treatment of choice since it focuses on how the personality of the individual reflects such environmental and sociocultural factors as family, activities, work, language, and habits. Rules and norms that are integrated into the personality structure, as well as behaviors, feelings, and thoughts, are seen to be operationalized within the individual's environment. His or her responses to environmental stresses, resources, and processes are seen as directly influencing perceptions, cognitions, memory, learning, and the activation of emotional responses. The individual's mental processes, distinctively organized toward the goals of self-regulation and social adaptation, lead him or her to respond in distinctive patterns to environmental stimulation.

Since the person is socialized by the total environment, it is assumed that:

1. The environment and culture affect the psychological functioning of the person.
2. Every culture is of paramount importance to its possessor.
3. One who functions in an environment is part of it, and every phase of his or her life and thought reflects that cultural environment.
4. Alien environments produce anxiety and stress (Fenlason, 1962; LeVine, 1973).
5. An individual's conception of self is generated from the social interactions that make up his or her life.

When the environment is contributing to the mental illness of the individual, the therapist modifies that environment so that it will offer the individual stimulation, comfort, cultural familiarity, and corrective interactions with others. Some of the modes of treatment are (1) foster home care for children and adults recently out of institutions; (2) day treatment care in which the person is directly placed in an environment with specific stimuli to produce specific responses; (3) halfway houses, which enable gradual change from large institutions to the client's own home; (4) group homes with persons of similar age; and (5) hospital or institutional placement.

Crisis Intervention

Individuals are frequently faced with emergency situations, both internal and external, that create a state of disequilibrium. The process by which the mental health professional helps restore balance is referred to as crisis intervention. Although the techniques and procedures used in crisis intervention are similar to those used in other psychotherapies, distinct differences exist, based on the definition of crisis and on crisis "theory."

Crisis theory—which has its primary roots in psychodynamic theory, stress theory, and learning theory—is not a formal theory in the sense of being an internally consistent set of verified hypotheses but is a body of knowledge gained from studies of death and dying, family crises, stress and shock, grief reactions, and acute and chronic illness. Crisis is usually perceived as an acute situational disorder that is self-limiting in time and often superimposed on healthy personalities or on long-term chronic conditions (Golan, 1979). Basic assumptions of crisis theory include:

1. An individual is subjected to various internal and external stresses and seeks to maintain a state of equilibrium by use of a series of adaptive maneuvers.
2. The stress creates disturbances in the person's homeostasis that increase if the adaptive maneuvers do not work to restore balance.
3. The stressful or hazardous event is perceived as a threat and creates anxiety.
4. The state of active crisis is time limited, depending on the nature of the hazardous event, the individual's patterns of perception, response, and coping, and the resources available to deal with the situation.
5. Usually within four to six weeks, a new equilibrium is reached, and a reintegration takes place.

Studies of mourning and loss, separation, acute physical disability, and chronic illness have validated some of these assumptions, showing that most people experience crisis in similar ways and that the person who has a series of stresses in a short period of time is more vulnerable to mental disturbance.

Early recognition of the crisis or situational disorder is important and requires specialized knowledge on the part of the mental health professional in identifying normal coping patterns in crisis and in determining when, and to what extent, the person requires intervention. Assessment includes inquiry about the stress, the events preceding the onset of the anxiety, and the individual's attempts at relieving the stress. Symptoms often presented are despair, lethargy, emotional instability, rapid change in social relationships or interests, and suicidal ideations.

The goals of the treatment process are to relieve the symptoms as soon as possible, restore the person to his or her former level of functioning, facilitate an understanding of the precipitating event, identify the way in which the person restored balance, recognize the current state of equilibrium, anticipate any recurrence, and reinforce the ability to cope. It is important that the client understand what happened in order to prevent recurrence of the symptoms and to allow the client to become aware of new behaviors and coping abilities that he or she can call upon when anxiety or stress recurs. According to crisis theory, this process involves four to six weeks of intense work with the client because of the acute nature of the anxiety and the client's sense of inadequacy to cope with the situation.

Techniques used in the process include any or all of those described earlier among the psychotherapies: cognitive, behavioral, affective, and environmental.

The person may need to be given direct advice or suggestions, may need to be put in touch with community resources (hospitals, relatives, support groups), or may need medication, reflection, clarification, rehearsal of new behaviors, thoughts, or social skills. Population groups making contact with crisis programs include all races, cultures, ages, and classes, although there do appear to be more females than males and more married people than single people.

The key factor in using crisis intervention is the identification of the distress as a crisis. At the time of presenting symptoms, the client appears often confused and sometimes disoriented. Examining critical life events at the time of the onset of symptoms is crucial to determining whether the symptoms are situational, and careful evaluation of the effectiveness of each applied intervention aids in confirming whether or not it is useful in that particular case. For example, reduction in tension and confusion as the result of medication, reduction of anxiety by cognitive awareness and reassurance, and follow-through contacts with family should each be evaluated to see if the expected results have been achieved.

Advocacy

Advocacy, a method of intervention not ordinarily perceived as part of the mental health clinician's repertoire, is used regularly in obtaining services for the client. Advocacy is essentially a method for making sure that the client receives the services offered inside and outside the mental health system and is particularly necessary with people considered at risk—the elderly, socially disadvantaged, poor, transient, or minority populations—who hold less powerful positions within the general population, remain in care longer, and have higher recidivism rates. This method is also useful with groups that have been identified as needing special kinds of mental health care but are not receiving the services they require. With the increasing bureaucratization of human service organizations, discrepancies between needs and services rendered are often great.

An assumption of this method is that the persons or groups are unable to handle the problem by themselves and need someone to act on their behalf. It further assumes that the mental health system is less responsive to certain groups or persons than to others and for various reasons discriminates against some people by identifying them as mentally ill more readily than others with the same symptoms—for example, double standards of mental health for men and women (Boverman and others, 1972) or the disproportionate number of hospitalized racial minorities.

The advocacy method involves a careful assessment of the above data, as well as an examination of the client's ability to act on his or her own behalf. If the person is unable to act in gaining needed services, the advocate works within the system to effect service delivery. The techniques used involve communicating needs to administration, gathering supporting evidence, consulting with professionals, appearing before decision-making groups on behalf of the client, and supporting the client during the process. The advocate may bargain with certain power groups within the agency or community to initiate service for special groups of persons or may act at times as a social broker, locating and making available to the client services within the community—for example, arranging an interpreter for a non-English-speaking client or assisting a client in gaining legal aid.

Consultation

Consultation and education, though not specific therapeutic techniques or methodologies, are yet integral functions of the mental health professional's responsibility. Mental health consultation, designed to extend information to individual and agency caregivers less knowledgeable in some aspects of mental health, is a cooperative relationship between two kinds of professionals—the mental health consultant, who is a human relations expert, and the consultee, who specializes in some aspect of human services or a related field (for example, teachers, welfare workers, family physicians, clergy, police, probation officers, media and advertising personnel). Specifically, the goals of consultation are to increase the consultees' effectiveness at work in handling specific clients or programs and to add to the consultees' knowledge so that they will be able to deal effectively with similar cases and problems in the future (Caplan, 1970).

The main thrust of consultation is education and communication, not therapy, supervision, or collaboration. Emotional and personal issues, therefore, are adroitly skirted by the consultant, who uses all his or her clinical skills to establish and maintain an objective, problem-solving atmosphere. The consultee is viewed as a professional of equal status to the consultant, whom the consultant does not confront or tell what must be done. The consultant acts in an advisory role only. He or she may provide differential diagnostic formulations, advise on treatment plans, provide clarifications, and suggest a host of alternatives for solving current work problems, but, unlike the therapist, supervisor, or collaborator, the consultant does not have authority or responsibility for implementing remedial action for the client or program. This authority or responsibility always rests with the consultee.

In addition to having good clinical observation and interviewing skills and effective problem-solving techniques for use in individual and group situations, the mental health consultant must acquire expertise in social systems, organizational theory, and administrative practice, as well as acquiring specialized skills in the particular field in which he or she is consulting. For example, consultation with the police requires familiarity with police organizations, the specific needs and problems associated with police work, and the actual work environment of police personnel. The mental health consultant must be sensitive to the social and political milieu of the consultee and must be clear about his or her function and role within the organization receiving the consultation. This involves attention to: the boundaries of his or her own expertise and knowledge; the consultee's expectations and goals for the consultation; the time frame within which the consultation is to occur; the interrelationship of a specific area of consultation to the total organization; resources within the organization available to the consultant, as well as to the consultee; the method or form the consultation will take; the fees involved for consultation; and the follow-up and evaluation procedure. These issues are often clarified in a contractual agreement.

Basically, there are four types of consultation: (1) client-centered case consultation; (2) consultee-centered case consultation; (3) program-centered administrative consultation; and (4) consultee-centered administrative consultation (Caplan, 1970). A consultation situation is more likely to be a mixture of these types than to fall neatly into any one category, but a brief definition of each type serves to highlight some of the responsibilities of the mental health consultant.

1. *Client-centered case consultation* involves analyzing the client's problems with the consultee, communicating a variety of means by which the client may be helped, and helping the consultee learn how to deal effectively with similar cases in the future.
2. *Consultee-centered consultation* is more educational than diagnostic, focusing on the consultee's difficulty in handling a specific case and helping the consultee remedy work problems related to lack of knowledge, lack of skills, lack of self-confidence, or lack of objectivity.
3. *Program-centered administrative consultation* involves a request from a manager or planning committee for assistance in diagnosing a problem in program development or organization, presenting an appraisal and a range of alternatives, and making recommendations for dealing with the problem.
4. *Consultee-centered administrative consultation* is similar to consultee-centered case consultation except that the focus is on analyzing programming and organizational problems—for example, poor leadership, communication blocks, authority problems, lack of skills, knowledge, and self-confidence—in order to help improve the problem-solving skills of staff.

The basic approach in consultation, then, is problem solving. Consultants try to understand the genesis of the problem by collecting data and then either provide consultees with a number of possible interventions or support them in exploring ways of solving the problems for themselves.

Clinical Evaluation

Clinical evaluation and the utilization of new knowledge and research are critical components of clinical practice, since no theory of behavior or treatment method can address all the problems presented by the large variety of clients seeking mental health services. In recent years, the clinician has been called upon to utilize a multitude of new knowledge and treatment technologies without an overall design for implementation. Nevertheless, empirical knowledge must be systematically collected and the clinician must acquire an empirical approach to practice (Jayaratne and Levy, 1979; Bloom and Fischer, 1981).

Through the use of single-subject design—which requires specifying and measuring the problem, collecting information both before and during intervention, and designing and implementing a specific program of intervention—the clinician is able to measure the change that a methodology produces (Jayaratne and Levy, 1979). Such systematic planning and collection of data develops a knowledge base for behavioral change and contributes to the refinement of treatment methodology theory and to the validation of certain treatment procedures. Such empirical knowledge, combined with the results of other research in the field, provides guidelines to treatment approach and program planning and allows a clearer definition of what is not known in practice.

Conclusion

This chapter has presented an overview, rather than an inclusive discussion, of treatment methodologies. The psychotherapies, crisis intervention, advocacy, and consultation have been described, but such techniques and procedures as social brokerage, case management, and drug therapies have not been included. Treatment methods and assessment have been conceptualized from the multidimensional perspective on human functioning, which includes cognition, behavior, emotions, physiology, and environment.

The development of treatment methods in the field of mental health continues to be influenced by untested theories, myths, superstitions, and political expediency. Knowledge about the cause, treatment, and prevention of mental illness is increasing, with the community mental health movement in the forefront of this progress. Helping the mentally ill to cope with their environment within the context of their community aids in counteracting the myths surrounding the mentally ill and allows for observation and documentation of the treatments involved. Such treatment also recognizes the multidimensional aspects of human functioning and can preclude the hazards of institutionalization.

References

Allen, A. *The Practice and Theory of Individual Psychology*. Paterson, N.J.: Littlefield, Adams, 1963.

Barnwell, J. E. "Gestalt Methods and Techniques in a Poverty Program." In J. S. Simkin (Ed.), *Festschrift for Fritz Perls*. Los Angeles: Celestial Arts, 1968.

Beck, A. T., and others. *Cognitive Therapy of Depression*. New York: Guilford Press, 1979.

Bloom, M., and Fischer, J. *Evaluating Practice: A Guide for Helping Professionals*. Englewood Cliffs, N.J.: Prentice-Hall, 1981.

Boverman, I. I., and others. "Sex-Role Stereotypes and Clinical Judgments of Mental Health." In J. Bardwick (Ed.), *Readings on the Psychology of Women*. New York: Harper & Row, 1972.

Caplan, G. *The Theory and Practice of Mental Health Consultation*. New York: Basic Books, 1970.

Corsini, R. J. (Ed.). *Current Psychotherapies*. (2nd ed.) Itasca, Ill.: Peacock, 1979.

DiLoreto, A. O. *Comparative Psychotherapy: An Experimental Analysis.* Chicago: Aldine-Atherton, 1971.

Ellis, A., and Grieger, R. *Handbook of Rational-Emotive Therapy.* New York: Springer, 1977.

Fenlason, A. F. *Essentials in Interviewing.* (Rev. ed.) New York: Harper & Row, 1962.

Fischer, J. "The Social Work Revolution." *Social Work,* 1981, *26* (3), 14–20.

Gambrill, E. D. *Behavior Modification: Handbook of Assessment, Intervention, and Evaluation.* San Francisco: Jossey-Bass, 1977.

Golan, N. "When Is a Client in Crisis?" *Social Casework,* 1979, *50* (7), 389–394.

Jayaratne, S., and Levy, R. L. *Empirical Clinical Practice.* New York: Columbia University Press, 1979.

LeVine, R. W. *Culture, Behavior, and Personality.* Chicago: Aldine, 1973.

McFall, R. M., and Marston, A. R. "An Experimental Investigation of Behavior Rehearsal in Assertive Training." *Journal of Abnormal Psychology,* 1971, *77* (3), 313–323.

Mahoney, M.J. "Cognitive Therapy and Research: A Question of Questions." *Cognitive Therapy and Research,* 1977, *1,* 5–16.

Mannino, F. V., and Shore, M. F. "Evaluation of Consultation: Problems and Prospects." In A. S. Rogawski (Ed.), *New Directions for Mental Health Services: Mental Health Consultations in Community Settings,* no. 3. San Francisco: Jossey-Bass, 1979.

Meichenbaum, D. H. *Cognitive Behavior Therapy.* New York: Plenum, 1977.

Moreno, J. L., and Enneis, J. M. *Hypnodrama and Psychodrama.* New York: Beacon House, 1950.

Perls, F. S. "Jane's Dreams." In F. S. Perls, *Gestalt Therapy Verbatim.* Moab, Utah: Real People Press, 1969.

President's Commission on Mental Health. *Report of the President's Commission on Mental Health.* Vols. 3, 4. Washington, D.C.: U.S. Government Printing Office, 1978.

Rogers, C., and Dymond, R. (Eds.). *Psychotherapy and Personality Change.* Chicago: University of Chicago Press, 1954.

Schlien, J., and Zimring, F. "Research Directives and Methods in Client-Centered Therapy." In J. T. Hart and T. M. Tomlinson (Eds.), *New Directions in Client-Centered Therapy.* Boston: Houghton Mifflin, 1970.

Shepherd, I. L. "Limitations and Cautions in the Gestalt Approach." In J. Fogar and I. L. Shepherd (Eds.), *Gestalt Therapy Now.* Palo Alto, Calif.: Science and Behavior Books, 1970.

Simkin, J. S. "Gestalt Therapy." In R. J. Corsini (Ed.), *Current Psychotherapies.* (2nd ed.) Itasca, Ill.: Peacock, 1979.

Zinker, J. C. *Creative Process in Gestalt Therapy.* New York: Brunner/Mazel, 1977.

ဦ 3 ဦ

Medications
Management

John R. Brinkley

Mental health administrators require a working knowledge of medications management in planning and implementing comprehensive mental health services. John R. Brinkley describes medications management and treatment planning components of the recently revised diagnostic and statistical manual of psychiatric classifications, the major types of psychotherapeutic drugs, and key management issues related to medications clinics.

The introduction of effective psychotherapeutic drugs has been a significant factor in shaping mental health care delivery in the United States and elsewhere. Since the 1950s, when medications were introduced to control the symptoms of schizophrenia, the population of psychiatric inpatient facilities, notably state mental hospitals, has dramatically declined. Indeed, the emergence of community mental health programs has been directly tied to the discovery of psychopharmacological agents. The progressive decrease in the number of chronically hospitalized psychiatric patients created an urgent need for expanded outpatient facilities for those individuals whose medication-induced improvement in functioning had spared them protracted or lifelong institutionalization.

Of course, psychotherapeutic drugs are neither curative nor a panacea. In some cases, they are totally ineffective or produce only minor symptom reduction; in other cases, they cause adverse effects that outweigh any benefits obtained. Nonetheless, their existence has immeasurably advanced psychiatric treatment from the pre-1950s era when insulin coma, electroconvulsive therapy, psychosurgery, and relatively nonspecific drugs such as barbiturates and scopolamine constituted virtually the sum total of available "medical" treatments. When skillfully and judiciously used, psychotherapeutic drugs have an enormous potential for enhancing the quality of life, markedly improving global functioning, and improving the effectiveness of other, concurrent modes of psychiatric treatment, such as psychotherapy. In some severe affective disorders—for example, the primary affective disorders, in which the lifetime risk of suicide is estimated to be 15 percent (Clayton, Rodin, and Winokur, 1968)—drugs are clearly lifesaving.

Some mental health practitioners vehemently question or even denounce the current prevalence of psychotherapeutic drug use. Without discussing the various facets of this controversy, we will view medications management as an integral part of community mental health services provided to a wide variety of patient populations.

The Role of Medications Management

A medications clinic in a typical community mental health program involves the prescribing, monitoring, and adjusting of psychotherapeutic agents in collaboration with a variety of clinical services. Such clinics are managed, according to legal mandates, by a licensed physician who is, ideally, a fully trained psychiatrist with both interest and competence in the areas of diagnosis and psychopharmacology. In most settings, the physician's services are complemented by those of a licensed nurse. Depending on state laws, nurses may be authorized, within varying limits, to carry out medical and psychiatric assessments, to dispense medications ordered by a physician, to exercise varying degrees of autonomy in altering prescribed regimens, or even to engage in prescribing medications independent of the physician.

Some community mental health programs have their own pharmacy staffed by a licensed pharmacist. Ideally, such a pharmacist serves as an active member of the clinic staff, providing other staff with current, readily accessible information on new drugs, drug interactions, and adverse drug reactions. In addition, the pharmacist may augment the drug information provided the patient and assess the patient's understanding of the drug regimen. With the use of individual drug profile recordkeeping, pharmacists can assist clinicians in monitoring a patient's medication compliance by noting whether the patient is picking up a new supply sooner or later than would be expected.

In mental health medications clinics affiliated with a teaching hospital or a department of psychiatry within a medical school, valuable training experiences can be provided for trainees in medicine, psychiatry, nursing, psychology, social work, and pharmacy. Since the typical outpatient population seen in a medications clinic represents a wider spectrum of psychopathology and severity of impairment than can be found on psychiatric inpatient units, the medications clinic experience provides psychiatric residents and others with an excellent opportunity to refine and integrate psychiatric, diagnostic, and psychopharmacological skills. Patients are usually referred for medications evaluations, conducted by psychiatrists, from all segments of a community mental health program, including inpatient, outpatient, day treatment, and transitional services. Referred patients are generally seen voluntarily, but patients may also be referred from agencies administering involuntary treatment services.

Medications assessment involves several important issues. First and foremost is the question of diagnosis: Has a patient been assigned a diagnosis or diagnoses congruent with the historical and clinical data available? In asking this, the physician is taking a diagnostic second look at the patient. Given a presumably accurate diagnosis, the physician must decide whether or not medications will contribute to a reduction in the severity of symptoms. The answer may be equivocal, since research may support the use of drugs in the case of a particular diagnosis even though such usage is not recognized by official organizations like the Food and Drug Administration. In this case, the physician's psychopharmacological experience and familiarity with current literature are critical variables affecting the decision to prescribe.

Second, even after concluding that the diagnosis represents an appropriate indication for medication, the physician is still confronted with the question: Should medications be prescribed for this particular patient? Indeed, contraindicating factors may exist, such as a patient's ambivalence about taking medication, a past history of poor response to certain medications, or medical problems that may involve a significant risk to the patient if drugs are prescribed. In general, no factor is an absolute contraindication to prescribing drugs; each factor must be weighed against the best estimate of potential benefit. For example, a patient's ambivalence about taking a psychotropic drug may be the result of an unpleasant experience with an inappropriately or unskillfully prescribed medication or may be based on erroneous preconceptions—that he or she will turn into a drugged zombie, for example—about the effects of such drugs. In such cases, reassurance, thoughtful explanation, and good rapport between patient, physician, and therapist may have a markedly ameliorative effect.

If the decision is made to prescribe, then the physician must decide which specific drug or drugs should be used and in what regimen—dosage, frequency of administration, and length of treatment course. This decision may be relatively straightforward—for example, lithium is clearly the drug of choice for preventing the manic and depressive episodes of bipolar disorder when the patient is not known to be a lithium nonresponder—or more complicated, as in the case of a patient with psychotic depression, where investigators are divided in their preferences for antidepressant and neuroleptic drugs.

A number of other factors must also be considered in making this decision: the patient's age (older patients metabolize and excrete drugs more slowly, and their nervous systems tend to be generally more sensitive to psychoactive drugs); known medical problems; general health; and, finally, current and past use of both prescribed and nonprescribed medications. In addition, attention must be paid to the patient's use of other substances, such as "street" or illicit drugs—for example, marijuana—and ethanol, since such use may have direct bearing on diagnostic issues, as well as medication response. It is also important to assess the patient's attitudes toward his or her psychiatric dysfunction and the use of medications.

Finally, the physician has an ethical and clinical obligation to explain the rationale for prescribing a medication and the hoped-for therapeutic—and possible adverse—effects. Such an explanation should be understandable, with minimal use of technical, medical vocabulary, and designed to promote compliance and minimal anxiety about possible side effects. Careful communication also includes an opportunity to educate patients about the nature of their dysfunction. For example, it may be very helpful to a depressed patient to have it clearly stated by the physician that depression (1) is distinctly different from the temporary unhappiness and disappointment everyone experiences as a part of daily life, (2) is a medical illness which affects many aspects of bodily function, and (3) can be appropriately treated with drugs. This may help patients who are ambivalent about taking drugs and may perceive medications as a crutch.

After the initial evaluation by a physician, a patient is referred for a follow-up appointment with a nurse or other staff member in the medications clinic. Ideally, patients should be seen frequently by medications clinic staff to provide adequate monitoring of the therapeutic and side effects of prescribed drugs, changes in the patient's symptoms or overall diagnostic picture, and global level of functioning. The staff may consult with a physician if problems or questions arise, and patients should be scheduled for regular visits with a physician to maintain an overview of the course of treatment, facilitate the process of revising the diagnosis, and prevent the continuation of a medications regimen beyond the point of necessity.

Diagnosis and DSM-III

The integration of diagnosis and medications management is a critical aspect of effective treatment. This axiom does not imply an absolute necessity for a specific diagnosis, since patients receiving the DSM-III designations of "unspecified mental disorder" or "diagnosis deferred" may still respond positively to drug treatment prescribed on the basis of the preponderant character of their symptoms (Croughan, Woodruff, and Reich, 1979). Heated controversy has raged over the role of diagnostic labels in delivering mental health services (Berlin and others, 1981). Suffice it to say that the medications clinic frequently remains the primary, or even sole, focal point for psychiatric diagnosis in community mental health programs.

The nosology or classification of psychiatric disorders has undergone significant evolution in the United States within the past fifteen years, highlighted by the efforts of Feighner and associates (1972) and, subsequently, those of Spitzer and others (1978). In an ever-increasing effort to move away from vague descriptive terms, psychiatric specialists have sought to develop explicit criteria for each diagnostic category, utilizing quantitative terminology whenever appropriate—for example, specifying that a given symptom must have persisted for at least a designated period of time before being considered diagnostically significant. They have also tended to utilize exclusion criteria—that is, to permit the application of a diagnosis only in the absence of certain other conditions. Finally, and perhaps most important, diagnostic criteria have increasingly been based on actual research-derived data, including longitudinal follow-up studies to establish validity and reliability, rather than simply being fashioned from the fabric of a particular theory structure.

The most recent and ambitious effort to revise the classification of psychiatric diagnoses is the third edition (1980) of the American Psychiatric Association's *Diagnostic and Statistical Manual of Mental Disorders* (DSM-III). DSM-III represents the end product of a five-year effort that involved committees of experts and field trials by volunteer clinicians. DSM-III introduced a so-called multiaxial descriptive system involving the use of five major axes, or areas of assessment. Axis I includes all of the mental disorders recognized by the American Psychiatric Association except personality disorders and specific developmental disorders, which make up Axis II. In addition, Axis I includes categories of dysfunction that are not deemed attributable to a mental disorder in the judgment of the assessing clinician—for example, "marital problem." Both Axis I and Axis II also include other coded categories, such as "unspecified mental disorder" ("atypical personality disorder" on Axis II), "diagnosis deferred," and "no diagnosis" (see Table 1).

Axis III includes physical disorders and conditions that are related to Axis I or Axis II diagnoses or are felt to be relevant in some other way to the assessment or management of the patient. The last two axes are designed to provide the clinician with an enhanced view of a patient's individual needs and vulnerabilities vis-à-vis treatment and other management issues. Axis IV rates the magnitude and contribution of the stress factors to which the patient has been exposed during the year preceding onset or exacerbation of psychological dysfunction. Ratings range from 1 ("no stressor perceived as contributory") to 7 ("catastrophic"), with 0 indicating "no information or not applicable." Data recording under Axis IV includes each relevant stressor accompanied by its numerical rating. Axis V consists of an assessment of the highest level of adaptive functioning, lasting at least a few months, achieved by the patient during the preceding year. This assessment takes into account the patient's social relations, occupational or academic functioning, and use of leisure time, rated on a range from 1 ("superior") to 7 ("grossly impaired"), with 0 indicating "no information."

Each diagnostic category that can be listed on Axis I or Axis II is designated by a unique five-digit code number of the form "000.00," with the fifth digit used to denote severity or a clinical subtype of the diagnostic category. Thus, the code number may be used to convey to service providers more treatment or prognosis information than just a diagnostic category. The manual itself also provides specific information about each category in a number of areas, including age of onset, prevalence, sex ratio, and predisposing factors, to the extent that such data are available.

The intent underlying the format of DSM-III is to provide a structured diagnostic system that is largely atheoretical with respect to etiology and reminds the clinician of the importance of focusing on more than just the current nature of a patient's psychological dysfunction. For the most part, DSM-III fulfills this intent, though clinicians should be aware that, despite extensive reliability assessment, the diagnostic categories vary widely in demonstrated validity. Validation is based primarily on the categories of previously validated diagnostic systems. Nonetheless, DSM-III represents a significant move toward greater precision and clinical utility in psychiatric diagnostic criteria.

Table 1. Major Components of DSM-III, Axes I and II.

I.   Disorders Usually First Evident in Infancy, Childhood, or Adolescence

   1. Mental retardation   6. Stereotyped movement disorders
   2. Attention deficit disorders   7. Pervasive developmental disorders
   3. Conduct disorders   8. Other disorders—physical
   4. Anxiety disorders   9. Other disorders—emotional
   5. Eating disorders

II. Organic Mental Disorders

   1. Dementias and senile onset
   2. Substance-induced disorders (alcohol, barbiturates, opioids, cocaine, amphetamines, phencyclidine, hallucinogens, cannabis, tobacco, caffeine, and other unspecified substances)
   3. Organic brain syndromes

III. Schizophrenic Disorders (Disorganized, Catatonic, Paranoid, Undifferentiated, and Residual)

IV. Paranoid Disorders and Unclassified Psychotic Disorders

V.   Neurotic Disorders

   1. Affective disorders (bipolar, major depression, and atypical disorders)
   2. Anxiety disorders (phobic disorders, anxiety states, post-traumatic stress disorder)
   3. Somatoform disorders (somatization, conversion, psychogenic pain, hypochondriasis, and atypical disorders)
   4. Dissociative disorders (psychogenic amnesia, psychogenic fugue, multiple personality, depersonalization, and atypical disorders)
   5. Psychosexual disorders (paraphilias, psychosexual dysfunction, and other disorders)
   6. Factitious disorders
   7. Other disorders of impulse control
   8. Adjustment disorders
   9. Psychological factors affecting physical condition
  10. Personality disorders

The Interface Between Diagnosis and Psychotherapeutic Drugs

Despite a steady increase in the number of psychotherapeutic drugs approved by the Food and Drug Administration for clinical use in the United States, their range of effects still falls within only four basic categories of pharmacological classification: antianxiety agents; antidepressants; neuroleptics; and lithium, which constitutes a category by itself. To an extent, the classification of a given drug implies the diagnostic category for which it is most therapeutically useful, with the exception of lithium, which is useful across a variety of diagnostic categories. The following is a brief overview of each of the four groupings.

Antianxiety Agents

Although various drugs have been used in the treatment of anxiety symptoms, most have significant drawbacks. Barbiturates, such as Seconal and Nembutal, are potentially lethal, rapidly induce tolerance by increasing the rate of their own metabolism, and pose substantial management problems because of the risk of addiction and withdrawal symptoms. The same problems exist, though to a lesser extent, with meprobamates, such as Miltown or Equanil. Antihistamines, such as Benadryl, Atarax, and Vistaril, are widely prescribed as antianxiety agents, often because they are thought to represent a benign alternative to the use of benzodiazepines, such as Valium. In fact, the antihistamines can produce significant adverse reactions—dry mouth, blurred vision, constipation, urinary retention—mediated primarily through their anticholinergic activity. Any therapeutic response is largely a function of sedation, as it is also in the use of antidepressant and neuroleptic drugs in treating anxiety syndromes that are primary rather than one facet of a depressive episode. The random prescribing of antihistamines, antidepressants, and neuroleptics for anxiety can subject patients to side effects that are of a higher order of magnitude than those produced by benzodiazepines.

The benzodiazepines (BDZs)—used largely in the treatment of generalized anxiety disorders and when anxiety is a significant aspect of another disorder—appear to produce their antianxiety effect by modulating the central nervous system (CNS) response to GABA, a neurotransmitter. They also tend to produce varying degrees of skeletal muscle relaxation and may produce some degree of sedation. Sedation is one of the more common BDZ side effects—but not a significant therapeutic effect—although generally fewer than 10 percent of BDZ takers experience it, and tolerance develops quickly. Other side effects include imbalance when walking, changes in coordination, and increased effects of CNS-depressing drugs. The lethal potential of the BDZs is extremely low and fatal doses are almost unknown, although the risk is clearly increased when other drugs or alcohol are used concomitantly.

Concern has been expressed, especially in the popular media, about the abuse and addiction potential of the BDZs. Although abuse undoubtedly exists, it certainly must be considered qualitatively different, in terms of public health and social cost, than the abuse of more powerful drugs. The administering of BDZ in large dosages is not intended over extended periods of time and requires careful monitoring, especially during periods of heavy dosage. Prolonged use of a large dosage of BDZ may lead to withdrawal symptoms when the drug is abruptly discontinued, but this is much more a function of injudicious prescribing and inattentive follow-up than of malevolent characteristics of the drugs themselves. (Recent research has uncovered this withdrawal phenomenon.) The cornerstone of therapy with BDZs is careful measurement of dosage and objective assessment of continued need for the drug.

Neuroleptic Drugs

The term *neuroleptic* is not ideal, since it erroneously implies that neurological side effects necessarily accompany these drugs' therapeutic effects. However, neuroleptic drugs are preferable to the other so-called antipsychotic drugs, including antidepressants and lithium, which can, under some circumstances, ameliorate psychotic symptoms. Included among the neuroleptics are phenothiazines, such as Thorazine and Haldol, and thioxanthines, such as Navane.

The traditional and primary use of these drugs has been the amelioration of the characteristic symptoms of schizophrenia. The therapeutic effect of the neuroleptics has generally been attributed to their ability to block certain CNS receptor sites for dopamine, a neurotransmitter. The more intricate aspects of this activity and its implications for the neurochemical underpinnings of schizophrenia remain the focus of ongoing debate (Alpert and Friedhoff, 1980).

It is common in acute care settings to use a rapid tranquilization regimen—the administration of fairly high doses of a neuroleptic at frequent intervals—to reduce symptoms quickly. Ideally, once a response has occurred, the dosage is immediately reduced to a low maintenance level. Although dramatic changes in a patient's symptoms may be seen in as little as twelve to forty-eight hours, many schizophrenic patients experience only gradual reduction in symptoms over a period of weeks or months. Unfortunately, once a patient has been started on neuroleptics, the medication tends to be prescribed at a larger dosage level and for a longer period of time than is necessary, based on the assumption that a schizophrenic patient's neuroleptic medication is essentially a "life sentence." Although it is true that many schizophrenics do require chronic maintenance and will predictably decompensate when their medications are stopped, a subgroup of patients—unfortunately, not identifiable by current methods of assessment—does exist that can discontinue neuroleptics indefinitely without relapsing. It can only be urged, however, that drug dosages be reduced over time and that, whenever feasible, patients be given the benefit of a drug-free trial.

The side effects of neuroleptic medication are closely correlated with its potency. Higher-potency drugs—those requiring a relatively small dose to produce a given therapeutic effect—are more likely to produce altered muscle and motor function, and less likely to produce such symptoms as dry mouth, blurred vision, constipation, and blood pressure changes, than lower-potency drugs. Muscle and motor function side effects can generally be ameliorated by the coadministration of an anti-Parkinson drug, such as Symmetral.

In recent years, increasing interest has focused on the potentially irreversible neurological disorder tardive dyskinesia (TD), which consists of involuntary movements, most commonly of the tongue, mouth, and jaw, though sometimes involving the extremities and trunk. The disorder usually appears after long-term treatment with neuroleptic drugs but may develop after a relatively brief period of use. A wide variety of interventions have been investigated in attempts to reduce the symptoms of TD, but none has been found to be consistently effective.

Whenever possible, both neuroleptics and anticholinergic agents should be tapered to the minimum dosage possible and ultimately discontinued. Clearly, prevention in the form of avoiding unnecessary or unnecessarily prolonged use of such medications is preferable to after-the-fact intervention—an important issue in a program where large numbers of chronic schizophrenic patients are treated.

Antidepressant Drugs

CNS-stimulant drugs, such as amphetamines and methylphenidate or Ritalin, were the first agents used on a sizable scale in the treatment of depressive disorders. These drugs were initially effective in many patients, but prolonged use often led to tolerance to the mood-elevating effects and sometimes to adverse reactions. Although some patients, especially the elderly, do experience a sustained positive response to stimulants, their utility as antidepressants is now largely limited to a brief trial of Dexedrine or Ritalin to predict treatment response to tricyclic antidepressants.

The tricyclics, the most commonly used antidepressants in the United States, are postulated to cause reversal of depressive symptoms through a variety of effects on certain biogenic amine neurotransmitters, notably serotonin and norepinephrine, which are thought to modulate mood function. The tricyclics differ among themselves with respect to the way they affect the biogenic amine system; a particular patient may experience marked differences in response when given sequential trials of various tricyclics. Exactly why tricyclics differ in effect, however, remains an unresolved area of investigation.

The tricyclics are most commonly used for treating patients with the major depression disorder and the depressed phase of bipolar disorder, although chronic and atypical forms of depression are more responsive to drug treatment than was previously assumed. These drugs have other established indications, such as prophylactic treatment of panic disorder, that are ostensibly outside the realm of the formally designated affective disorders. Treatment of a depressed adult is generally instituted with around 50 mg. per day of imipramine or an equivalent dose of another drug—a dosage that is then maintained for several days to ensure that the patient is not unusually sensitive to adverse effects. Ideally, the dose should be increased rapidly to minimize the time required for a therapeutic plasma level to be achieved. This rapid increase is especially important in administering antidepressants, as there is usually a lag of a week or more before a response begins to appear even at a dosage that subsequently proves to be effective. The ultimate determinant of dosage is the patient's response, which in some cases may require dosage regimens three or more times the usual effective level.

Once a response occurs, current data suggest, the drug should be continued for at least another eight months, since earlier discontinuation is associated with an increased relapse rate. Some patients require longer-term regimens, perhaps even continued maintenance, but the features distinguishing such individuals are not well established. The usual side effects of the tricyclics are dry mouth, blurred vision, constipation, sedation, and changes in blood pressure or in the electrophysiology of the heart—though this last is rarely of clinical significance except when unusually large doses are taken, as in the case of tricyclic overdose.

The other established class of antidepressant drugs is the monoamine oxidase inhibitors (MAOIs). The MAOIs available in the United States are Nardil, Parnate, and Marplan. Also available is Eutonyl, which is not marketed as an antidepressant but is demonstrably effective as such. These drugs produce therapeutic response in depressed patients through effects on biogenic amines similar to the effects produced by tricyclics, although by a significantly different mechanism.

The traditional belief, held until recently, that the MAOIs were not as effective as the tricyclics was based largely on studies whose validity is now in question, since the MAOI dosages employed tended to be significantly below what is now viewed as generally necessary for a therapeutic response. In addition, a number of investigators have suggested that there are identifiable subpopulations of depressed patients who are specifically responsive to MAOIs. In any event, there has been a marked resurgence of interest in these drugs—a fortunate trend, since clinicians need to have available a broad range of drug modalities in treating a condition like depression, which is associated with such a high mortality rate.

Lithium

Lithium salts, such as Eskalith and Lithionate, have been heralded as a major tool in the treatment of affective disease, in particular, bipolar disorder. Lithium is recognized as being the most specific treatment available for mania, as well as being highly effective prophylactically in preventing manic-depressive swings. It is variably effective in the acute treatment of depression—frequently depressed patients will also require antidepressants to experience complete remission—and has been effective in a variety of other disorders, including aggressive dyscontrol and cyclothymic subaffective disorder.

Lithium serum levels are easily measured, and it is standard practice during long-term maintenance of a patient on lithium to obtain levels regularly—generally twelve hours after the most recent dose every two to three months—in order to check on compliance and ensure that the body's excretion of the drug has not changed, as might occur with a recent, unreported use of diuretics or alterations in the patient's kidney function or sodium intake. Although rough therapeutic ranges have been established, clinical assessment, rather than laboratory results, should determine dosage decisions. In addition to the lithium level, thyroid function tests and indices of renal function should be obtained at regular intervals. Lithium has a well-documented potential for producing hypothyroidism, and concern has increased in the past several years over possible kidney damage due to long-term use.

More common adverse reactions to lithium include nausea (usually prevented by taking the drug after eating), hand tremor (treated with Inderal), and increased frequency of urination (which usually subsides spontaneously after several weeks).

Other Medications Management Issues

The role of a medications clinic clearly extends beyond an established protocol for diagnostic evaluation, follow-up monitoring, and prescribing of psychoactive agents in conformity with good clinical practice. As one part of a functioning whole, the medications clinic necessarily interfaces with other service areas on patient care issues, administrative problems, and other points of common patient concerns.

The staff of a medications clinic can provide constructive assistance to clinical staff by disseminating practical information concerning medications issues in order to encourage clinicians to take an active role in monitoring the therapeutic response and side effects of their patients who are on drug regimens. Such monitoring facilitates the referral process for medications evaluations. In settings where clinicians reflect antimedications and antidiagnosis sentiments, however, the medications clinic staff may find itself isolated and in adversarial relationships with other staffs. Physicians may thus find themselves as mere prescription writers instead of members of treatment teams. In such situations, patients pay a heavy penalty, since they are likely to be subjected to conflicting and even hostile messages about use of prescribed drugs and may get the impression that medications are used only when all else fails.

The medications clinic staff can also have a positive impact beyond the immediate domain of an inpatient or outpatient program. A mental health agency can provide consultation, educational, and follow-up services to congregate care or intermediate care facilities so as to improve awareness of medications issues on the part of the facilities' residential staff, and then may directly or indirectly upgrade the psychotropic prescribing practices of the facilities' attending physicians, most of whom are apt not to be psychiatrists. Similarly, patient care can be enhanced through liaison between the staffs of the medications clinic and the inpatient units of local general or psychiatric hospitals, and a smoother transition can be provided for a patient being discharged from inpatient to outpatient services if medications follow-up is promoted with some degree of congruence between the prescribing practices and protocols of the two programs. For example, if an inpatient is being started on lithium, the inpatient unit's prelithium lab workup should incorporate all the tests that were included in the medications clinic's routine follow-up studies, so that baseline reference points are available.

Conclusion

Through the integration of diagnosis and judicious prescribing of psychoactive drugs, a medications clinic measurably enhances the therapeutic scope of clinical mental health services. The advent of effective psychotherapeutic drugs—although it revolutionized mental health services and promoted a shift from inpatient to outpatient treatment—was accompanied by the potential problems of indiscriminate drug use and the occurrence of significant side effects. However, a mental health medications clinic that adheres to rigorous diagnostic standards and well-defined medications management practices and is staffed by a psychiatrist with adequate training in psychopharmacology can help to circumvent or minimize these problems. In addition to its clinical function, the medications clinic's staff can serve as a clinical and educational resource for mental health staff members both inside and outside community health agencies.

References

Alpert, M., and Friedhoff, A. "An Un-Dopamine Hypothesis of Schizophrenia." *Schizophrenia Bulletin,* 1980, *6,* 387–390.

American Psychiatric Association. *Diagnostic and Statistical Manual of Mental Disorders.* (3rd ed.) Washington, D.C.: American Psychiatric Association, 1980.

Barchas, J. D., and others. *Psychopharmacology from Theory to Practice.* New York: Oxford University Press, 1977.

Berlin, R., and others. "The Patient Care Crisis in Community Mental Health Centers: A Need for More Psychiatric Involvement." *American Journal of Psychiatry,* 1981, *138,* 450–454.

Bernstein, J. G. *Clinical Psychopharmacology.* Littleton, Mass.: PSG Publishing Company, 1978.

Clayton, P. J., Rodin, L., and Winokur, G. "Family History Studies, III. Schizo-Affective Disorder, Clinical and Genetic Factors, Including a One to Two Year Follow-up." *Comparative Psychiatry,* 1968, *9,* 31–49.

Croughan, J. L., Woodruff, R. A., and Reich, T. "The Management of Patients with Undiagnosed Psychiatric Illness." *Archives of General Psychiatry,* 1979, *36,* 341–346.

Feighner, J., Robins, E., and Guze, S. B. "Diagnostic Criteria for Use in Psychiatric Research." *Archives of General Psychiatry,* 1972, *26,* 57–63.

Goodwin, D. W., and Guze, S. B. *Psychiatric Diagnosis.* (2nd ed.) New York: Oxford University Press, 1979.

Spitzer, R. L., Endicott, J., and Robins, E. "Research Diagnostic Criteria: Rationale and Reliability." *Archives of General Psychiatry,* 1978, *35,* 773–782.

Spitzer, R. L., and Klein, D. F. (Eds.). *Critical Issues in Psychiatric Diagnosis.* New York: Raven Press, 1978.

Mental Health Policy
and Patient's Rights

Richard A. Weatherley

Richard Weatherley focuses on some of the policy issues and dilemmas that currently face mental health practitioners and on professional and organizational constraints that influence and limit the range of practice alternatives available to those in the field. Special attention is given to distortions of policy and practices as well as to strategies for limiting their negative impact on clients. Ethical considerations may require a willingness to question agency policies and practices, to seek to change them, and, under some conditions, to refuse to implement them. The chapter discusses (1) problems raised by various forms of treatment, including the use of psychoactive drugs (especially by criminal offenders), behavior modification, and aversive therapy; (2) right to refusal of treatment; (3) day-to-day policy and financial constraints; and (4) choices available to practitioners and managers seeking to reconcile demands for humane treatment, on the one hand, and the constraints emerging from new policies and unrealistic work settings, on the other.

The mental health field is now in the midst of a paradigm shift or, perhaps more precisely, a series of shifts. Prevailing attitudes about the treatment and processing of the mentally ill are increasingly being questioned and legally challenged. Underlying these changes is a growing recognition that many of the reforms of the past, although undertaken with the best humanitarian motives, have produced unspeakable injustices. We hear even today of men and women subjected to lifelong confinement in institutions because of an initial misclassification. Juveniles have been subjected to severe punishments, lengthy confinement, and a denial of due process for "crimes"—truancy, incorrigibility, running away—that do not exist for adults. Mind-altering operations, resulting in basic

The author wishes to acknowledge the valuable contribution of Steven Eckstrom, who served as research assistant for this project.

personality changes and in loss of functioning, have been performed on prisoners and mental patients without their informed consent.

The changing approaches in the treatment of the mentally disordered are perhaps most apparent on the boundary between treatment and punishment, where legal and medical systems intersect. Although the discovery of rehabilitation and treatment as a response to deviance can be traced back to the eighteenth century, rehabilitation has been most pervasively applied in this country since the early part of this century. As Kittrie (1971) demonstrates, increasing numbers and categories of deviants—the mentally ill, juveniles, alcoholics, and drug addicts— have been shifted from criminal law sanctions to systems emphasizing treatment and rehabilitation instead of confinement and punishment. This "divestment of criminal law," as Kittrie terms it, "has not been motivated, on the whole, by societal willingness to begin tolerating the conduct or condition previously designated as criminal. Instead, divestment has most frequently indicated a shift from criminal sanctions to a different system of social controls" (p. 4). Because the agents of the state were presumed to be acting in the interests of their charges, the due process protections of the criminal justice system were presumed to be unnecessary. As recent history has amply demonstrated, however, this presumption of benign intervention was unwarranted, and great harm has often been inflicted by those seeking to help.

These are indeed difficult times for the helping professions. Shrinking budgets are forcing administrators and practitioners to search for new means of accommodating increasing work loads with declining resources. The concern for the civil rights of those processed through the helping agencies presents new dilemmas for the human service practitioner, who can no longer assume that doing one's job well is sufficient—we now learn that our therapeutic, helping agencies are capable of doing harm in the guise of doing good. Nor are our professional ethics sufficient to prevent us from participating in what may subsequently be identified as unethical treatment. Many of the humane reforms of the past—the development of a separate juvenile court system, the institutionalization and, more recently, the deinstitutionalization of the mentally ill, various rehabilitation programs, indeterminate sentencing of offenders—have become today's problems. Who can say with any assurance whether the solutions of today will not become the problems of another era?

The purpose of this chapter is to identify for practitioners and administrators the dilemmas created by various mental health policies. A brief examination of the ethical and practical issues raised by changing practices should help those charged with implementing those practices become more self-conscious about the choices available to them and the broader implications of their actions. The selected issues are among those currently receiving attention in the literature; they are meant only to illustrate the dilemmas thrust on practitioners by changing standards of treatment and patient rights. Since these issues are so ideologically charged, our analysis will be short on prescription, seeking instead to identify the range of choices and their consequences.

A secondary focus will be on the professional and organizational constraints that influence and limit the range of practice alternatives available to
those in the field. Discussions of policy frequently proceed as if selection of a
"correct" policy were sufficient. Implementation tends to be taken for granted, as
if it were enough simply to decide what to do without considering how it is to be
done. There is now an abundant literature, much of it based on examples from
mental health, demonstrating that policies may become distorted even as they are
implemented. These deviations from the desired goals are not necessarily the
result of any evil intent or neglect, but may occur as an unintended result of the
zealous pursuit of professional and organizational goals. Our discussion will seek
to identify the kinds of policy distortions that may occur in the implementation
process and the actions that policy makers and practitioners may take to limit the
negative impact on clients of these constraints.

The discussion of policy will first be concerned with treatment issues,
including the use of drugs, behavior modification, and psychosurgery. Next, the
right to treatment and the right to refuse treatment will be considered, along with
the issues of involuntary treatment and dangerousness. In addition, attention will
be given to the day-to-day constraints facing administrators and practitioners as
they seek to carry out policies in a manner consistent with public attitudes, professional standards, organizational imperatives, and available resources. Such shifting policies, together with the societal values underlying them, and the
constraints to implementing them, confront conscientious practitioners with ethical dilemmas that their superiors, administrators, policy makers, and legislators
have often failed to address. The concluding section further elucidates the choices
available to the practitioner or administrator seeking to reconcile the sometimes
conflicting demands for humane treatment with the realities of a work setting
which does not afford the necessary conditions for such treatment.

Psychoactive Drugs

The use of psychoactive drugs, especially the phenothiazines, has revolutionized the treatment of the mentally ill over the past twenty-five years. Since
they were first introduced in the early 1950s, widespread use of such drugs has
been associated with the deinstitutionalization of the mentally ill, although some
argue that drug use merely exaggerated an earlier trend begun in response to
increasing costs (Sterling, 1979). In any event, drug therapy is now the prevailing
treatment for mental disorders in the United States (Scheff, 1976). Other factors
associated with the rapid proliferation of drug therapy include the aggressive
marketing of the drug companies and the eagerness of psychiatrists for a more
distinctly "medical" treatment to ward off encroachment from such nonmedical
therapists as social workers, psychologists, and nurses, who offer a form of professional intervention, "talk" therapy, that is similar to psychiatry. Tranquilizers
and antidepressants offer a fast and inexpensive way to arrest symptoms and make
institutionalized patients more manageable, and the use of chemotherapy has

given impetus to studies of the relationship between the biochemistry of the brain and mental disorder.

Whereas the obvious benefits of chemotherapy in the treatment of mental disorders have received considerable attention, the associated costs and risks have not, at least until very recently. Several court cases have signaled the beginning of what is likely to be a reexamination of drug therapy for the maintenance of mental patients not only in mental hospitals but in the community as well.

In *Rennie* v. *Klein* (1978), the U.S. District Court of New Jersey ruled that "refusal of drugs, even by a patient who is psychotic, can be prompted by a rational desire to avoid unpleasant side effects and a realistic appraisal that the medication is not working" (Sterling, 1979, p. 14). In *Rogers* v. *Okin* (1979), the U.S. District Court of Massachusetts ruled that those committed to a mental institution, even as involuntary patients, were not to be considered incompetent per se and therefore had the right to refuse medication (Annas, 1980). The president of the American Psychiatric Association, Alan Stone, called the ruling "the most impossible, inappropriate, ill-considered judicial decision ever made in the field of mental health law" (quoted in the *Boston Globe*, Nov. 21, 1979, p. 13). The ruling did provide for the nonvoluntary medication of patients in an emergency—defined as a situation where there is "a substantial likelihood of personal injury to the patient, other patients, or staff members"—and the medication of incompetent patients against their will in nonemergency situations with the prior consent of the court or a court-appointed guardian (Annas, 1980, p. 21). Most significantly, the court found that antipsychotic drugs, "such as Thorazine, Mellaril, Prolixin, and Haldol, are powerful chemical agents with serious and severe side effects" (Annas, 1980, p. 21).

The most common side effect of the phenothiazines used in the treatment of schizophrenia is tardive dyskinesia, affecting a substantial proportion of those who receive long-term "maintenance" doses. Scheff (1976) cites studies showing this reaction in as many as 40 percent of the cases. It is characterized by "slow, rhythmical movements in the region of the mouth, with protrusion of the tongue, smacking of the lips, blowing of the cheeks, and side-to-side movements of the chin, as well as other bizarre muscular activity. More careful examinations of patients on long-term drug therapy revealed that not only the mouth but practically all parts of the body could exhibit motor disorders" (Crane, 1973, cited by Scheff, p. 304).

Shapiro (1974, p. 245) cites the 1971 Owens case where Thorazine, a phenothiazine antipsychotic drug, was used on juveniles "without careful medical review . . . for controlling conduct, and perhaps for purely punitive purposes." The court ruled that the drug was "used as a behavior control device for episodes of aggressive, assaultive, and destructive behavior" and ordered that "no intramuscular injection of Thorazine or other tranquilizer be administered 'except as part of a treatment for medical or emotional illness or disorder.'"

Sterling (1979), a University of Pennsylvania brain researcher who testified for the plaintiff in the *Rennie* case, likens the social effects of some phenothiazines to those resulting from a frontal lobotomy—namely, the blunting of consciousness, motivation, and the ability to solve problems. He asserts that "a psychiatrist would be hard put to distinguish a lobotomized patient from one treated with chlorpromazine" (p. 17). He further claims that in fact most patients released from hospitals on maintenance drugs have not made a successful readjustment. Scheff (1976, p. 303), examining conflicting findings from postrelease studies, concludes that the phenothiazines "are effective in some cases, especially in the beginning of treatment, not effective in others, and actually harmful in others."

In 1974, 250 million prescriptions for psychotropic drugs were filled. That magnitude of drug usage requires a close examination of practice. Such an inquiry raises a number of issues. One broad controversial issue is whether hospitalized patients can be forced to accept drug treatment against their will. Other issues involve matters of discretion, such as monitoring proper dosages, the appropriateness of any drugs for some patients, or discerning in individual cases whether the use of drugs will do more harm than good in the long run.

Behavior Modification

Behavior modification techniques are based on the assumption that unwanted behavior may be unlearned and desired behavior learned through the controlled application of rewards and aversive conditioning. The underlying psychological problem is not one of relevance in addressing the behaviors one wishes to change. Behavior modification techniques in one form or another are widely used in institutions; by therapists in the community working with individuals and groups on a variety of adjustment problems; and in programs to help persons stop smoking, lose weight, and control eating and drinking habits. They have become part of the classroom routine of elementary schools and the preferred technique in assisting various categories of handicapped children.

There is nothing inherently good or bad about the use of behavioral techniques; as Bandura (1975, p. 19) has stated, "Behaviorism is a system of principles and procedures which can produce diverse moral outcomes." However, ethical issues arise when such treatment is imposed on one person "to satisfy the wishes of others" (Halleck, 1974, p. 381). It is important to consider some of the ethical issues implicit in the use of behavioral techniques, particularly on nonvoluntary or institutionalized clients.

Token economies, whereby individuals gain tokens redeemable for material rewards (cigarettes, candy, special food) or nonmaterial rewards (trips, entry to special programs, extra leisure time), are widely used in correctional and mental health institutions. Although such programs appear to be benign, since they do not provide punishments, they do in fact raise serious moral issues. The basic problem is that such schemes may hold out as rewards to be earned "items and activities that basic principles of dignity—and of law—would demand as a matter of absolute, noncontingent right" (Wexler, 1972, p. 297). Wexler cites the example of a "positive control" program at Patton State Hospital in San Bernardino, California, in which all patients start in a minimally furnished "orientation group" and must exhibit "proper behavior" to earn wanted items and be elevated to a better environment:

> This group sleeps in a relatively unattractive dormitory which conforms to bare minimums set by the State Department of Mental Hygiene. There are no draperies at the windows or spreads on the beds, and the beds themselves are of the simplest kind. In the dining room, the patient sits with many other patients at a long table, crowded and somewhat uncomfortably. The only eating utensil given him is a large spoon. . . . He is not allowed to wear his own clothes and cannot go to activities which other patients are free to attend off the unit. . . . During this time, the patient learns that his meals, his bed, his toilet articles, and his clothes no longer are freely given to him. He must pay for these with tokens. . . . These tokens pay for all those things normally furnished and often taken for granted [Bruce, 1966; cited by Wexler, 1972, p. 298].

Such token economy systems have been used with drug addicts, alcoholics, and juveniles, as well as the mentally ill.

At the other end of the continuum are procedures, clearly and explicitly aversive, that raise constitutional questions about the Eighth Amendment prohibition against cruel and unusual punishment. For example, the drug Anectine (or succinylcholine) is a muscle relaxant that has been used in aversion therapy and "rapidly produces complete paralysis of the skeletal muscles, including those which control respiration" (Schwitzgebel, 1972, p. 267). It has been administered to alcoholics just prior to offering them a drink, in an effort to condition them against drinking: "Just as the patient is about to drink the alcohol, paralysis occurs, producing great fright about being unable to breathe and a fear of suffocation" (Schwitzgebel, 1972, p. 299). The drug has also been used on both unwilling and "consenting" inmates in California institutions, sometimes without prior warning, "as a means of suppressing hazardous behavior. The drug . . . was selected for use as a means of providing an extremely negative experience for association with the behavior in question. . . . It was hypothesized that the association of such a frightening consequence (respiratory arrest, muscular paralysis) with certain behavioral acts would be effective in suppressing these acts" (Mattocks and Jew, n.d., p. 3). The practice was "to administer 20 to 40 mg. of succinylcholine intravenously, with oxygen and an airway available, and to counsel the patient while he is under the influence of the drug that his behavior is dangerous to others or to himself, that it is desirable that he stop the behavior in question, and that subsequent behavior of a nature which might be dangerous to others or to himself will be treated with similar aversive treatments" (Wexler, 1972, p. 299).

Aversive conditioning is "an attempt to associate an undesirable behavior pattern with unpleasant stimulation to make the unpleasant stimulation a consequence of the undesirable behavior" (Rachman and Teasdale, 1969, p. vii). When translated from the aseptic language of the clinician, "unpleasant stimulations" have included the use of a 200-volt electric shock to discourage self-destructive behavior in retarded children, electric cattle prods to control chronic schizophrenics, the total withholding of food, sublethal injections of chemical poisons, and the use of "draconic versions of the 'hole'" (Opton, 1975, p. 26).

One might argue that even such drastic punishment is justified to "cure" or control certain kinds of deviant and dangerous behavior. But objections may be raised on practical as well as ethical grounds. In addition to possibly producing unintended and undesired side effects, particularly in institutional applications, such behavioral techniques are of questionable effectiveness in bringing about the changes desired. Often the sole criterion of success is whether the treatment makes the patient more placid or makes him or her act in a way that is approved by his or her institutional guardians. The treatment may produce behavioral repertoires more suitable to adjusting to institutional life than to adapting to the real world. Moreover, the elimination of an undesired behavior, even if successful, does not necessarily produce a "better" way of behaving. The elimination of deviant behavior may leave underlying drives unaffected and may simply lead to new undesirable behavior (Naon, 1978). Standards of effectiveness tend to be related to subjective clinical judgment, which is rarely neutral; there have been few, if any, controlled, double-blind evaluation designs. Although clinical results are inconsistent, there is some evidence that aversive conditioning is especially ineffective and sometimes counterproductive in treating aggressive behavior (Bandura, 1962). Side effects include "pain, increased aggressiveness, arousal, anxieties, somatic and physiological malfunctions, and the development of various unexpected and often pathological operant behaviors" ("Conditioning and Other Technologies. . . ," 1972, p. 616).

Another troubling issue is that of who shall decide what therapies are to be applied to whom. Institutional administrators are not neutral observers; they may be expected to favor measures that enable them to control the behavior of patients. Those who sanction punitive "therapies" are frequently not involved in the day-to-day administering of them. As Opton (1975, p. 24) observes, "the language of behavior modification is marvelously suited to soothe the consciences of institutional administrators." The inmates of institutions are generally the poor and minority group member, for whom less intrusive "talk" therapies are held to be less effective, and who are, consequently, more likely to be subjected to intrusive, behavior-changing interventions.

What categories of deviant behavior should be treated? The act of diagnosis carries profound implications. One commentary states that there is no reason why one "could not use aversion therapy to treat armed robbery or any other crime as easily as homosexuality" (Singer, 1970, p. 432). Why then not speeders, truants, or draft resisters? The concept of mental illness is an elastic one which may be stretched to accommodate almost any type of deviant behavior. An extreme example is the incarceration, with the collusion of mental health professionals, of political dissidents in mental hospitals in the Soviet Union. Could it never happen here? Some psychoanalysts have contended that members of the John Birch Society may be paranoid schizophrenics (Wexler, 1972) or that Richard Nixon, Ronald Reagan, Edmund Muskie, or others are deranged (Reich, 1980).

Psychosurgery and Electrical Stimulation of the Brain (ESB)

Psychosurgery has been defined as "surgical removal or destruction of brain tissue or the cutting of the brain tissue to disconnect one part of the brain from another with the intent of altering behavior" (National Institute of Mental Health, 1973, p. 7). Electrical stimulation of the brain (ESB)—stimulation of specific areas of the brain in order to alter violent, aggressive, or sexual behavior—is accomplished through the implantation of electrodes or through direct application of drugs to selected brain areas by means of microimplants. The traditional form of psychosurgery has been lobectomy, the surgical removal of the frontal portion of the temporal lobe. "A more modern technique, however, is stereotactic surgery, which involves, through the use of a surgical drill and other special instruments, implanting electrodes in the brain, determining through stimulation and recording procedures which brain cells are misfiring, and destroying a small number of cells in a precisely determined area by passing heat-generating currents through the appropriate electrode" (Wexler, 1972, p. 300).

These exotic procedures have staunch advocates, among them those who emphasize an electrobiochemical origin of behavior. The central hypothesis of this view is that thought and behavior are consequent to electrical and chemical activity of the brain. As one observer put it, "behind every crooked thought there is a crooked molecule" (Remmen, 1962, p. 32). Therefore, the administration of psychotropic drugs, ESB, and psychosurgery can produce predictable, replicable alterations in thought and behavior.

Critics point out that the outcomes of psychosurgery are unpredictable, alleged benefits have yet to be scientifically demonstrated, and the side effects are ignored by advocates of these practices. As one critic argues, psychosurgery at best "blunts the individual and at worst destroys all his highest capacities" (Wexler, 1972, p. 300). Some advocates consider that even if such procedures result in permanent personality changes and loss of intellectual functioning, the benefits are worth the price.

At issue in the application of such irreversible, intrusive procedures are what behaviors, if any, might justify their use and who is to decide when and under what circumstances they may be used. Before we address these concerns, it is worth noting the kinds of applications that have been made or contemplated. The California Department of Corrections has used stereotactic surgery on inmates subject to episodes of uncontrollable violence (Shapiro, 1974) and has contemplated performing brain cauterizations on inmates they considered to present serious management problems (Wexler, 1972). In another instance, Breggin (1972, p. 118) noted that homosexuals were "allegedly turned straight . . . through destruction of part of the brain called Cajal's nucleus—the supposed 'sexual switchboard.'" Breggin also reported that, in Mississippi, children as young as five labeled hyperactive have been subjected to psychosurgery. On the drawing boards are specific, detailed proposals for "making the release of prisoners and mental patients contingent on their acceptance of implantation of electrodes both for direct control of behavior and for monitoring or on their agreement to use psychotropic drugs in prescribed ways" (Shapiro, 1974, p. 248).

Mark, Sweet, and Ervin (see Shapiro, 1974) also propose a neurobiological explanation for, and intervention to prevent, urban violence. They attribute the riots of the late 1960s in part to "brain dysfunction in the rioters who engaged in arson, sniping, and physical assault" and recommend studies "to pinpoint, diagnose, and treat those people with low violence thresholds before they contribute to further tragedies" (Shapiro, 1974, p. 249, Note 25). Studies undertaken at the behest of the Kerner Commission, however, effectively dispose of the notion that riot participants were either deranged or drawn predominantly from a criminal underclass, as those seeking to deny the political significance of the riots were prone to believe (Lipsky and Olson, 1974).

Wexler (1972, p. 316) comments as follows on the pitfalls of neurological screening to predict violent behavior:

> Some physicians, drawing upon neurological knowledge to the effect that violent behavior attributable to brain pathology can often be detected by electroencephalogram (EEG) readings, have recommended that violent offenders with demonstrated abnormal electrical brain activity be removed from society until their EEG's become normal. Only an aggressive adversary proceeding, however, would enable a deviant to demonstrate some of the flaws of EEG interpretation—that, for example, a sizable proportion of the normal population has abnormal EEG's and that an abnormal EEG, instead of being a cause of violence, may be the result of a violent episode involving a head injury.

The Right to Refuse Treatment

Given the intrusive nature, questionable benefits, and potential hazards of some of the treatment procedures currently being used on criminal offenders, juveniles, and the mentally ill, one may reasonably ask what rights these persons have to refuse treatment. In addition to citing recent court cases on the right of persons confined in mental institutions to refuse drugs, we must consider the legal issues relating to the client's right to refuse various kinds of treatment.

Surprisingly, in view of the fundamental issues involved, few states have laws specifying the conditions under which various kinds of treatment or confinement (seclusion, use of restraints) may be employed. Some procedures are subject to regulation by public administrative bodies, although such guidelines vary considerably from state to state. Stone (1975, p. 100) cites the example of electroshock therapy, which is defined in some localities as "accepted therapy"— thus requiring no consent—and in others as requiring the permission of a "legally responsible person." Formerly, persons who were mentally ill were considered, by definition, to be incompetent to make decisions about their treatment; treatment was invariably considered to be in their best interest and the obligation of the state to provide (Ennis, 1971). However, as established in *Rogers* v. *Okin* (one of the cases pertaining to the administration of psychotropic drugs), commitment to a mental institution cannot in itself be taken as proof of incompetence. Moreover, certain kinds of treatment may constitute cruel and unusual punishment and may impinge on constitutionally protected rights, including "the right to think and communicate, the right to privacy, and the right against illegal search and seizure" (Naon, 1978, p. 124). In *Kaimowitz* v. *Department of Mental Health,* the Michigan circuit court cites these considerations in determining that an involuntarily committed patient could not be subjected to psychosurgery: "In the hierarchy of values, it is more important to protect one's mental processes than to protect even the privacy of the marital bed. . . . Intrusion into one's intellect . . . is an intrusion into one's constitutionally protected right of privacy. If one is not protected in his thoughts, . . . then the right of privacy becomes meaningless" (Naon, 1978, p. 124).

A related issue is whether a person confined involuntarily in a prison or mental health hospital can indeed give uncoerced, informed consent to a proffered treatment or therapy. The argument may be made that the pressures on the inmate and the coercive atmosphere of the institution effectively negate informed consent, and, in fact, this was the finding of the court in *Kaimowitz* v. *Department of Mental Health.* The court held:

> It is impossible for an involuntarily detained mental patient to be free of ulterior forms of restraint or coercion when his very release from the institution may depend upon his cooperating with the institutional authorities and giving consent to experimental surgery. . . . Although an involuntarily detained mental patient may have a sufficient I.Q. to intellectually comprehend his circumstances, . . . the very nature of his incarceration diminishes the capacity to consent to psychosurgery. He is particularly vulnerable as a result of his mental condition, the deprivation stemming from involuntary confinement, and the effects of the phenomenon of "institutionalization" [Shapiro, 1974, p. 316].

It should be noted that the court only limited "experimental surgery," specifically exempting, although not defining, "accepted neurosurgical procedures." Banning certain procedures altogether denies to some inmates the right to elect treatment that they may deem beneficial. If one accepts the principle of personal autonomy, the inmate should have the same right to accept treatment as to refuse it. "To deem any therapy to be impermissibly coerced on its face may, it is argued, interfere with an individual's 'freedom of mentation'" (Wexler, 1975, p. 133). And as Opton (1975, pp. 27–28) reasons, "To respond to a request for help from a person who asks for it is a matter entirely different from imposing 'help' on a group of people." Shapiro (1974, p. 252) argues that "the conflicting aims of freedom from madness and freedom from state incursions upon personal autonomy are substantially accommodated by the requirement of informed consent. Prisoners who competently reject organic therapies will be free of them; those who give their informed consent may venture such therapies; and those who lack the capacity for informed consent are guaranteed an informed adjudication which is intended to restrain the arbitrary or improper exercise of state power."

The Right to Treatment

The involuntary confinement of juveniles and the mentally ill under the *parens patriae* power of the state is predicated on the assumption that individuals so detained will receive some kind of remedial or rehabilitative treatment. With the recent emphasis on civil rights, there has been a significant increase in state legislation and federal judicial activity, particularly with respect to involuntarily committed mental patients and sexual psychopaths. In fact, half the states enacted some type of right-to-treatment legislation during the ten-year period from 1966 to 1975, probably in response to judicial actions (Grant and Donaldson, 1976, p. 604).

The criminal justice system focuses attention on the determination of the guilt or innocence of the individual and provides due process safeguards for the protection of the accused. For juveniles and the mentally ill, however, since the state is presumed to be intervening for the good of the individual, less attention has been given to the safeguarding of individual rights. The result has been a gross disparity, whereby persons detained under juvenile and civil commitment law have sometimes been confined indefinitely for behavior which would bring a minor penalty or no penalty under the criminal statutes. This fact, coupled with the absence of any meaningful treatment, presented for those so confined the worst of both worlds—indeterminate detention, poor or nonexistent treatment, and an abrogation of procedural, due process safeguards.

The juvenile system clearly illustrates the limitations of a rehabilitation model. Because a separate juvenile court system has been established to promote rehabilitation and avoid criminal stigmatization of children, proceedings were informal and nonadversarial. A series of Supreme Court decisions beginning in 1966 significantly changed the procedures for processing juveniles, extending to juveniles some of the protections available to adult offenders. In *Kent* v. *United States,* the Court ruled that the juvenile hearing in the District of Columbia must satisfy "the essentials of due process and fair treatment" and noted that "there may be grounds for concern that the child receives the worst of both worlds; that he gets neither the protections accorded adults nor the solicitous care and regenerative treatment postulated for children" (Simpson, 1976, p. 992).

In the next case, *In re Gault,* the Court considered the procedural protections afforded juveniles by the Constitution. Gerald Gault, accused by a neighbor of making lewd or indecent remarks during a telephone call, had been found to be a delinquent following an informal hearing. Whereas the state provided a maximum penalty of a fifty-dollar fine and two-month prison term for adults making obscene telephone calls, fifteen-year-old Gault was committed to the state industrial school "for the period of his minority (that is, until age twenty-one) unless sooner discharged by due process of law" (Simpson, 1976, p. 992). In its decision, the Supreme Court held that "notice of charges, the right to counsel, the right to confrontation and cross-examination of witnesses, and the privilege against self-incrimination" were "essentials of due process and fair treatment" alluded to in *Kent* and were therefore "constitutionally required" (Simpson, 1976, p. 993).

Since the rationale for a separate juvenile court system and for the continuing denial to juveniles of the same due process safeguards afforded adult offenders has been, at least in part, the notion that juvenile offenders should receive rehabilitation that would prevent them from becoming hardened criminals, one may ask how well this intent has in fact been realized. The statutory standard of care for juveniles is in most states "custody, care, and discipline, as nearly as possible equivalent to that which should have been given by his parents" (Simpson, 1976, p. 996, Note 69). Yet even this minimal standard far surpasses the appalling conditions found in many facilities for juveniles.

Asserting a constitutional right to treatment for juveniles, several district courts have held that the "failure to provide juveniles the procedural protections constitutionally required in criminal proceedings, combined with a lack of treatment, is a denial of due process" (Simpson, 1976, p. 997). In *Morales* v. *Turman*, the federal district court stated: "The commitment of juveniles to institutions under conditions and procedures much less rigorous than those required for the conviction and imprisonment of an adult offender gives rise to certain limitations upon the conditions under which the state may confine the juveniles. This doctrine has been labeled the 'right to treatment,' and finds its basis in the due process clause of the Fourteenth Amendment" (Simpson, 1976, p. 997).

The first cases outside the juvenile justice system dealing with the right to treatment were brought on behalf of civilly committed sexual psychopaths. For example, in *Miller* v. *Overholser*, the Supreme Court held that the state could not legally confine a person to a facility for the violently insane under a state statute promising treatment when the facility in fact offered no treatment. *Rouse* v. *Cameron* is frequently cited as maintaining that the right to treatment has constitutional force; the Court found that even though Rouse—who had been confined after a finding of "not guilty by reason of insanity"—was receiving what was loosely termed "environmental therapy" the alleged treatment was inadequate because there was no individual treatment plan and no individual treatment.

In *Wyatt* v. *Stickney* (also known as *Wyatt* v. *Anderholt* and *Wyatt* v. *Hardin*), a class-action suit that focused attention on the situation of the mentally ill in large state hospitals, the court ruled that the failure to provide adequate treatment following an individual's involuntary confinement for ostensibly humane and therapeutic reasons violates the very fundamentals of due process.

Of particular significance is the fact that the Court stipulated specific and detailed standards of treatment and established a seven-member citizen advocacy group to monitor progress in attaining them. The standards covered such things as "rights to privacy, presumption of competency, communication with outsiders, compensation for labor, staff/patient ratios, educational opportunities, floor space, sanitary facilities and nutrition, individual treatment plans, written orders, and restraint orders" (Miller, 1977, p. 106). As Stone (1975, p. 88) observed, "The *Wyatt* decree was far from a generalized array of commands arbitrarily arrived at. It was formulated from testimony of institutional personnel, outside experts, and representatives of national mental health organizations appearing as *amici*." Critics of right-to-treatment decisions cite *Wyatt* as an example of undue judicial interference that forces the state to spend money it cannot afford on unproven reforms that do not make any difference anyway. As a result of *Wyatt*, Alabama civil commitment policies have been revised so that the overall hospital population has been reduced and the majority of admissions are now voluntary (Miller, 1977, p. 117). As Stone observes, a sad and ironic consequence of right-to-treatment litigation is that it may simply accelerate the "dumping" of chronic patients from hospitals into the community, where treatment is not available to them and resources are not sufficient to meet their basic needs.

Stone (1975, p. 94) likens such dumping of the mentally ill to the Renaissance practice of consigning them to "ships of fools." According to Foucault (1973, p. 9), "They did exist, these boats that conveyed their insane cargo from town to town. Madmen then led an easy wandering existence. The towns drove them outside their limits; they were allowed to wander in the open countryside, when not trusted to a group of merchants and pilgrims. . . . Frequently they were handed over to boatmen. . . . Often the cities of Europe must have seen these 'ships of fools' approaching their harbors. . . . It is possible that these ships of fools, which haunted the imagination of the entire early Renaissance, were pilgrimage boats, highly symbolic cargoes of madmen in search of their reason."

Involuntary Commitment and the Processing of Dangerousness

A 1966 account of lunacy commission hearings of one California county described the proceedings as informal and speedy (Miller and Schwartz, 1966). The average length of the hearings was four minutes, the median less than three. Of fifty-eight cases which were observed, in only one was the defendant served by a defense attorney, and that case was dismissed. Several of the defendants were non-English-speaking Mexican-Americans who showed little awareness of what the hearing was all about. The commission was comprised of two local doctors (one a psychiatrist) and a superior court judge, and the medical examinations conducted prior to the hearings were as cursory as the hearings themselves. The observers concluded: "The short period of time spent on each prepatient and the fact that there was often no one (including himself) to speak on his behalf contributed to a definite feeling that here was a presumption of insanity held by the commission members. . . . One is tempted to conclude that the judgment about mental illness was made earlier in the commitment process, and that the hearing was a rubber stamp to this earlier decision" (Miller and Schwartz, 1966, p. 34).

Under the pressure of court challenges, such procedures are becoming less frequent, although, as we shall see, serious problems persist in protecting due process rights for persons subject to involuntary commitment proceedings. In *Donaldson* v. *O'Connor*, the court ruled that if they are dangerous to no one and can live safely in freedom, there is no constitutional basis for detaining and confining against their will persons who are mentally ill.

In *Lessard* v. *Schmidt*, the U.S. District Court ruled that a patient was entitled to "notice of the judicial proceedings, to a privilege against self-incrimination vis-a-vis the examining psychiatrists, to a relatively prompt judicial hearing, to retained or appointed counsel who is to function as an advocate, and to a commitment determination meeting a beyond-a-reasonable-doubt test" (Wexler, 1972, p. 316). Stone (1975, p. 52) asserts that *Lessard* "would invalidate the provisions of commitment laws in virtually all states and would, if followed exactly, put a virtual end to involuntary confinement." In the state of Washington, after a civil commitment law containing the provisions of *Lessard* was passed, there was an immediate decline in civil commitments, but the number of commitments has since steadily increased, as has the number of commitments under criminal statutes. On the legislative front, over the past ten years a number of states have adopted civil commitment laws modeled on California's 1969 Lanterman-Petris-Short (LPS) Act. This law—described as including "the broadest changes in the procedures for the involuntary commitment of the mentally disordered since the process began in the early 1800s" (Urmer, 1978, p. 137)—contains the following major provisions:

1. Limits involuntary hospitalization to individuals who are observed to be dangerous to others, dangerous to self, or gravely disabled as a function of their mental disorder.
2. Permits involuntary treatment without court review for a maximum of seventeen days, with provisions for an additional fourteen days of involuntary commitment for individuals who are suicidal.
3. Requires court approval to allow an additional ninety days of treatment for persons who are found dangerous to others.
4. Appoints a conservator for one year for individuals who are considered "gravely disabled"—"a condition in which a person, as a result of mental disorder, is unable to provide for his basic personal needs for food, clothing, or shelter" (p. 137).
5. Defines the rights of patients who are involuntarily committed, including a habeas corpus hearing, retention of personal property, right to refuse shock treatment, and right to maintain their own clothes.
6. Shifts control of state mental health funds from the state department of mental hygiene to the local communities.

The traditional rationale for involuntary commitment has been to permit treatment of those who pose a threat of violence to themselves or to others, those who are gravely disabled such that they are unable to care for themselves, and those whose bizarre or disruptive behavior is troublesome to their families or to the community. The judicial and legislative reforms of the past decade have sought to limit commitment to the dangerous and disabled and exempt those who are merely troublesome. As Stone (1975, p. 46) points out, the confinement of this latter category serves a "convenience function" which cannot be justified under either the police or *parens patriae* powers of the state: "This convenience function has seldom been explicitly acknowledged; rather, it has been hidden behind a promise of technical treatment, although at some points during the past century it has been the only goal actually achieved. Its implementation all too obviously calls for a macrosocietal policy judgment of a type which a free society is unwilling to confront in an open forum. It is therefore a typical instance of the clandestine decision-making role of mental health practitioners, which allows society to do what it does not want to admit to doing, that is, confining unwanted persons cheaply."

There is evidence that, despite legal reform, this convenience function continues to be an implicit goal of involuntary commitment. Furthermore, the imprecision of the definitions of mental illness, disability, and dangerousness, together with the dismal record of those purporting to be able to predict dangerousness, had led some to advocate abolition of involuntary commitment altogether. For example, Miller (1976, p. xii) argues that his own clinical work, research, and review of the research of others "leads me to believe that civil commitment for mental illness is wrong. It is wrong in that it is practiced in a highly selective fashion; it frequently involves the violation of individual rights; it is predicated on false premises; it usually does not achieve its avowed purposes; and it is wasteful of resources and damaging to the mental health profession."

One study shows that behavior not seeming to warrant confinement according to the criteria of California's LPS Act is, in practice, commonly defined by the courts as falling within the category of "gravely disabled." "Dancing in the street, parading around in uniform, yelling and screaming, moving furniture, reciting on a streetcorner, standing on the streetcorner trying to hail a taxi, being obese, being transient, and having a dirty home were among the folkway violations used as evidence of grave disablement. . . . Grave disablement standards dealt less with food, clothing, shelter, and finances—functioning within the community—than with functioning inside the family and the mental health system" (Warren, 1977, p. 638).

As this evidence suggests, psychiatric labels such as "mentally ill" and "dangerous to oneself or others," as well as the legal tests used to assign them, are vague and inherently elastic, squeezing in an almost unlimited range of behavior. According to Wexler (1972, p. 294), *"danger to others* can run the gamut from a serious risk of homicide, through a propensity to drive carelessly, to simply offending the sensibilities of others. Indeed, one court found a probable 'check bouncer' dangerous to others."

Abundant evidence attests to the fallibility of mental health professionals who attempt to make predictions of dangerous behavior. For example, one investigator summarized this literature as suggesting that "present ability to predict suicidal and assaultive behavior of psychologically abnormal persons is, to understate the matter, poor. Present systems using a dangerousness criterion almost certainly are unnecessarily institutionalizing a high proportion of involuntary patients, probably as many as half" (Dix, 1976, p. 332). Another investigator, commenting on the tendency of psychiatrists to overpredict, finds that "psychiatric testimony, to the extent that it overextends the reasonable boundaries of dangerousness, reflects an amalgam of ignorance, zeal, and self-protectiveness" (Brooks, 1978, p. 44).

The following hypothetical example illustrates the severe consequences of incorrect predictions of dangerousness: "Assume that one person out of a thousand will kill. Assume also an exceptionally accurate test is created which differentiates with 95 percent effectiveness those who will kill from those who will not. If 100,000 people were tested, out of the 100 who would kill, 95 would be isolated. Unfortunately, out of the 99,900 who would not kill, 4,995 people would also be isolated as potential killers" (Livermore and others, 1968, as cited by Stone, 1975, p. 28).

The 4,995 innocent persons isolated as a result of this 95 percent accurate test are what social scientists refer to as false positives. No techniques or procedures now in existence or even contemplated could claim a predictive accuracy anywhere approaching 95 percent; consequently, it can be safely assumed that a large proportion of those presently confined as dangerous are in fact false positives—persons incorrectly identified as dangerous. Their continued confinement can only be considered an unjustifiable form of preventive detention. Underlying such considerations is the question, How many harmless persons are we willing to confine in order to protect ourselves against the few who are in fact dangerous?

It is commonly assumed by mental health professionals, and by the general public as well, that those confined to institutions ought to be there. Goffman (1961) uses the phrase "automatic identification of the inmate" to describe the tendency of professionals to ascribe to their patients behaviors and characteristics that justify their deviant status, whether or not they in fact exhibit such behaviors. In other words, a mental hospital patient is by definition crazy, otherwise he or she would not be there.

An interesting demonstration of this phenomenon was provided by Rosenheim (1973) and his associates, who were voluntarily admitted to mental hospitals reporting a fabricated precipitating incident but factual personal histories. Once admitted, they behaved normally. Other hospital inmates immediately discerned their normality and questioned their presence in the hospital. The staff, however, interpreted their normal behavior as symptomatic of their alleged illness—for example, note taking was described in the charts as "compulsive writing behavior." In a deceptive follow-up, which would not be permitted under today's human subject review standards for research, Rosenheim told hospital administrators that a second group of normal subjects would be seeking admission. Hospital staff, believing they had correctly identified these normal subjects, rejected a number of applicants for admission, only to discover later that in fact none had been sent.

A special category of individuals confined against their will in mental hospitals is made up of those charged under criminal statutes and found "not guilty by reason of insanity." Such individuals are frequently worse off than if they had been found guilty and imprisoned. Generally, on a finding of not guilty by reason of insanity (NGRI), the individual is automatically hospitalized without the same procedural safeguards available to those who are civilly committed and subjected to confinement for longer than if convicted under the criminal charge. Once confined, the patient must often demonstrate that he or she is sufficiently recovered to justify release, a difficult case to make for someone in a mental hospital.

The Supreme Court case *Jackson* v. *Indiana* illustrates the problem. Jackson, a retarded deaf mute, was committed to a state mental institution after being found incompetent to stand trial for a criminal charge, and his mental functioning was not likely ever to improve to the point where he might be found competent to stand trial. Therefore, his lawyers argued, the finding of incompetence was tantamout to a life sentence to a mental institution, even though he had not been convicted of a crime. The Court ruled that his due process rights had been violated. "At the least, due process requires that the nature and duration of commitment bear some reasonable relation to the purpose for which the individual is committed" (German and Singer, 1976, p. 1016). Such commitments are predicated on a presumption of dangerousness unsupported by the available evidence. In fact, many who plead insanity did not commit a violent crime.

Mental health professionals would do well to ponder their role in mental health programs that may operate to deprive persons of their rights. As some observers have noted, if professionals did not studiously ignore the literature demonstrating the dismal record at prediction, they could not persist in making predictions of dangerousness—unless simply to maintain their professional status as experts (Shah, 1978). As Shah (1978, p. 185) concludes, "Mental health professionals need . . . to consider very carefully the roles that they find themselves playing as agents of social control with respect to various categories of the mentally ill, rather than as caregivers and therapists."

Moral Dilemmas in Mental Health Practice and Administration

This chapter has included a range of mental health policy issues that have been subject to recent legal challenge and professional debate and could easily have been expanded to include others as well—the use of physical restraints, seclusion and time out, electroshock therapy, inmate labor or penal servitude, and the prioritization of access to various kinds of treatment programs. All of these policies illustrate a fundamental tension between the basic rights of individuals and professional concerns for effective and humane treatment, on the one hand, and societal concerns for social control and efficient response to social problems on the other. One legacy of the social reforms of the progressive era is a belief that human service professionalism provides sufficient protection for those processed through the helping bureaucracies. However, as recent legal activism and scholarly and professional debate demonstrate, progressive policies, professional ethics, and administrative rules are insufficient guarantors of client rights (Rothman, 1980; Larson, 1977). In view of the constantly evolving standards of practice, there are no absolute rules to guide professional decision making—one may follow administrative directives and apply the ethical guidelines of one's profession yet still participate in the implementation of punitive or harmful practices.

The enactment of an appropriate policy—if such a thing is possible—does not resolve the dilemmas of professional practice. As this discussion has shown, we cannot know with certainty that any given policy will not be subsequently called into question as legal and professional standards change. In addition, the enactment of a "good" policy does not in itself offer any guarantee against harmful results. There are often unintended and unanticipated consequences of reform policies. An example, already cited, is the shifting of deviants to criminal justice sanctions in the wake of civil commitment reforms that restrict the involuntary hospitalization of persons deemed mentally ill and either dangerous to self or others or gravely disabled.

Various implementation problems limit the ability of administrators and practitioners to faithfully translate policy into practice, including conflicting professional ideologies and roles, differing organizational missions, interorganizational and jurisdictional competition, spatial and temporal frameworks, and work load and resource constraints. Chronic shortages in staff and treatment resources constantly force workers and administrators to compromise the policies they implement, as well as their own standards of humane and effective treatment (Weatherley, 1979, 1980).

Recent events at Washington's Rainier School, an institution for the developmentally disabled, illustrate the dilemmas created by enacting ostensibly humane policies but implementing them with insufficient resources. In the wake of an inmate death, the newly appointed administrator ordered a sharp curtailment in the use of restraints. A call for the collection of restraint devices yielded hundreds covering a six-by-ten-foot room to a depth of three feet. Staff, though acknowledging an overreliance on restraints, nonetheless defended their use as necessary to protect residents and staff in view of staff shortages exacerbated by appallingly low pay. But even the director acknowledged that staff increases were unlikely in view of legislative sentiments to reduce social program expenditures. The director's goal of reducing the resident census was also limited by the opposition of parents and the lack of less restrictive community alternatives. For the individual worker, the progressive policies of the reform-minded administrator had somehow to be reconciled with a day-to-day reality in which there was too much work and too few resources (Jones, 1980). The conflict between policy goals and insufficient resources is a chronic problem in the human services that the frontline worker is generally given little guidance in resolving. But when public attention is focused on program deficiencies and abuses, most often in the wake of some particularly poignant tragedy, the frontline worker and administrator serve as convenient scapegoats—it is easier to blame individuals than to correct an inoperative system.

The activities of individual human service workers are subject to a moral division of labor. The processing of clients through our mental health and criminal justice systems entails numerous decisions and activities which individually may appear logical and benign but cumulatively may produce abuses. The worker in the Rainier School, for example, is not asked to choose between policies for or against the use of restraints; he or she faces the more immediate and practical issue of how to watch over a group of potentially violent and self-destructive residents without enough backup help. Restraints or drugs may seem the least of evils.

Similarly, the hospital emergency room social worker is not required to take a stand on civil commitment policy but must quickly decide what to do with a disoriented person who has no place to go and no one to look after him or her. The community mental health worker does not decide the agency's policy on drug therapy but may recommend medication because there are no treatment alternatives available. Potentially long-term ill effects may seem insignificant when weighed against the client's current crisis. Individual decisions that appear to conform to professional ethics and to be in the best interests of the client can, in the aggregate, contribute to systematic client abuse. The worker thus becomes an unwitting participant in abusive systems, even while striving to conform to ethical maxims of service and respect for the individual.

There is no tradition of whistle blowing in the human services. Professionalism, it has been thought, controls abuse. The human service professions operate on the assumption that whatever one does must, by definition, be beneficial to clients. This analysis suggests the need for practitioners and administrators to examine and assess their individual interventions in terms of the long-term and cumulative effects on clients. There are no well-developed ethics for administering and practicing in unjust and harmful systems. Yet ethical considerations may require a willingness to question agency policies and practices, to seek to change them, and, in some circumstances, to refuse to implement them.

References

Annas, G. J. "Refusing Medication in Mental Hospitals." *Hastings Center Report,* Feb. 1980, *10,* 21–22.

Bandura, A. "Punishment Revisited." *Journal of Consulting Psychology,* 1962, *26,* 298.

Bandura, A. "Ethics and Social Purposes: Behavior Modification." In C. Franks and G. Wilson (Eds.), *Annual Review of Behavior Therapy.* New York: Brunner/Mazel, 1975.

Breggin, P. R. "The Return of Lobotomy and Psychosurgery." 92nd Congress, 2d session. *Congressional Record,* Feb. 24, 1972, E1602, E1610.

Brooks, A. D. "Notes on Defining the Dangerousness of the Mentally Ill." In C. J. Frederickson (Ed.), *Dangerous Behavior.* DHEW Publication No. (ADM) 78-563. Washington, D.C.: U.S. Government Printing Office, 1978.

Bruce, W. R. "Tokens for Recovery." *American Journal of Nursing,* 1966, *66,* 1800–1801.

"Conditioning and Other Technologies Used to 'Treat?' 'Rehabilitate?' 'Demolish?' Prisoners and Mental Patients." *Southern California Law Review,* 1972, *45,* 616–617.

Crane, G. E. "Clinical Pharmacology in Its 20th Year." *Science,* July 13, 1973, *181,* 124–128.

Dix, G. E. "Civil Commitment of the Mentally Ill and the Need for Data on the Prediction of Dangerousness." *American Behavioral Scientist*, 1976, *19*, 318–334.

Ennis, B. J. "Civil Liberties and Mental Illness." *Criminal Law Bulletin*, 1971, *1*, 101.

Foucault, M. *Madness and Civilization: A History of Insanity in the Age of Reason.* New York: Random House, 1973.

German, J. R., and Singer, A. C. "Punishing the Not Guilty: Hospitalization of Persons Acquitted by Reason of Insanity." *Rutgers Law Review*, 1976, *29*, 1011–1086.

Goffman, E. *Asylums.* Garden City, N.Y.: Anchor Books, 1961.

Grant, J. E., and Donaldson, K. "Dangerousness and the Right to Treatment." *Hastings Constitutional Law Quarterly*, 1976, *3*, 599.

Halleck, S. L. "Legal and Ethical Aspects of Behavior Control." *American Journal of Psychology*, 1974, *131*, 381–382.

Jones, M. "Rainier School Changing: Morale Hurting." *Seattle Times*, Sept. 1, 1980, p. 1.

Kittrie, N. N. *The Right To Be Different.* Baltimore: Johns Hopkins Press, 1971.

Larson, M. S. *The Rise of Professionalism: A Sociological Analysis.* Berkeley: University of California Press, 1977.

Lipsky, M., and Olson, D. *Riot Commission Politics: The Processing of Racial Crisis in America.* New Brunswick, N.J.: Transaction Books, 1974.

Mattocks, L., and Jew, A. "Assessment of an Aversive Treatment Program with Extreme Acting-Out Patients in a Psychiatric Facility for Criminal Offenders." Unpublished manuscript prepared for the California Department of Corrections, on file at the University of Southern California Law Library, undated.

Miller, D., and Schwartz, M. "County Lunacy Commission Hearings: Some Observations of Commitments to a State Mental Hospital." *Social Problems*, Summer 1966, *14*, 26–36.

Miller, H. L. "The 'Right to Treatment': Can the Courts Rehabilitate and Cure?" *Public Interest*, Winter 1977, *46*, 96–118.

Miller, K. S. *Managing Madness.* New York: Macmillan, 1976.

Naon, B. *Issues to Treatment and Rehabilitation in Mental Hospitals and Penal Institutions.* Olympia, Wash.: Office of Program Research, Washington House of Representatives, Aug. 11, 1978.

National Institute of Mental Health. *Psychosurgery: Perspectives on a Current Problem.* Washington, D.C.: Department of Health, Education, and Welfare, 1973.

Opton, E. "Institutional Behavior Modification as a Fraud and Sham." *Arizona Law Review*, 1975, *17*, 20–28.

Rachman, S., and Teasdale, J. *Aversion Therapy and Behavior Disorders: An Analysis.* Coral Gables, Fla.: University of Miami Press, 1969.

Reich, W. "The Force of Diagnosis: Opportune Uses of Psychiatry." *Harper's*, May 1980, *260*, 20–32.

Remmen, E. *Psychochemotherapy: The Physician's Manual.* Los Angeles, Calif.: Western Medical Publications, 1962.

Rosenheim, D. L. "On Being Sane in Insane Places." *Science,* Jan. 1973, *179,* 250–251.

Rothman, D. J. *Conscience and Convenience: The Asylum and Its Alternatives in Progressive America.* Boston: Little, Brown, 1980.

Scheff, T. J. "Medical Dominance: Psychoactive Drugs and Mental Health Policy." *American Behavioral Scientist,* Jan./Feb. 1976, *19,* 299–317.

Schwitzgebel, A. "Limitations on the Coercive Treatment of Offenders." *Criminal Law Bulletin,* 1972, *8*(4), 267–320.

Shah, S. A. "Dangerousness and Mental Illness: Some Conceptual, Prediction, and Policy Dilemmas." In C. J. Frederickson (Ed.), *Dangerous Behavior.* DHEW Publication No. (ADM) 78-563. Washington, D.C.: U.S. Government Printing Office, 1978.

Shainberg, L. *Brain Surgeon: An Intimate View of His World.* Philadelphia: Lippincott, 1979.

Shapiro, M. H. "Legislating the Control of Behavior Control: Autonomy and the Coercive Use of Organic Therapies." *Southern California Law Review,* 1974, *47,* 237–356.

Simpson, A. L. "Rehabilitation as the Justification of a Separate Juvenile Justice System." *California Law Review,* 1976, *64*(4), 984–1017.

Singer, J. L. "Psychological Studies of Punishment." *California Law Review,* 1970, *48,* 405–443.

Sterling, P. "Psychiatry's Drug Addiction." *The New Republic,* Dec. 8, 1979, *181,* 14–18.

Stone, A. A. *Mental Health and the Law: A System in Transition.* DHEW Publication No. (ADM) 76-176. Washington, D.C.: U.S. Government Printing Office, 1975.

Urmer, A. H. "An Assessment of California's Mental Health Program: Implications for Mental Health Delivery Systems." In C. J. Frederickson (Ed.), *Dangerous Behavior.* DHEW Publication No. (ADM) 78-563. Washington, D.C.: U.S. Government Printing Office, 1978.

Warren, C. A. B. "Involuntary Commitment for Mental Disorder: The Application of California's Lanterman-Petris-Short Act." *Law and Society,* Spring 1977, *11,* 629–649.

Weatherley, R. A. *Reforming Special Education: Policy Implementation from State Level to Street Level.* Cambridge, Mass.: M.I.T. Press, 1979.

Weatherley, R. A. "Implementing Social Programs: The View from the Front Line." Paper presented at the annual meeting of the American Political Science Association, Washington, D.C., Aug. 1980.

Wexler, D. B. *Criminal Commitments and Dangerous Mental Patients: Legal Issues of Confinement, Treatment and Release.* Washington, D.C.: U.S. Government Printing Office, 1972.

Wexler, D. B. "Reflections on the Legal Regulation of Behavior Modification in Institutional Settings." *Arizona Law Review,* 1975, *17,* 132–143.

ॐ 5 ॐ

Planning and Administering Services for Minority Groups

Joseph S. Gallegos

An understanding of the mental health of minority groups must include a knowledge of cultural history, minority group strengths, and attitudes of minority families and communities. Imposing mainstream mental health standards on minority communities creates stress and resistance to the use of mental health services, especially when they are perceived as inaccessible or irrelevant. Joseph Gallegos describes the problems of differential treatment and unresponsive services for minority groups and of premature termination and underutilization of services by minority clients. Also emphasized are the role of affirmative action programs, expansion of the mental health treatment perspective to include environmental and cultural factors, and examination of institutional barriers to service. The recognition of cultural diversity is also related to role expectations of minority staff and minority administrators.

Minorities continue to be overrepresented among those of our nation's impoverished. Many of these minorities are in need of mental health services but are unable to gain access to them due to racism and barriers to effective cross-cultural communication. The purpose of this chapter is to enhance the effectiveness of administrators and planners who find themselves working with minority individuals and communities by promoting an awareness of minority issues in mental health administration and by considering practice principles. We will focus on the differences in meaning attached by minorities to the terms *mental health, planning,* and *administration* and will use a cross-cultural framework to generalize a minority perspective for American Indian, Asian, black, and Hispanic groups.

Central to this discussion will be the notion of empowerment, which refers to a process as well as a goal. As a process, empowerment involves the exchange of resources between two systems to enhance or increase the functional capability of one or both systems. For example, a nonminority administrator is empowered when he or she acquires increased sensitivity to minority perspectives or access to minority communities through the contribution of a minority colleague. Similarly, a minority staff member is empowered when he or she is given the authority to develop a new minority approach to services delivery. As a goal, empowerment refers to the increased functional capability of a given person or system. Solomon (1976) refers to empowerment as the development of an ability to effectively use resources to achieve individual or collective goals. The notion of empowerment refers to the development of a true working partnership between minority and nonminority staff members, who cooperate to provide services that in turn empower clients and communities to meet their needs.

Although the issues related to racism and prejudice are important, they tend to focus on pathology within either the majority or minority cultures. For the purpose of understanding minority issues in mental health planning and administration, other concepts—especially *pluralism, socialization,* and *sociocultural dissonance*—provide a more useful perspective on cultural difference. *Pluralism* refers to the variety of ethnic cultures and cultural value systems that constitute the American social structure. This concept gives credence to the equal importance of minority views by suggesting that there is no one national value system but rather a multitude of competing values. The notion is expressed in mental health public policy by the mandate that services must be provided to all citizens. *Socialization* refers to the learning process by which persons discover who they are and how they must behave within the cultural norms of a society. Many socializing institutions, based on majority white norms and values, devalue minority cultural values, especially those related to self-esteem and self-concept. Finally, *sociocultural dissonance* refers to the conflict that arises for the minority group member who attempts to respond and be accountable to two different cultures. Although not unique to ethnic minorities of color, *sociocultural dissonance* is crucial in understanding the minority experience.

Pluralism, socialization, and sociocultural dissonance provide a context for answering two fundamental questions: Why is there such a great discrepancy between the well-meaning intentions of traditional mental health practitioners and policy makers and the continuing, unmet need of ethnic minorities of color? And what are the consequences and implications of this discrepancy for mental health administrators?

Cultural Differences and Terminology

Throughout this chapter, we are considering ethnic and cultural differences—if there were no differences, we would not need to consider minority perspectives at all. One significant area of difference is in meaning. Whether expressed through culture, custom, or language, social communication is the basis for all human understanding and misunderstanding. Therefore, a consideration of terms used in this chapter is in order.

The following terminology highlights subtle and not so subtle differences in interpretation of seemingly neutral terms. By understanding and accepting these differences, we can begin to establish effective mental health services for minorities. Without such an understanding, we can only perpetuate an unresponsive system.

Minorities

We use the term *minority* in our discussion to refer to ethnic minorities of color—American Indians, Asians, blacks, and Hispanics—because they share unique life issues not necessarily experienced by other ethnic or nonethnic minorities—for example, women, handicapped persons, homosexuals, American Jews, or Italians. Of course, numerous differences exist even among ethnic minorities of color, but the following commonalities make general consideration of these groups appropriate: (1) these groups share in a history of discrimination and oppression based primarily on differences in culture and color, (2) they share non-Western or non-European historical antecedents (American Hispanics represent a blend of Indian or African and Spanish heritage), and (3) they share an experience of sociocultural dissonance.

Minority Mental Health

A definition of minority group mental health has yet to be agreed on. Our intent is not to provide such a definition but to point out some of the ways in which minority attitudes and perceptions about mental health differ from those of the majority—particularly those who control policy making and disbursement of funds.

In general, the minority perception of mental health agrees with the notion of holistic health as outlined by Tager (1978, p. 3): "Primarily, this is a dynamic state of personal health which is maintained and fostered through the use of a wide range of health-giving practices: it encompasses biological, intellectual, and spiritual well-being. Advocates of holistic health, therefore, suggest that no aspect of life can be ignored as a component in the health process." In particular, a recognition of natural support systems is critical for understanding the help-seeking behaviors of minorities, and any definition of mental health for minorities must include the relationship of the individual to his or her family, community, culture, and history. Quite often the narrowness of traditional majority definitions of mental health creates compliance problems for the minority agency; for example, in order to secure certain public funds, minority practitioners—who may be uncomfortable in using psychiatric terms unfamiliar to clients and practitioners alike—must conform to established mental health standards and terminology. The result is that the treatment situation may suffer from externally imposed rules and norms.

Among minority groups, there remains significant resistance to the notion of mental health as a service area. Minorities find it more palatable to consider using social services, including housing and employment services, than to consider seeking help for mental dysfunction. In fact, however, mental dysfunction transcends color lines, and the stress of living has devastating effects on minorities and nonminorities alike.

Planning

Research indicates that, in their approach to planning and problem solving, minorities differ from white males in cognitive style and in the locus of control. For example, Ramirez and Castandea (1974) found that minority groups were more group conscious, more cooperative, more field dependent, and less hierarchical in their thinking than their white counterparts. Maruyama (1974) found that the minority approach to planning is more attuned to seeing the gestalt or holistic design and less facile in the compartmentalization of problems.

In their attitudes toward planning, minorities appear to see power as something held by others and therefore external to their own control. Growing up in this country, minority individuals know that certain power lies outside themselves, their families, and even their communities. Minority groups exhibit a tendency toward fatalism in their religious beliefs and customs and in their response to a state of powerlessness. "It is God's will"; "things happen for a reason"; "decisions will come when their time is right"—these maxims are commonly heard in minority circles. This attitude implies a resistance to imposing structured plans on future events or, when plans are made, there is a tendency to view them with a degree of pessimism. "Don't count your chickens before they hatch," or "Don't put all your eggs in one basket," cautions the minority planner who seeks to develop contingency plans. Finally, the importance of face saving among minorities further inhibits risk taking in the planning process. Planning for or by minorities is a cautious undertaking, designed to respond simultaneously to two cultural mind sets.

Administration

The concept of administration conjures for minorities images of power and influence, of white males controlling large bureaucracies. The white administrator is socialized in the ways of power and influence and thereby drawn into leadership roles. Administration is a new role for minorities, however, who sometimes erroneously define it as a method for gaining power and influence over resources for the empowerment of ethnic groups.

Client-Therapist Relationships

The development and delivery of mental health services to minorities differs from the development and delivery of such services to the rest of society. America is a pluralistic society, and the diversity of cultures demands a diversity of treatment approaches—a premise that refutes two beliefs deeply rooted in the

American ethos. The first is the belief in the assimilation of various peoples into one culture or melting pot, bound together by common goals, beliefs, and values—a direct contrast to the concept of pluralism. The second belief suggests that, since we are a nation of one culture, we should treat one another as if we were all one color. This notion posits that, since people are people regardless of their ethnic or cultural background, a humanistic approach will suffice for all.

Research clearly points to a different standard for minorities by documenting the disparities between majority and minority mental health services. Owan (1980) finds different standards evidenced in four areas: treatment, outcomes, utilization, and compliance. It also should be acknowledged that minority clients are neither financially rewarding for an agency nor professionally rewarding for clinicians.

Differential Treatment

Owan (1980) provides substantial documentation that minority clients receive different treatment. Accuracy of diagnosis and specificity in treatment planning are directly correlated to the degree of sociocultural difference between the therapist and the client. The type of treatment appears to be racially linked, with insight-oriented therapy for whites and crisis intervention modalities for minorities. In addition, nonminorities are more likely to be accepted for mental health services in the first place (Owan, 1980).

The data cited by Owan (1980) leave no question that minorities receive differential treatment, if in fact they receive any treatment at all. An administrator wishing to address this issue must first become aware of the practices in his or her own agency, then seek out and change discriminative and restrictive policies. Equally as important as policy analysis is an investigation of actual treatment practices. Such an assessment should include the treatment process from beginning to end. Are minorities deterred by intake screening procedures or personnel? Does the case assignment procedure shunt minorities to less-qualified professionals? Does the clinical staff have a repertoire of treatment approaches necessary to meet the needs of a culturally varied population? Can clinicians count on administrative support to effectively serve minorities?

Negative Outcomes

Premature termination of treatment occurs more frequently among clients who are poor, working class, and minority. Owan (1980) attributes dissatisfaction with mental health services—the reason most often given for termination by minorities—to a miscommunication of expectations. Minorities seem to expect from counseling concrete advice for coping with social problems, rather than insight and changes in personality. Owan (1980, p. 445) reports the following findings on dropout rates:

Considerable research points to the class-bound nature of psychotherapy as a factor in the high dropout rate among lower-class clients (Garfield, 1971; Goldstein, 1962; Lorion, 1973; Fiester and Rudestam, 1975). Padilla, Ruiz, and Alvarez (1975) reported that culture- and class-bound therapists constituted major problems in the psychotherapy of ethnic clients. Although studies of long-term follow-up of treatment and outcome are rare, there are substantial findings indicating that race and ethnicity are very important variables in predicting outcome. For example, Yamamoto, James, and Palley (1968) and Sue and others (1974) found greater treatment dropout rates among blacks than whites, where 52.1 percent of blacks dropped out after the first session, as compared to only 29.8 percent of whites (Sue and others, 1974). Sue (1977) found in his study of seventeen community mental health centers in the greater Seattle area over a three-year period that dropout rate after the initial intake session for Asian patients was 52 percent, or almost twice the dropout rate for white patients. Yamamoto and Going (1965) and Krebs (1971) found that blacks attended fewer sessions than whites. Karno (1966) has also documented high dropout rates among Mexican-Americans and Puerto Ricans.

It is as though we have two systems of mental health, one of which provides little service to minorities, and one in which the outcomes are woefully inadequate when service is provided. A common response to this discrepancy is to label clients who terminate early as resistive and lacking in motivation.

An administrator concerned with this problem must consider the treatment expectations of client, therapist, and agency. To understand the client's expectations, an administrator must have an awareness of that client's culture. Equally as important is an awareness of the culture—whether ethnic or professional—from which the therapist derives his or her therapeutic expectations. Is the therapist a psychiatric nurse? A psychiatrist? A social worker? Will the professional culture or other variable inhibit the therapist's ability to share therapeutic expectations with the client? Knowledge of client expectations, when matched with a clinical capacity to accommodate those expectations, would result in more positive therapeutic outcomes.

Understandably, most clinicians avoid clients who are resistive and lack motivation. If, however, an administrator is concerned with the minority population, accommodations must be made. Are incentives provided to work with difficult cases? Are there procedures for sharing these cases, or do the minority cases get channeled to minority staff? Is training and consultation made available to staff for culturally specific issues such as Indian alcoholism? Are minority cases monitored to determine if there is a discrepancy between outcomes for minorities and for nonminorities? Such procedures will ensure a responsiveness to minority clients and their communities. Without this responsiveness, agencies will continue to experience negative outcomes in their efforts to serve minorities and will continue to be underutilized by minority communities.

Underutilization

Underutilization of mental health services by minorities continues to be a serious problem and has been documented in every state. Owan (1980) reports various analyses of utilization rates by American Indians and by Hispanic and Asian Americans that found that only a fraction of a percent utilized mental health services—numbers that did not reflect the proportion of minority group members in the general populations surveyed (Abad, Ramos, and Boyce, 1974; Hatanka, Watanabe, and Ono, 1975; Karno and Edgerton, 1969; Sue, 1977; President's Commission on Mental Health, 1978). Various authors have speculated on the causes of this phenomenon and have noted in-cultural factors, such as natural support systems, and external factors, such as inaccessibility of services and linguistic and cultural differences between client and therapist. The mental health administrator must understand the problem of underutilization and consider steps to reverse this trend. An administrator must first be concerned with providing effective services to minority clients—services that cannot be provided by a culturally insensitive or unaware staff. The ideal situation is to have bicultural and, if necessary, bilingual staff, but this is not always possible. Therefore, a second line of action is to ensure that the agency has the resources to respond to the culture-specific needs of clients by securing sensitivity and cultural awareness training for staff and by using culturally specific consultation and minority community resources.

For example, agencies can broaden their response capabilities by utilizing nontraditional consultation. Mental health agencies have successfully used *curanderos* (Mexican-American folk healers) in the Southwest, *espiritualistas* (Puerto Rican folk healers), and American Indian medicine men. Minority mental health consultants are usually available, although they may not hold traditional mental health degrees, and minority mental health organizations are available for consultation and training.

A word of caution regarding the use of minority resources: these resources should not be used on a critical need basis only. A more effective and fruitful approach is to develop an ongoing collegial and peer relationship that fosters mutual respect, enhances the effectiveness of consultation, and sensitizes the agency in its interaction with minority clients and their communities.

To deal with the disparities between services to minorities and services to nonminorities, then, administrators must begin with an assessment of their own and their agencies' level of awareness of, and sensitivity toward, minorities. Second, an assessment of the agency's capabilities to respond to minority needs is in order. In each case, minority consultation is necessary, and is usually available from local minority mental health professionals or from minority agencies and organizations. Cultural assessment should cover every sphere of agent activity, and the process of remediation must be ongoing.

Compliance Issues

The Civil Rights Act of 1964 mandates that "no person in the United States shall, on the ground of race, color, or national origin, be excluded from participation in, be denied the benefits of, or be subjected to discrimination under, any program or activity receiving federal financial assistance" (Title VI, 42 U.S.C. S2000d).

The federal government has issued regulations designed to ensure the equal treatment of all qualified persons under programs receiving federal financial assistance (45 C.F.R. S 80 et seq.) by forbidding:

- Denial of any service, financial aid, or other benefit to an individual because of the individual's race, color, or national origin.
- Provision to an individual of any service, financial aid, or other benefit that is different or is provided in a different manner from that provided to others because of the individual's race, color, or national origin.
- Separate or unique treatment of an individual because of the individual's race, color, or national origin in any matter relating to his or her receipt of any service, financial aid, or other benefit.
- Restriction of an individual's enjoyment of any advantage or privilege enjoyed by others because of the individual's race, color, or national origin.
- Differential treatment of an individual in determining eligibility because of the individual's race, color, or national origin.
- Denial to an individual of the right to participate in programs on the same basis as other participants because of the individual's race, color, or national origin.
- Discrimination against an individual resulting from the utilization of criteria or methods of administration that have the effect of defeating or substantially impairing the objectives of federally assisted programs.

Despite the existence of these regulations, extensive discrimination against non-English-speaking (NES) and limited English-speaking (LES) individuals persists. In part, the problem relates to the lack of effective use of bilingual staff and printed matter. An approach to combatting the problem can be seen in the New York City "Chinatown Project," where a branch office of the Social Security Administration was staffed entirely by Japanese, Chinese, and Filipino workers and used bilingual literature and signs. A study of that office clearly demonstrated that the utilization of indigenous bilingual/bicultural staff members can significantly improve productivity, quality of services, and the overall effectiveness and efficiency of services delivery (Owan, 1978).

Owan (1980) further notes the 1975 federal legislation that seeks to ensure racial and ethnic minorities equal benefits and equal opportunities to receive services. For example, the Community Mental Health Act (1963) and the amendments (1975) make reference to ethnic minorities as follows:

The [community mental health] center's services . . . shall be available and accessible to the residents of the area promptly, as appropriate, and in a manner that preserves human dignity and assures continuity and high quality care and that overcomes geographic, cultural, linguistic, and economic barriers to the receipt of services [Sec. 301 (b) (2)].

An application for a grant under this part . . . shall contain or be supported by assurance . . . that . . . in the case of a community mental health center serving a population including a substantial proportion of individuals of limited English-speaking ability, the center has (i) developed a plan and made arrangements responsive to the needs of such population for providing services to the extent practicable in the language and cultural context most appropriate to such individuals and (ii) identified an individual on its staff who is fluent in both that language and English and whose responsibilities shall include providing guidance to such individuals and to appropriate staff members with respect to cultural sensitivities and bridging linguistic and cultural differences [Sec. 206 (c)].

Further, the National Institute of Mental Health (1977) has developed nonbinding standards for the quality of clinical services provided by federally funded mental health centers, among which the following are relevant to the issue of cultural diversity:

Program Administration—Policy and Procedures Manual, Criteria G: Written policies and procedures shall be maintained for . . . handling major language/cultural population subgroups.

Program Administration—Program Evaluation, Criteria A: Demographic characteristics (for example, age, sex, ethnicity, income, language, and subarea of residence) of persons served shall be monitored and compared with the demographic characteristics of the catchment areas [1977, p. 31].

Services—Availability and Accessibility of Services, Standard #2 Criteria 6: Bilingual/bicultural advertising materials shall be used in communities where there are heavy concentrations of minorities [1977, p. 37].

Services—Availability and Accessibility of Services, Standard #4: The center shall minimize social and cultural barriers to the receipt of mental health services. . . . Service staff shall be familiar with the culture of major population subgroups in the catchment area. . . . Written policies and information for clients shall be written in languages appropriate to the catchment area.

The demographic characteristics of the service population shall reflect those of the population at risk in the catchment area and those projected in the comprehensive plan for services. . . . For centers with major population subgroups in the catchment area, there must be designated bilingual/bicultural staff with service ability for these subgroups. . . . Service staff shall be as representative as possible of the racial, ethnic, and cultural characteristics of the catchment area [1977, p. 39].

Federal legislation and standards clearly mandate that federally funded mental health centers provide equitable mental health services to racial and ethnic minorities. Yet in 1974, out of a total of 98 community mental health centers in one region of the country, 42 were serving nonwhites at lower rates than whites. Although they received technical assistance for a period of three years (1974-1977) to improve their services to nonwhites, the 42 showed little or no improvement (Windle and Wu, 1977).

Affirmative action policy compliance in the field of mental health provides yet another example of the disparity between the ideal and the real. All minority groups are underrepresented in the area of mental health administration (Wheeler, 1980). Bush (1977) notes that the issue of affirmative action goes beyond the hiring of minorities and must include the retention and career development of minority administrators. Due to the considerable job stress experienced by minority administrators, special attention needs to be given to the role of organizational survival, minority community expectations, and the dilemmas of rapid career advancement.

The identification of differential treatment, negative outcomes, underutilization, and noncompliance issues requires mental health administrators to continuously monitor policies and conduct detailed evaluations of mental health services in order to substantially improve access for, and utilization by, racial and ethnic minorities. The pluralistic nature of our society, the diversity of needs, and the inequities of mental health services substantiate the critical importance of meeting the mental health needs of minorities. If culture is such an important variable in mental health treatment, it must also be an important element in administration and planning.

Administrative and Planning Implications

The many issues related to a minority mental health perspective threaten to overwhelm even the most conscientious of administrators. However, a number of issues demand particular attention, and the remainder of this chapter is devoted to the implications of those issues within the context of a number of external and internal factors.

External—Mental Health Programming
- Minority community perspectives of mental health agencies
- Service planning: environmental and cultural factors
- Service barriers
- Board membership

Internal—Agency Administration
- Interagency communications
- Internal agency communications, accountability, and organizational change issues from a minority-group perspective
- Staff recruitment and deployment

- The role of affirmative action in mental health agency personnel management
- The role of a minority administrator
- The role of a nonminority culturally sensitive administrator

Minority Community Perspectives

From a minority perspective, the planning process is the most crucial point at which to include minority participants and perspectives. Each of the stages in the planning process—including problem identification, issue analysis, alternatives selection, implementation, and evaluation—requires the solicitation and inclusion of minority perspectives on planning for mental health services.

The first stage, needs assessment and problem identification, requires intensive minority input. The nonminority administrator, seeking credibility and acceptance for his or her plans, should give special attention to this first stage in order to ensure fewer problems with later stages. For example, consider the problem of defining a minority community for services delivery when mental health catchment area boundaries are developed according to geographical and population boundaries. If one wished to develop Asian mental health services in the city of Seattle, for example, one would probably think first of the International District. However, Seattle Asians acknowledge that their community is really dispersed throughout the Seattle area. Therefore, ethnically sensitive services focusing solely on the International District would miss numerous Asians who live outside its boundaries. Seattle Asians do, however, acknowledge the International District as the symbolic center of their community. Thus, a more responsive service plan might be to base services in the International District and locate outreach services in other parts of the city. Such a conclusion requires an awareness of the Asian minority perspective and the active participation of Seattle Asians in assessing needs. This example further illustrates that minority communities are more accurately described by social connections than by geographic or political boundaries.

The potential for cross-cultural misunderstandings is probably greatest at this stage of need determination and problem identification. Once defined, the problem will determine alternative solutions, implementation strategies, and, finally, the type of program evaluation strategy to be used. Minority input is best achieved by the use of key minority informants, community surveys, community advisory groups, and minority staff and board members.

Service Planning

Planning of mental health services must take into account that the middle-class values of the larger society may not be relevant in minority communities. For example, mental health administrators need to be aware of the economic realities in minority communities when they develop program plans for their clients. Special attention needs to be given to altering the economic system that reinforces poverty among minorities (Mayfield, 1972).

A crisis intervention program is the type of service utilized most frequently by minority populations. The initial request for professional help may involve a major role change—from that of an independently functioning person to that of a person who needs help in dealing with the problems of day-to-day living (Wolkon and others, 1974). The sooner clients receive services after the request for services, the more likely it is that they will be successfully treated. Wolkon and others (1974) state that the critical issue in establishing agency priorities is assuring continuous input from the client population regarding their needs and demands.

Service planning also needs to take into account the environmental factors of overcrowding and substandard housing that trouble most minorities. The psychological consequences of being raised in such an environment are increased stress and fewer opportunities for self-expression. Another environmental factor is unemployment, which tends to deprive people of their social standing, their self-respect, and the respect of their friends and family. Out of these environmental factors emerges a sense of powerlessness that causes individuals to feel unable to control or significantly alter their life situations (Mayfield, 1972).

Mental health service planning must recognize the unique cultural dimensions of a minority community, including linguistic patterns, socioeconomic standards, and points of view (Abad and others, 1974). When a minority individual goes to school, for example, the white-controlled school system tends to deny his or her uniqueness, thereby producing serious conflicts between family and societal values. Extended families and support systems are survival mechanisms by which minorities survive in white-dominated society (Saunders, 1969). The network of mental health services is seen by minorities and low-income individuals as inflexible, possessing too much red tape, and therefore unable to successfully and immediately offer relevant services (Cameron and Talavera, 1976).

Service Barriers

Blatant institutional racism is one of the major barriers to the delivery of effective mental health services in the minority community, discouraging and angering minority individuals in their search for services. Another barrier to the delivery of mental health services, attributable to institutional racism, is the location of agencies outside minority communities or away from bus lines, which often discourages individuals from seeking services (Golden, 1965).

The structure and programs of an organization can also serve as a barrier to the delivery of mental health services. Minority individuals and lower socioeconomic group members—discouraged from seeking services by the formality of an agency and the expression of middle-class values—often become accustomed to living with chronic problems until they are acute emergencies requiring emergency services, an attitude that is not conducive to preventive and follow-up programs (Abad and others, 1974).

Labeling people also serves as a barrier to the delivery of mental health services. Labels such as *culturally disadvantaged* and *deprived* are often used to describe minority communities. Such descriptions assume that these groups lack a culture or that whatever culture exists is of little value. Also, the description of these groups as nonwhite is a projection of white supremacy (Burgest, 1973). Even the concept of equality in its white American version is often seen as racist in that it implies that blacks and other minorities should become more like whites. Such an attitude is truly a barrier in the delivery of mental health services to minority populations.

Boards of Directors

The responsibilities of agency board members include seeking and responding to client input as well as being sensitive to their needs and being accountable to the community (Coulson, 1969). The policies affecting an agency are formulated by the board and implemented by its staff. Often boards of mental health agencies serving minority populations do not include minority members or include only a few token representatives, who are frequently chosen because they get along with white board members (Coulson, 1969). Many boards view tokenism as a painless way to meet the problem of minority representation. In fact, however, to effectively serve minorities, the board of a mental health agency must represent equally providers and consumers from all walks of life and all racial backgrounds, thus ensuring input from all elements of the community.

Mental health programming, then, must incorporate a planning process that exhibits a commitment to seeking the varying viewpoints needed to reflect service priorities. Minorities must be included in the planning process, and the goals of services must be consistent with minority goals. Environmental factors, cultural values, and service barriers must be approached by a mental health administrator with the interactional skills needed to communicate with the minority community. When dealing with minority communities, the successful administrator must know how to dress and how to talk and with whom. Unlike the analytical skills of needs assessment or program evaluation, which are most easily learned from books, these planning skills are best learned from experience and exposure to addressing minority needs.

Agency Administration

In addition to being sensitive to the issues of clients and minority communities, the mental health administrator must be cognizant of issues of cultural differences within the agency itself, including the issues of staff communication, role expectations, and supervision.

Interagency Communications

Interagency communications and the communications of staff members with their clients are critical components in mental health service delivery. In discussing communications, one must realize that mental health treatment methods reflect the dominant culture (Trader, 1977). Furthermore, most mental health practitioners are not aware of the racist implications of everyday language or of mental health treatment approaches. Burgest (1973) defines racism as a conscious or unconscious desire on the part of whites to destroy, castrate, and exploit others, both physically and psychologically, based in part on a desire for feelings of superiority. Consciously or unconsciously, language can be used to exploit minorities psychologically by using the negative connotations of a word or name associated with minorities; by attaching positive, favorable, and superior connotations to the word *white* and, by implication, to white people; and by expressing the view that all characteristics of minority cultures are inferior and white American culture is superior. Language not only expresses ideas and concepts but actually shapes them (Burgest, 1973).

Maruyama (1974) expands on this notion and notes that minorities of color share in a non-Western world view, which is less oriented to classifying phenomena, less competitive, more harmonious, and less hierarchical than its Western counterpart. For example, Native Americans did not use a hierarchical system of governance until the federal government imposed the use of tribal councils. Those Indians who accepted leadership roles in this new system were cultural deviants within their own native communities.

Effective interagency communication also requires an understanding of subtle linguistic cues, voice tones, gestures, and expressions in order to avoid misinterpretation (Hall and Whyte, 1960). In addition, the utilization of formal and informal communication networks within the minority community is essential for the success of mental health programs in minority communities (Golden, 1965).

Staff Recruitment and Deployment

In addition to recruiting minorities for entry-level jobs, mental health agencies are increasingly seeking skilled minority group members for managerial positions (Parker, 1976). Golden (1965) states that hiring minority workers not as tokens but on the basis of their qualifications demonstrates that an agency is willing to serve minorities and to provide new experiences for their white staff. Minority staff can expand the range of staff skills by introducing cross-cultural communication skills and knowledge. For example, research has indicated that black social workers were addressing themselves to the profession's perceived racial needs long before others in their profession and were incorporating their own insights about race into their practice (Brown, 1976). Even more important is the fact that minority staff members serve as bridges between their community and predominantly white mental health agencies (Abad and others, 1974).

Minority staff members can also utilize the informal communication system that exists within their particular community, as well as serve as role models for clients and fellow workers. Minority staff can also serve as successful role models for minority students entering the mental health field and thereby compensate for the student's previous discouraging experiences with educational institutions (Leavitt and Curry, 1973).

A minority perspective on staff supervision should include an assessment of the cultural differences that influence supervisor effectiveness. How do the experiences of minority supervisors differ from those of nonminority supervisors? Do minority supervisors need to approach the traditional supervisory role differently? While research indicates that minority supervisors are often more qualified for promotions than their white colleagues (Parker, 1976), in order for minorities to survive in the system, they must perform far better than their white coworkers. A mental health administrator needs to be sensitive to the unique skills, talents, experiences, and potential limitations of minority applicants for supervisory positions (Vargus, 1980).

Affirmative action continues to be an issue, since the number of minority supervisors and administrators has not appreciably increased. Aggressive and well-planned recruitment at competitive salaries remains the most reasonable approach—minorities must be recruited and retained to gain balanced staffing patterns that include bilingual supervisors. Once a minority staff member is hired, a commitment to his or her professional development is important, as is training that addresses minority needs and increases cross-cultural awareness of all staff members (Kautz, 1976). When minority staff members share experiences with white coworkers and supervisors, communication among staff members is increased and white supervisors gain first-hand insights into the needs of minority clients.

Expectations of Minority Administrators

Once a minority professional administrator has been hired, the unique demands made on him or her need to be taken into account. Such an individual experiences a variety of role expectations, such as (1) agency demands to be a spokesperson for minority staff, clients, and community; (2) pressures from minority and nonminority colleagues for support, interpretation, and expertise; (3) pressures for accountability from members of the minority community; (4) conflicting commitments to self, minority community, agency, and profession; and (5) pressures to live up to the traditional administrative role model and to personal ambitions for career advancement.

Herbert (1974) provides a graphic description of the multiple role demands on a minority administrator in Figure 1. These role demands often prove overwhelming for minority individuals who enter positions of leadership unprepared to cope effectively with administrative pressures. Furthermore, cultural differences influence how minority staff members accommodate to such pressures—for example, whereas a nonminority administrator might try harder, a minority administrator might quit. This is a critical factor in the retention of staff and reflects the importance of understanding cultural differences.

Role of Nonminority Administrators

The role of the nonminority administrator carries its own set of responsibilities for understanding minority issues and continuously acquiring and main-

Figure 1. Role Demands on Minority Administrator.

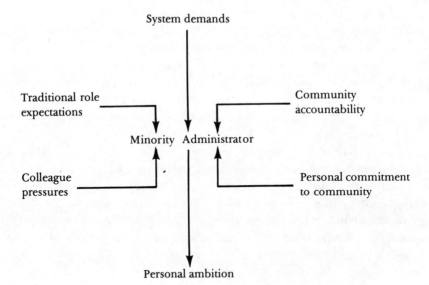

taining cultural awareness. The nonminority administrator must be able to recognize the special pressures experienced by minority colleagues and thereby support and enhance the special qualities of minority staff.

Unless culturally aware administrators are ready to risk rocking the boat in confronting institutional and personal racism in the system, the issue will never be addressed (Kautz, 1976). The desire for maintaining the status quo is often a barrier to improving an agency's own service delivery to minorities. The quality of both the majority and minority cultures' needs must be recognized in order for individuals to be black or brown or white and yet work together on a free and equal basis within a mental health agency, thereby promoting the mental health of all staff.

Conclusion

The minority perspective on mental health administration and planning includes an understanding of the concepts of pluralism, socialization, and sociocultural dissonance. This chapter has explored a variety of definitions, including minorities of color, minority mental health, orientations to planning, and administration. It has devoted particular attention to an elaboration of the administrative issues involving client-therapist relationships, differential treatment, negative service delivery outcomes, underutilization of service, and compliance with federal legislation.

To acquire a minority perspective, program managers need to understand the dynamics of minority communities that affect the planning of mental health services—such as environmental and cultural factors, barriers to service delivery, and the importance of minority representation on agency boards of directors. Similarly, the administration of programs and agencies serving minority communities requires sensitivity to the issues of interagency communication, staff recruitment and deployment, and the roles of both minority and nonminority administrators.

To sum up, it is important for mental health program managers to keep in mind the many ways in which the social and economic systems affect minorities—for example, by limiting the flow of resources to minority communities, by promoting policies that fail to account for minority concerns, and by failing to involve minority group representatives in decision-making activities (Cameron and Talavera, 1976). Mental health administrators can help in the process of empowering minorities to utilize their own community networks to gain power and resources, provided that administrators have sufficient awareness of the cultural diversity, history, and socioeconomic status of minorities in need of relevant and appropriate mental health services.

References

Abad, V., Ramos, J., and Boyce, E. "A Model for Delivery of Mental Health Services to Spanish-speaking Minorities." *American Journal of Orthopsychiatry*, 1974, *44* (4), 584–595.

Brown, P. A. "Racial Social Work." *Journal of Education for Social Work*, 1976, *12* (1), 28–35.

Burgest, D. R. "Racism in Everyday Speech and Social Work Jargon." *Social Work*, 1973, *18* (4), 20–25.

Bush, J. A. "The Minority Administrator." *Journal of Education for Social Work*, 1977, *132*, 15–22.

Cameron, J. D., and Talavera, E. "An Advocacy Program for Spanish-speaking People." *Social Casework*, 1976, *57* (7), 427–431.

Coulson, R. "The Black Voice and the Board Member." *Child Welfare*, 1969, *48* (8), 456–458.

Fiester, A. R., and Rudestam, K. E. "A Multivariate Analysis of the Early Dropout Process." *Journal of Consulting and Clinical Psychology*, 1975, *43* (4), 528–535.

Garfield, S. "Research on Client Variables in Psychotherapy." In A. Bergin and S. Garfield (Eds.), *Handbook of Psychotherapy and Behavior Change*. New York: Wiley, 1971.

Golden, J. "Desegregation of Social Agencies in the South." *Social Work*, 1965, *10* (1), 58–67.

Goldstein, A. P. *Therapist-Patient Expectations in Psychotherapy*. Oxford: Pergamon Press, 1962.

Hall, E., and Whyte, W. "Intercultural Communication: A Guide to Men of Action." *Human Organization*, 1960, *19* (1), 5–12.

Hatanka, H., Watanabe, B., and Ono, S. *The Utilization of Mental Health Services in the Los Angeles Area*. San Diego: Service Delivery in Pan Asian Communities, 1975.

Herbert, A. W. "The Minority Administrator: Problems, Prospects, and Challenges." *Public Administration Review,* 1974, *34* (6), 556–563.

Karno, M. "The Enigma of Ethnicity in a Psychiatric Clinic." *Archives of General Psychiatry,* 1966, *14* (5), 516–520.

Karno, M., and Edgerton, R. B. "Perceptions of Mental Illness in a Hispanic Community." *Archives of General Psychiatry,* 1969, *20,* 223–238.

Kautz, E. "Can Agencies Train for Racial Awareness?" *Child Welfare,* 1976, *55* (8), 547–551.

Krebs, R. L. "Some Effects of a White Institution on Black Psychiatric Outpatients." *American Journal of Orthopsychiatry,* 1971, *41* (4), 589–596.

Leavitt, A., and Curry, A. "Training Minority Mental Health Professionals." *Hospital and Community Psychiatry, 24* (8), Aug. 1973, pp. 543–546.

Lorion, R. P. "Socioeconomic Status and Traditional Treatment Approaches Reconsidered." *Psychological Bulletin,* 1973, *79,* 263–270.

Maruyama, M. "Paradigmatology and Its Application to Cross-Disciplinary, Cross-Professional, Cross-Cultural Communication." *Cybernetica,* 1974, *17* (2), 149–157.

Mayfield, W. G. "Mental Health in the Black Community." *Social Work,* 1972, *17* (3), 106–110.

National Institute of Mental Health. *National Standards for Community Mental Health Centers.* Rockville, Md.: National Institute of Mental Health, 1977.

Owan, T. "Improving Productivity in the Public Sector by Use of Bilingual Bicultural Staff." *Social Work Research and Abstracts,* Spring 1978, pp. 74–81.

Owan, T. "Neighborhood Based Mental Health: An Approach to Overcome Inequities in Mental Health Service Delivery to Racial and Ethnic Minorities." Unpublished manuscript, National Institute of Mental Health, Rockville, Md., 1980.

Padilla, A. M., Ruiz, R. A., and Alvarez, R. "Community Mental Health Services for the Spanish-speaking/surnamed Population." *American Psychologist,* 1975, *30* (9), 892–905.

Parker, W. S. "Black-White Differences in Leader Behavior Related to Subordinates' Reactions." *Journal of Applied Psychology,* 1976, *61* (2), 140–147.

President's Commission on Mental Health. *Report to the President from the President's Commission on Mental Health.* Washington, D.C.: U.S. Government Printing Office, 1978.

Ramirez, M., and Castandea, A. *Cultural Democracy, Bicognitive Development, and Education.* New York: Academic Press, 1974.

Saunders, M. S. "The Ghetto: Some Perceptions of a Black Social Worker." *Social Work,* 1969, *14* (4), 84–88.

Solomon, B. *Black Empowerment.* New York: Columbia University Press, 1976.

Sue, S. "Community Mental Health Services to Minority Groups." *American Psychologist,* 1977, *32* (8), 616–624.

Sue, S., and others. "Delivery of Community Mental Health Services to Black and White Clients." *Journal of Consulting and Clinical Psychology,* 1974, *42,* 794–801.

Tager, M. *Whole Person Health Care.* Portland, Ore.: Victoria House, 1978.

Trader, H. P. "Survival Strategies for Oppressed Minorities." *Social Work,* 1977, *22* (1), 10–13.

Vargus, I. D. "The Minority Administrator." In F. D. Perlmutter and S. Slavin (Eds.), *Leadership in Social Administration.* Philadelphia: Temple University Press, 1980.

Wheeler, W. H. "Developing and Administering Mental Health Services to Minorities." Rockville, Md.: National Institute of Mental Health, 1980.

Windle, C., and Wu, I. "The Impact of Data-Based Technical Assistance to CMHCs Underserving Ethnic Minorities." Pamphlet, National Institute of Mental Health, Rockville, Md., 1977.

Wolkon, G. H., and others. "Ethnicity and Social Class in the Delivery of Services: Analysis of a Child Guidance Clinic." *American Journal of Public Health,* 1974, *64* (7), 709–712.

Yamamoto, J., and Going, M. "Social Class Factors Relevant for Psychiatric Treatment." *Journal of Nervous and Mental Disease,* 1965, *142,* 332–339.

Yamamoto, J., James, Q. C., and Palley, N. "Cultural Problems in Psychiatric Therapy." *Archives of General Psychiatry,* 1968, *19,* 45–49.

Yamamoto, J., and others. "Racial Factors in Patient Selection." *American Journal of Psychiatry,* 1967, *124,* 630–636.

❦ 6 ❦

Women in Mental Health Administration

Theresa Aragón Valdez

Problems experienced by women seeking administrative careers—including late career decisions, difficulties in career advancement, stereotyping, and limited access to top management positions—are discussed in this chapter. Informal networks, mentors, and support systems are suggested as methods for lowering internal barriers to advancement, and affirmative action policies and procedural and structural changes in mental health programs are examined as approaches to eliminating external barriers. In addition, strategies for developing constructive plans for combating institutional sexism are identified.

A key affirmative action issue for women during the past decade has been their lack of representation in the managerial levels of business, education, and health and social services. In the area of health and social services, the issue goes beyond advancement to include more general concerns regarding quality of services and services delivery for women. The underrepresentation of women in social and health services management influences problem identification and definition, policy development, and resource allocation, often resulting in policies and practices that do not effectively address the needs and concerns of women.

The underrepresentation of women in management and the concerns of women managers in mental health are of sufficient significance to merit special attention. Some may argue that these are not issues in the mental health field, because women are in fact visible in the managerial ranks and because the admin-

Note: The author wishes to acknowledge all of the participants in the Women and Social Services Management Seminar who interviewed women mental health managers, as well as the women managers who gave freely of their time to share the information on which this chapter is based.

istrative problems unique to mental health administration are the same for male and female managers. However, preliminary research indicates that the lack of proportional representation of women in management is as much an issue in mental health as it is in social services in general, and the issues confronting women managers in mental health—such as the use of power and authority, the combatting of stereotyping, risk taking, and exclusion—parallel those encountered by women managers in other fields.

Effective management is not gender specific. However, men have traditionally been the managers, and they have defined boundaries and set the rules for participation, achievement, and success. These rules and boundaries often work in concert to keep women out of management or to limit their effectiveness and mobility once they have management positions. In addition to having an administrative knowledge base and managerial skills, a woman needs to understand how she as a woman affects the organization and how she in turn is affected by it. The primary purpose of this chapter is to facilitate that understanding.

The Underrepresentation of Women

Fairly recent arrivals in the upper echelons of mental health administration, women have also grown in number in middle management in recent years—a time when women have been pressuring for equal rights in all areas and at all levels of work. Although national figures on the number of women professionals employed in the mental health field and on the numbers of these women in middle or top management positions are not available, cursory examination would suggest that women are well represented at all managerial levels. However, closer examination shows that, given their numbers in the pool from which mental health professionals and managers are drawn (social work, nursing, clinical psychology, and psychiatry), women as a group are underrepresented in top management positions. For example, only 13 percent of the directors of mental health clinics, hospital units, and agencies in the Pacific Northwest are women (Vandervelde and Patti, 1978). In addition, a national survey of 868 social agencies directed by social workers found that only 141 (16 percent) of these agencies were directed by women (Szakacs, 1977). Other findings indicate that men outnumber women five to one in social services management (Curlee and Raymond, 1978).

Several theories advanced to explain the underrepresentation of women in the managerial ranks of other fields, especially business, can be of value in explaining similar phenomena in the mental health field. The focus of these theories ranges from the individual to the organizational or institutional structure. These theories and related research have been based on one or a combination of three basic observations, all of which are applicable to the mental health field:

1. The socialization of women can limit aspirations for leadership, power, and authority and may not impart the qualities essential for effective management.
2. Institutional and societal sexism can be a major obstacle to the advancement of women, regardless of their ability.

3. The structure of organizations can impede the upward mobility of workers in certain worker classifications, most of whom are women.

In addition to the problem of the socialization of women and its impact on job performance and success, incidents of direct discrimination, sexist behaviors among male clinicians, and the elitism of some disciplines have compounded the problem of women managers in the mental health field. Other problems include lack of credibility for women, stereotyping, salary discrimination, and limited opportunity for advancement. This chapter provides an overview of these issues. Stereotyping is explored in relation to its impact on a woman's self-perception. The discussion of organizational context focuses on both internal and external barriers to women and pays particular attention to informal networks, mentors, and support systems as they relate to a woman's advancement in management. Assertiveness and risk taking are considered as problems resulting from women's socialization and ones that can be resolved by women. Affirmative action policy is briefly reviewed in order to apprise women of their rights.

Patterns in Career Decisions Among Women

Defining a career as "a conscious commitment to advancement over the long term," Hennig and Jardim (1977) discovered three major patterns among women in their various studies of career concepts among male and female managers. First, women make late career decisions. Not until they have been working for ten years or more do most women see work as something other than a temporary job and start thinking of their work as a career with potential for advancement. Second, most women have a generally passive attitude toward career advancement, crediting their promotions to good luck rather than to their own ability. This passivity tends to keep women from assessing their strengths and abilities for the purpose of directing their own careers (Safilios-Rothschild, 1979). Third, many women strongly believe that the most critical factor in determining career advancement is individual self-improvement. This belief renders many women blind to the role played in career advancement by the organizational environment and by the network of informal relationships.

These patterns were distinct from those found among the male managers studied—they had made early career choices, were active in the pursuit of advancement, credited themselves, rather than external factors, for their success, and were very much aware of the role of both formal and informal factors in their advancement. Another important difference to emerge between male and female managers was in their concepts of what a career in fact is. According to Hennig and Jardim (1977, p. 14), "Women see a career as personal growth, as self-fulfillment, as satisfaction, as making a contribution to others, as doing what one wants to do. While men indubitably want these things too, when they visualize a career they see it as a series of jobs or a path leading upward, with recognition and reward implied."

Many women mental health managers prefer clinical practice to advancement in management. Hennig and Jardim (1977) and others have found that women prefer to invest themselves in their area of expertise or to serve as the specialist's specialist—usually first-line supervision—rather than deal with the ambiguities and unknowns of top management. This reluctance to move away from specialization or to use specialization as a foundation for advancement in management results in part from women's perceptions of careers and of management. When faced with the decision of whether or not to aspire to a position in middle management, a woman, Hennig and Jardim (1977) note, is often afraid to be cut off from what she knows, from the comforting familiarity of an area she has mastered in depth, from the basis of her sense of legitimacy and security, only to confront new and quite different people in a setting where she may now be the only woman in a managerial position. On the other hand, a man worries about being able to put a team together, whether subordinates will be capable, and whether his new boss will help him grow and advance. A man's perceptions of possible problems tend to focus outward, whereas a woman's tend to focus inward.

These findings suggest that women need to be more conscious of the impact of their socialization on their present lives and to modify their behavior when that impact has been a negative one.

Self-Perception and Stereotyping of Women

Women need to understand the social myths and stereotypes about women that have developed in our society and that coincide with societal role expectations. In this way, women can understand how they contribute to their own oppression by conforming or adapting to those expectations. Until recently, women have had little, if any, reason to believe that their role boundaries could extend beyond those society has defined for them. The women's movement has provided the climate and support women need to begin the process of self-identification and self-definition. The first step in this process is to distinguish between realities and myths about women. The second step is for a woman to make conscious decisions about how she wishes to shape her behavior—whether according to society's role expectations or according to her own perception of self.

Stereotypical adjectives used to describe women in order to rationalize their exclusion from many professions and to limit their access to management in most areas include: passive, dependent, other-directed, sensitive, emotional, nurturing, weak, unassertive, unintelligent, and lacking in motivation. These traits have been taken from behavioral observations and then generalized to women as a group; some writers have even claimed that these traits are biologically determined. As we will see, women do manifest some of these qualities but were not born with them. They are learned behaviors that can be shown to be a direct result of women's socialization (Safilios-Rothschild, 1979). A closer look at some of these stereotypes is presented in Table 1.

Table 1. Common Erroneous Stereotypes About Women.

1. Women are intellectually inferior.

    Research shows that women are not intellectually inferior (Stead, 1978). However, society's stereotype of the ideal woman and the ways in which it rewards or sanctions according to that stereotype discourage a woman from acknowledging or demonstrating her abilities.

2. Women are emotionally unstable.

    Research does not support this stereotype (Stead, 1978). Studies suggest that one of the major reasons for its currency is that, in this society, women are freer than men to express emotions other than anger. By contrast, male managers report the strain of "staying in role"—that is, being unemotional, aggressive, and competitive. Both men and women need to feel free to express themselves emotionally and to share feelings with each other.

3. A woman's place is in the home. When women work, it's temporary. Work is something to fill in the time before they marry, a hobby, or a way to provide luxuries. Women do not value achievement, advancement, or meaningful work.

    This combination of stereotypes and directives has been used to limit women's access to the work force as well as their opportunities for advancement once they are working. In addition, these generalizations serve to foster other myths about women, including that women should stay out of the work force because they take jobs away from men and that their employment contributes to juvenile delinquency because mothers are not home to mind the children. Research also refutes these myths (Stead, 1978).

4. Women are inherently unassertive and passive.

    Women are not born passive or unassertive. Passivity among women is a learned behavior that is strongly reinforced by society. Closing management ranks to women because it is feared they will be passive or incapable of exerting leadership is not justified, given contemporary research findings (Stead, 1978).

5. Women lack achievement motivation.

    Even though one cannot generalize and say that women fear success—the most they may fear is the rejection of men if they are successful—many women do experience achievement anxiety. Such anxiety may stem from socialization emphasizing that a woman should not achieve or excel and that a woman is, paradoxically, equal but inferior (Stead, 1978).

6. Good management is male management.

    This myth, although not a stereotype of women, has the net effect of excluding women from management—a field viewed as the exclusive preserve of men with the management attributes of aggressiveness, competitiveness, and directness. However, the traits needed for good management—the ability to be flexible and to have situationally adaptable leadership styles—are not biologically determined (Stead, 1978). Leadership studies have shown that men do not inherently possess all leadership traits, nor are women born without them. In fact, the only testable difference between men and women seems to be women's greater ability in interpersonal relationships . . . "the manager of the future will need to be more people-centered, more able to work with people than to exercise position power" (Stead, 1978).

    It is understandable that some women find the costs of not staying in the role prohibitive. Certainly, being both a woman and a manager involves conflict and some women managers will exhibit role strain (Hanlan, 1978). Male workers often relegate female managers to stereotypically convenient roles—such as daughter, mother, hostess, tease, piece, dumb broad, and bitch—in order to make it easier to interact with them (Curlee and Raymond, 1978). These role expectations have to be challenged if a woman is to become a successful manager.

A woman needs to make conscious choices about her behavior based on her own self-perception. If she chooses to be passive, it should be because that is what she wants and not because it is what society has preordained for her. Women can and should support each other's efforts to free themselves of these stereotypes.

The Organizational Context

Understanding the organization is a prerequisite for success for both male and female managers. A woman's ability to move into the managerial ranks is often inhibited by lack of understanding and misperceptions of organizational structure and functions. Organizations and positions within organizations are often formally structured in such a way as to define women out of the managerial ranks. In addition, the informal network and norms of many organizations function quite effectively—even though unconsciously in some instances—to keep women in their "organizational place." A realistic working knowledge of the organization, the rules of the game, and even the jargon is necessary for women who wish to break through organizational barriers to their success.

Harragan (1977) has likened the organizational structure of corporations to that of the military. In fact, the rules and strict hierarchical structure of the military, in which positions and roles are well defined and fairly rigid, are readily applicable to many organizations, including large mental health organizations. Harragan further suggests that the operation of an organization is similar to that of a sports team—the rules and norms of organizational functioning and structure coincide. For example, a first baseman does not routinely try to cover third base as well as first base. The jargon of organizational life is often filled with sports terminology, and expressions typically reflect the preferences of the boss or upper-echelon managers. Changes are definitely needed in the rigid hierarchical structure and competitive and dehumanizing environment of some organizations.

Analyzing the structure and functioning of a corporate entity, Kanter (1977) found that the range of behaviors for each of the established roles within an organization was very limited. In assessing power and opportunity within the organization, Kanter was able to demonstrate how women are shunted to the side and have limited opportunity for involvement in the mainstream/line staff. The lack of opportunity and the lack of potential for significant upward mobility structured into many organizational positions result in low self-esteem and in limited aspiration and commitment on the part of the persons in those positions. Kanter uses persuasive evidence to argue that the structure of the organization is the major barrier to women's advancement.

Even when women do become managers, they must battle both internal and external organizational barriers to success and advancement. Among these barriers are personnel policies (especially recruitment and promotion), task and position assignments, relationships with peers and subordinates, lack of mentors, and exclusion from informal communication networks.

Some of the complaints expressed by women managers include tokenism, evaluation of affirmative action in terms of an individual woman's success or failure, peer pressure, isolation, and problems with subordinates (Harlan, 1976). These problems seem to be exacerbated the higher a woman moves in the hierarchy. "Unlike men, women who improve their positions by increasing their expertise, by moving up occupationally, or by moving into positions of authority may also run the risk of losing friendship and respect, influence, and access to information. They can expect that the strains created by the work might increase, and almost none of this will improve with time" (Miller, Labovitz, and Fry, 1975, p. 378).

On a more positive note, however, women are taking up the challenge in greater numbers and are in many cases providing the mutual support necessary to relieve some of the tensions and strains exclusive to women managers. The higher a woman goes, the greater the threat she presents to many men, a threat foisted on men by social stereotypes—for example, that in order to be a man one must be better than a woman (Wells, 1973).

The Informal Network

Although assessing and participating in the informal network in an organization has long been considered critical to advancement, women are often unaware that an informal network exists. For example, the creator of *Cathy*, a syndicated cartoon strip, depicts a woman manager as completely astonished when a recently hired male peer acquires twice as much information through the informal network in his two days on the job as she has in all the time she has been there. If women do recognize the existence of the informal network, they often identify it with politics or gossip and say that they prefer not to get mixed up in it.

In fact, informal networks emphasize interpersonal relationships, the sharing of timely information, survival strategies, advancement tactics, and tricks of the trade and may be related to profession or status. Women are well advised to move into that aspect of the network aligned with their own position or profession and to maintain open lines of communications with superiors as well as subordinates. However, this is easier said than done. Waiting to be asked to join an informal group may last forever. In addition, although women are often excluded by men, they also self-exclude by accepting the perception that they are being excluded (Albrecht, 1978). Women in traditionally male professions find exclusion from the informal networks even more costly because along with information go the signs of belonging and recognition that are part of the reward of achieving professional status. Women mental health managers with backgrounds in psychiatry and psychology find that the exclusion experienced in graduate school is often continued in the work place.

The only woman in an area will have more difficulty breaking into the informal network than will the woman who is one among many in her profession or position. Experimental studies on interactions between men and women have shown that a lone woman interacting with all men in a professional peer group is ostracized and isolated (Walman and Frank, 1978). When more equal proportions of men and women exist in the same group, the nature of the interaction becomes more sharing and less competitive and isolates the women less.

Participation in the informal network can provide women with access to significant others who can facilitate their mobility in the organization. These significant others are important because they control resources ranging from power over promotion, budgeting, or project assignment discussions to information and knowledge meaningful to job performance and advancement (Albrecht, 1978).

Mentors and Support Networks

For a woman to succeed in an organization, it has been said, she must think like a man, work like a dog, and act like a lady. A woman manager needs a working knowledge of the formal and informal networks and communications systems of the organization in order to succeed. Securing a mentor and establishing support networks are the first steps in obtaining this knowledge. Mentors can provide their proteges with the special knowledge, opportunities, and skills necessary for upward mobility, including coaching, feedback, and tasks and situations that develop the protege's abilities. Aspiring women need to seek out persons to serve as mentors and to develop the mentor relationship by using the following guidelines:

1. *Assess the persons who presently fill the positions to which you aspire.* What significant resources are controlled by these persons? Which of these resources are important at this stage in your career? Which of these persons would feel least threatened by an ambitious woman? Which of these persons is more respected by those higher in the organization? Which of these persons do you respect? Which do you like? (Liking a mentor is not essential, but it helps.)
2. *Assess the resources and positions held by potential mentors in relation to your career, rank potential mentors, then select one.*
3. *Identify yourself as a potential protege to your selected mentor.* A number of subtle methods may be employed to make yourself visible to your prospective mentor—for example, having coworkers bring your work to his or her attention, indicating a deep interest in his or her area of expertise, admiring his or her achievements, and making it a point to emphasize positive similarities in your respective backgrounds. Remember, if the mentor is to be effective, he or she will consider you as a protege primarily in terms of your potential success.
4. *Determine whether you have succeeded in getting yourself a mentor or should move to your second choice.* This step may seem gratuitous, but discussion with many women regarding mentors has demonstrated sufficient confusion to warrant this step. Many women mistake the advice or suggestions of prospective mentors for criticism or interference. Some see ulterior motives in offers of help. Since the prospective mentor is usually male, women are war-

ranted in their concern about motives or about ways in which the relationship may be perceived by coworkers.

5. *Remember that mentor-protege relationships are two-way streets.* Because women have been socialized all their lives to wait and be chosen, they tend to have some difficulty in assertively seeking a mentor. Some women have further difficulty in that they consider the mentor-protege relationship manipulative if they are the ones who purposefully identify and use the mentor. However, the mentor is not the only one who is giving in this relationship—the protege, through learning and subsequent advancement, reflects well on the mentor's abilities.

6. *Move on to another mentor.* A mentor may exhaust his or her usefulness to you as a protege—not necessarily your respect or friendship. Some mentors will be willing and able to help connect you with your next mentor.

7. *Recognize when you no longer need a mentor.* You may be pressured by a mentor to remain loyal to a relationship long past its utility for you. This does not mean that a friendship cannot continue, but does mean that you should not be constrained by loyalty to staying with your mentor. At some point, you will need to move out on your own, and you are the best judge of when that time has come (Williams, Oliver, and Gerrard, 1977).

8. *Become a mentor to a woman in your organization.* You do not have to be at the top to be a mentor. You can share what you have learned each step of the way with women who are below you in status or position but who also aspire to middle and top management. You can help introduce others to organizational support networks and can be a source of personal support. Women managers need to determine the nature and extent of the personal, career, and organizational support necessary for them to function effectively.

Many women report building organizational support networks with women in similar management positions or, if this is not possible, with women in similar positions in related organizations. Organizational support networks are important for job effectiveness by providing visibility inside and outside the organization and can lead to important information about opportunities for advancement or additional training (Harragan, 1977).

Mentors play a critical role in career support networks, as do members of both organizational and personal support networks. At least three factors ought to be considered in identifying persons for a career support network. First, include persons who hold positions similar to yours or have the expertise to which you aspire, preferably persons in organizations or areas outside your own with whom you can openly share your aspirations and who are willing to share their experiences and expertise. These persons can also play an important role in helping with career planning and providing praise and enthusiasm for your achievements. Second, choose persons who are able and willing to provide you with visibility in your professional area, including persons who are in a position to discuss your abilities with others in the profession. Persons who can provide access to presentations at professional conferences and opportunities to serve on local and statewide committees, experts in your area of work, and editors and publishers are also important. Third, assess whether or not the person might be threatened by your career plans. If he or she is threatened by you, you run the risk of having your confidences exploited or shared in ways detrimental to your career.

Women who are changing their thinking and behavior to coincide with their own perception of self are moving away from socially dictated roles and stereotypes. Persons who have grown to rely on such predictable, stereotypical behavior will feel threatened by the implicit demand that they change the way they relate to women and will tend to respond with fear or anger. As members of their support network, women need persons who will be supportive, not persons who will make them feel guilty. Many women have found that other women going through a similar experience are the best sources for sharing and personal support.

Assertiveness and Risk Taking

The socialization of women accounts to a large degree for their unwillingness to take risks. Women see risk taking as an opportunity to fail, rather than an opportunity to succeed. Since childhood they have been cautioned about the negative outcome of all behaviors, including assertiveness, that might involve risk. They are seldom given an opportunity to consider the potentially positive outcomes of risk-taking behavior and then to assess whether the risk is worth it—and what would be truly lost if they did not succeed. For example, in physical activity, little boys are encouraged to push to their limit. Little girls, on the other hand, are told not to climb trees because they might fall; not to play baseball or football because they might get hurt or be perceived as tomboys; not to run because it is not ladylike; and, when they are older, not to win or excel, especially in competition with boys, because they might not be admired. Studies have also found that, when and if women do take risks, they require a lack of ambiguity—that is, a high degree of certainty—regarding the outcome. However, risk taking and ambiguity are both inherent in mental health administration. Hence, increasing the willingness to take risks is of major importance for women in management.

Much of the current literature on assertiveness—which often includes specific steps and suggestions for dealing with such situations as exercising authority, interviewing, and risk taking—relates to women but rarely focuses primarily on management assertiveness. Some adaptation of the basic assertiveness training model is useful for women managers who have already achieved a significant level of assertive behavior but find their assertiveness accompanied by a significant degree of discomfort and anxiety (Gambrill and Richey, 1975). Other adaptations have included relaxation exercises, cognitive methods for anxiety reduction, and material on deciding when to be assertive.

Psychology has provided us with studies of the risk-taking behavior of women. The most frequently used instrument for studying risk taking is the Choice Dilemma Questionnaire (Kogan and Wallach, 1959), which differentiates risk choices by sex. They found that, where women are more certain of their judgments (low-ambiguity outcome), they are more extreme in taking risks. In general, they found that women are not more conservative than men in risk taking but that their risk taking is dependent on the level of certainty and the subject matter. Kogan and Wallach (1959, p. 561) attribute this to the socialization process, noting that "fear of punishment for inappropriate behavior in new situations is likely to be more severe for girls than for boys in American society."

We know that women are willing to take risks in situations of low ambiguity. We also know that administration in mental health is conducted in an ambiguous context characterized by multiple funding sources, uncertainties about funding and the political climate that affects it, and the inability to measure output in most instances. However, women managers and students have been able to utilize several of the following techniques to expand their risk-taking behavior:

1. Begin by learning and practicing assertive behavior. Women often perceive situations requiring assertive behavior as risk taking. They usually need to confront the risks of assertive behavior—for example, the refusing of a request—before they are ready to expand risk taking into personal, career, or programmatic decisions.
2. Attempt a preliminary assessment of your own orientation to risk taking. List those decisions you have previously made that involved risk. What was the degree of ambiguity involved? Are there decisions you have avoided or put off because of uncertainty of outcome? Were you afraid? Try to pinpoint the reasons for your fear.
3. Develop your own method for assessing the costs and benefits of risk taking in your personal and professional life, reviewing your values and priorities in each of the spheres of your life. Then determine what you stand to gain and what you can afford to lose in given situations.
4. Keep a log of what you perceive to be your risk-taking behaviors and the degree of ambiguity of outcome related to each. If possible, note the actual outcomes.
5. Practice risk taking in low-risk environments. This can range anywhere from bluffing and upping the ante in penny poker to giving oral presentations to a supportive group.
6. Role play risk-taking behaviors with someone from your personal support network or in a low-risk supportive group.

Women who wish to develop assertive and risk-taking behaviors have a number of resources at their disposal but must take the first step themselves—in itself a risk for many women. That step is the decision to change accustomed and often comfortable behavior patterns.

Affirmative Action

Affirmative action in organizations runs the gamut from strictly legal compliance on paper to training and internship programs geared to making viable opportunities out of legally required ones. Legal recourse and advocacy organizations are now available for women in combating sexual discrimination in the work place. Not readily available, however, are resources that will assist women in identifying and selecting strategies for pursuing their rights that are congruent with the organization and with their own personal goals.

A major side effect of affirmative action is tokenism, which results from an organization's effort to identify a "woman's position" on a management team. Token positions are often disguised as promotions, and women should be able to analyze potential positions in the context of their own organization, distinguishing between positions that can lead to goal achievement and positions that lead nowhere.

In any case, women cannot depend on affirmative action policies to open doors for them—they need to take the initiative. Affirmative action policies will not implement themselves, and many employers spend more time trying to avoid compliance than gearing up to comply. Nonetheless, affirmative action and fair pay policies do give women legal redress. The Equal Employment Opportunity Commission (EEOC) and the Civil Rights Office of the Department of Health and Human Services (HHS) can be utilized in pursuing discrimination complaints. In some cases, women have found that the hint or threat of filing a complaint or commencing a legal suit is sufficient for gaining redress.

EEOC has developed a series of responses to the most commonly asked questions about the complaint process. This list and other publications regarding sexual discrimination in employment practices and pay scales can be readily obtained at your regional EEOC office. Other local sources of advice and assistance in these areas are the women's rights office in city government, local university women's resource centers, and local working women's organizations, which usually offer the following types of suggestions for those contemplating a sexual discrimination suit (Stead, 1978):

1. Make every effort to resolve your situation outside the complaint process.
2. Be sure you or a trusted representative go to the top of the organization (and even beyond) with your complaints.
3. Bear in mind the stakes of the battle, and be sure of your specific goals.
4. Consider your weapons.
5. Expect to do large amounts of research and statistical analysis.
6. Collect documentation on the good quality of your work and job performance.
7. Prepare your complaint with energy and enthusiasm in order to receive justice under the law.
8. Get together with other female employees who may have experienced similar problems.
9. Understand the full meaning of sexual discrimination:
   - Discrimination does not have to be deliberate or in any way intentional to be actionable.
   - Sexual discrimination must involve a comparison of male to female.
   - Discrimination is not necessarily limited to issues of equal pay for equal work.

- A pattern of discrimination should be established.
10. Expect employers to ignore you, drag their feet, and hope the situation will go away; to fire you or harass you in the hopes of forcing you to leave; or to persuade you that your analysis of the situation as discriminatory is incorrect.

Many women know that they have legal recourse, but the costs of pursuing legal redress are high, both financially and psychologically. The costs of winning may also be high, particularly if you are hired or promoted in an agency or program that fought vehemently to keep you out. In many instances, women can avoid being discriminated against in the first place by knowing and diligently exercising their rights.

How well do you know your rights and related employer requirements? The Equal Employment Opportunity Commission has developed a quiz (see Table 2) that assists women in assessing their knowledge of their rights. Since women as a group carry the major burden of exercising and protecting their hard-won rights under affirmative action policies, knowing your rights is essential. However, the strategies you pursue in exercising your rights are also important and should be based on your best assessment of the reasons your employer may have had for denying or infringing on your rights.

Table 2. Equal Employment Opportunity Commission Quiz.

An employer can:	True	False
1. Refuse to hire women who have small children at home.	___	___
2. Generally obtain and use an applicant's arrest record as the basis for nonemployment.	___	___
3. Prohibit employees from conversing in their native language on the job.	___	___
4. Rely solely on word of mouth to recruit new employees when the majority of employees are white or male.	___	___
5. Refuse to hire women to work at night because he or she wishes to protect them.	___	___
6. Require all pregnant employees to take leave of absence at a specified time before delivery date.	___	___
7. Establish different pension, retirement, insurance, health plans for male employees than for female employees.	___	___
8. Hire only males for a job if state law forbids employment of women for that capacity.	___	___
9. Attempt to adjust work schedules to permit an employee time off for a religious observance.	___	___
10. Disobey the equal employment opportunity laws whether intentionally or not.	___	___

Answers: All answers are false.

Conclusion

The profile of women in mental health administration suggests that (1) it is less difficult now than in previous years for women to move into middle management and (2) women are more aware of their rights in the work place. The problems experienced by women mental health managers are similar to those identified by women managers in other fields, including stereotyping, exclusion from informal networks, lack of career support systems, limited access to top management, and unequal pay for equal work. This chapter has considered a number of these issues in the hope that women who wish to pursue management careers in mental health will overcome barriers to success.

Women may feel that they should not be solely responsible for freeing themselves from internal and external constraints. However, men have only recently begun to be interested in advocating changes that benefit women, recognizing that many of these changes will also benefit men. Ultimately, every woman is faced with the task of helping to effect these changes in herself and in the organization—for her own sake and for the sake of other women.

References

Albrecht, S. "Informal Interaction Patterns of Professional Women." In B. A. Stead (Ed.), *Women in Management*. Englewood Cliffs, N.J.: Prentice-Hall, 1978.

Curlee, M., and Raymond, F. "The Female Administrator: Who Is She?" *Administration in Social Work*, 1978, *2* (3), 307–318.

Gambrill, E., and Richey, C. "Assertiveness Training: An Assessment and Research." *Behavior Therapy*, 1975, *6*, 550–561.

Hanlan, M. S. "Women in Social Work Administration: Current Role Strains." *Administration in Social Work*, 1978, *1* (3), 259–265.

Harlan, A. "Career Differences Among Male and Female Managers." Paper presented at National Academy of Management conference, Kansas City, Mo., March 1976.

Harragan, B. L. *Games Mother Never Taught You: Corporate Gamesmanship for Women*. New York: Ramson Associates, 1977.

Hennig, M., and Jardim, A. *The Managerial Woman*. Garden City, N.Y.: Anchor Books, 1977.

Kanter, R. M. *Men and Women of the Corporation*. New York: Basic Books, 1977.

Kogan, N., and Wallach, M. "Sex Differences and Judgment Processes." *Journal of Personality*, 1959, *27*, 555–564.

Miller, J., Labovitz, S., and Fry, L. "Inequities in the Organizational Experiences of Women and Men." *Social Forces*, 1975, *54* (2), 378.

Safilios-Rothschild, C. *Sex Role Socialization and Sex Discrimination: A Synthesis and Critique of the Literature*. Report prepared for National Institute of

Education. Washington, D.C.: Department of Health, Education, and Welfare, 1979.

Stead, B. A. (Ed.). *Women in Management.* Englewood Cliffs, N.J.: Prentice-Hall, 1978.

Szakacs, J. "Survey Indicates Social Work Women Losing Ground in Leadership Ranks." *NASW News,* 1977, *22* (4), 12.

Vandervelde, M., and Patti, R. J. *Management Preparation for Women: A Report of the Social Welfare Management Curriculum Development Project.* Seattle, School of Social Work, University of Washington, 1978.

Walman, C., and Frank, H. H. "Gender Deviance in Male Peer Groups." *Proceedings of the 81st Annual Meeting of the American Psychological Association,* 1978.

Wells, T. "The Covert Power of Gender in Organizations." *Journal of Contemporary Business,* Summer 1973, *2* (3), 53–68.

Williams, M., Oliver, J. S., and Gerrard, M. *Women in Management: A Bibliography.* Austin: Center for Social Work Research, University of Texas at Austin, 1977.

❧ 7 ❧

The Program Manager
as Planner

William E. Hershey

As an action-oriented, collaborative process involving many participants at various levels inside and outside the organization, planning defines an agency's direction and details the means for reaching its goals and objectives. This chapter presents a trifocal view of planning: internal program planning, including project-level planning; interagency planning; and long-range planning. Case studies are provided to illustrate planning principles and practices, and coordination and negotiation are discussed as critical skills in the planning process.

In the midst of rapid social change and inconsistent government mandates for managing mental health services, planning provides a sense of program coherence and direction for the community mental health system. An orderly process for setting goals and solving problems helps to establish programs that are more effective in meeting emerging community needs. From a manager's perspective, the planning role is trifocal; the program manager must (1) look down into the program's internal planning; (2) look out into the community, focusing on interagency program planning; and (3) look ahead to future trends and social indicators. Although program managers may focus on only one area at a time, they need to be aware of the other planning perspectives. In this chapter, we will describe all three perspectives and the skills required of mental health program managers to implement them.

Internal Program Planning

This discussion of internal program planning includes the agency's overall plans, plans for a particular program, and plans for projects within specific programs. Before planning for the future, however, the mental health program manager first needs to monitor the present state of agency program operations. How does the current program fit into the overall mission of the agency?

The agency's mission statement, often hidden away in articles of incorporation and not necessarily current, tends to reflect general hopes for bettering the human condition. A useful mission statement describes the key responsibilities of the organization and the parameters of service—that is, what the organization does and does not do. For example, the mission of a crisis outreach agency might be "to provide immediate, twenty-four-hour access and response, primarily by telephone, to persons in King County encountering emotional crisis or stress and to link those persons with key community resources." This statement of purpose, a clear signal to the community of the availability of a crisis phone service, may be used as the keystone for internal program planning, frequently developed collaboratively between the staff and the board and ultimately approved by the board.

A major reason for examining the agency's mission statement is to raise several basic questions: Are the goals of my program still relevant to the overall mission of the agency? How have client populations and community needs changed? Have funding sources set new priorities? Sometimes programs are created to meet a certain need and then, years later, a proliferation of services to meet similar needs creates the dilemma of programs competing for the same clients. A mission statement should be reexamined at least every five years in the light of client needs assessments, community service systems studies, and service trends. Even if the mission statement itself does not change, goals for carrying out individual programs will probably require modification.

Whatever the process of analysis, the criteria for program assessment presented in Table 1 prove helpful. Items to be examined include: program-planning and goal-setting processes; staff participation and coordination; leadership and direction; purposes and objectives; financial issues; and community relations. A manager needing a more specific set of criteria for assessing his or her agency would do well to examine the new *Consolidated Standards Manual* for psychiatric, alcoholism, and drug abuse reentry facilities for children, adolescents, and adults (Joint Commission on Accreditation of Hospitals, 1981).

In addition to this formal monitoring process, some managers periodically conduct a thorough study of similar programs in the field by scanning the literature and making site visits to other agencies in order to stimulate new program ideas and motivate themselves and their staff. Such visits often provide documents, plans, and training ideas for setting future agency program directions and help managers engage in a personal analysis of their own leadership styles.

Planning with Goals and Objectives

Once the mission statement has been reviewed and operations assessed, a set of program goals and objectives should be established. The program manager uses the mission statement as a guide in designing program goals that state specific methods for achieving broad agency purposes. A program goal is a statement that describes a desired condition to be reached some time in the future. Program goals, usually few in number, generally reflect a long-term perspective; specific objectives

Table 1. Criteria for Program Assessment.

	Yes	Yes, But Needs Work	Uncertain	No

A. *Planning and Goal Setting*

1. Staff have established operational goals that reflect program purposes.
2. Staff have determined objectives for administrative and program operations that are time limited and are reviewed—and revised, if warranted—periodically.
3. Objectives are used as management tools to evaluate progress toward goals.
4. Staff members utilize a program-planning process that involves volunteers and client representatives in determining program plans and implementation.
5. Program strategies specify:
   a. Problem to be addressed.
   b. Objectives to be accomplished.
   c. Time needed to achieve goals.
   d. Resources required.
   e. Implementation steps planned.

B. *Decision Making/Problem Solving*

1. Staff have sufficient policies, procedures, and standards to guide decision making.
2. The program manager has established rules determining procedures for presenting information to the executive or board for action.
3. Staff debates and decides issues, and program manager facilitates discussion and decision making.
4. Policy recommendations are basically limited to setting new goals and to establishing new directions or new or improved standards.

C. *Evaluation*

1. Staff members conduct periodic internal evaluations of administrative program effectiveness and program outcomes.
2. Staff has predetermined standards for measuring job effectiveness.
3. Board regularly monitors administrative and program activities to determine progress toward meeting objectives.
4. Staff maintains appropriate statistics for evaluation purposes.
5. Services are accessible and responsive to clients most in need of services.
6. Unit costs are appropriate for services and clientele.

	Yes	Yes, But Needs Work	Uncertain	No

D. *Public and Community Relations*

1. Program has system for obtaining feedback from individuals and groups regarding service planning, delivery, and results.
2. Collaboration and cooperation exist between the agency and other agencies delivering similar programs in the same service area.
3. Staff members participate actively in other community planning activities.
4. Staff maintains regular communications with other community groups and private and government organizations that affect its operation.
5. Staff effectively presents its accomplishments to the community.

E. *Resource Development*

1. Staff members participate with board representatives in developing a resource plan to ensure that the agency has adequate financial resources to meet objectives.
2. Agency has a financial plan for the securing of alternative, time-limited funding if resources expire and for orderly phaseout when funds are no longer available.
3. Agency has a diverse funding base, thereby minimizing disruption with the withdrawal of one resource.
4. Staff is innovative in generating new funds.
5. Staff is effective in grant writing.

indicate how the goals will be achieved. For example, three program goals for a crisis phone service might be:

1. To have six telephone lines staffed by volunteer phone workers and supervised by six master's-level social workers from December 30, 1981, to December 30, 1982.
2. To answer 45,000 calls for assistance from persons in emotional stress by December 30, 1982.
3. To provide an information and referral resource for linking clients with appropriate services.

Managers need to ask: Will a particular goal help the organization achieve its purpose? A broad program goal should therefore contain key approaches to its implementation, which usually reflect the professional judgments of the manager and staff. For example, the first goal in the preceding list focuses energy on recruiting volunteers and hiring competent staff to supervise them, as well as on having appropriate phone equipment. Goals, in summary, may be defined as broad, time-anchored statements that describe how major program components will be developed.

Program objectives are milestones or targets on the way to reaching a goal; they are time limited, measurable, and specifically related to goals. For example, objectives related to volunteer staff recruitment and training might call for the recruitment of thirty volunteers per month and for six training sessions per quarter, each of three hours' duration, on the subjects of crisis intervention, communications, and suicide prevention. Whereas goals set direction, objectives tell managers when and how goals are to be reached. Managers link staff members to program objectives by assigning key jobs and job performance standards, enabling managers to evaluate staff performance in terms of progress toward accomplishing objectives. This results-oriented approach—which aims to provide for systematic and orderly organizational growth by exacting performance standards for all employees with respect to specified goals and objectives—is popularly known as management by objectives (MBO).

The manager can also start with the line staff and build program objectives from the bottom up—for example, by using a written job description that includes a staff member's major responsibilities within the program area. In the case of a line worker responsible for doing intake in an organization's outpatient service, key areas of responsibility might include: answering the telephone and doing intake by phone; seeing clients in person; supervising volunteers who will also do phone intake and see clients; scheduling next-day appointments for emergency clients and appointments to other services, where appropriate; referring clients to other services, if necessary; assisting in training volunteers; and completing necessary administrative tasks. However, performance standards—often lacking in formal job descriptions—are needed for each area in order to indicate how the key responsibility is to be accomplished. For example, a performance standard might read: "The worker will staff the phone room and be available to receive calls three hours per day. Three shifts will be scheduled each week."

In summary, internal program planning serves to define financial, personnel, and public relations activities, as well as to establish a management-by-objectives framework for planning and implementing an agency program. The board of directors is ultimately responsible for establishing the mission or purpose of the organization, from which goals describing broad program outcomes are derived. Objectives are then set to outline the activities necessary to meet those goals. Linked to each level of this MBO system are performance standards and objectives for all staff members, and by monitoring staff performance level, a manager can judge how efficiently and effectively a program is accomplishing its purpose.

Another major strength of the MBO method is that it is not another top-down planning process. Staff members at all levels of the organization are involved in setting objectives, providing performance standards, and assessing degrees of success. Workers do not need to be told that they are not performing

well—they themselves have agreed to standards of performance and know when
and at what pace those standards are being met. Such a high degree of staff
self-monitoring frees program managers to provide support and creative reinforcing activities for their staff.

Project Planning

A project is a strategy, usually requiring a special concentration of effort,
for implementing or improving one aspect of an organization's program. As such,
a project most often begins with a proposal for policy clearance and funding.
Even though a project, once established, should be able to stand by itself, it still
needs to be related throughout its existence to its parental program, lest it become
the tail that wags the program dog. For example, the manager of an agency's
referral system believes the system can be improved by changing from a manual to
a computerized storage and retrieval process. This belief is translated into a
proposal to the agency administration and board of directors, who may decide that
the project is worth pursuing or reject it if it appears to be leading in a direction
contrary to agency purpose. A proposed computerized information and referral
system, for example, has the potential of doubling agency staff, moving the
agency into a new services delivery mode, and incurring great expense in the
leasing or purchasing of equipment. Program staff have the obligation to spell
out as many of the costs and benefits of such a proposal as possible. If, after a
careful analysis, the board decides to give the go-ahead, the program manager
then begins the complex process of project development.

The first step is usually a detailed project proposal—frequently a grant
proposal or request for proposal (RFP)—for the purpose of raising new funds. A
project proposal prospectus includes a statement establishing the credibility of the
project agency and its proposal, a problem statement, a statement of project
objectives, a statement of methods for reaching those objectives, and a statement of
costs. At this stage, such a project prospectus might serve as an adequate base for
marketing the program idea. Program managers, agency administrators, and
interested board members then move about the community with the proposal in
hand, ascertaining the level of interest and solicitive cosponsorship of the project
in order to increase the chances of being funded. If a number of prospective public
and private funding agents express interest, an informational meeting is held to
discuss the feasibility and viability of the project. If the project is seen as a
community venture, an ad hoc advisory committee is formed. The manager then
develops the proposal further in the format suggested in Table 2 (Kurtz, 1979).

Interagency Planning

The mental health manager's second planning focus is on interagency
planning—the activity that links the agency's internal plans with external
organizational strategies. At this point, the manager looks outward and asks: How
do we plan with others?

Table 2. Project Proposal Check List.

Face Sheet: Summary

1. Name of agency and program where project resides _____
2. Brief statement of position _____
3. Statement of objectives _____
4. Brief description of implementation strategies _____
5. Total cash summary _____

Problem Statement or Needs Assessment

1. How project is related to mission of agency _____
2. Evidence—such as statistics or survey of need by an authority—to be used to justify project _____
3. Problem to be addressed, stated in terms of client need _____
4. Specific forms of client involvement in proposal _____

Program Objectives

1. Objective to meet need 1 or to solve problem 1 _____
   Objective to meet need 2 or to solve problem 2 _____
2. Expected outcomes of project _____
3. Client population that will benefit _____
4. Objective will be accomplished by: Objective 1 (date) _____
   Objective 2 (date) _____

Implementation

1. Statement of how one moves from problem to objectives _____
2. Activities needed to accomplish objectives _____
3. Sequence of activities: Objective 1
   Activity a (dates accomplished) _____
   Activity b (dates accomplished) _____
   Activity c (dates accomplished) _____
4. Staff members responsible for: Activity a _____
   Activity b _____
   Activity c _____

Evaluation

1. Brief statement of plans for evaluation:
   a. Of entire project _____
   b. Of degree to which outcomes were reached _____
   c. Of methods used in operations _____
2. Criteria for success _____
3. Who will conduct evaluation, and when? _____
4. List of evaluation instruments, questionnaires, and so on _____
5. Description of evaluation reports to be produced, with dates _____

Future Funding

1. Summary of plan to continue funding once grant expires _____
2. Description of how maintenance and future program costs will be obtained (if capital expenditures involved in project) _____
3. Extent of reliance on future grant support _____
4. Letters of support and possible future commitment to buttress project from:
   1. _____
   2. _____
   3. _____

Budget (Attached to project proposal and including the following:)
1. Direct relevance to substance of proposal _____
2. Detailed presentation of all proposed income and expenditures _____

Table 2, cont'd.

3. Project costs that will differ at time of service delivery if different from time of proposal writing _____
4. All items asked for by funding sources _____
5. Description of how other items not paid for by funding sources will be covered _____

6. Volunteer time _____
7. Fringe benefits separate from salary _____
8. Consultant costs _____
9. Direct and indirect costs _____

Coordination is not always a natural tendency, despite the fact that coordinated activities may be more economical and in the community's best interests (Lauffer, 1978). Cooperation often means that some of the parties involved must give up something they have and are familiar with in return for yet-to-be-realized gains and an uncertain future. The major payoffs of cooperation are increased service availability, accessibility, efficiency and effectiveness, and accountability (Lauffer, 1978).

Just as they assessed the internal environment of their agency, program managers must evaluate the interagency environment, assessing such community factors as suppliers of resources, personnel, funds, equipment, and workspace; consumers of the agency's services; competitors for both resources and consumers; and those regulatory groups that provide auspices and legitimation or legislative rules and procedures regarding the agency's operations (Lauffer, 1978). Funding sources may announce to the agency that, unless there is a coordinated plan for the delivery of services to children, for example, no funds will be released. Such an outside prod often serves as an impetus for coordinated planning. Similarly, the announcement of available funds for a coordinated system of services to youth might bring together a collection of agencies both to plan and, hopefully, to implement such a program, once funded. Moreover, regulatory agencies at times necessitate coordination by setting new standards for service delivery that no single agency can carry out in isolation—as in the case of federal legislation setting accessibility standards for services to the handicapped.

Or clients might demand services that exceed the mental health agency's capacity and therefore require the manager to seek outside resources. Transportation services for an elderly program, for example, might require coordination with the transportation resources of the other agencies. Finally, proliferation and duplication of certain kinds of services may inhibit an agency in carrying out its mission. For example, the competition for funding and duplication of services as a result of the proliferation of crisis and information hotlines in the 1960s and 1970s caused allocators to call a halt and publish RFPs for single, centralized agencies. Indeed, competition may cause an organization to assess its general mission statement and ask if it should continue to exist at all.

Each of these elements in the task environment might influence the mental health manager in deciding with whom to coordinate planning and for what purpose. As the shortage of funds becomes more acute and accountability requirements increase, this approach to interorganizational planning will become increasingly critical. Program managers need not be totally reactive, however. The following case study illustrates the positive, active role agency board members and managers can play in interagency planning.

Crisis Clinic, Inc.: A Case Study

Crisis Clinic, Inc.—concerned with the delivery of crisis services, primarily by telephone hotline—found itself blocked in carrying out its primary mission, which was defined as "providing immediate access, primarily by telephone, to persons in crisis or suffering from emotional stress." The board and staff had established the goal of the crisis telephone subprogram: "To provide a comprehensive, centralized twenty-four-hour-per-day telephone service in King County for persons in crisis and to link clients with problems to appropriate community resources." This subprogram goal presented two problems: *Comprehensive* and *centralized* implied a single crisis emergency service network with community recognition and organization that made the intake process both comprehensive in terms of a system of emergency service and centralized in terms of an agreed-upon process for organizing crisis calls; *linkage* implied available resources appropriately linked to the central phone network. Such a system, however, did not exist.

At a long-range planning meeting, the organization's board of directors had established this relatively new subprogram goal, with its emphasis on words like *centralized* and *comprehensive,* because of the staff's frustration in meeting the agency's primary mission and in carrying out internal agency plans without adequate coordination with other community agencies; the other agencies had either competing, parallel, or uncooperative emergency resources. The board, executive director, and program manager saw two choices before them: (1) to go on as before, maintaining a major, but not the only, telephone crisis service; coordinating with other crisis and emergency service resources when informal agreements could be made; providing hit-and-miss referrals based on linked-agency whims to deliver resources or not; patching together a staff of volunteers, CETA trainees, professionals, and paraprofessionals to staff phone lines that were increasingly netting calls from severely disturbed people; or (2) to undertake plans to coordinate with other emergency services agencies for the development of a comprehensive network of emergency services in which the crisis phone component would play a systematic, centralized role. The board of directors and staff opted for the second choice.

The program manager immediately contacted the county mental health planning coordinators, who had been concerned for some time about the lack of coordination of emergency mental health services, and was invited to join a task force of private and public agencies similarly concerned about the lack of a definitive emergency services system. The goal of the task force was to design a comprehensive model for the delivery of emergency services. Other groups invited to participate—fire aid, police, mental health center outreach teams, and involuntary treatment teams—represented divergent interests and territories but overlapped considerably in the services they delivered. For example, outreach teams staffed crisis phones and were often not available for outreach. Both involuntary treatment teams and mental health center outreach teams saw voluntary and involuntary clients, and it was often not clear who should go on a specified outreach. Crisis phone workers frequently could not get mental health center outreach teams to respond unless the outreach worker knew and trusted the crisis phone supervisor, since there were no formal agreements between the two organizations. Fire aid and police responded in some cases; in others, they did not—again, it depended on trust and previous rapport. Finally, persons with emergencies could not be scheduled for appointments the next day at a mental health center. In short, no viable system existed.

The task force divided the proposed model into three parts—intake, outreach (both voluntary and involuntary), and next-day appointments—and assigned a subcommittee with representatives from all participating agencies to work on each part. The subcommittee on intake agreed almost at once that since the continued funding of multiple phone lines was wasteful, there should be one central, twenty-four-hour phone service with a single number advertised throughout the county. This agreement was buttressed by the fact that the crisis service agency had at the same time obtained cooperation and funding from city, county, and state officials for a comprehensive community information and referral (I&R) line, with which a single emergency services intake hot line could be linked. The subcommittee and the full task force made this centralized community crisis line the center of the emergency services model.

The subcommittee working on outreach services agreed that there should be a single countywide outreach component as well. Although the subcommittee did not decide whether the component would be stationed at one or a number of geographical locations, it did agree that the outreach component should be either stationed with, or at least dispatched from, the central phone service, with the majority viewpoint being that the teams should be located throughout the county and dispatched by the phone service. The subcommittee resolved the issue of the relationship between involuntary and voluntary outreach services by combining both functions in one large team (mobile or stationary). Finally, the subcommittee on next-day crisis appointments delegated the responsibility for making appointments to the central crisis phone service.

The task force approved the model in outline form only, with general principles established for a single centralized phone line and a single centralized outreach team. The proposal was accepted by the county mental health board in this form. Two key things happened next: (1) the seven mental health centers undermined their own power by trying to compete for the outreach team contract, and (2) the power and persuasiveness of the single phone line concept caused the county to contract with the Crisis Clinic. Next the county took the competitiveness of the centers as a signal that the county would need to manage the outreach team function of the plan. These two components were then attached to newly formed emergency units at each of the mental health centers. Although there was dissension over the plan, ultimately it succeeded because everyone achieved something: clients, better access; the CC, a centralized phone contract; the county, an integrated system of emergency services; and the centers, some emergency service units (Figure 1). The main role of the crisis services program manager throughout this process was to argue for the central point of the fiscally efficient and service-effective benefits of centralized phone services. At the same time, she was working on coordinating her efforts with agency plans in contracting for city, county, and state I&R services, which once in place made the co-location of a crisis line even more appropriate, if not outright necessary.

Figure 1. Crisis Clinic, Inc., and the Emergency Services Program.

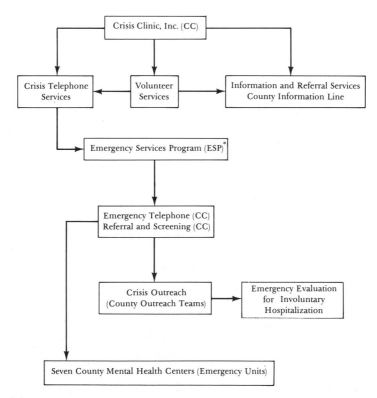

*The emergency services program (ESP) includes:

—A one-number response unit with twenty-four-hour counseling, evaluation, and referral services.
—Countywide dispatch service for crisis outreach services.
—Countywide twenty-four-hour crisis outreach services to respond to all appropriate requests for emergency counseling and resolution.
—Catchment area emergency counseling and case management services.

Cooperation and Negotiation in Interagency Planning

Interorganizational planning can make use of formal interagency contracts or agreements or can rely on informal plans formulated by ad hoc committees. Of course, collaboration has its problems; skills need to be learned and pitfalls avoided. Managers entering into cooperative efforts need to clarify the varied assumptions and preconceptions they bring regarding the purpose and outcome of those efforts. Hidden agendas need to be revealed in order to facilitate cooperation. If the goal of a meeting is to advise or plan or implement, then the implications of advice, planning, or implementation should be addressed.

Most important, clear agreement must be reached on the responsibilities and roles of participants. Participants need to select leaders, or at least know who is leading and why. Confused roles often mean dissipated energies as participants struggle to decide who has what piece of the action. Fear of merger or loss of identity is another potential obstacle; in collaborative efforts, there is often the sense that participating agencies will be pushed into an unwanted conformity (Schindler-Rainman and Lippitt, 1975). Sometimes groups within the collaborative framework have hidden agendas that would result in loss of identity for another agency if the implications of suggested changes are not made clear.

Negotiating is not a way to avoid conflict but rather a means to resolve it. Skills in negotiation and the bargaining process can assist managers in the interagency planning, since the consummation of interagency planning is often a contract or agreement for services to be delivered by the program manager's agency and other cooperating organizations. Focusing on conflicting issues, rather than on personalities, can help make negotiating less painful. Further, if all parties are committed to reaching an agreement, compromise is to be expected—not as a sign of weakness, betrayal of ideals, or surrender of moral principles, but with the recognition that, to reach an agreement, each party will have to concede something. Finally, the use of power (defined as the capacity to influence the actions of others) is an important aspect of negotiation—knowing how much power you have, how much you are willing to use, and how your power is perceived by others (Cormick, 1977).

Negotiating requires the use of technical skills (such as the ability to interpret applicable regulations and other contracts and to engage in fact-finding and policy analysis), public relations skills, and social and communication skills (such as the ability to build group cohesiveness; to engage in active listening, leadership, and assertiveness; and to make effective use of one's self). Finally, the manager needs to know exactly what the negotiation process is to entail—the agency's goals for the process and the strategies to be used. An appropriate list of strategy questions and negotiating guidelines is included in Table 3.

In summary, the interagency planning focus involves mental health program managers in the community—seeking allies, assessing competition and resources, and developing opportunities for program services—and links the mental health program with other components of the human services system. Because the

Table 3. Questions to Be Asked Before Negotiating.

1. What do you want to achieve?
2. Are all relevant parties involved? If not, how can you involve them?
3. Which of your demands are most important?
4. What power do you have to make the other side give you what you want?
5. How powerful do you think the other side thinks you are (remember, it is not how strong you think you are, but how strong your opponent thinks you are)?
6. What possible allies and other added sources of power might you be able to tap?
7. What kinds of financial or political limits are there on the power you have?
8. What positive benefits can the other side get by meeting your demands? Can the demands be made legitimate and reasonable in their terms?
9. What do you really expect to gain?
10. What do you think your opponent expects to give up?
11. What is the least that you will settle for?

Negotiation Guidelines

- Take positions consistent with your values.
- Do not negotiate for the fun of it.
- Use negotiation skills to recognize what others are doing to you.
- Know what you are trying to achieve. For example:
    - Counter the moves of others.
    - Stall for time.
    - Obtain more and better information.
    - Develop allies.
    - Reassess objectives.
    - Work out intragroup issues.
    - Soften a position.
    - Determine your opponent's position.
    - Press toward an agreement.

skills necessary for interagency planning require trust and open communication, one must engage in the process with care and patience.

Future-Oriented Planning

Whereas internal agency planning has a program focus and interagency planning has a community focus, future-oriented planning requires managers to look to the future by attending regional, national, and international conferences and reading relevant journals, new publications, and research reports. Such an active processing of new information enables a manager to recognize recurring themes or particularly imaginative approaches to delivering services.

Community needs assessments may also be used to serve as predictors of future community trends in demands for services. For example, at a public forum held in one community to involve lay people and professionals in assessing future needs for services, a program manager of a local youth counseling agency asked a key question: Where should our agency be going in the future, since the original purpose of the agency, drug abuse counseling, is no longer as significant as initially conceived? This program manager subsequently brought together other youth service agency managers and representatives from the mental health field, the schools, public welfare, city government, and other civic groups to collectively seek some answers. This ad hoc group engaged a community consultant, held a series of community forums to identify the future problems of youth, and produced a set of community goals for schools, city and state government agencies, and volunteer organizations. In the process, the program manager who asked the original question gained a new set of goals that served to revitalize his staff and maintain agency program relevance (Hershey, 1971).

Key-informant studies have been used to predict future economic and social development, as in the prospectus *Washington Future—1990.* Community forums were used extensively in the 1963-1965 "Planning for Planning" period by state mental health authorities anticipating the Comprehensive Mental Health Center (CMHC) program. Another useful tool in future planning is a data system called the mental health demographic profile system (MHDPS), which can be used to implement the social indicators approach discussed in Chapter Twenty. The complete system includes 130 standard census items from the 1970 U.S. Census, including 6 indicators of population size, 48 socioeconomic status variables, 5 ethnic composition variables, 36 household composition and family structure indices, and 35 housing variables. This system produces data that permit the statistical comparison of each federally defined mental health catchment area with county, state, national, and other catchment areas, but does not attempt to establish the service implications of demographic profiles. Experience with the application of the MHDPS has led to selection of those indicators deemed useful in predicting the existence of populations at high risk for mental illness and thus the need for mental health services (National Institute of Mental Health, 1975a). Data on social class, life-style, ethnicity, and other social characteristics can be combined with data on health and mental health status and on services utilization to make inferences about future mental health needs.

Program managers might use these social indicators to develop scenarios for the future and then extrapolate from and analyze them for program planning. For example, using the social indicator "percent of all families below poverty level," one could develop a future scenario reflecting an increase in that indicator of 25 percent in the next five years due to inflation. Such an increase might lead to increases in youth crime, homicide, and mental illness and result in an increased demand for services from persons unable to pay. At the same time, future federal anti-mental health views would result in an unwillingness to fund this increased need. After studying the scenario, the program manager would begin to develop prospective strategies to meet the need: lobbying to get state legislators to pick up the slack caused by lack of federal spending; redesigning fees for counseling programs so that clients who can pay will pick up a bigger share of costs; developing grant requests for private foundations; approaching local United Ways to ask for their leadership in developing private business-supported grant programs.

Another future scenario might involve an increase of 50 percent over the next five years in the number of disabled persons not in institutions or schools. Such an increase would mean an expanding handicapped population needing services from agencies now only equipped to serve those who are not disabled. Based on that scenario, a program manager might plan to install teletype machines for deaf persons on all emergency telephone lines, to prepare the agency building for handicapped accessibility, and to develop training programs for staff in serving handicapped persons. All of these strategies require that a manager look to the future and not simply be content with either internal or interagency planning alone.

The mental health manager can also use local statistical reports on trends in suicide, crime (particularly crime related to family violence), child abuse and neglect, marriage and divorce rates, hospital and nursing home admissions, youth and adult probation and parole, and accident and drunk-driving arrests. Such data might indicate what new programs should be developed or provide background information for future research needs. Population trends in a local community might indicate where services should be delivered and under what circumstances—as populations shift to suburban areas, for example, agencies might need to decentralize their programs.

Some managers might not be satisfied with merely adjusting or accommodating programs to probable future outcomes but would prefer to plan to create future events themselves. For example, certain reports, such as the Club of Rome description of the future limits of human and physical world resources, can be transformed into action plans for preventing the predicted scenario. Still other planners might create networks of planners, clients, managers, and staff to interact and spell out together the intended shape of the future (Friedman, 1973). At the very least, mental health program managers need to work in partnership with others in the social and health services fields, to regularly assess community needs, with the conviction that the quality of life in the future is undetermined and thus open to human choice and that planning directed in this way is both an opportunity and a challenge.

Conclusion

Effective mental health program planning necessitates a trifocal perspective. Internal planning focuses on agency program and project activities, requiring the manager to assess a program's goals and objectives in terms of the agency's purpose and relate program goals to staff performance and program outcomes. Since programs interact with others in the community, interagency planning requires negotiating skills—managers need to represent their agencies' goals and needs and seek cooperation from competing and at times hostile organizations in the communities. Finally, the program manager needs to anticipate potential changes by using forward-looking scenarios to plan for, and perhaps even help to create, future mental health organizations.

References

Cormick, G. W. "Power, Strategy, and Process of Community Conflict: A Theoretical Framework." Unpublished doctoral dissertation, University of Indiana, 1977.

Friedman, J. *Retracking America*. Garden City, N.Y.: Anchor Books, 1973.

Hagedorn, H. *A Manual on State Mental Health Planning*. Rockville, Md.: National Institute of Mental Health, 1977.

Hershey, W. E. "Futures Planning for Youth in Puyallup, Washington." Unpublished paper, United Way of Pierce County, Tacoma, Washington, 1971.

Joint Commission on Accreditation of Hospitals. *Consolidated Standards Manual for Child, Adolescent, and Adult Psychiatric, Alcoholism, and Drug Abuse Facilities*. Chicago: Joint Commission on Accreditation of Hospitals, 1981.

Kurtz, N. "Proposal Checklist and Evaluation Form." *The Grantsmanship Center News*, 1979, 5(4), 42–45.

Lakein, A. *How to Get Control of Your Time and Your Life*. New York: McKay, 1973.

Lauffer, A. *Social Planning at the Community Level*. Englewood Cliffs, N.J.: Prentice-Hall, 1978.

Miller, S. "Organizations, Values, and the Mental Health Manager." Unpublished paper, National Institute of Mental Health Staff College, Rockville, Md., 1981.

National Institute of Mental Health. "A Typological Approach to Doing Social Area Analysis." Series C, No. 10. National Institute of Mental Health, Rockville, Md., 1975a.

National Institute of Mental Health. "Catchment Areas with Unusually High Proportions of Some 'High Risk' Groups: Region X." Unpublished working paper No. 20. National Institute of Mental Health, Rockville, Md., 1975b.

Rothman, J. "Three Models of Community Organization Practice." In *Social Work Practice*. New York: Columbia University Press, 1968.

Schindler-Rainman, E., and Lippitt, R. "Toward Interagency Collaboration." In E. Schindler-Rainman and R. Lippitt (Eds.), *The Volunteer Community: Creative Use of Human Resources* (2nd ed.) San Diego: University Associates, 1975.

Schoderbek, P. P. *Personnel Administration in the Voluntary Agency*. Alexandria, Va.: United Way of America, 1980.

❦ 8 ❦

Analyzing
Agency Structures

Rino J. Patti

The systems, the structural, the political perspective—in this chapter, descriptions of each provide an analysis of organizational behavior and implications for mental health management practice. Such organizational analysis allows insights into a number of critical management issues and concerns, including (1) resource development and allocation; (2) staff management, including output, morale, and cooperation; (3) interdepartmental and interorganizational coordination; (4) agency governance; (5) the benefits and limitations of staffing hierarchies; (6) the advantages and disadvantages of departmentalization, job specialization, centralization, and formalization; and (7) societal ambivalence toward the goals of mental health agencies. Depending on the problem at hand, a manager can employ one or another of the perspectives described, in order to understand what is occurring in his or her organization and its environment, as well as to choose the appropriate organizational change strategy.

Most experts agree that there is no comprehensive, unified theory of organizations, in general, or of mental health organizations, in particular. Instead, many different theoretical approaches to understanding organizational behavior exist, each addressing a certain truth but never the whole truth. Theoretical perspectives in the organizational field may be likened to the transparent overlays frequently employed to illustrate features of the human anatomy—one overlay details the skeletal structure, another the circulatory system, a third the musculature, a fourth the nervous system, and so on. Not until each of these overlays is finally superimposed upon the basic human form can we appreciate the full complexity of the human anatomy. In the same way, each theoretical perspective on organizations provides a certain insight, but only when all of them are brought to bear do we begin to appreciate the full complexity of the organizational anatomy.

We must be careful, however, not to overextend this analogy. Unlike anatomical overlays, which illustrate physically demonstrable attributes, theoretical perspectives on organizations are largely hypothetical models. Some of these models are supported by empirical evidence; others are constructs imposed on reality by perceptive observers; still others are ideologically inspired statements that derive from some conception of how things should be. Theoretical perspectives also differ in that they are in part a product of historical context. If the major problem of a historical period is how to build efficient and productive organizations, then theoretical perspectives that bear most directly on such outcomes are likely to be central to that era. If a major problem, on the other hand, is how to reduce worker alienation and increase employee commitment to organizational objectives, the model is likely to include quite different variables.

One need only look to scientific management and human relations theories of this century to illustrate this point. In the early 1900s, one of the major concerns was how to increase the efficiency of workers in the developing American industrial plant. Not surprisingly, a scientific management theory emerged during this period that emphasized concepts like specialization, authority, and compliance. Somewhat later, when the industrial work force was beginning to show signs of restlessness and the specter of organizational conflict and potential unionization emerged, a human relations theory of organizations developed that had as its central feature the concepts of communication, cooperation, participatory democracy, and informal organization. In other words, whereas the human form remains relatively constant over time, perceptions of organizational form differ in accord with the issues and dilemmas that characterize a particular historical period.

Unlike social scientists, mental health administrators are concerned with how to change, manipulate, or maintain processes and events in order to achieve organizational objectives. Therefore, a theoretical perspective must deal with actionable referents, that the manager can see and do something about, as well as potential courses of action. The concerns of managers are far ranging and defy neat categorization, but, for purposes of discussion, let us mention several areas that typically occupy a great deal of a manager's time and attention.

1. How to obtain resources and support for agency operations.
2. How to gain the cooperation, commitment, and compliance of subordinates.
3. How to increase the output, efficiency, and effectiveness of staff.
4. How to build and maintain the morale of staff.
5. How to foster staff acceptance of needed changes in programs, procedures, and technologies.
6. How to facilitate interunit and interpersonal coordination and minimize unproductive conflict.

Organizational theory, to be of practical value to the manager, must illuminate these and related issues. This chapter includes an assessment of three theoretical perspectives on mental health organizations: systems theory, structural theory, and political theory. With each perspective, we will (1) describe its essential features; (2) identify the major variables or phenomena with which it is concerned; and (3) suggest ways in which the manager might find it useful. Before discussing these theoretical perspectives and their implications for management, however, we will define some of the distinctive features of the mental health organization and describe the groups and factions comprising it and their roles in influencing agency behavior.

Distinctive Features of Mental Health Organizations

Although mental health administration and general administration draw upon many of the same fundamental sources of organization and management theory, mental health administration is increasingly considered to be a distinctive area of management practice. This view is based largely on the observation that the characteristics of organizations condition the ways in which managers order their priorities, allocate their time and energy, and choose their strategies and tactics.

A growing literature deals with the factors that distinguish mental health agencies from business and industrial organizations (Hasenfeld and English, 1974). Among the attributes and processes thought to influence mental health management practice are the following:

1. Societal ambivalence toward the goals of mental health agencies often results in tenuous political support, especially in times of funding cutbacks or political reaction. Mental health administrators consequently devote a good deal of their time and energy to advocating the need for programs and justifying the continuance of those in existence. They also must become adept at strategies for buffering external threats that may be harmful to agency operations.
2. The "raw materials" that mental health agencies seek to modify are human beings, whose cooperation in the delivery of services is usually vital. Managers must attend to the needs, interests, rights, and values of clients by becoming informed about and remaining sensitive to their preferences and by developing ongoing processes to assure that decision making reflects those preferences.
3. There is seldom widespread agreement regarding the goals of mental health agencies. Goals are, by and large, value statements about which disagreements are likely, both within the agency and among groups and organizations in the community. The task of building a level of consensus and mediating between conflicting conceptions of agency purpose thus becomes a central function of administration.
4. Mental health agencies rely heavily on a labor force of professionals whose values, ethics, norms, and conventions sometimes run counter to organizational expectations. Negotiating and accommodating these differences is a major part of the administrator's responsibility.
5. Since many of the services provided in mental health organizations are non-routine, particularized responses to individual client needs, discretion must often be exercised by front-line workers in delivering services. As a result,

administrators must often strike a precarious balance between maintaining equity and reliability in the administration of programs, on the one hand, and allowing workers sufficient autonomy to be responsive to individual needs, on the other. This balancing act complicates the process of monitoring, controlling, and evaluating performance and poses special problems for the administrator.

6. Lacking a market mechanism to determine the value of services to clients, mental health agencies must often turn to other mechanisms for evaluating program effectiveness. The development of valid and reliable measures of effectiveness that are at the same time feasible to implement is a continuing concern to administrators.

This list of factors is hardly exhaustive—one might add the governance and funding arrangements found in the mental health field, the extraordinarily diverse array of community agencies offering some form of mental health services, and the heavy reliance on community participation in policy decision making. Suffice it to say that these factors raise special issues and problems that require managers to selectively draw from, adapt, and even modify the theories and technologies available from general administrative and organizational theory.

Roles of Board and Staff in Agency Decision Making

Mental health agencies vary greatly in purpose, organization, and program, but they share certain basic group characteristics. As a point of departure, the major groups and factions that generally comprise these organizations are described, followed by a discussion of how each may influence agency decision making.

Governing Body

Each mental health organization is created and controlled by a governing body to which it is ultimately accountable. The fundamental purpose of this body, which sponsors the agency and sanctions it to perform certain functions or activities, is to represent and protect the interests of the community, in general, and the clients or consumers of the agency, in particular. The members of this body or board serve essentially as trustees, acting on behalf of the community to ensure that the agency serves that community's vital interests as defined by the board. Governing boards have responsibility for approving policy regarding the basic purposes, scope, and character of the organization, monitoring performance to see that policies are implemented in accord with the board's intent, and assisting in the acquisition of resources the agency needs to carry out its purposes.

Governing bodies take a variety of forms. In voluntary agencies, a board of directors normally has this responsibility, with its authority and composition generally set forth in the agency's articles of incorporation. Public agencies are ultimately accountable to elected legislative bodies such as the city council or state legislature, although operational control is usually shared with an official, such as the mayor or governor, who heads the executive branch of the government unit. In some instances, governing arrangements may be more complicated, as, for example, in the case of agencies that are sponsored by several units of government or conjointly by agencies in the government and voluntary sectors.

In recent years, funding patterns have obscured the issue of who governs mental health agencies. For example, a number of agencies are partially or wholly supported by public monies through purchase of service contracts and federal medical assistance reimbursements. In many instances, such agencies have become so totally dependent on public funds for their continued existence that they are in fact not controlled by their own boards of directors. Rather, such governing bodies serve largely to "pass through" public funds and increasingly find it necessary to defer to government agencies on matters of fundamental agency policy. Although the boards of such agencies can choose not to accept public monies and the conditions that go with them, this is often done at some risk to agency survival. In practice, then, many voluntary mental health agencies are controlled not by their legally constituted board but by government policies. The term *quasi-public agency* is often used to describe the status of voluntary agencies that operate under such circumstances.

A similarly mixed picture may be found in the public sector. Human services agencies created at one level of government are often funded in full or in part by another level of government. Under these increasingly common circumstances, it is very difficult to determine where the ultimate control for agency operations resides.

Administrative Staff

The executive of an agency is delegated authority and responsibility by the governing board for implementing the policies according to which the agency operates. Basically, he or she is responsible for translating these policies into operational plans and seeing that the plans are carried out. The executive director is accountable to the governing body for achieving goals and directives, expending funds, and supporting and facilitating the work of subordinates in providing intended services effectively and efficiently. For purposes of discussion, we may suggest three levels of administration and corresponding management functions.

1. The *executive management level* includes those persons in the agency who carry the overall responsibility for directing the organization. Directors, assistant directors, and heads of major divisions in large agencies comprise the personnel at this level. These administrators carry major responsibility for interpreting policy mandates and translating them into organizationwide goals and objectives. They are heavily involved with policy and funding bodies, accounting for their agency's performance, justifying requests for funds, seeking authorization for new agency initiatives, negotiating agreements, and generally attempting to get favorable consideration for the organization's needs and accomplishments. In addition to representing these interests, however, managers at this

level also play a vital role in identifying emerging changes and opportunities in the environment that may have long-range implications for their agencies. By sensing these changes, assessing the likely consequences, and translating them into potential courses of action, executive-level managers help to keep their organization in tune with external realities. Finally, executive managers provide overall leadership and direction to the agency, deciding on major allocations and programs, issues concerning organizational structure, and questions of agency priority.

2. The *program management level* includes those persons who are directly responsible for departments, bureaus, programs, and other major operational units. This middle-management group converts the directives received from executive-level management into specific program objectives, chooses among alternative program strategies for achieving those objectives, procures and assigns staff and materials to various program elements, develops internal operating procedures, and monitors, coordinates, and assesses program activities. Program managers play a major role in mediating technical front-line personnel and top management. On the one hand, they explain, interpret, and convey the wishes of those at upper levels to their subordinates; on the other hand, they serve as spokespersons and advocates for the ideas, requests, concerns, and needs of front-line personnel. Where the interests and the aspirations of subordinates conflict with those of top management, the program administrator works to reconcile those differences. The middle manager also carries responsibility for representing and negotiating the interests of his or her program with heads of other units of the agency at the same organizational level and for maintaining cooperative relations with those units—no easy task when there is competition for resources. Finally, the program manager has the critical task of developing and maintaining conditions conducive to worker morale, efficiency, and effectiveness by facilitating the flow of communication vertically and horizontally within and between departments; resolving interpersonal and intergroup conflicts; maintaining a normative system that rewards risk, innovation, and problem solving; and encouraging growth and development.

3. *Supervisory-level management*—those administrative personnel who have direct day-to-day contact with front-line staff—are responsible for overseeing program implementation, for maintaining work flow, for delegating and assigning work, and for seeing that services are provided in a manner consistent with policies and procedures. They will ordinarily carry the responsibility for consulting with front-line staff on case-level decisions. *Unit supervisor, coordinator, team leader,* are some titles commonly given to managers at this level. A distinctive feature of supervisory management is the maintenance of relatively intense relationships with professional and technical workers on a day-to-day basis. In this context, the supervisory manager provides advice and instruction on technical aspects of work, identifies areas of knowledge and skill that need to be developed, and evaluates individual performance. To perform these duties, the supervisory manager must usually have some firsthand knowledge of methods and techniques that are employed by subordinates. Indeed, such managers are often recruited from

the ranks of professional employees precisely because they have shown expertise and proficiency in this area of practice. Where this has occurred, the manager may serve as a kind of senior practitioner. Like those at the program level, supervisory managers also serve as a linking agent, advocating and representing the interests of subordinates to superiors but also communicating, clarifying, and enforcing the directives of superiors. Because of the close relationships and often intense loyalties that develop with staff, supervisory managers sometimes experience dissonance when they are required to enforce organizational policies that their subordinates oppose.

All these levels of administration are normally referred to as *line management*—those persons in the chain of command vested with the authority to see that the organization's major functions are carried out. In addition, most organizations have administrative personnel devoted to *staff* functions. Such persons provide assistance and support to the line and, as these terms imply, are not ordinarily in positions of formal authority with respect to line personnel— although it often happens that they exert a good deal of informal authority when the director allows them to borrow on his or her power. Staff personnel normally perform activities that require specialized knowledge and skill or that cannot be easily integrated into line operations. Some common examples are planning and budgeting, program auditing, evaluation, staff development and training, and citizen participation and public relations. As organizations grow large and complex, these functions tend to be delegated to special organizational units.

Front-line Staff

Front-line staff members are responsible for delivering the service or product that justifies the agency's existence. They are administratively responsible to their superiors for carrying out officially designated duties, but, because of the nature of such tasks in human services organizations, front-line staff members exercise a good deal of judgment and discretion in carrying out these responsibilities. In so doing, the front-line staff collectively creates, modifies, and elaborates agency policy. Sometimes referred to as "street-level bureaucrats," the practitioners in mental health agencies may enrich and improve or, under some circumstances, undermine the implementation of agency policy. The informal power of staff in this regard is a critical organizational dynamic.

Front-line staff members can be characterized in terms of their tenure in the agency and their degree of professionalization. Theory suggests that, as the average length of tenure in an organization increases, employees are more likely to value and maintain continuity in program operations, routine, and employment security. Thus, when the majority of front-line staff members have been employed in an agency for an extended period of time, they tend to act as a conservative influence on the agency. This influence need not be negative but may become problematic if the agency is required to significantly change its modes of operation or adapt to new and innovative policies and procedures.

Again, theory suggests that the more professionalized the staff, the more likely they are to value autonomy, to be innovative in their work, and to resist administrative detail and routine. Therefore, front-line workers may be at once a vital force for improving agency practices and a source of considerable resistance to management. In either case, when the manager is confronted with a professionalized staff, he or she will ordinarily find it necessary to adopt management tactics that allow for staff participation, two-way communication, and joint problem solving. Research indicates that where these processes are not implemented frontline practitioners tend to become alienated, dissatisfied with their work, and generally less effective in their treatment role.

The Task Environment

Mental health agencies typically exist in a task environment consisting of groups and organizations—for example, legislators, planning and funding bodies, professional schools and associations, and other agencies that provide parallel or complementary services—from which they receive resources, cooperation, and support. These groups and organizations likewise depend upon the agency for certain resources and therefore have a vital interest in how it operates. To varying degrees, the agency maintains an interdependent relationship with this network, exchanging money, program resources, information, personnel, and clients.

One common problem facing mental health administrators is that groups and organizations in the task environment tend to have divergent and sometimes conflicting expectations regarding the agency's proper function, including the issue of who should be served, to what ends, and in what manner. For example, a legislative body may require that an agency emphasize the treatment of the chronically mentally ill, while at the same time other groups in the community may insist that it do much more in the way of prevention, crisis-oriented treatment, and community education. Although the legislature may be more powerful in pressing its expectations upon the agency, the organization must also be attentive to the preferences of other, less-influential groups in order not to antagonize the community and thereby precipitate strikes, organized protests by consumer groups, and the withdrawal of cooperation by other service agencies. Of course, for an agency to maintain relationships with the task environment by simply reflecting such diverse expectations would inevitably lead to its own set of problems. However, these relationships do exert an influence on administrative decision making.

Having discussed some of the characteristics that distinguish mental health agencies and the groups that tend to be influential in determining organizational behavior, we can now turn to three theoretical perspectives on organizations and their implications for the manager.

The Social Systems Perspective

Perhaps no perspective on organizations enjoys greater popularity than social systems theory (Churchman, 1968; Etzioni, 1978; Gummer, 1980; Katz and

Kahn, 1967; Miringoff, 1980; and Monane, 1967). Such popular concepts as input, feedback, maintenance, and equilibrium, commonly used to describe organizational processes, are derived from social systems theory. This perspective seeks to describe the processes that are common to a wide array of social phenomena, including groups, families, associations, communities, and, most pertinent to our purposes, formal organizations.

Basic Notions

The social systems perspective on organizations involves several basic notions. First, organizations are seen as facing several imperatives—goal attainment, adaptation, integration, and pattern maintenance—that must be addressed if the system is to remain a viable entity. Organizations must achieve certain goals that are valuable to the surrounding environment. They must adapt to changes in the external environment in order to acquire the resources necessary for goal attainment. They must develop means for achieving interdependence and complementarity among their membership and maintain continuity of operations through the commitment of members to a common set of norms. A system that devotes itself exclusively to goal attainment and neglects pattern maintenance, integration, and adaptation functions will sow the seeds of its own undoing. The systems view suggests that organizations pursue multiple goals, some of which are unofficial, and survive in the long run only if they give balanced attention to these various imperatives.

Second, organizations are seen as open systems constantly interacting with and being influenced by the external environment. What occurs internally in an organization is, in this view, largely determined by external forces—ideas, values, people, and social conditions—that inevitably penetrate the system's boundaries. In addition, organizations seek to counteract the processes of gradual deterioration, disorganization, and death (negative entropy) by importing and storing more energy and resources than they expend in generating their products or services.

Third, organizations are seen as consisting of the patterned activities of individuals and subsystems, all of which are complementary or interdependent with regard to some output or outcome. Among other things, the concept of interdependency suggests that a change occurring anywhere in a system will affect other parts of the system as well. No action of any significance is without secondary consequences, positive or negative.

Fourth, organizations are seen as governed by the principle of dynamic equilibrium, according to which forces internal and external to the system that disrupt recurring patterns of activity, modes of interaction, or the distribution of power tend to be counteracted by processes within the system that work to restore the organization as closely as possible to its original state. Dynamic equilibrium does not mean that organizations remain in a steady state, but rather that they resist dramatic changes in their character. Real change tends to occur incrementally and is absorbed in the ongoing fabric of agency life.

Fifth, systems theory suggests that organizations have a natural tendency to become increasingly complex and internally differentiated over time. As they grow older, systems tend to develop sharply differentiated authority levels, to spawn specialized functions, and to generate rules and procedures. The norms governing behavior become increasingly crystallized and serve to reinforce existing modes of behavior. The forces for equilibrium become more powerful with age.

The notions of multiple goals, interaction with the environment, negative entropy, interdependence, dynamic equilibrium, and the tendency toward complexity provide the basic building blocks of the systems perspective. They also provide a context for understanding the following generic processes.

1. Organizations constantly import energy and information from the environment in the form of people, ideas, money, artifacts, technology, and so on. These inputs are the raw materials with which the system functions.
2. Organizations transform these inputs into a service or product. The process of marshaling these inputs and applying them to the task of service or production is often called throughput.
3. Organizations export a product or service to the environment and receive feedback regarding the nature of this output.
4. Organizations maintain internal and external feedback loops that provide the system and its parts with information regarding their performance, the acceptability of their products or services to the external environment, and changes that need to be made in internal operations.

Functional Subsystems

Organizations are also composed of functional subsystems responsible for achieving organizational goals. In larger organizations, these functions tend to be lodged with separate identifiable units and people. In smaller systems, they are more likely to be broadly shared. Each of the five major subsystems noted in Table 1—production, maintenance, management, adaptation, and support—is necessary, but none is sufficient unto itself. All functions must be performed, and all are interdependent. For example, if the adaptive subsystem is ineffective, the organization loses touch with how well or how poorly it is serving the public and therefore has no way of anticipating what changes should be made. The service goals of the organization are likely to lose relevance over time, resulting in a loss of external support. If the supportive subsystem fails, the organization will lack the vital resources it needs to deliver services. The management, maintenance, and production subsystems must modify the internal operations to reflect external constraints that are encountered by the supportive subsystem. Alternatively, the adaptive and supportive subsystems must be aware of the constraints, preferences, and capabilities of these internal subsystems if the organization's needs are to be adequately represented.

Table 1. Five Major Organizational Subsystems.

1. *Production or technical subsystem.* This subsystem includes all those activities directly concerned with achieving the product goals of the organization. In mental health organizations, this subsystem would refer to people and processes used to maintain, restore, or control the psychosocial functioning of clients. Front-line staff, referred to earlier, are the central agents in this functional system.

2. *Maintenance subsystem.* This subsystem is concerned with coordinating, integrating, and facilitating the activities of persons within the technical subsystem, functions performed largely by supervisory management personnel, often with the assistance of staff development and training specialists. The general purpose of this subsystem is to see that programs and services are properly implemented by variously socializing, educating, rewarding, punishing, and coordinating front-line personnel. The primary systems goal served by this functional subsystem is pattern maintenance.

3. The *managerial subsystem* includes those functions concerned with determining the operational objectives of the organization, allocating resources, determining priorities, and coordinating the activities of several programs or divisions. These functions are ordinarily the province of middle and subexecutive levels of management, usually aided by such staff personnel as planners, program evaluators, budget and fiscal analysts. This subsystem is primarily concerned with the systems goal of integration.

4. The *adaptive subsystem* is concerned with monitoring changes, trends, and developments in the outside world, projecting the implications of this information for the agency, developing long-range strategic plans, and formulating goals. These functions ordinarily fall to top management, often with the assistance of public relations personnel, advisory committees, and research departments. Adapting the organization to its environment is the principal aim of this functional subsystem.

5. The *supportive subsystem* transacts with the organizations and groups in the task environment for the inputs needed by the agency. Activities like community education, bargaining, fund raising, and resource exchange are central to this function. Top and middle management are the central agents in this subsystem, but lobbyists, grantspersons, and fund raisers also play a vital role. Achieving the adaptation and production goals is the primary aim of this subsystem.

Source: Katz and Kahn, 1967.

Practice Implications

The systems perspective has a number of useful applications for the mental health manager, perhaps the most important of which derives from the dependence of organizations on the environment in which they operate. Administrators working at the organization-environment interface are responsible for reaching out to the environment, collecting and interpreting information, and then conveying this information to members of the organization so that policies, practices, and programs can be adjusted to minimize threats and exploit opportunities. This boundary-spanning role requires the manager to be an intermediary between the environment and the agency, becoming involved with, and well informed about, external events and developments and translating and disseminating that information for internal use. Most of us are familiar with executives who spend a great deal of time in the community developing linkages with other groups and organizations but relatively little time keeping their agency abreast of these developments, helping subordinates to understand their meaning, and feeding that information into policy deliberations. Such administrators are often chagrined when agency staff members are slow to respond to the need for changes suggested by external trends. They are, in effect, leaders without followers.

The effective performance of this boundary-spanning role also requires that the manager selectively determine which social, political, and economic factors in the environment are critical to decision making. The administrator obviously cannot attend to everything and therefore must define a "relevant environment" crucial to the agency's purpose and operation by setting some implicit priorities regarding what is important to agency survival and development. Unless this is done, boundary-spanning functions are likely to be hopelessly diffused. Worse yet, agency personnel will become confused about which environmental cues are important and therefore uncertain about how to apportion their time and energy.

A second major set of practice implications derived from systems theory involves the recognition that administrators must address internal maintenance and integration needs as well as the imperative of goal attainment. Managers should not focus exclusively on the attainment of the agency's formal service goals without also devoting organizational resources to building and maintaining internal capability through the use of training and staff development, supportive supervision, conflict resolution, and effective communication. Unless some portion of the organization's energy is directed toward sustaining these processes, productivity and effectiveness will suffer. Such problems as staff absenteeism, turnover, low morale, and burnout inevitably undermine an agency's ability to achieve its service goals.

A third set of practice implications relates to the role of the manager as change agent and to the principle of dynamic equilibrium, which suggests that managers can expect resistance to both the acceptance and the implementation of directives that seek to significantly modify agency operations. Incremental changes consistent with prevailing norms and values are likely to be more readily received than those that introduce major discontinuities. Moreover, a strategy of intermittent change, in which the administrator allows the organization time to reintegrate and renew itself between modifications, would tend to be less disruptive than a series of significant changes in rapid succession.

Finally, the concept of systems interdependency draws the manager's attention to the importance of considering secondary, unanticipated consequences of decisions. Most managers learn through experience that seemingly straightforward decisions can set in motion unintended and often undesirable side effects. Changes in personnel, program modifications, or new fiscal or accountability procedures intended to solve one problem often end up generating a series of secondary issues that can be more critical than the original problem. For example, a manager in an agency serving low-income multiproblem families was able to substantially lower caseloads so that clients could be provided more individualized, intensive services. Several months later, he became concerned when he heard that the number of service contacts had declined and that staff morale seemed to be dipping. On investigating, he learned that, although staff members had been initially enthusiastic about the opportunity to work more intensively with clients, they had later come to feel that they did not have the knowledge and skill required to provide these more sophisticated services. Moreover, there was a feeling that the failure to meet heightened service expectations would reflect badly in staff performance evaluations. Fortunately, this manager was able to initiate an in-service training program and develop more reasonable service expectations. Had he not understood the relationship between the caseload decision and the subsequent decline in productivity and morale, the consequences for the organization and its clients could have been disastrous.

The Structuralist Perspective

The structuralist perspective, commonly associated with the theory of bureaucracy, is principally concerned with designing organizations to most effectively achieve their purposes. This theoretical tradition owes much to such social scientists as Max Weber, Frederick Taylor, Henri Fayol, and Lester Gulick, who sought to understand how human effort might best be organized in the interests of efficiency, productivity, and effectiveness. Unfortunately, many of the central ideas in the structuralist perspective, such as hierarchy, specialization, and span of control, have come to be associated with the pathological, dehumanizing aspects of organizational life. Nevertheless, this approach to organizations and the concepts it encompasses remain central to current thinking about organizations (Etzioni, 1964; Fayol, 1949; Gerth and Mills, 1946; and Hage and Aiken, 1968).

What Is Organizational Structure?

In the simplest terms, organizational structure can be defined as the established pattern of relationships among components or parts of the organization. More specifically, structure consists of those formal, relatively stable arrangements that prescribe how the functions and duties of an organization are to be divided and then coordinated, how authority is to be distributed, and how work responsibilities are to be carried out. Structure does not encompass relationships, sentiments, and norms that emerge spontaneously in the course of interaction between members of an organization, although it is important to acknowledge that these informal processes do much to influence the nature of formal relationships. Organizational structure is less a description of what is than a blueprint of how activities should be orchestrated to achieve desired objectives.

Because organizations seldom, if ever, function in precisely the manner formally prescribed, there is a tendency to minimize the influence of structure on behavior, and to regard it as window dressing that obscures, rather than illuminates, what really happens in organizations. Although structure alone does not account for all organizational behavior, considerable evidence suggests that structure exerts significant influence on a wide variety of processes and outcomes, including morale, job satisfaction, attitudes and behavior toward clients, efficiency, turnover, and absenteeism. A review of this evidence would take us far afield, but suffice it to say that designing a formal structure for an organization may prove to be one of the manager's most consequential tasks.

Perhaps the most common way of depicting structure is the organizational chart—usually a rough, simplistic representation of the major functional subunits and administrative positions in an organization and their hierarchical relationship to one another. Most organizational charts focus more on lines of authority and communication between superiors and subordinates and less, if at all, on the horizontal and diagonal relationships between agents in parallel subsystems (see Figure 1). Typically, this kind of chart is supplemented with detailed descriptions of the functions of various subunits, position descriptions for each class of employee, an operations manual containing rules, regulations, and procedures, and an assortment of explanatory memos and directives.

In organizational structure, four variables are particularly relevant to organizational reliability, efficiency, and internal accountability. The first two, job specialization and departmentalization, refer to the degree of complexity or horizontal differentiation to be found in an organization—the extent to which labor is divided among participants. Centralization and formalization, the other two variables of structure, measure vertical differentiation—the manner in which authority is distributed among positions in the administrative hierarchy. Each of these four variables may be visualized on a continuum from little to much, or low to high, and the manager must determine how much or how little of each is to be designed into the structure of the organization. After defining each of these variables, we will define some of the factors managers might consider in making these choices.

Horizontal Differentiation

Job specialization is reflected in the number of positions or job classes that have distinct responsibilities—the greater the number of functionally distinct positions, the greater the specialization. Thus, for example, a residential treatment program for disturbed children may divide its front-line staff into two job classes, social workers and childcare workers, with employees in each class carrying essentially the same responsibilities. However, a second program of similar size and purpose may adopt a more complex division of labor. Social workers, for example, might be assigned to several job classes, including intake and assessment workers, individual and family therapists, and community placement supervision specialists. Childcare functions might similarly be separated into specialties like recreation, group life coordination, and custody. The more specialized the job responsibilities, the more complex the organization's division of labor.

Several arguments are advanced for job specialization in organizations, most of which derive from the experience of industry. First, the more narrowly defined the responsibilities of workers, it is argued, the more easily the worker can master the skills and activities required of the job. Relatedly, as the worker spends more time with fewer activities, the efficiency with which he performs those activities should increase. Second, the narrower the range of job responsibilities, the

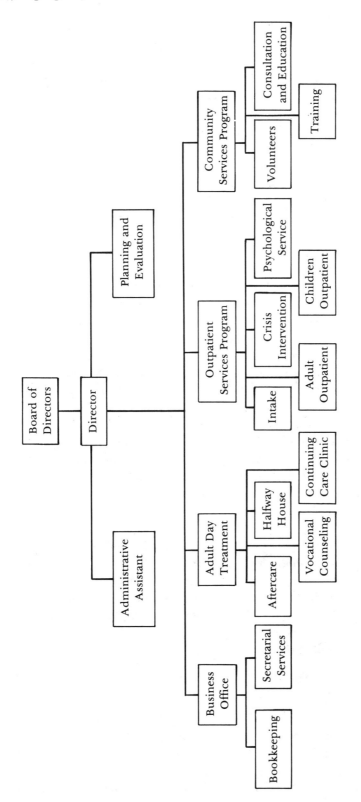

Figure 1. Organizational Chart for Community Mental Health Clinic.

more easily the manager can define performance standards and therefore control and evaluate the work of employees. Third, since jobs that are broadly defined are likely to require varying levels of knowledge and skill, advantages are thus likely to be gained by ordering positions in accordance with the level of technical expertise required. In this way, employees with more training and experience can concentrate on those activities that require their expertise, whereas employees with less training and experience can be assigned less-demanding duties. Finally, dividing labor into defined specializations enables the organization to flexibly deploy employees to make best use of their interests and aptitudes.

Departmentalization, the second dimension of complexity, concerns the degree to which the activities of a program are grouped into distinct administrative units (departments, bureaus, offices), each with its own leadership and areas of responsibility. As programs increase in size, they tend to become more departmentalized, if for no other reason than that a single manager finds it increasingly difficult to oversee and effectively relate to the activities of a large number of subordinates. Departmentalization, then, reduces the manager's span of control, or the number of subordinates to be supervised. Clearly, a manager with thirty-two employees will find it much more manageable to relate to four supervisors, each of whom is responsible in turn for seven subordinates, than to deal directly with all thirty-two employees.

The size of an organization is only one of several reasons for departmentalization. A second reason lies in the desirability of clustering related activities into subunits to facilitate interaction and coordination of workers whose jobs are highly interdependent—for example, the formation of project teams to design and implement an experimental service. Subunits such as budget and planning offices, research departments, and training and staff development units may also be formed in order to concentrate technical expertise and create a critical mass of specialists who perform support functions for an entire program. Further, the types of clients served by the program may provide a basis for departmentalization. Such factors as age, ethnicity, or type and severity of problem may result in client groups with sufficiently distinct service needs to justify the formation of separate units. Processes or technologies used may also serve as criteria for internal differentiation; intake may be separated from ongoing treatment, day treatment from inpatient services, or consultation and education from emergency services. Finally, some programs are separated into geographical units in order to ease client access or foster responsiveness to unique cultural or social characteristics in the various communities or regions.

Vertical Differentiation

Discussions of authority and compliance tend to evoke images of the classical pyramidal hierarchy, starting at the top with the administrator and fanning out symmetrically to all employees in a network of superior-subordinate relationships. Such pyramidal representations reflect the span of control of administrative personnel at each level in the organization—the greater the span of control, the fewer the administrative levels and the flatter the hierarchy. Conversely, the smaller the span of control, the more numerous the administrative levels and the steeper the hierarchy.

However, the hierarchical configuration, although it indicates how authority is distributed, reveals little about how authority is actually exercised. For approaching this question, the concepts of centralization and formalization are useful. *Centralization* may be defined as the degree to which the authority to make decisions is concentrated in a few persons in an organization—the greater the number of decisions made at upper levels of the organization, the greater the centralization. Conversely, the more authority for decisions is delegated downward, the more decentralized the organization. Of course, the extent of an organization's centralization or decentralization may vary with the kinds of decisions under consideration. For example, budget and personnel decisions may be reserved for the administrator, decisions regarding services delivery methods may be delegated to program managers and supervisors, and treatment decisions may be made at the front line.

Formalization refers to the degree to which the organization relies on rules and procedures to govern employee behavior. Administrative regulations, procedural manuals, forms, job descriptions, and memos are among the most frequently used instruments for conveying rules, but less formal means such as custom, tradition, and verbalized agreements also serve this purpose. The more detailed these prescriptions and the more consistently they are enforced, the more formalized the organization. Formalization may vary in activity areas. In determining client eligibility, conducting employee evaluations, or processing grievances, for example, procedures to be followed may be quite explicit and formally enforced. In other areas, such as the frequency of supervisory conferences, coordination between workers, or the conduct of treatment interviews, rules and procedures may be less specific or even lacking.

Formalization is essentially a mechanism for reducing discretionary behavior or routinizing decision-making processes in order to increase the reliability and consistency of subordinates' performance. Rules and procedures are often criticized for promoting inflexibility and undermining initiative and creativity; however, they can also serve to reduce role ambiguity, clarify interrole expectations, and constrain the arbitrary use of authority.

Practice Implications

What are the implications of the structural perspective for the managers of human services organizations? Let us take up each of the major concepts in this perspective and explore the intervention issues that are raised for the administrator.

The principle of dividing labor to increase productivity, efficiency, and expertise is by no means new or foreign to human services organizations. In larger agencies, especially, job specialization tends to be emphasized, a trend which is, if anything, increasing, for many of the reasons already mentioned. At the same time, the manager who is contemplating how best to divide labor in his or her organization must weigh the potential benefits of job specialization against such potential problems and dysfunctions as the boredom, monotony, and fatigue experienced by workers in narrowly defined, repetitive jobs; the development of parochial perspectives on client needs among agency workers and a consequent tendency to atomize client problems; the diminished use of worker discretion and judgment in responding to client needs; the diverse and inconsistent demands placed on clients as a result of having to relate to diverse specialists; and the difficulties of coordinating the work of numerous specialists. In recent years, approaches such as case management, case advocacy, and treatment teams have developed in part to offset some of the negative consequences of extensive specialization, but the costs and benefits of these solutions in terms of increased time and energy devoted to group processes and coordination must also be assessed. As antidotes to employee dissatisfaction with highly specialized, routine work, some organizations, most notably in the business sector, have adopted job enlargement and job rotation strategies. The benefits and limitations of these approaches to excessive specialization have yet to be systematically investigated in mental health service organizations, although some research evidence shows a correlation between job content and worker burnout in the mental health field.

Despite its potential advantages, departmentalization, like job specialization, frequently involves tradeoffs. The increased number of program management and supervisory personnel necessary to oversee agency departments often results in added administrative overhead. The greater the number of subunits, the greater the time and energy managers and others must spend in maintaining departmental communication and coordination, resolving conflicts, and attending to work flow. In addition, employees frequently develop deep loyalties to their departments that cause them to give higher priority to departmental objectives than to the overall goals and objectives of the organization. When this occurs, the accountability and control that theoretically follow from departmentalization tend to suffer. Among the most important negative consequences of departmentalization may be the discontinuity and fragmentation experienced by clients. Although these difficulties are often attributed to a lack of interagency coordination, two or more units in a single organization will not uncommonly provide overlapping services, fail to coordinate their interventions, and disseminate inconsistent messages about eligibility for services. These and other problems are more likely to occur as the organization is divided into subunits that share responsibility for dealing with the client group.

These problems of departmentalization and job specialization have prompted a search for organizational forms that can at once allow for a rational division of labor and at the same time prevent the difficulties such a division of labor frequently generates. One such structural alternative is the matrix organization, where parallel subunits of an organization operate in the traditional hierarchical manner, with specialists from each of these departments assigned to functional teams to work on some common task or problem. Each specialist continues to be administratively responsible to his or her departmental superior but also works with representatives of other departments under a team leader in order to develop a coordinated approach to the problem or clientele at hand. Team members must carry out the policies and procedures of their respective departments while at the same time articulating those departmental requirements at the team level in order to produce an organic, internally consistent approach to their common task.

The structure that emerges resembles the grid displayed in Figure 2; the staff members of four departmental units in a mental health agency are assigned to teams, with each team responsible for a number of clients in need of mental health services. The team assumes the entire responsibility for each case, including initial assessment, outpatient treatment, day treatment, and other services. However, the matrix structure, although it appears to have some utility in addressing the dysfunctions of organizational complexity, is no panacea. The worker is placed at the intersection of the vertical and horizontal systems in an organization and must be skilled at mediating their respective demands and expectations—a situation almost certain to produce some dissonance and role strain for the individual worker and at least occasional conflict among workers from several departments. Immersion in team group processes and a commitment to team effectiveness must be balanced with a need to be responsive to the directives and norms of the home department. From the departmental manager's point of view, such arrangements may serve to weaken control over subordinates and reduce the upward flow of information needed for accountability. Evaluation of subordinates may also prove problematic, since much of the primary data about the workers' performance will be provided by the team leader, who may have different criteria from those of the administrative superior for judging the quality of work. From his or her vantage point, the team leader will often perceive the lack of line authority as a constraint. If a worker is unable or unwilling to cooperate with other team members and has the support of his or her departmental director, the team leader may have few formal options, such as reassignment or dismissal, available to correct this situation.

Figure 2. Matrix Structure for Mental Health Agency.

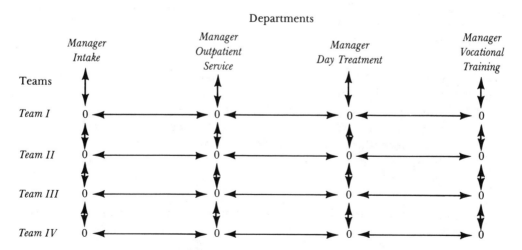

The use of centralization and formalization as structural means for ensuring the compliance and cooperation of subordinates also raises a number of questions for the manager. What kinds of decisions will be made by subordinates, and under what circumstances? What means could be employed to ensure that decisions, once made, are carried out in a reliable and consistent manner? In what area should rules and regulations be formulated to guide subordinates' behavior? How will such rules be enforced? How can the manager ensure his or her ability to monitor staff performance? The manner in which these and similar questions are answered by the administrator does much to determine the nature of the authority structure employed in an organization.

Given the complex staffing arrangements and multiple therapeutic approaches, along with uncertain funding sources, most mental health organizations are not readily adaptable to highly formalized and centralized structures. And since a high degree of centralization and formalization tends to produce undesirable secondary consequences such as lowered morale, job dissatisfaction, and strain in relations with professionals who desire autonomy, a manager obviously must proceed carefully in building an appropriate authority structure. Even taking into account the manager's responsibilities for coordination and accountability, delegation and discretion may actually enhance rather than erode the manager's authority.

The Political Perspective

Although the political perspective is not as fully developed or as widely employed as the systems and structuralist perspectives, it offers a promising approach to understanding organizational behavior at a time when resource cutbacks and program survival have become critical issues (Cohen and others, 1972; Gummer, 1978). Unlike the systems and structuralist views (which stress the themes of common goals, interdependence, integration, and coordination), the political perspective rests on the assumption that organizations are composed of distinct interest groups, each of which seeks to establish control over organizational resources in order to protect and advance its own interests. Thus, in this view, the central motivating force in organizational behavior is not the search for concerted action on behalf of higher common goals but the acquisition of power and influence that enable each interest group to maximize its impact on the allocation of resources and the policies of the organization. Multiple groups seeking to promote their interests has been referred to as a negotiated system, in which the operative goals of an organization at a given point in time emerge out of the struggle for dominance. Central to this conception of organizational behavior are the processes of conflict, competition, trading, and compromise.

Before proceeding, let us define some of the central concepts of this perspective:

- *Power* may be defined as the ability of a person or persons to gain control over resources in an organization to influence or change the behavior of other persons who are dependent on those resources. Five sources of power are commonly noted: coercion, or the ability to withhold or deprive another of something he needs; reward, or the ability to give another something he values; expertise, or a special knowledge or skill that is relevant to the tasks or problems facing an organization; legitimacy, or the formal authority that derives from an official position in the organization; and referent, or power based on such personal characteristics as charisma, honesty, and dependability. In practice, these sources of power often overlap and interact.

- *Resources* are the means employed by the organization to achieve its purposes—for example, personnel, clients, community support, and information.
- *Interest groups* take a variety of forms but are usually associated with departments or units in an organization (day treatment, outpatient), levels in the hierarchy (front-line workers, management), or functional specializations (nurses, psychiatrists, social workers). Whatever the locus of special interest groups, they are characterized by awareness of their shared fate and common goals with respect to certain issues. When several interest groups consciously combine their resources and coordinate their activities in order to pursue a common end, they may be defined as a coalition.

Special Interest Groups

What special interest groups does one find in mental health organizations? Each organization tends to develop its own configuration of interest groups in response to agency history, programmatic structure, and funding arrangements, but some commonalities exist. Bacharach and Lawler (1980), for example, argue that special interest groups tend to parallel levels in the administrative hierarchy, such that lower-, middle-, and upper-level personnel tend to develop similar vested interests and values. Kouzes and Mico (1979), in a similar vein, have posited three domains that seem to characterize human services agencies: the policy domain, the management domain, and the service domain. The authority and responsibilities associated with these domains differ, but what is more pertinent for Kouzes and Mico is that each of these domains tends, over time, to become a social entity with its own distinctive set of norms, assumptions, and goals. Members of the policy domain—which ordinarily consists of an elected or appointed board of directors functioning as something of a legislative body—tend to conceive of themselves as representatives of the community and therefore responsible for rendering fair and equitable policy decisions on behalf of various constituencies. Internally, boards are likely to use such processes as negotiation, trading, and compromise to arrive at decisions regarding the distribution of agency services.

Members of the management domain, which is comprised of those at upper and middle administrative levels, tend to think of themselves as controlling and coordinating the organization, with responsibility for rationally determining how the organization should operate and directing the work of subordinates accordingly. They are likely to measure organizational success in terms of cost efficiency and the achievement of program objectives. Therefore, they usually stress the development of accountability mechanisms and tend to see the compliance of subordinates with administrative directives as a preferred mode of organizational performance.

The service domain consists of professional service providers, who are likely to believe that, because of extended training and experience, they are best equipped to determine how services should be provided to clients. Unlike those in management, who tend to assume the necessity of hierarchical control, personnel in the service domain prefer self-regulation and professional autonomy and judge organizational success by the quality of care and professional practice provided. Professionals tend also to favor a collegial mode of interaction in relationships among organizational members.

Each of these domains and interest groups has a reasonable view of organizational reality based largely on what it deems necessary to perform its tasks and responsibilities. The problem, as Kouzes and Mico point out, is that the norms, assumptions, and goals associated with each of these domains can be sufficiently divergent to serve as barriers to the development of organizationwide agreement. Differences in language, philosophy, and organizational priorities create conditions for conflict and discordance and frequently result in adversary relationships among the various interest groups. The conflicts that divide domains are not simply matters of poor communication or insensitivity that can be resolved through greater intergroup understanding—though such understanding is beneficial. They result instead from staff members in each domain interpreting organizational reality from a perspective consistent with the roles they play. For example:

- Agency managers often find it necessary to resist or neutralize policy initiatives from the board out of a concern that such initiatives will be unfeasible or disruptive to agency operations. What may appear to the board to be a perfectly reasonable change in policy (for example, a greater effort in primary prevention) may represent for the manager a diversion of resources to non-revenue-producing programs that will threaten the integrity of the agency. The board may see the manager as recalcitrant and conservative. The manager may see the board as naive and fiscally irresponsible.
- The services staff of an agency that prides itself on providing intensive and highly sophisticated mental health services may come under criticism by the board on grounds that too few people can be served with this kind of treatment approach. The staff argue that quality is more important than quantity. The board insists that the agency cannot afford a "Cadillac" program in the face of widespread, unmet community need.
- The manager who initiates additional reporting requirements in a mental health agency in order to meet the demands of funding bodies may come into conflict with subordinates who view paperwork as a diversion from their primary service responsibility. The manager is likely to see the staff as naive regarding political and fiscal realities. The staff may see the manager as insensitive to the demands of clinical practice.

These and similar situations are seldom resolved by recourse to some seemingly objective, rational solution. Rather, they are more likely to be resolved through an implicitly political process in which contending interest groups seek to achieve their preferences through a process of negotiation and exchange.

Practice Implications

The political perspective on organizational behavior has a number of potential applications for mental health managers. First, viewing the organization from this perspective tends to "depathologize" some of the causes of conflict and disagreement among groups. Too often in organizational life, conflicts between parties are explained in terms of individual motives, traits, and behaviors. For example, the treatment staff in an agency may attribute a new management policy or procedure to the personal needs of the administrator—to punish, to control, to deal with insecurity. Conversely, a manager may discount a proposal made by subordinates as indicating their childlike dependence or their dislike of authority. Such factors may be operative in selected situations, but the political perspective suggests that the actions of a group or faction in the agency are likely to be quite rational, given their role in the organization and the goals they are pursuing. Such a perspective makes the conflict no less real but tends to shift the focus to areas of substantive disagreement.

Modern management theory has an implicitly anticonflict bias. Conflict, although generally recognized as inevitable, tends to be seen as a sign of organizational dysfunction that needs to be quickly resolved so that a "normal" state of complementarity can be restored. In this view, the organization is functioning well when there is widespread commitment to agency goals and cooperation among individuals and subunits in the interest of achieving common objectives. To the extent that the manager accepts this normative model as a standard against which to measure organizational behavior, the persistence of tension and conflict between groups must be seen as an undesirable state of affairs. Perhaps more important, those to whom the manager is responsible may interpret such a condition as evidence of poor administration. In any event, the manager often feels under some pressure, both internal and external, to get his or her house in order, the implicit assumption being that, if the manager is an effective problem solver, conflicts between interest groups will be resolved. But if discordance and tension between groups is intrinsic to the nature of mental health organizations, the expectation that the manager should reconcile differences among contending interest groups may be unrealistic. The political perspective can enable managers and others to more realistically determine what degree of harmony and complementarity among members of an organization is both feasible and desirable.

The political perspective may also have important implications for managerial behavior. In traditional management practice, organizational conflict calls forth one of two types of interventions. The first might be referred to as the human relations campaign, in which the manager seeks to open lines of communication, solicit input regarding problems, and create mechanisms for wider participation in administrative decision making. The assumption here is that conflict can be resolved through increased mutual understanding, information exchange, and attitudinal change. The human relations campaign may in fact improve the interpersonal climate in an agency and thus take the edge off disagreements between contending parties, but it may also create a veneer of agreement that obscures real differences on fundamental issues. A second kind of intervention commonly employed in conflict situations is the assertion of authority, in which the manager seeks to resolve differences by using the resources and power at his or her disposal to force compliance. Such a "you-do-it-or-else" strategy can be an effective short-term way of dealing with dissident groups that controls and suppresses but seldom resolves conflict. The consistent use of this strategy frequently gives rise to pervasive ill will and informal resistance to administrative initiative and promotes a passive, reactive posture among subordinates and a concomitant hesitancy to introduce new ideas or innovative practices.

Both of these strategies for dealing with conflict have their place in the management armamentarium but have severe limitations when the issues that divide groups in an organization are attributable to fundamental self-interest. The political perspective suggests a third strategy, which we shall refer to as negotiation. This strategy assumes a diversity of positions and seeks to fashion agreements among contending parties that allow each to protect or advance its interest. Rather than the win-win strategy associated with human relations, this strategy is one of win-lose for both parties—that is, each party to an agreement gives some and takes some. The negotiation posture acknowledges that although power is unevenly divided in organizations even the least-powerful groups can utilize the resources at their command to undermine management decisions if their interests are being disregarded. Negotiation therefore requires that managers solicit and deal directly with the preferences of the various groups that make up the political economy of the agency. At the heart of this process is the mechanism of exchange, in which the manager provides some resource that is important to the contending interest groups (for example, recognition, training funds) in return for a resource that he or she needs to accomplish a task (for example, expertise, energy, cooperation). The following case example helps to illustrate the role that the exchange process serves in helping interest groups resolve their differences.

>   In anticipation of funding cutbacks, the director of the Rainy
> City Mental Health Center instituted a policy calling for increased
> productivity in all the agency's nine programs. To make up for
> revenue losses, the director told the staff, it would be necessary for
> the agency to serve ten percent more clients than it had previously.
> The decision was discussed with program supervisors before it be-
> came policy, and the case was made that, unless more revenues were
> generated, it would not be possible to maintain the agency's existing
> level of operation. Program supervisors reacted negatively to this
> demand for increased productivity on the grounds that the staff was
> already working to capacity and that the quality of service would
> almost certainly decline. The director responded that fiscal realities
> dictated the move and reminded program supervisors that, unless
> more income was generated to meet the expected shortfall, personnel

cutbacks would be necessary. Over the objections of program supervisors, the new productivity standards were instituted.

In the next several months, the number of clients seen at the agency did in fact increase, but the program supervisors reported that the morale of staff was deteriorating. Several resignations of valued staff members were attributed to increased work pressures and reductions in program quality. Four months after the new policy was put into effect, the annual management retreat was held. Program supervisors took this occasion to present their concerns about the impact of the productivity policy on them and their staffs. Particular attention was focused on the lack of support and assistance they had received from management in dealing with the increased demands. Among other things, program supervisors recommended that the director appoint a director of clinical services who would be responsible for helping them to plan and administer their programs, monitor and improve service quality, and promote interprogram coordination. The supervisors felt isolated; a director of clinical services would, in their view, help them balance a need for increased productivity with service quality and staff morale.

The director opposed this plan during the course of the retreat on the grounds that such a new position would reduce his control over agency programs and further divide management and program personnel. The retreat ended with the director and program supervisors in open disagreement. Some minor concessions had been made, but the program supervisors left feeling that their need for support had not been fully responded to. It seemed to them that unless this conflict was resolved, working relationships between the supervisors and the director would be seriously affected.

In this case, the director failed to engage in negotiation and on basic issues. In return for cooperation with the new productivity policy, the program supervisors were asked for additional resources to help them deal with problems the policy created. The director could have used additional supervision, support, and technical assistance as negotiable points, but he was adhering to a management philosophy stressing centralized control. If he had conceded to the demands of program supervisors, he might have lost some administrative control—but meaningful negotiations could not have occurred without compromise on this issue. Instead of taking a posture of negotiation based on recognition of the program supervisors' interests, the director chose to simply assert his authority. In the short run, this strategy achieved the intended result. By the time of the retreat, however, it was clear that there would be costly, long-term consequences. The supervisors' sensitivity to their common plight was molding them into a strong interest group. Thereafter, the task of negotiating an agreement between management and program personnel would be increasingly difficult.

Conclusion

The organizational perspectives addressed in this chapter are only some of those potentially useful to the mental health agency manager. Systems theory, structural theory, and political theory each provide an insight about certain aspects of organizational behavior. Depending on the managerial problem at hand, these perspectives can help the manager better understand what is occurring and which interventions to choose. Instrumentally employed, they become valuable tools for problem solving. In this sense, the manager will find that nothing is quite so practical as a good theory.

References

Bacharach, S., and Lawler, E. *Power and Politics in Organizations: The Social Psychology of Conflict, Coalitions, and Bargaining.* San Francisco: Jossey-Bass, 1980.

Churchman, C. W. *The Systems Approach.* New York: Dell, 1968.

Cohen, M., March, J., and Olsen, J. "A Garbage Can Model of Organizational Choice." *Administrative Science Quarterly,* March 1972, *17,* 1–25.

Etzioni, A. *Modern Organizations.* Englewood Cliffs, N.J.: Prentice-Hall, 1964.

Etzioni, A. "Two Approaches to Organizational Analysis: A Critique and a Suggestion." In J. Shafritz and P. Whitbeck (Eds.), *Classics of Organization Theory.* Oak Park, Ill.: Moore Publishing Company, 1978.

Fayol, H. *General and Industrial Management.* London: Pitman Publishing, 1949.

Gerth, H., and Mills, C. W. *From Max Weber: Essays in Sociology.* London: Oxford University Press, 1946.

Gummer, B. "A Power Politics Approach to Social Welfare Organizations." *Social Service Review,* September 1978, *52,* 349–361.

Gummer, B. "Organization Theory for Social Administration." In S. Slavin and F. Perlmutter (Eds.), *Leadership in Social Administration.* Philadelphia: Temple University Press, 1980.

Hage, J., and Aiken, M. *Social Change in Complex Organizations.* New York: Random House, 1968.

Hasenfeld, Y., and English, R. *Human Service Organizations.* Ann Arbor: University of Michigan Press, 1974.

Katz, D., and Kahn, R. *The Social Psychology of Organizations.* New York: Wiley, 1967.

Kouzes, J., and Mico, P. "Domain Theory: An Introduction to Organizational Behavior in Human Service Organizations." *Journal of Applied Behavioral Science,* December 1979, *15,* 449–469.

Miringoff, M. *Management in Human Service Organizations.* New York: Macmillan, 1980.

Monane, J. *The Sociology of Human Systems.* New York: Appleton-Century-Crofts, 1967.

ꙮ 9 ꙮ

Managing
Interdisciplinary
Teams

Kermit B. Nash

In this chapter, Kermit Nash addresses the definition and function of inter-disciplinary teams in the mental health services, as well as the specific management functions of working with these teams and the role of group process and team leadership. The unique problems encountered in the use of professionals and paraprofessionals with widely different cultural, socio-economic, and racial backgrounds are discussed, as are broad issues of lead-ership, status, power, authority, roles, conflict, communication, team composition, accountability, and negotiation. Managers who wish to take advantage of the increased use of interdisciplinary teams in mental health settings need to establish a sound knowledge base in effective team management—including skills in group process, communication, decision making, conflict resolution, and self-awareness.

The goal of this chapter is to equip managers with the knowledge and skills to manage interdisciplinary teams in mental health settings. The impetus for fuller utilization of the interdisciplinary team in meeting the immense demand for individual therapeutic services developed as a result of the comprehensive Mental Health Services Act of 1963 (Berg, 1979). We will not address the economics of team-delivered services but will focus on the definition and function of interdis-ciplinary teams within the context of inpatient and day treatment programs.

An interdisciplinary team in mental health services is defined as a group of professionals and paraprofessionals from different disciplines who share the com-mon goal of effective patient care. The team members utilize a single record and participate in an organized decision-making process regarding treatment, con-sciously utilizing the various approaches, skills, and knowledge of the different team members. Authority, decision making, and accountability for the services provided rest with each professional; ultimate responsibility for patient care remains with the team. In contrast, the intradisciplinary team is a work group composed of specialists and paraprofessionals from the same general discipline who are working interdependently to deliver a service.

Given the interdisciplinary nature of the team, it is important to recognize the distinct skills and needs of each member, as well as the skills and needs that are shared by all. Among shared skills differences may exist; for example, a master's-level social worker with several years of postgraduate experience in a mental health setting may have better assessment skills than a master's-level nurse who is new to the field. In any case, overlap in areas of expertise is an integral feature of interdisciplinary work in mental health settings. Frequently, members of different disciplines view such overlap as professional encroachment on the range of services for which they have been trained. In fact, however, overlap may have great functional utility for a team, as indicated in the petal model in Figure 1. Each petal represents the unique expertise of a particular discipline; the circular area in the center represents territory where expertise is shared. Such territory may include specialized knowledge of the client population, or particularly strong skills in building client relationships or working with a team.

Current widespread use of the interdisciplinary team model is based on the belief that professionals and paraprofessionals of widely different socioeconomic and racial backgrounds and philosophical persuasions can combine their personal and professional expertise to provide more effective services to patients. The team can share the burden of immediate response to crisis, promote the effective involvement of family, and develop programs which keep patients out of hospitals by providing effective services in the community setting. The interdisciplinary team also allows team members to share the responsibility for difficult patients and thereby generates psychological support for team members who are struggling with difficult and sometimes unrewarding cases. In addition, the interdisciplinary team model increases opportunities for growth and development, as each team member gains insights from others based on the sharing of treatment issues and the self-disclosure of personal doubts or areas of confusion. Many mental health professionals who have operated in isolation value the mutual respect that can be engendered by the interdisciplinary team. Such a team can promote quality control, since team members work with, but are not subservient to, other mental health professionals and are continually involved in describing and reformulating their approaches. In fact, the team itself can be a creative force in the development of new approaches to treatment of different populations.

The interdisciplinary mental health team offers advantages for patients, as well as for professionals. Services received are frequently better coordinated than in other approaches and represent a wider range of skills focused on a particular problem or set of interdependent problems. Duplication of services is avoided, and a systems approach increases the effectiveness of problem solving.

Opponents of the interdisciplinary approach, who seek to retain the traditional approach to mental health services delivery, argue that the use of interdisciplinary teams poses disadvantages for patients, professionals, and paraprofessionals, including interference with the one-to-one relationship between

Figure 1. Interdisciplinary Sharing of Territory

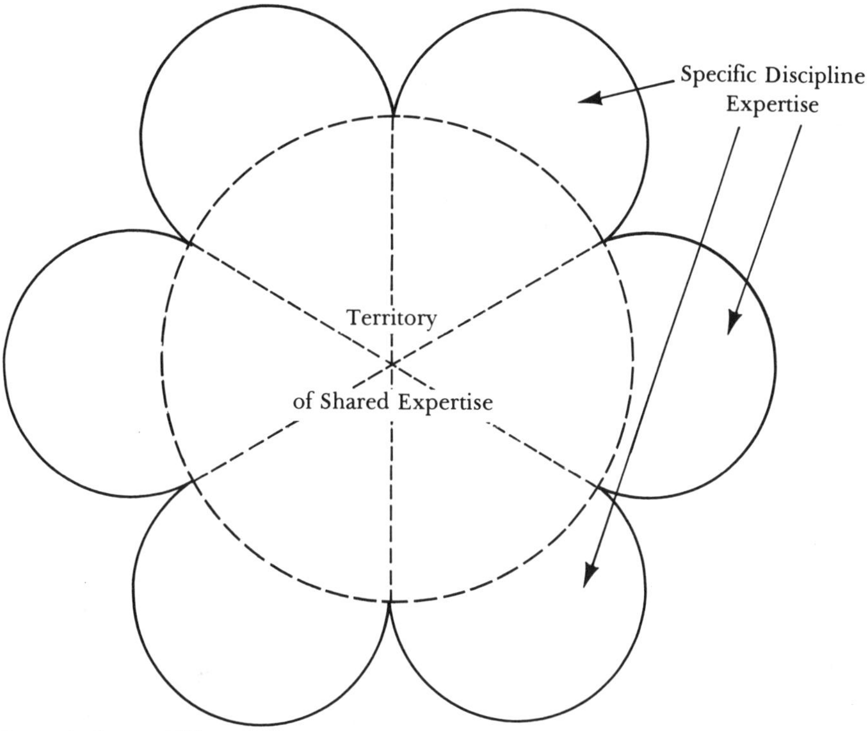

Source: Anderson, 1977.

professional and patient, the negative impact of team miscommunication, the involvement of too many professionals with no one assuming ultimate responsibility, and the inability of professionals to fully accept paraprofessionals as full-fledged team members. The paraprofessional, they argue, is faced with the problem of the caste system created by educational degree requirements in the mental health professions, which serves to block advancement (Bayes and Neill, 1978). Such restrictions may require the paraprofessional to leave the agency and enter a professional training program for several years in order to reenter the service system at a higher level. Dressler and Nash (1974), however, argue that the advantages of team-delivered community mental health services outweigh the disadvantages. The team model is seen as a vehicle to enhance continuity of care and coordination of services based on an understanding of social systems theory and small-group process. The team approach is seen as a practical framework for efficiently deploying mental health specialists, as well as for including representatives of other, nontraditional mental health disciplines in accomplishing certain patient-centered tasks.

Historical Origins of the Interdisciplinary Team

The team approach to treating mental illness evolved from the late-nineteenth-century belief that harmful social influences could lead to mental illness (Berlin, 1979). It was believed that, through public education, the environment could be modified, leading to the amelioration or prevention of mental illness. As therapists began to recognize the importance of the patient's complete social adjustment as a criterion of cure, the team concept in mental health emerged with the addition of social workers to hospital psychiatric wards managed by doctors and nurses. In 1905, Richard C. Cabot, a prominent internist, utilized the services of social workers to treat psychosomatic patients at the Massachusetts General Hospital (Berlin, 1979). The influence of Cabot, among others, established psychiatric social work as a specialty and marked the beginning of the team approach.

In 1912, E. E. Southard, the first director of the Boston Psychopathic Hospital, established a psychiatric social service department headed by Miss Mary C. Jarret. Dr. Southard directed his treatment to the complete social adjustment of his patients (Berlin, 1979). In a similar development, the child guidance movement, beginning in 1909 in Chicago, led to the formation of clinics where the team approach was used for the first time and usually included a psychiatrist, social worker, and psychologist who pooled their knowledge and observations for diagnosis and treatment (Berlin, 1979). Their roles were clearly delineated, with the psychiatrist treating the child, the psychologist doing the testing, and the social worker meeting periodically with the parents. These stereotypical roles endured for many years and still prevail in many mental health settings.

The need for interdisciplinary work in the field of mental health was formally recognized in 1923 by nine psychiatrists, working in different clinical settings, who saw the need to develop treatment methods based on the interaction of psyche, behavior, and society. Faced with a psychiatric establishment unresponsive to their concerns, they founded the American Orthopsychiatric Association, dedicated to treating the individual within the context of the community. Recognizing the need for a knowledge base broader than psychiatry, social workers, psychologists, sociologists, educators, and criminologists, among others, were soon involved in developing interdisciplinary team practice of the treatment of children and their families.

In the period between world wars, the increasing emphasis on specialization among mental health workers, the findings of ego psychology, and a growing patient population contributed significantly to the expansion of interdisciplinary teams. Hunt, Menninger, and O'Keefe (1947) noted that their experience with a psychiatric team in World War II marked the first time that a physician shared his treatment responsibilities with others on the team. They also suggested that the team approach might elicit a maximum of services with a minimum of staff, especially if specialists working together helped each other gain a more mature grasp of their work and offered supplementary information and assistance to patients.

By the beginning of the 1960s, a well-established hierarchy and status de-marcation had emerged among team members in the various disciplines—psychiatry, psychology, social work, and psychiatric nursing (Banta and Fox, 1976). The structure of the team followed the medical model, with the psychiatrist in charge and with fees for services based on the physician's status and on the perceived value of the tasks performed by each discipline. Bloom and Parad (1976) found that interdisciplinary functioning was the rule rather than the exception in community mental health centers in the 1960s. However, by the early 1970s, atti-tudes toward the desirability of interdisciplinary practice varied among the mental health disciplines studied: social workers and nurses expressed the greatest support for interdisciplinary practice, psychologists were the least impressed with inter-disciplinary functioning, and practicing psychiatrists reflected a high degree of interdisciplinary interaction (Bloom and Parad, 1976).

As early as the late 1950s, it was apparent that manpower would need to be used more efficiently and effectively to provide different types of mental health services (Albee, 1959). Welfare workers, clergy, probation officers, general physi-cians, and others were recruited to receive additional training in order to provide direct mental health service (Pattison and Elpers, 1972). The number and variety of nonprofessionals recruited into the mental health system also increased with the arrival of the indigenous nonprofessional in the wake of the social and politi-cal changes of the 1960s (Gartner, 1969). Consequently, by the middle of the 1960s, in order to meet the needs of a variety of patient populations (including former state hospital patients and racial and ethnic minorities), the interdisciplinary team had expanded to include paraprofessionals who often challenged traditional approaches to delivering services (Nash and Jacobs, 1977).

Management of Interdisciplinary Teams

The management of interdisciplinary teams in the delivery of mental health services has been increasingly complicated by the expansion in the number of teams, the introduction of new techniques for the delivery of services, a shift in teamwork focus from the traditional medical model to a psychosocial model, the varying degrees of commitment by professionals to interdisciplinary teamwork, and the entry of different client populations into the mental health system, includ-ing the previously unserved, the underserved, the poor, and racial and ethnic minorities. With professionals other than physicians serving as team leaders, ap-preciation of the difficulties of the management function has increased. The prob-lems confronting team leaders are illustrated by the following examples, gleaned from the personal experiences of team leaders from a variety of disciplines:

1. All members of my team, including those with B.A. as well as M.A. degrees, want to do intensive, one-to-one therapy with patients. However, this is not desirable for sound therapeutic and professional reasons—for example, many try to refer patients to their private practices. How does one address these issues and still retain staff?

2. Various members of my team resist using their particular skills: the psychologist does not want to administer psychometric tests, and the psychiatrist does not want to medicate patients and sign insurance forms.

3. Conflict on my team has emerged between the psychologists, who focus on interventions with the individual (medication, day treatment, hospitalization) that reinforce a patient's illness-and-dependency approach, and the social workers, who focus on family and community interventions and on reinforcing expectations for patient change and independent functioning using family therapy and community support systems.

4. Covert and often unexpressed differences in feelings of self-worth exist between team members with differing levels of education and practical expertise.

5. Too much time is spent in meetings, rather than in direct service; staffing needs to be structured to speed up the decision-making process; and therapists complain that the group note recordkeeping needs to be simplified.

6. I manage an interdisciplinary team serving adults in an outpatient community mental health center that offers outpatient therapy and emergency services. Our task is to do clinical case consultation, share information, and announce and discuss new policies and procedures. I experience problems of lack of participation (team members seem reluctant to bring up cases to discuss or to provide feedback on cases), and excessive deference to the psychiatrist and clinical psychologists (team members don't use each other as resources).

7. Staff members have various degrees. Recent graduates with M.A. or Ph.D. degrees consider themselves experts because of their ability to cite books and research; other staff members, often with lesser degrees, may have more experience in the field. Consequently, the staff has split into two separate factions, each of which feels threatened by the other. In addition, half of the staff members consider themselves specialists, whereas the other half consider themselves generalists.

8. I am currently managing an informal interdisciplinary team of alcoholism, mental health, and drug counselors. Problems I experience with this team that I anticipate would continue if a more formal team were developed include: reaching a consensus on treatment planning; establishing mutual respect among counselors; facing strong differences in philosophy of treatment and a fair amount of emotional investment by these philosophies; and facilitating the use of physicians.

9. I manage an interdisciplinary team in a community setting that includes adult therapists, child therapists, a child protective service worker, a police worker, a lay volunteer, and homemakers. I have difficulty engaging them all in treatment planning for child abuse families because of the issues of confidentiality, ethnic and cultural differences, and testimony in court.

10. I have experienced the following problems in managing an interdisciplinary team: lack of coordination and communication regarding the treatment plan (even if the treatment plan has been agreed on, various professionals do not follow the plan but do what they think best); psychiatrists unilaterally

making the decisions in treatment planning; and role conflicts (for example, team members stereotype each other in relation to who is qualified to do therapy).

11. The most frequent and troublesome problems I have faced in team management have involved the process of redefining roles within the team. The issues in this area occur in many different forms—for example, the physician is seen as the leader, regardless of administrative structure or personal desires; or the members begin to overlap functions because of increased information sharing, leading to territorial issues and, at times, to decreased quality of service. The solution is to restructure the process of team interaction. The question is how.

Team management is further complicated by the inadequate training of all professions in interdisciplinary teamwork, by the changing statuses of team members, by lack of consensus on which type of problems are best answered by the team approach, by location of services in settings where resources may be scarce, and by the influence of broader societal issues such as ageism, sexism, and racism. The complexities tend to obscure issues of patient care and frequently compound the primary task of services delivery. In addition, such conflicting mental health services priorities as providing reimbursable services, training students, keeping beds filled, conducting research, and realizing a profit can complicate the lives of team managers who are unclear about the service priorities of the organization.

Although management of interdisciplinary teams in a mental health setting usually includes the traditional management functions of planning, organizing, staffing, directing, and controlling, the approach taken in this chapter involves a shift from a hierarchical to a more egalitarian model. Of course, a pure model does not exist, and the model proposed here has some hierarchical elements. However, the value base presented is predicated on group decision making, flexible role definition, and open communication—all aspects of collegial relationships and participatory management.

According to this model, the manager determines the extent to which team members participate in organizational matters and has the responsibility to sanction and foster teamwork by creating a climate of cooperation conducive to accomplishing organizational goals. In doing this, the manager of the interdisciplinary team usually follows these broad guidelines: (1) ensures commitment to a common, overall organizational goal; (2) recognizes that the goals and the means of accomplishing them may differ between the organization and the interdisciplinary team; (3) provides specific channels for communication; (4) provides for autonomous exercise of judgment; and (5) provides for accountability and evaluation. Team leaders also grapple with issues of leadership, status, power, authority, dual roles, conflict, communication, team size and composition, accountability, negotiation, skill building, and team expansion or contraction.

More specifically, the functions of the manager include: representing institutional goals and policies; planning and organizing; directing and socializing staff; orchestrating and coordinating; monitoring and evaluating; handling boundary and ceremonial matters; nurturing and stimulating staff growth and development; providing resources; handling disturbances that interfere with the task; and promoting staff creditability in the wider arena.

This management approach assumes that interdisciplinary teams are constituted on the basis of the skills needed to deliver the services required by a particular patient population. The team leader is often responsible for enhancing organizational effectiveness and services delivery to patients through the following activities:

1. Clinical and administrative care of patients assigned to the team.
2. Knowing the total treatment plan for each patient.
3. Delegating responsibilities to team members.
4. Leading and planning to achieve treatment goals.
5. Transmitting pertinent information to appropriate persons.
6. Monitoring the relationships of the team in negotiations with other units and outside agencies and monitoring how services are described to the patient.
7. Knowing the resources available to the team and awareness of its needs.
8. Attending to group dynamics and monitoring boundaries between task and maintenance activities of the group and preventing any interference with team functioning.
9. Evaluating team members' performance.
10. Establishing the collaborative working relationship among team members.

In contrast with team leaders, the program administrator is involved in developing and monitoring the organizational structure in order to facilitate the work of the teams. Special attention needs to be given to the nurturing role of the administrator in helping teams to function effectively. The administrator who supervises interdisciplinary team leaders in mental health settings needs to be able to recognize and differentiate the three levels of leadership within the organization (see Figure 2): the administrator, who oversees several teams; the team leader, who oversees one team responsible for direct patient care to several patients; and the clinician, who works directly with the patient, mobilizing the resources of team members to meet the patient's needs (see Figure 3).

Knowledge Base for Interdisciplinary Team Management

Mental health professionals who lead interdisciplinary teams in a mental health setting need to acquire the knowledge and skills of effective team management. The remainder of this chapter focuses on the following key areas of knowledge, which are critical to the operation of interdisciplinary teams: (1) the values, training, and customs of professionals and paraprofessionals; (2) group process; (3) human behavior in organizations; (4) team functions; (5) decision-making processes; (6) conflict resolution, including the use of power and influence; (7) verbal and nonverbal communication; (8) components that foster growth and

Figure 2. Three Levels of Leadership in Mental Health Organizations.

1. Program Administrator (Inpatient, Outpatient, Day Treatment)

2. Interdisciplinary Team Leader

3. Primary Clinicians

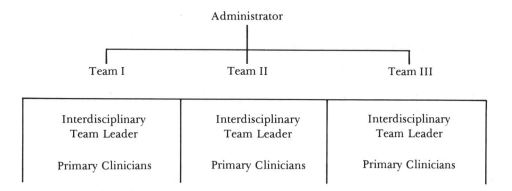

Figure 3. Sample Team Structure.

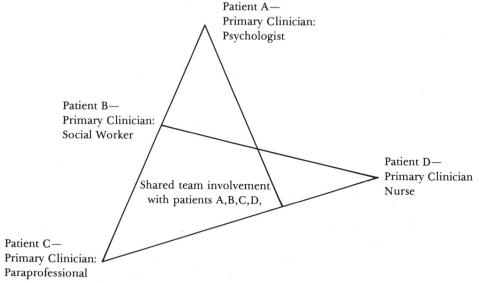

development; (9) the impact of race, ethnicity, sexism, and social interaction on teams; (10) development of self-awareness on the part of the team leader.

Values, Training, and Customs of Professionals and Paraprofessionals. The leader of an interdisciplinary team needs to have knowledge of the value base of each discipline and paraprofessional area represented on the team. Mental health professionals are socialized in different ways and hence acquire values and goals that may differ. For example, physicians and nurses are trained to intervene, to value acting on the presenting problem; social workers value the right of the patient to self-determination; and some professionals and paraprofessionals in all areas are committed to ensuring that poor and minority group clients receive services and to educating team members about the needs, aspirations, and culture of such clients (Boyette and others, 1972). Since these values and goals may conflict, awareness of competing values provides a knowledge base for handling personal and professional differences within the interdisciplinary team. In addition, sharing knowledge of the expertise of team members can increase the credibility of their diagnostic and treatment recommendations within the team.

The team manager also needs to know how the customs of different professions can detract from the ability of the team to function efficiently. Some professions, for example, have requirements relating to the need for senior clinicians to supervise novice clinicians. Social workers under close supervision sometimes need to discuss their activities with a social work supervisor, which can reduce a team member's effectiveness in team decision making (Banta and Fox, 1976). The team leader needs to understand how specific professions are organized and what degree of autonomy workers need in order to be effective team members.

Group Process. An understanding of group dynamics is important for the team leader because of frequent breakdowns in team group process. Interdisciplinary cooperation often improves when team leaders acquire techniques and skills in expediting group dynamics for effective problem solving. Research indicates that a small group promotes interaction at many levels, serves as the focal point for developing responsible participation, fosters learning by exchange and experience, and facilitates the development of leadership (Odhner, 1970).

The resources of interdisciplinary team members must be shared if the team is to provide effective services. The team cannot survive on the omnipotent authority of one member or on the evaluation of members' contributions according to professional status. Each member's contribution to the team must be evaluated in terms of its relevance to the task; stereotyped expectations are destructive to effective communication (Brill, 1976).

Human Behavior in Organizations. The team leader needs to know how organizational structure affects human behavior and how staff members use formal and informal organizational channels of power and authority. Classical organizational issues include power, responsibility, division of labor, specialization, and interdependence (Davis, 1967; Wells, 1972). Organizational structure influences the amount of power held by staff members, as well as staff members' perceptions of their roles. Although those with centralized power at the top of the organizational hierarchy may provide staff members with support for carrying out their tasks, the reverse is too often the case.

The team leader's knowledge of organizational structure should be helpful in structuring relationships with regard to the use of authority, the development of influence, and the reduction of dependence (Lewis, 1969). The division of work into levels and functions is an important concept for the leader of interdisciplinary teams. Dividing tasks according to the expertise, interests, and available time of staff helps to distribute authority and responsibility for special functions (Davis, 1967).

Team Functions. The tasks of a mental health treatment team include establishing a relationship with the patient in order to understand his or her needs, managing distress through medication and/or hospitalization, involving significant persons in the patient's environment in the treatment process, and identifying and strengthening the patient's coping mechanisms to deal with future stresses. Unless the tasks and priorities of the mental health team are clearly defined, necessary skill areas and, therefore, appropriate team members cannot be identified and selected. In addition to clinical psychologists, psychiatrists, social workers, and nurses, treatment teams may include landlords, lawyers, welfare workers, and ministers, since environmental intervention and manipulation are often necessary for effective treatment. Once the goals of treatment are determined, the team is then in a position to determine the skills and the particular team members necessary to accomplish those goals. Services provided by the mental health system are limited, and team members' time must be carefully meted out in order to serve as many people as possible.

Stages of Team Development. Development of the treatment team begins with the selection of a team member as primary clinician (Dressler and Nash, 1974). The primary clinician, who can be a professional from any of the disciplines or a paraprofessional, is usually the person who has the best understanding of the unique needs of the patient. Use of the primary clinician as leader of patient care can promote the integration of clinical and administrative activities (Dressler and Nash, 1974).

Assessment is the initial task of the primary clinician. The assessment of the patient's presenting problems determines the treatment plan and the composition of the patient's treatment team. Once the patient's needs have been determined, the individuals possessing the skills necessary to meet those needs are brought together to comprise the treatment team, and treatment objectives and task assignments are delineated. A timetable for the completion of tasks is prepared, and team members begin to work on their assignments. Regularly scheduled team meetings are held, at which problems and progress are discussed. The team organization maintains standards of quality by means of peer accountability. Status, power, and authority issues affect the efficiency or effectiveness of teamwork. Successful team functioning means investing authority on the basis of an individual's role on the team, rather than on the basis of power or professional status. Treatment team members must recognize and respect one another's competence, values, and shared authority.

Team development progresses through the following phases: pregroup phase; group formation phase; phase of integration, disintegration, reintegration, or reorganization; group functioning and maintenance phase; and termination phase (Thelen, 1961). In the pregroup phase, the leader assists the team in coming into being, making important decisions about the composition of team membership that have an effect on what happens when the team forms. In the group formation phase, new relationships form, and the team begins to discern common goals and to perform the tasks necessary to achieve those goals. Team members begin to define themselves in the group and to establish roles and patterns of behavior (Hartford, 1972). After the team begins to form, there is a period of testing in this second phase of team development. During the third phase, integration, disintegration and conflict, reintegration, or reorganization occurs. The struggle in this phase is related to a redistribution of power and control and to competition for a redefinition of leadership. Frequently, the disintegration is slight, and, after briefly focusing on its own functioning, the team realigns its structure, restates its goals, and moves ahead to accomplish its tasks. If the conflict goes unresolved, the group disintegrates.

During the group functioning and maintenance phase, the team accomplishes its tasks. The culture and style of group behavior are established and observable. Interpersonal relationships usually stabilize in the form of dyads and triads based on personal affection, shared interests, or other forces. The stabilization of leader-follower patterns and the firming of the status hierarchy based on skills appropriate for the purpose of the team are observable aspects of this phase. If the team loses or adds members or has failures or special successes in its operations, it may need to reintegrate itself during this phase.

The termination phase consists of three parts: pretermination, or the period of preparation for the actual ending; termination, or the recognized ending; and posttermination, or the plan for follow-up. Pretermination includes planning for the ending, enumerating and evaluating team accomplishments and failures, planning for recognition of individual team members and leaders, and working through the difficulties that some members may feel in breaking team ties. Termination of the team in the last meeting of the group sometimes includes a summary, a ritual closing ceremony or party, or plans for the posttermination or follow-up evaluation. At this time, team members release whatever control they have had over each other, resolve their relationships, and dissolve the team.

Decision Making. Decision making has both structural and substantive aspects. For the interdisciplinary team, the substantive aspect of decision making involves reaching agreements and resolving disagreements among individuals with differing perceptions, concepts, methods, philosophies, and treatment modalities. The structure of decision making involves the distribution of roles and authority and is organized according to either a hierarchical or an egalitarian model.

The interdisciplinary team follows the hierarchical model in that authority is associated with specific positions; the leader must have the capacity to exercise authority and to make decisions. For a team leader, authority means the use of agency procedures to guarantee appropriate follow-up to decision making, ensure coordination, and define individuals' responsibility. The interdisciplinary team also follows the egalitarian approach in holding that interdisciplinary teams should be composed of professional members deliberately selected to bring complementary knowledge, skills, and expertise to the group (March and Simon, 1958). In a mental health setting, interdisciplinary team members approach patient care on the basis of joint concern for amelioration, data collection, problem solution, outcome prediction, and the determination of the activities necessary to achieve those ends. All activity must be integrated so that the team is responsible for the outcome. Unless an integrated strategy is developed by the interdisciplinary efforts of the personnel involved, conflict will threaten cooperation and collaboration.

The differences and limitations of hierarchical and egalitarian approaches to decision making within the interdisciplinary team may be illustrated by the gatekeeping decisions that control the admission or rejection of clients for services. Predominantly hierarchical teams assign these decisions to a team member who determines who will receive services. This gatekeeper must be able to recognize problems that fall within the domain of professions other than his or her own. In a team with a predominantly egalitarian pattern of decision making, all team members have the opportunity to interview or examine patients and to determine the presence or absence of problems that fall within their professional domain. The limitation of this approach lies in the possible tendency for team members to overdiagnose as a means of protecting their domain by demonstrating the significance of their expertise to the team—thereby serving their own interests rather than those of the patient.

Conflict Resolution. Conflict results when there is a breach in expected attitudes and behavior leading to a breakdown in the standard mechanism of decision making (Given and Simmons, 1977). Conflict occurs when communication and interaction patterns are disrupted; norms become confused or do not apply, role conflicts emerge, and social controls become meaningless or ineffective. When status relationships become confused or unacceptable, conflict escalates. On an interdisciplinary team, a variety of these factors work together to disrupt prescribed patterns of interaction. Symptoms of conflict include competition, tension, rivalry, and the discrediting of other team members.

Although social conflict is generally viewed as something to be avoided, it can have positive consequences, focusing attention on issues that need to be resolved if the team is to function effectively. Conflict can unite the members of a group for a common purpose, stimulate changes in interactional, interpersonal, and group patterns, and resolve differences in values, perceptions, attitudes, and approaches. In interdisciplinary mental health teams, the growing role of paraprofessionals and the use of leaders other than physicians are graphic examples of changes in the established pattern that can create conflict. Ways of dealing with conflict include: remaining neutral, neither encouraging nor discouraging conflict but simply accepting it as it occurs, allowing it to resolve itself, and viewing conflict as essentially desirable as long as it is controlled.

Conflict and its resolution can be ordered so that they follow fairly regular and predictable patterns. To accomplish this, mental health teams must create numerous means of effectively managing and resolving conflict whenever it occurs. Typical management procedures involve: bringing together and promoting full communication between opposing sides of a conflict; achieving mutually satisfactory compromises or other solutions to conflicts; developing compensatory mechanisms to deal with threatening stresses and strains; enabling all of those affected by a change to make necessary adjustments in their own activities; and limiting the power that any one individual can exercise over the team. The extent and success of these management precedures largely determine the kinds of conflicts and resolutions that can occur within the team setting. If the team suppresses conflict and resists change, conflict will occur sporadically and unexpectedly and usually go unresolved. If conflicts, pressures, or stress are allowed to build up within a team, they will become uncontrollable, erupt into sharp conflicts involving abrupt changes, and seriously disrupt, alter, or destroy the effective functioning or working existence of the team.

In contrast, if the team leader and team members encourage the expression of conflict through established procedures and allow as much change as possible, then conflict, along with its expression and resolution, will occur continuously. No single conflict or change will be disruptive or extensive, but, over time, the cumulative effects of many minor alterations should produce lasting change and stability. Conflict is an inherent aspect of interdisciplinary team functioning and must be faced and dealt with if the team is to function at its optimum effectiveness.

Verbal and Nonverbal Communication. The team leader needs to have an understanding of the communication process, both verbal and nonverbal. A single communication between two persons may appear to be innocent enough but is actually complicated by such factors as selection of words, delivery, reception, translation, consideration, and a number of other related and influential factors that affect the entire communication process. Communication is a dynamic process, and team leaders need to be familiar with the following concepts (This, 1972): communication-space, which addresses issues of spatial relationship, distance between communicators, and equal access to the communication-space, rather than domination by one person; the filter-system, in which the receiver of a message filters it through his or her own values, prejudices, biases, and stereotypes; information-space, which includes shared language, experience, values, and goals (research suggests that effective communication varies directly with the size of this space); and total sensory input, which recognizes that all subjective responses are a function of the totality of sensory inputs.

Communication is a two-way interaction in which each person is trying to influence the other. Forces influencing the communication process include organizational position, commitment to certain ideas, cultural conditioning, resistance to influence, situational orientation, and the symbolic nature of communication (This, 1972). Communication among team members can be further complicated by differing orientations regarding the importance of service. For example, the treatment-oriented values of social work practitioners may be opposed by the more diagnostic orientations of clinical psychologists. The conditions under which differing orientations affect communication and cohesion, as well as the direction and extent of those effects, remain largely unexplored.

Finally, the manager must be aware of the nonverbal dimension of communication. When the verbal and nonverbal dimensions of communication are incongruent, the nonverbal message takes priority for the receiver of the communication. Nonverbal phenomena are signs of culture, values, and assumptions about the topic being discussed.

Creating Climate for Growth. Using the ability to assess organizational climate and to determine whether personnel are operating at an existence, relatedness, or growth level, team leaders can consciously promote the personal growth of staff members. The levels of existence, relatedness, and growth represent a realignment of Maslow's hierarchy of needs, translated into the institutional setting of Alderfer (1972, 1974, 1976). The existence level corresponds to Maslow's physiological and safety needs, relatedness to needs for love and esteem, and growth to the need for self-actualization. By understanding their motivations and needs, the team leader can help team members move beyond the existence level and can facilitate relatedness and growth. The goal of the team leader, then, is to integrate and coordinate staff self-actualization behavior to allow for growth and upward mobility for all team members.

Impact of Race, Ethnicity, Sexism, and Social Interaction. The team leader needs to be aware of the impact of race, ethnicity, sexism, and social interaction on the operation and makeup of the teams. Inequity needs to be understood—especially the way in which it is manifested by stereotypical roles and the way in which women and minorities tend to be "used" by the organization.

The entry of minorities into the treatment system has led to an increase in the hiring of minority professionals and paraprofessionals. Conflicting opinion exists as to whether minority staff members should work only with minorities to serve as bridges to the minority community; in any case, language, culture, and socioeconomic class of minorities need to be fully understood (Wesson, 1975). The team leader also needs to address the problem of staff resistance to incorporating a minority group member into the team. An example of a lack of sensitivity to minority group issues is the assignment of a patient to a clinician on the basis of seeming compatibility of race or sex or ethnic origin, without consideration for the other reasons for which the patient came for help (Nash, 1980).

Self-Awareness. In order for team leaders to become more effective, they need to understand themselves as well as their jobs. For team leaders to identify their own needs and to understand why they are what they are, why they do what they do, and how they can best accomplish their goals, they need to be introspective, open to feedback, and aware of their impact on others. This increased self-awareness should lead to insights that enhance responsiveness to the pressures and dilemmas of the job.

One way of increasing self-awareness is through the use of the Johari window, which helps people acquire information from others about their behavior, thereby expanding their self-awareness (Luft, 1963). The visualization of the four quadrants representing the window serves as the model for examination. Quadrant I represents behavior known to self and others—for example, smoking. Quadrant II represents behavior of which the individual is unaware but others are aware—for example, grinding the teeth. Quadrant III is an area of secret activities or thoughts an individual knows about himself or herself but does not reveal to others—for example, a hidden agenda. Quadrant IV is the unconscious area, which eventually surfaces as a small group works together.

Change in any one of the quadrants will affect the other quadrants if the individual is willing to accept feedback. In fact, the importance of feedback to increased self-awareness and behavioral change cannot be overemphasized. Useful feedback is descriptive rather than evaluative; is specific rather than general; accounts for the needs of both individuals involved; is directed toward behavior that the individual can do something about; is asked for rather than imposed; is well timed after the given behavior; is checked to ensure clear communication; and is checked with others in the training group.

Managerial Skills for Team Leaders

Interdisciplinary team leaders must acquire managerial skills to complement their clinical skills. The emphasis on skill building is imperative—only through practice and feedback in real or simulated situations can appropriate skills be acquired. Mintzberg's (1975) description of managerial work suggests that the following skills have relevance for the leaders of interdisciplinary teams:

1. Developing peer relationships with those within and outside the organization.
2. Carrying out negotiations with colleagues, superiors, and subordinates.
3. Motivating subordinates within the team.
4. Resolving conflicts between team leaders.
5. Establishing informational networks and subsequently disseminating information within the organization, the team, and the community.
6. Making decisions in conditions of extreme ambiguity.
7. Allocating resources.
8. Introspecting about their work as managers.

These management skills require the integration of all the knowledge areas into a managerial style necessary to function as a team leader. Mintzberg (1975) has identified fourteen self-study questions (see Table 1) that address the issue of integration.

Team leaders' recognition and understanding of their role in a group can be facilitated by participation in small study groups such as those developed at the Tavistock Clinic in England (Rioch, 1970). The orientation in the Tavistock groups is psychoanalytical; unconscious forces, projection, anxiety, hostility, authority relations, and power relations are examined. Conflict growing out of the context of defined legitimate authority, for example, is considered in light of projections, their antecedents, and their consequences. Depending on his or her goals, the manager can use these small groups to acquire skills in a task focus, in role relations, in the assessment of the impact of structure on the task, in relationships to authority and power, in covert and overt issues in group process, and in the understanding of group, intergroup, and organizational processes.

Table 1. Team Leader Self-Study Questions.

Question 1

1. From what source do I get my information, and how?
2. Can I make greater use of my contacts to get information?
3. Can other people do some of my scanning for me? In what areas is my knowledge weakest, and how can I get others to provide me with the information I need?
4. Do I have powerful enough mental models of those things I must understand within the organization and its environment?

Question 2

1. What information do I disseminate in my organization?
2. How important is it that my subordinates get the information I have?
3. Do I keep too much information to myself because dissemination is time-consuming or inconvenient?
4. How can I get more information to others so that they can make better decisions?

Question 3

1. Do I balance information collecting with action taking?
2. Do I need to act before information is in?
3. Do I wait so long for all the information that opportunities pass me by and I become a bottleneck in my own organization?

Question 4

1. What pace of change am I asking of my organization?
2. Is this change balanced so that our operations are neither excessively static nor excessively disrupted?
3. Have we sufficiently analyzed the impact of this change on the future of our organization?

Question 5

1. Am I sufficiently well informed to pass judgment on the proposals that my subordinates make?
2. Is it possible to leave final authorization for more of the proposals with subordinates?
3. Do we have problems of coordination because subordinates in fact make too many decisions independently?

Question 6

1. What is my vision of direction for this organization?
2. Do these plans exist primarily in loose form in my own mind?
3. Should I make them explicit in order to better guide the decisions of others in the organization?
4. Do I need the flexibility to change those decisions at will?

Question 7

1. How do my subordinates react to my managerial style?
2. Am I sufficiently sensitive to the powerful influence my actions have on them?
3. Do I fully understand their reactions to my actions?
4. Do I find an appropriate balance between encouragement and pressure?
5. Do I stifle their initiative?

Question 8

1. What kind of external relationships do I maintain, and how?
2. Do I spend too much of my time maintaining these relationships?
3. Are there certain types of people whom I should get to know better? If so, why?

Table 1, cont'd.

Question 9

1. Is there any system to my time scheduling, or am I just reacting to the pressures of the moment?
2. Do I find an appropriate mix of activities, or do I tend to concentrate on one particular function or one type of problem just because I find it interesting?
3. Am I more efficient with particular kinds of work at particular times of the day or week?
4. Does my schedule reflect this?
5. Can someone else (other than my secretary) take responsibility for much of my scheduling and do it more systematically?

Question 10

1. Do I overwork?
2. What effect does my workload have on my efficiency?
3. Should I force myself to take breaks or to reduce the pace of my activity?

Question 11

1. Am I too superficial in what I do?
2. Can I really shift moods as quickly and as frequently as my work patterns require?
3. Should I attempt to decrease the amount of fragmentation and interruption in my work?

Question 12

1. Do I orient myself too much toward current tangible activities?
2. Am I a slave to the action and excitement of my work, so that I am no longer able to concentrate on issues?
3. Do key problems receive the attention they deserve?
4. Should I spend more time reading and probing deeply into certain issues?
5. Could I be more reflective?
6. Should I be more reflective?

Question 13

1. Do I use the different media appropriately?
2. Do I know how to make the most of written communication?
3. Do I rely excessively on face-to-face communication, thereby putting all but a few of my subordinates at an informational disadvantage?
4. Do I schedule enough of my meetings on a regular basis?
5. Do I spend enough time touring my organization to observe activity at first hand?
6. Am I too detached from the heart of my organization's activities, seeing things only in an abstract way?

Question 14

1. How do I blend my personal rights and duties?
2. Do my obligations consume all my time?
3. How can I free myself sufficiently from obligations to ensure that I am taking this organization where I want it to go?
4. How can I turn my obligations to my advantage?

Conclusion

The use of the interdisciplinary team in the delivery of mental health services is increasing. The interdisciplinary nature of assuring quality patient care requires the continuous assessment of the contribution of the team concept to meeting the psychosocial needs of patients. Teams need to be expanded to include landlords, merchants, police, employers, and others in the community who may affect the well-being of the patient needing mental health services.

Interdisciplinary team leaders must adapt their knowledge and skills to the ever-changing nature of mental health services delivery. The implications for the team leader include the need to work with varying organizational arrangements and with continual change. In this sense, the team leader must have the knowledge and skills necessary to act as a change agent both inside and outside mental health agencies.

References

Albee, G. W. *Mental Health Manpower Trends.* New York: Basic Books, 1959.

Alderfer, C. P. *Existence, Relatedness, and Growth: Human Needs in Organizational Settings.* New York: Free Press, 1972.

Alderfer, C. P. "Change Processes in Organizations." In M. Dunnette (Ed.), *Handbook of Industrial and Organizational Psychology.* Chicago: Rand McNally, 1974.

Alderfer, C. P. "Boundary Relations and Organizational Diagnosis." In H. Meltyer and F. R. Wickert (Eds.), *Humanizing Organizational Behavior.* Springfield, Ill.: Thomas, 1976.

Anderson, J. R., Jr. *Some Issues and Problems Inherent in Efforts to Implement the Concept of the Health Care Team.* Paper presented at the annual Social Work Forum, Issaquah, Wash., Oct. 28, 1977.

Banta, H. D., and Fox, R. C. "Role Strains of a Health Care Team in a Poverty Community." *Social Science and Medicine,* 1976, *6,* 697–722.

Bayes, M., and Neill, T. K. "New Roles for Paraprofessionals in Mental Health Services." In K. B. Nash, N. Lifton, and S. E. Smith (Eds.), *The Paraprofessional: Selected Readings.* New Haven: Advocate Press, 1978.

Berg, L. K. "Coordination of Service: The Interdisciplinary Team and Social Work Practice in Community Mental Health." In A. Katz (Ed.), *Community Mental Health.* New York: Council on Social Work Education, 1979.

Berlin, R. "The Team Approach in Hospital Treatment as a Defense of the Psychiatrist." *Comprehensive Psychiatry,* March 1979, *11* (2), 147–157.

Bloom, B. L., and Parad, H. J. "Interdisciplinary Functioning: A Survey of Attitudes and Practices in Community Mental Health." *American Journal of Orthopsychiatry,* Oct. 1976, *46* (4), 669–677.

Boyette, R., and others. "The Plight of the New Careerist: A Bright Horizon Overshadowed by a Dark Cloud." *American Journal of Orthopsychiatry,* July 1972, *42* (4), 596–602.

Brill, N. I. *Team Work: Working Together in the Human Services.* Philadelphia: Lippincott, 1976.

Davis, K. *Human Relations at Work: The Dynamics of Organizational Behavior.* New York: McGraw-Hill, 1967.

Dressler, D. M., and Nash, K. B. "Project Team Organization and Its Application to Crisis Intervention." *Community Mental Health Journal,* Apr. 1974, *10,* 156–162.

Gartner, A. "The Use of the Paraprofessional and New Directions for the Social Service Agency." *Public Welfare,* 1969, *27* (2), 117–124.

Given, B., and Simmons, S. "The Interdisciplinary Health Care Team: Fact or Fiction?" *Nursing Forum,* 1977, *16* (2), 165–184.

Hartford, M. *Groups in Social Work.* New York: Columbia University Press, 1972.

Hunt, M., Menninger, W., and O'Keefe, D. "The Neuropsychiatric Team in the U.S. Army." *Mental Hygiene,* 1947, *31,* 103–119.

Lewis, J. M. "The Organizational Structure of the Therapeutic Team." *Hospital and Community Psychiatry,* July 1969, *20,* 36–38.

Luft, J. *Group Processes: An Introduction to Group Dynamics.* Palo Alto, Calif.: National Press Books, 1963.

March, J., and Simon, H. *Organizations.* New York: Wiley, 1958.

Miller, E. J., and Rice, K. *Systems of Organization: The Control of Task and Sentient Boundaries.* New York: Tavistock, 1970.

Mintzberg, H. "The Manager's Job: Folklore and Fact." *Harvard Business Review,* July–Aug. 1975, *3* (4), 49–61.

Nash, K. B. *Cross-Cultural, Cross-Class, and Cross-Racial Issues in Working with Black Americans: From a Psychiatric Perspective.* Paper presented at the Transcultural Colloquium, University of California-San Francisco, Fresno, Calif., Apr. 1980.

Nash, K. B., and Jacobs, S. C. *The Non-Physician Clinician on an Inpatient Psychiatric Service: Recruitment, Selection, Utilization and Training.* Paper presented at the First Regional Congress of Social Psychiatry, Santa Barbara, Calif., Sept., 1977.

Odhner, F. "Group Dynamics of the Interdisciplinary Team." *American Journal of Orthopsychiatry,* Oct. 1970, *24* (7), 484–487.

Pattison, M. E., and Elpers, J. R. "A Developmental View of Mental Health Manpower Trends." *Hospital and Community Psychiatry,* Nov. 1972, *23* (11), 325–328.

Rioch, M. J. "The Work of Wilfred Bion on Groups." *Psychiatry,* 1970, *33,* 56–66.

Thelen, H. A. "Intergroup Conflict." In *Forces in Community Development.* Washington, D.C.: National Training Laboratories, 1961.

This, L. E. Personal Communication. Washington, D.C.: Leadership Resources, Inc., 1972.

Wells, L., Jr. "Toward a Comprehensive Approach to Organizational Diagnosis: Ten Diagnostic Domains for Understanding Organizations." Unpublished manuscript, Yale University School of Administrative Science and Management, 1972.

Wesson, A. K. "The Black Man's Burden: The White Clinician." *The Black Scholar,* July/Aug. 1975, 13–19.

❦ 10 ❧

Facilitating
Productive
Staff Meetings

Herman B. Resnick

In this chapter, Herman Resnick identifies approaches for managers to use in improving staff meetings and dealing with staff resistance, fears, and objections. A model for effective staff meeting management—including premeeting, meeting, and postmeeting phases—and a five-step model for constructive problem solving are described in detail; roles and norms contributing to productive staff meetings are discussed; and several guidelines and techniques drawn from the fields of group dynamics and organizational management are delineated. Topics discussed include agenda setting and building, problem clarification, decision making, and action planning.

"Staff meetings are a drag."

"My stomach turns to mush whenever I walk into that large staff meeting room on Mondays."

"Nothing ever happens that means anything."

These reactions to staff meetings probably represent the feelings and attitudes of many mental health practitioners and administrators. The staff meeting is typically viewed as an obstacle to organizational effectiveness, yet staff meetings can provide the support and direction needed by staff to carry out their complex and demanding jobs.

The primary purpose of this chapter is to identify principles and practices that can lead to more effective staff meetings. Meetings are often dreaded by participants for a number of reasons: fear of looking foolish, unresolved conflict, boredom, general inefficiency, and poor leadership. Staff meeting leaders may be able to alter these perceptions by focusing on the following purposes and functions of staff meetings: to provide information; to make decisions; to establish identity and affirm that one organization is made up of many parts, all working together; to confirm statuses, so individuals know and understand their specific roles in the organization; and to provide a forum for promoting and managing change. The staff meeting, then, is a reflection of the whole organization. Meetings that are dreaded and inefficient suggest the need for organizational self-assessment; meetings experienced as democratic, efficient, and positive indicate organizational strength.

Football teams practice on the average of six hours per day, five days per week, for a weekly, two-hour game. In mental health organizations, the staff meeting is the two-hour game, yet administrators fail to invest much time in understanding or practicing for their organizational game. Nearly everyone has been involved in the meetings of a club, a church, a business, a school, or a professional organization; experience gained from such organizational meetings should be organized to facilitate agency team work. Practice for agency staff meetings, then, should be considered as crucial as practice for a weekly football game. This chapter offers a number of group process models that, when practiced and internalized by the participants, can enhance staff meetings and possibly lead to the improvement of other aspects of the agency, as well.

This chapter is based on several assumptions about administrative styles and staff meeting activities. First, it is assumed that managers of mental health agencies, in response to the values and treatment principles of the mental health field, identify with the philosophy and procedures of an egalitarian and participative mode of management and recognize the needs of staff for autonomy, involvement, and influence. Many mental health managers seek to demonstrate subordinate-centered leadership—for example, freedom to function within defined limits—rather than boss-centered leadership, in which managers assume total authority for making and announcing decisions. Second, the following assumptions have been made about the structure and function of staff meetings:

1. A staff meeting is a prototype of the agency social structure.
2. The staff meeting exists at the intersection of three systems: the agency social system, the agency service system, and the agency administrative system.
3. Administrators and staff are engaged in building long-term working relationships, and staff meetings occur regularly, two to four times per month.
4. Staff meeting composition typically ranges from five to twenty-five participants.
5. Administrators and staff are willing and able to learn new approaches to staff meeting management.

These assumptions are crucial building blocks needed to help managers and staff facilitate more productive staff meetings. The next section describes the **PDP** (pre-, during-, and postmeeting phases) model of staff meeting management, which consists of the following distinct but interrelated parts: a preparatory phase; a during-meeting phase; and a postmeeting phase. Related to these phases are the following processes: problem solving, norm setting, role clarifying, message sending and receiving, and decision making.

PDP Model of Staff Meeting Management

The PDP model is built on the assumption that each phase of the staff meeting process is as important as any other and that the success of one is linked to the effectiveness of the others. The three phases will be discussed in order.

Premeeting Phase

Of primary importance to effective staff meetings is preparation. A direct relationship probably exists between the amount of time spent on the premeeting preparation and the effectiveness of the meeting. Although most managers are intuitively aware of this phase, they usually prepare only themselves and fail to create conditions for the staff to prepare themselves. This oversight leads to the perception that managers own the meeting, rather than the perception that the meeting is jointly owned by managers and staff. Activities that help to prepare management and staff prior to a staff meeting include setting the agenda, selecting the place and space for the meeting, and deciding on appropriate food and drink.

Agenda Setting. Agenda setting is necessary for an effective staff meeting, and much care and attention should be given to the development and distribution of an agenda. Items should be solicited from all levels of the agency, and the agenda presented at the meeting should reflect that participative effort. Agenda items provide continuity from previous meetings and assure participants of an active role in decision making.

In addition, agenda items need to be prioritized so that sufficient time can be allotted to important items. Experience suggests that the more important items should come in the middle of the meeting, rather than at or near the end. Prioritizing agenda items also requires the manager to think through the issues involved with each item, the facts pertinent to those issues, and the action that may need to be taken. Moreover, an effective manager needs to be sensitive to the attitudes and potential reactions of staff to the issues and plan the meeting strategy accordingly. For example, if managers expect negative staff reaction to a position taken by management, they should: prepare themselves psychologically to deal with that difference without being personally affronted or threatened and prepare themselves to learn from the differences; present relevant information and a carefully considered rationale based on value or pragmatic considerations; have a plan designed to obtain a fair hearing for their position; and promote an atmosphere conducive for staff presentations of alternative positions. Finally, the careful construction of agenda items may suggest the involvement of resource persons who need to be notified sufficiently in advance to allow them time to prepare relevant reports.

Selecting Space and Refreshments. Since the effects of the physical environment on interaction and morale are now well documented (Mehrabian, 1976; Proshansky, 1970; Summer, 1969), managers should take note of the following suggestions for enhancing the effectiveness of staff meetings:

1. *Room size.* The room should be large enough to contain a square or round table with comfortable upright chairs for each member but should not be so large as to give the group the feeling of being a small group in a huge room. A small room, despite the cramped feeling that may occur, does provide a sense of heightened interaction, clarity of communication, and an intimacy that can sometimes contribute to a more interesting meeting.
2. *Light.* The room should be airy and bright, with light coming from windows as well as electrical fixtures.
3. *Ambience.* An ambience suggestive of both work and pleasure, although difficult to attain, sends the message that both organizational and staff needs will be addressed at the meeting.
4. *Access.* Ease of access for handicapped persons should be provided.
5. *Resource materials.* The presence of an easel, markers, and flip charts signals to participants that work will be recorded and conducted in an efficient, systematic manner.
6. *Food and drinks.* Coffee should be available before, during, and after a staff meeting. Some managers organize a rotation system whereby each staff member takes responsibility for bringing a treat to go with the coffee.

Meeting Phase

The major activities of this phase are completing the agenda, taking the minutes, conducting the meeting, and reviewing the meeting and assigning tasks.

Agenda Building. As a result of the premeeting activities, a tentative agenda consisting both of follow-up items from previous meetings and of new items proposed by management or staff should be distributed two or three days in advance of the meeting. The agenda should be kept tentative to allow for important last-minute items. The beginning of the meeting should be devoted to establishing the final agenda by deciding which items should be added or deleted, sequencing the items, and allotting appropriate time to each. Although necessary for the meeting to proceed smoothly and for staff to feel responsible for its process, agenda building should not take more than five to ten minutes.

Taking the Minutes. Minutes should be read, amended where necessary, and accepted by staff. Agenda building and the approval of the minutes should be led by the facilitator of the previous meeting. Following these activities, a new recorder of the minutes and a new meeting facilitator should be selected. Managers do not need to chair or record the minutes of every meeting—rotation of both responsibilities provides the opportunity for all staff to acquire experience in these two processes.

Recording of the minutes, although often seen as an onerous task, can be crucial to the agency's sense of history and continuity. Considerable summarizing and conceptualizing skill is required to capture the essence of decisions made without recording unnecessary detail. Norms about whether names are to be recorded in connection with decisions should also be agreed on in advance.

The facilitator role requires the use of problem-solving and decision-making skills that are as important to the effectiveness of the staff meeting as the subjects being discussed. In addition to fulfilling his or her role as staff member, the facilitator should follow and protect the agreed-on agenda; pay attention to covert events and nonverbal communication; aid in creating a climate of trust; remind the group of its procedures and processes; and facilitate some brief activity at the end of the meeting to help the group examine its processes through a debriefing discussion or a postmeeting reaction sheet that can be tallied, posted, and briefly discussed (see Table 1).

Conducting the Meeting. A number of strategies can increase the likelihood that meeting work will be accomplished effectively. At the beginning of the staff meeting, for example, it is important to start the meeting on time, establish time limits for the length of the meeting, identify agenda items and order them according to their importance, ask participants to contribute additional topics for discussion, and specify ground rules for conducting the meeting. Factors in the opening phase that can hinder the attainment of staff meeting goals are tardiness, absenteeism, lack of clarity about the expected length of the meeting, ambiguity as to the meeting's purposes or goals, a lack of review of previous discussions or decisions, and ambiguity regarding the responsibilities to be assumed by facilitator and staff.

The discussion of each agenda item should be handled separately and should be opened, channeled, and closed in the following manner:

1. *Opening.* Define each issue to be discussed and identify the goals of the discussion—for example, to give information, to collect information for future decision, to make a decision.
2. *Channeling.* Make sure that everyone talks who has important information to give, that rules of discussion are not excessively or insufficiently enforced, that extraneous topics do not interfere with the purpose of the discussion, and that important ideas are restated and clarified. Factors that can hinder the attainment of goals during the channeling phase include: too little or too much conversation; introduction of too many topics; failure to notice or respond to key nonverbal cues; and failure to define confidentiality—namely, what is public and what is confidential information.
3. *Closing:* Make sure discussion does not go overtime, summarize the conclusions reached or not reached, clarify what is going to happen next and who will take responsibility for working on the issue or implementing a decision, and evaluate how well the discussion reached its goal. Factors that can hinder the attainment of goals during the closing phase include not keeping within time limits, not clarifying or defining homework responsibilities, not evaluating how well the meeting achieved its purpose, not answering questions, and not defining or clarifying the problems.

Postmeeting Phase

Some activities in this phase take place immediately after the meeting or on the same day—for example, a thank you to staff for a courageous vote, clarifica-

Table 1. Analyzing Team Effectiveness.

Analyze your team by rating it on a scale from 1 to 7 (7 being what you would consider to be ideal) with respect to each of the dimensions indicated. Then, with the rest of the team, discuss in depth the situation with respect to each dimension, paying particular attention to those for which the average rating is below 5 or for which the range of individual ratings is particularly wide. Formulate some ideas as to why these perceptions exist. The whys are likely to be quite different for different dimensions.

1. *Degree of Mutual Trust*

High suspicion	1 2 3 4 5 6 7	High trust

2. *Degree of Mutual Support*

Every man for himself	1 2 3 4 5 6 7	Genuine concern for each other

3. *Communication*

Guarded, cautious	1 2 3 4 5 6 7	Open, authentic

4. *Team Objectives*

Not understood by team	1 2 3 4 5 6 7	Clearly understood by team

5. *Handling Conflicts Within Team*

Deny, avoid, or suppress conflicts	1 2 3 4 5 6 7	Confront conflicts and work them through

6. *Utilization of Member Resources*

Abilities, knowledge, and experience not utilized by team	1 2 3 4 5 6 7	Abilities, knowledge, and experience fully utilized by team

7. *Control Methods*

Control is imposed on us	1 2 3 4 5 6 7	Control ourselves

8. *Organizational Environment*

Pressure toward conformity, restrictive	1 2 3 4 5 6 7	Free, supportive, respect for individual differences

tion about what was really happening in the meeting, or a brief meeting to set up future meetings in order to ensure that decisions are implemented. Managers may ask staff members for reactions to the content or process of the meeting either directly, as they leave the meeting room enroute to their offices, or through the use of postmeeting reaction forms. The manager may also work with a small group of staff members to analyze the meeting, discuss the follow-up tasks, and allocate assignments. Additional tasks may include writing thank you notes to guest resource people, developing implementation plans, contacting staff members who missed the meeting, making phone calls, and preparing minutes. It is in this phase that management demonstrates the level of its commitment to effective staff meetings.

CITDA Model for Effective Staff Meetings

Staff meetings can sometimes be inhibited by the lack of an explicit, agreed-on, problem-solving model. For example, some staff persons address a problem by seeking to understand its nature, others are more interested in its relevance to the organization, and yet others direct their energy toward thinking of solutions. Each of these approaches has utility if it is part of an overall problem-solving model that the staff can identify and agree on. However, when these approaches to problem solving are not recognized or understood, meetings may result in poor problem solving and sometimes interpersonal conflict.

The following problem-solving model, developed by the London School of Business and amplified by the author, consists of five major steps or components, which will be described in terms of the major activities of each step, typical obstacles to problem solving occurring in each step, and strategies for overcoming those obstacles. The five components of the CITDA model are clarification, information giving, testing, decision making, and action planning.

Clarification: Problem Identification and Selection

This first step focuses on clarifying and understanding the particular problem by asking the following questions: (1) What are the facts pertaining to the problem? (2) How do we evaluate these data? (3) What is the source of the problem? (4) How serious is the problem? (5) Who or what is adversely affected by the problem now and in the future? (6) Who or what benefits from the problem?

These questions and their answers serve to clarify the basic issue: What is the problem situation that needs remedying? This diagnostic activity is no different in quality or purpose from a clinician's attempts to understand the nature and extent of a patient's illness. Developing a problem statement—according to guidelines such as those presented in Table 2—is an important part of clarifying the problem in order to select a solution.

Obstacles to the clarification process include the false assumptions that everyone agrees on the definition of the problem, that the problem is not definable in specific terms, and that discussion of solutions takes place before the problem is fully identified. Another obstacle to clarification is an overly abstract definition of the problem. Often groups reach agreement about a problem at such a general level that they move into the solution phase before dealing with the complexities of the problem. Such a false sense of shared understanding can inhibit questions about specific issues that need to be understood for informed problem solving to take place. In addition, staff meeting participants, in this early stage, frequently spend too much time on specific solutions before having thought through how they would like the situation to be when the problem is reduced or solved. Groups should delay discussion of detailed solutions in order to complete this stage of the clarification process.

Table 2. Four Guidelines for Writing a Problem Statement.

The following four questions can serve as guidelines for writing a problem statement:

1. *Who is affected?* Consider these possibilities before deciding what you want to say about this: Is it you? Is it one other person? Is it a small group of people? Is it an entire organization? Is it the community or society at large?

2. *Who is causing it?* We frequently speak of problems as though they were caused by circumstances that did not relate directly to people, but this is almost never the case. Almost always, some person or persons could make a difference.

3. *What kind of a problem is it?*

   • Lack of clarity or agreement about goals?
   • Lack of clarity or agreement about the means of achieving goals?
   • Lack of skill needed to address the means?
   • Lack of material resources?
   • Inaccurate communication or too little or too much communication?
   • Different understanding of the same thing?
   • Insufficient time or schedule conflicts?
   • Roles lacking or inappropriate?
   • Norms restrictive, unclear, or misinterpreted?
   • Lack of clarity or agreement about decision making, resulting in power struggles?
   • Inappropriate or inadequate expression of feelings?
   • Conflict related to individual differences or ideologies?

4. *What is the goal for improvement?* Ideally, this goal should be stated so clearly that anyone reading your statement would know how to determine when the goal had been reached. The statement should tell exactly who will be doing what, where, how, and to what extent. Until you know where you are going, it is very difficult to make and implement plans to get there.

The following strategies and tactics are useful in reducing obstacles and facilitating movement through the clarification stage: (1) encourage members to ask questions; (2) establish a temporary devil's advocate role or period of time when members can freely challenge or question agreements or understandings; (3) establish a norm of fighting the tendency for early and easy agreement about a problem; and (4) ask group members for their understanding of the problem to see if that understanding is shared.

Idea Giving

At some point, when the problem seems to be understood, the group needs to engage in an idea-generating session in order to explore ways and means of solving the problem. The premium here is on spontaneity and individuality of ideas. The group often possesses ideas that can be helpful in problem solving, but an atmosphere must be created that encourages the emergence of these ideas. Obstacles to idea giving include lack of group experience, inadequate knowledge of a particular problem, or, more frequently, a negative group climate that tends to reduce the sharing of information and smother innovative ideas.

In order to offset these obstacles to the expression of relevant and original ideas, the following strategies should be considered:

1. Divide large groups into smaller groups to reduce formality and threat.
2. Use the brainstorming technique, which is based on the notion of separating the giving from the evaluation of ideas. This technique will not only help the emergence of original notions but also contribute to a satisfying and energy-creating climate.
3. Search other systems, including the literature, for relevant ideas.
4. Consider engaging a consultant whose area of expertise matches the group's interest.

Testing

The third step in this problem-solving process involves testing the feasibility of the ideas advanced in the second step and replacing interesting but impractical ideas with more realistic notions. Many obstacles to this phase of group problem solving exist. For example, lack of experience with a problem may prevent effective reality testing. Without hard data, a group may give opinions disguised as facts—especially inimical to problem solving if these opinions are given by influential persons in the group. Another obstacle is the unwillingness of the group to fully consider the implications of alternatives. In addition, groupthink hinders problem solving by preventing people from bringing up problems that must be faced if an idea is to prove useful to the organization. Janis (1973) outlines eight symptoms of groupthink:

1. *Illusion of invulnerability.* Nothing to lose, take excessive risks. Complacency leads to being unprepared and to feeling secure.
2. *Shared stereotypes.* When stress to reach a decision arises, groups increase their "we" feeling.
3. *Rationalization.* "Explaining away" the issues confronting the group.
4. *Direct pressure on the deviant member.* Groups pool resources to increase individual investment.
5. *Illusion of morality.* Enables members to maintain self-esteem.
6. *Self-censorship.* If you counter the group, you will get censored by the group so you do not counter the group.
7. *Illusion of unanimity.* All members feel they are a cohesive unit. Doubters do not express doubts.
8. *Mind-guarding.* Keeps leader and others in the group from hearing divergent opinions.

Strategies that can be used to overcome these obstacles are: role playing to test the feasibility of an idea; tabling the agenda until another committee has an opportunity to gather more information; and establishing a devil's advocate role, which legitimizes criticism, helps to surface ideas that reflect the worst possibilities, and allows for thorough exploration of alternatives.

Decision Making

Since groups often feel some pressure to arrive at a decision prematurely, it is important that the final decision be made only after the first three steps have been taken. At this point, the group selects the solution that seems to have the greatest probability of solving or reducing the problem, based on the information the group has been able to obtain. One of the obstacles to this phase is the tendency to use majority vote as the primary decision-making technique. However democratic it may sound, this approach tends to alienate losing members from the majority and may lead to lack of commitment to the decision on the part of those who voted against it.

As an alternative, consensus decision making, however time-consuming and difficult to effect, has potential not only for reaching the best decision possible from the group but also for creating the widest and deepest commitment to that decision. Consensus requires a climate that actively values differing viewpoints; a sense that each person's ideas are listened to and acknowledged, although not necessarily accepted as the idea the group will adopt; and some commitment from each person to the agreed-on decision.

Action Planning

Group members tend to assume that decision making, rather than action planning, is the final phase of problem solving and therefore may leave a meeting thinking that action planning will be taken care of by others. In order to prevent this misunderstanding, specific action planning should occur immediately after the decision-making phase so as to involve staff members directly. A further obstacle to action planning is a lack of sufficient reality testing or data gathering in earlier phases. A thorough planning phase may reveal the inadequacy of earlier phases and may force the group to reformulate the problem and the solution, perhaps requiring a recycling of the whole process. In action planning, as in other phases of the process, the consensus method, however time-consuming, increases commitment to the ultimate goal—in this case, plan implementation. Some of the strategies for overcoming these obstacles to action planning include brainstorming, role playing to test the plan, and dividing into small groups to devise plans to be shared with the larger group and combined into an overall plan.

By following these five steps to effective problem solving—clarification, information giving, testing, decision making, and action planning—the staff can move toward a shared course of action based on agreement and clarity as to who will take what action when. This course of action is based on a shared evaluation of the goals sought and the problem to be solved, as well as on a shared understanding of the data used in the problem definition and the terms used in the discussion. Ideally, this shared course of action will contribute to mutual trust among staff members and administration, enabling each person in the agency to contribute his or her resources to managing the staff meeting.

Norms for Effective Staff Meetings

A major ingredient for effective staff meetings is the establishment of and adherence to a set of ground rules that serve as a substitute for Roberts' Rules of Order in small, informal meetings. These norms, if selected and developed consciously and collectively by the staff, can contribute to orderly staff meeting process, to efficient use of staff time and resources, and to a sense of accomplishment and group satisfaction. The following list presents a number of possible norms:

1. Members check to make sure they know what a speaker means before they agree or disagree. This norm helps the group separate understanding from evaluation. When paraphrased and closely but not judgmentally examined, ideas that at first seem unclear often prove useful.

2. Members express their own reaction to an event or interaction or idea and do not attribute that reaction to others or give the impression that they are speaking for others.

3. All contributions are viewed as belonging to the group and are to be used as the group decides. A member who makes a suggestion does not need to defend it; instead, all accept responsibility for evaluating the suggestion as the joint property of the group.

4. All members participate, but in different and complementary ways. Some members are more task-oriented, whereas others are more concerned about interpersonal dimensions. Therefore, while some members are providing information, others should be making sure that information is understood by the group. Some members are adept at identifying points of agreement or disagreement; others are skilled at facilitating communication between members who might tend to disagree. Also, a given member does not always participate in the same way—each member's role changes appropriately from situation to situation.

5. Whenever the group senses it is having difficulty getting work done, it tries to find out why. Symptoms of difficulty include excessive repetition of the same points; suggestions being offered but not considered; private conversation in subgroups; the domination of the conversation by two or three people; members continually taking sides and refusing to consider compromise; members' ideas being attacked before they are completely explained; and apathetic participation. When such symptoms occur, the group is able to shift from working on tasks to discussing the interpersonal or problem-solving processes that may be causing these problems. Occasional discussions of interpersonal issues clear the air, allowing the group to work more effectively on the task.

6. The group recognizes that it accomplishes what it has chosen to accomplish—no group can avoid making decisions. Thus, an effective group makes decisions openly, rather than by default. Decisions by default are felt as failures by group members and can create tension. A group grows more by openly agreeing not to act than by not acting because they cannot agree.

7. Members recognize that conflict is inevitable in interaction and deal with
    conflict openly, rather than letting it get out of control by disguising it.
8. The group takes the view that behavior that hinders its work is allowed or
    welcomed by the group and is not just the result of a so-called problem
    member.

Typical Staff Meeting Roles

The work ethic, the demand for productivity in social agencies, and the
general reluctance of professionals to disclose their doubts and worries about their
work have contributed to overly task-oriented staff meetings in many mental
health agencies. These meetings are usually characterized by a long agenda, limited time, and a pressure to make decisions. The very human needs of staff
members and administrators are rarely addressed; indeed, the pressures of these
meetings sometimes add to the woes and worries of the staff. However, administrators need to recognize the importance of attending to the social and emotional
needs of staff by gaining more awareness of the individual and social aspects of
staff behavior. Table 3 describes three types of behaviors employed both by administrators and by staff members: work roles, maintenance roles, and blocking roles.

Blocking behaviors may occur in response to an excessive task orientation
at the staff meeting or to a failure to meet some of the social and emotional
concerns of the members. Work roles include several different subroles that can
help a group complete a task at hand. Maintenance roles include a range of
subroles that help support the social and psychological needs of members. Administrators and staff members who effectively and sincerely demonstrate work and
maintenance roles in a staff meeting are contributing to the accomplishment of
organizational goals and the needs of staff. Most individuals are socialized in early
life to be either task-oriented or maintenance-oriented, but rarely both. However,
one can widen one's repertoire of roles through awareness and practice—task-
oriented persons can increase their maintenance behaviors, and maintenance-
oriented persons can increase their task-directed behaviors. In contrast, the
blocking behavior may indicate to the administrator and the rest of the staff that
time and energy need to be directed to meeting the social and psychological needs
of the staff.

Effective Decision Making

In this section, we will explore several aspects of group decision making for
managing staff meetings, including the problems encountered in decision making, some types of decision making, conditions that facilitate effective decision
making, and ways of engaging in decision making.

In order to achieve its goals, a staff meeting must engage in making decisions: big decisions, little decisions, easy decisions, hard decisions, right decisions,
wrong decisions—but inevitably decisions. Thus, decision making reflects a continuous pattern of relationships among staff members over which every individual

Table 3. Roles Assumed by Administrators and Staff Members.

Work Roles

1. *Initiator.* Proposing tasks, goals, or actions; defining group problems; suggesting a procedure.
2. *Informer.* Offering facts; expressing feelings; getting an opinion.
3. *Clarifier.* Interpreting ideas or suggestions; defining terms; clarifying issues before the group.
4. *Summarizer.* Pulling together related ideas; restating suggestions; offering a decision or conclusion for the group to consider.
5. *Reality tester.* Critically analyzing an idea; testing an idea against data to see whether the idea would work.

Maintenance Roles

1. *Harmonizer.* Attempting to reconcile disagreements; reducing tensions; getting people to explore differences.
2. *Gatekeeper.* Helping to keep communication channels open; facilitating the participation of others; suggesting procedures that permit sharing of remarks.
3. *Consensus tester.* Asking to see if the group is nearing its decision; sending up a trial balloon to test a possible solution.
4. *Encourager.* Being friendly, warm, and responsive to others; indicating by facial expressions or words the acceptance of others' contributions.
5. *Compromiser.* Offering a compromise that sacrifices his or her own status; admitting an error; modifying a position in the interest of group cohesion or growth.

Blocking Roles

1. *Aggressor.* Deflating others' status; attacking the group or its values; joking in a concealed way.
2. *Blocker.* Disagreeing and opposing unreasonably; stubbornly resisting the group's wish for personal reasons; using a hidden agenda to thwart the movement of the group.
3. *Dominator.* Asserting authority or superiority to manipulate the group or certain group members; interrupting the contributions of others; controlling by means of flattery or other forms of patronizing behavior.
4. *Play person.* Making a display in playful fashion of one's lack of involvement; "abandoning" the group while remaining physically present; seeking recognition in ways not relevant to the group task.
5. *Avoidance behavior.* Pursuing special interests not related to task; staying off a subject to avoid commitment; preventing the group from facing controversy.

member has influence. A bit of information, a loud objection, an expression of approval or hostility, envy or admiration, contempt or condescension, can influence an impending decision. Therefore, it is little wonder that group after group has difficulty making decisions. Some become paralyzed or argue interminably when confronted with a decision; others rush into a vote only to reverse a decision later or fail to carry it out; others appoint a committee or look for a savior (sometimes the chairperson) to avoid making a collective decision. The reasons for difficulty in decision making are manifold, and the following list includes only a few:

- *Fear of consequences.* What will people think if we decide to walk out?
- *Conflicting loyalties.* What position will the finance committee, for example, want me to take in the meeting of the building committee?

- *Interpersonal conflict.* Often we find ourselves disagreeing regularly with the ideas of someone we dislike.
- *Procedural blundering.* A group may be so bound by rigid procedures that there is little chance for free expression or real differences of opinion.
- *Inadequate leadership.* Members of the committee may be coerced into acceptance of the chairperson's pet ideas.

The following types of decisions reflect the most common actions made in staff meetings:

1. *Plops.* A decision suggested by an individual to which there is no response. Plopping often occurs in a new group confronted by many problems; in a group where a number of members have fairly equal status; when a member is overaggressive; when a member has difficulty articulating the decision; or when a low-status member makes a suggestion.
2. *Self-authorized decisions.* A decision made by an individual who assumes the authority to do so. When such a decision is proposed, the group as a whole often finds it easier to accept than reject, even though some individuals may not be in agreement. Such decisions are made by default.
3. *Hand clasping.* A decision made by two members of the group joining forces. Such a decision, emerging suddenly, may catch the other members off guard and at the same time present them with the additional problem of dealing with two people at once. But it may also be perceived that the two members are giving leadership to the group and are actually moving the group forward.
4. *Topic jumping.* A decision cut short by the inappropriate intrusion of another topic. Topic jumping confuses the issue confronting the group and thus changes the nature of the decision.
5. *Majority rule.* A decision made by some form of voting. The traditional procedure of taking a vote often seems to be the only way to reach a decision under the given circumstances. Nevertheless, the minority may oppose the decision despite the vote and are therefore not likely to act in support of it.
6. *The clique.* A decision by several members of the group based on advance collaboration. Cliques exist in almost every group, and their prearranged decisions may be positive, but often the effect of this activity is to destroy group cohesion and trust.
7. *Fear of disagreement.* A decision made as a result of pressure not to disagree. When confronted by such pressure, several persons who strongly disagree or have not had the opportunity to express their opinion on the issue might show reluctance to voice opposition in the absence of apparent support.
8. *We all agree, don't we?* A decision made by pressure to agree. Again, persons who really disagree or have not had the opportunity to express their opinions would probably be reluctant to voice opposition by themselves.
9. *Unanimity.* A decision made by overt and unanimous consent. The pressure to conform may be strong enough to win apparent one hundred percent agreement, but a majority of the members may actually disagree.

10. *Consensus.* A decision made after allowing all aspects of the issue, both positive and negative, to be put forward and ensuring that everyone openly agrees. Dissenters, if they have been clearly heard, will usually go along with the decision and act on it with commitment.

Decision-making groups perform more effectively when the following five conditions are present: democratic leadership that checks out issues with the group is employed; flexible patterns of communication are used, in which minority opinions are encouraged; a collaborative approach is used, in which members seek to build on each other's ideas, rather than put each other down; atmosphere is open, candid, and accepting of differences; and shared decision-making techniques are used to protect the rights of individuals against the power of the dominant few. In addition, the decision-making method itself influences what decisions are reached. Table 4 presents six decision-making methods commonly used by individuals and groups.

Table 4. Six Approaches to Group Decision Making.

I. *Intuitive.* Emphasizes the feeling component of decision making but tends to be haphazard and risky.

Stages: 1. A felt problem bothers an individual.
2. Individual links up with others, and they ventilate their feelings in an informal group.
3. All search individually for some appropriate action.
4. They attempt to share ideas and produce group feeling.
5. They attempt to act together.
6. They look back.

Difficulties: Tends to be haphazard and may not produce results.

II. *Structuralist.* Emphasizes determining who is responsible for what and assumes that each group member will carry out his or her own responsibilities.

Stages: 1. A set of tasks is allocated to different staff members.
2. Some of these tasks are reallocated by others.
3. Each person carries out his or her responsibilities.
4. The measure of success is the degree to which everyone completes the activities for which he or she has authority.
5. If this approach is not working, the solution is to change the structure.

Difficulties: 1. Some tasks are always left unallocated, since it is difficult to think of everything.
2. People assigned responsibility may sabotage the decision-making process.
3. This approach requires extensive control over every activity.
4. The prejudices of individuals who delegate authority and those who receive authority are reinforced and reflected in the decision-making process.

III. *Dialectic.* An analytical method involving confrontation over a wide range of topics using argumentation and lengthy discussions.

Stages: 1. Examine the ostensible problem.
2. Define what the real problem is.
3. Record all the relevant facts and ideas.

Table 4, cont'd.

4. Explore alternative solutions. Swap views and ideas.
5. Test alternative solutions.

Difficulties: 1. Slow and time-consuming and therefore not to be used for all decisions.
2. The definition of the problem itself may solve the problem, so that further action is not necessary. However, this approach may proceed too narrowly, with focus on one single problem to the neglect of related problems.
3. Tends to ignore the organizational context of decision making.

IV. *Incrementalist.* A pragmatic, opportunistic approach that emphasizes learning by doing and taking quick, arbitrary actions.

Stages: 1. No use looking for problems—look for opportunities to get something done.
2. Proceed step-by-step, making small, minor changes wherever possible.
3. Select the most convenient and apparent problem. If too much resistance or too many constraints arise, drop the problem.
4. Look carefully at strengths and weaknesses; build on strengths. Do not bother recouping on failures or weaknesses.
5. Plan strategies for making use of opportunities, and identify those people most likely to resist.
6. Take action and define problems as you go along. "Chaotic action is preferable to orderly inaction."

Difficulties: Doing what comes easiest is not always the best approach; it can lead to chaos and a lack of coordination.

V. *Microrationalist.* Managing by objectives, with careful attention to specifying anticipated outcomes.

Stages: 1. Each individual specifies objectives for the organization from his or her own perspective.
2. Each individual also defines personal objectives related to his or her own needs and skill requirements.
3. Look at potential obstacles and predict what will happen when resistance arises.
4. Take action on the objectives.

Difficulties: Preoccupation with specific details can blind one to the larger realities.

VI. *Macrorationalist.* Seeks to gain a total picture of the organization's goals and objectives.

Stages: 1. Where are we coming from?
2. Where do we want to go?
3. Define the criteria of success in assessing problem solution.
4. Define the problem, its potential causes, and the necessary decisions.
5. Determine all possible courses of action.
6. List possible advantages and disadvantages. ("The more we attempt to predict, the more we will be able to forestall failure.")
7. Specify ideas regarding the decision to be made.
8. Take action.
9. Evaluate the action.

Difficulties: 1. This process is very time-consuming.
2. It must be carried out well for all subsequent decisions to fall into place.
3. The process requires considerable coordination and staff involvement.

Conclusion

Group leaders and group members alike must meet the challenge of conducting effective and satisfying staff meetings. This chapter is based on the assumption that staff meeting management can be improved by sensitizing all participants to the roles played by leaders and followers and to the group processes that underlie staff meeting activity. Guidelines have been drawn from the field of group dynamics to provide mental health managers with the knowledge and skills necessary for conducting effective and enlivening staff meetings.

References

Janis, I. *Group Dynamics—Group Think*. Film, University of Washington Instructional Media Center, 1973.

Mehrabian, A. *Public Places and Private Spaces*. New York: Basic Books, 1976.

Proshansky, H., and others (Eds.). *Environmental Psychology: Man and His Physical Space*. New York: Holt, Rinehart and Winston, 1970.

Summer, R. *Personal Space*. Englewood Cliffs, N.J.: Prentice-Hall, 1969.

ℨ 11 ℨ

The Manager
as Problem Solver

William E. Hershey

In the daily administrative activities of mental health program managers, group process skills are critical. This chapter examines how differing values, politics, communication and leadership styles, and interpersonal skills of mental health administrators influence the problem-solving process. Distinguishing between the process and the content of problem solving, William Hershey presents a useful, composite framework that divides the content into five major phases: (1) problem identification, (2) formulation of action alternatives, (3) feasibility testing, (4) selection of strategy for implementation, and (5) implementation, adoption, and diffusion of solution. An analytical process for problem definition is offered, the major problem-solving issues faced by program managers are addressed, and hypothetical case studies are presented and analyzed.

The program director at a community mental health center is faced with a difficult problem. Space in the center is at a premium; a new computer will be installed within the year; new program staff will be added in six to nine months; and renovations are needed to comply with federal regulations on handicapped accessibility. The problem is whether to move, to acquire new space, or to renovate present space. Where should she begin?

Another mental health administrator is confronted with a crisis. The program manager of the center's day treatment services has just resigned, giving as cause the inability to function under prevailing conditions—the third resignation of a day treatment manager in a year and a half. The staff is demoralized, and the quality of services delivery is slipping. In addition, there has been pressure to hire more minority staff members in administrative positions. Something must be done. Should the process of hiring be approached differently?

In order to manage problem solving and decision making in mental health settings, program administrators need to master the interplay of content and process in those two key management functions. In addition, administrators are expected to manage the communication process, giving due consideration to the influence of values, politics, personal communication styles, leadership preferences, and key interpersonal skills. This chapter will examine content—including problem-solving frameworks, decision-making grids, and other basic tools of analysis needed for this role—as well as process—interpersonal communication skills, values clarification, political considerations, and leadership styles.

Problem solving is a process whereby a problem is identified and alternative solutions are proposed. Decision making is the process of developing criteria for selecting among the proposed alternatives and developing and implementing the selected strategy (Maple, 1977). In this chapter, the term *problem solving* will be used to encompass all aspects of the process, from the rational and developmental (moving in a smooth, orderly fashion from problem definition to alternative solutions to implementation) to the crisis-oriented (requiring quick reactions and constant incremental adaptations of problem definitions and alternative solutions) (Cyert and March, 1963).

How program managers approach problem solving depends on a combination of personal disposition, patterns of dealing with life/work tasks, values conditioned by education and training, political concerns, choices of communication style, and leadership preferences. Managing the process requires attention to each of these elements.

Personal Disposition and Values

Every manager has a particular style or disposition for approaching problems, as well as a set of values that condition how the problem is defined and solved. Managers view problems and alternatives through a screen that is shaped by their own personal training, values, disposition, and personal goals (Mannheim, 1952). Situations are perceived as right or wrong, true or false, preferred or not preferred, desirable or undesirable, depending on the patterns of action and thought developed by managers for dealing with conflicts and challenges in their personal or work lives. These patterns, formed through a combination of circumstances involving family socialization, education, and life experiences, regulate a person's tendency to prefer structure or looseness, give or take, inclusion or exclusion, control or passivity, and can be evaluated by managers with measures like FIRO-B (Schutz, 1977), which measures disposition for inclusion-exclusion and control. In the crisis of needing to employ a new day treatment manager, for example, no affirmative action plan could be implemented successfully in the hiring process unless the personal preferences of the administrator confirmed that minorities or handicapped persons were important additions to the agency.

Administrators of mental health centers should recognize that the staff and board members of the agency also have personal dispositions toward problems and use value screens reflecting interests, preferences, choices, and goals that may vary from those of the administrator. These values often remain hidden unless addressed directly. For example, the administrator who adopts a consensus style for defining problems will bring issues of value to the surface and provide a process of clarification for reaching a consensus on those issues. Such a manager believes that, unless such a consensus is reached, unresolved value issues may block even simple decisions. For example, the process of recruiting, interviewing, and selecting a candidate for a management position may meet with multiple problems. Recruitment and selection processes may be confounded by some staff members wanting to apply for a vacant position while the board wants a nationwide search in order to select someone from outside the agency. Such decision making may be further confounded by the larger value issue of whether the center's services should be expanded, as the staff might believe, or reduced and made more cost effective, as the board might believe. Therefore, the failure to reach consensus on such value concerns related to the agency's mission and program may block an otherwise simple replacement process.

An administrator whose view of organization is political might not try to reach consensus but rather use the various perspectives as counterpoints for negotiating or for adjusting power between factions within the agency. For example, an administrator in the midst of a struggle for unionization might not be able to find a consensus between staff and board values but instead might see to it that the values inherent in each point of view were exposed at the beginning of the negotiations. Regardless of how value screens are used, one must recognize that the personal values of key individuals do influence the decision-making process.

The manager's personal preferences in working with others in approaching problems is another key to how the problem will be defined and solved. Is he or she more concerned with people or production? The individual manager must assess his or her own approach to people-process matters and to the accomplishment of a task (Blake and Mouton, 1978). How one responds to the feelings of others and how one communicates make a difference in problem solving. In the case of hiring the day treatment manager, the administrator who is concerned about people's feelings would extend the time frame for hiring by including in the process adequate samplings of staff and board views. Approaches to ensure this feedback would include staff representation on screening committees, a board committee to help develop more realistic job descriptions and performance standards, and a board-staff search committee designed to expand the candidate pool. A manager more attuned to production would tend to shorten the hiring process by setting clear objectives for completion with a minimum of staff and board involvement.

At every level of problem solving, the manager's value screen is in operation. In deciding the criteria for selecting one alternative over another, an administrator must determine what values are relevant to the problem being analyzed and on what basis they are to be considered. For example, one such value question in the first case cited at the beginning of this chapter would involve a choice between moving and renovating. How costly would it be to move, and how costly to stay? Is the manager by nature frugal, cautious, and conservative? A crisis-oriented manager might seek to cut costs related to a particular solution without looking too long or hard at the effects of the cuts. A more fiscally conservative manager might push for cost controls, with specific targets set, performance reviewed in accord with predetermined standards, and nothing left to chance. A manager who valued a more rational, developmental approach might call for a comparison of the cost effectiveness of moving with the cost effectiveness of staying. An entrepreneurial manager would seek to influence the decision making by emphasizing potentially valuable outcomes to be derived from moving while deemphasizing other options. In each case, the value screen introduced by the manager influences the problem-solving and decision-making process (National Family Planning Management Institute, 1972).

In the recruiting, screening, and selecting of new staff, a manager's personal values and preferences are especially evident. Managers often feel anxious when faced with the selection of a new supervisor with whom they will be working closely, who performs similar administrative tasks, and who may have a similar background and family history. Interactional rituals similar to courting take place (Goffman, 1973), and numerous subjective judgments are involved.

Leadership Styles

An administrator's style of leadership and communication also affects the decision-making process. Managers who have an authoritarian leadership style will attempt to persuade others that their point of view is correct and, if possible, enforce and dominate the decision-making process, keeping the problem definition and the choice of alternative solutions to themselves. For example, in our first case study, an authoritarian manager might seek to control the definition of the problem early in the process by establishing a property search committee. On the other hand, a manager with a more accommodating and compliant leadership style would allow staff and board to participate equally in the problem-solving process, soliciting their reactions to problem definition and encouraging a variety of alternative solutions. This approach can be quite productive if a purposeful planning process is provided to assist problem solving. However, if a person with such an open style exerts too little leadership, the problem may grow to crisis proportions as problem definitions and alternative solutions proliferate.

Evidence also suggests that managers who adopt a participative, democratic leadership style tend to be successful in stimulating board and staff involvement in organizational decision making and usually establish communication patterns that allow for an open, informative, exploratory problem-solving process. The primary value of this style of leadership is that it usually ensures a higher degree of commitment to the problem's solution than do other leadership styles and allows numerous conflicting viewpoints to contribute to problem definition and the development of alternative solutions.

Some managers might tend to avoid problems or, worse yet, tend to be defensive when problems or disturbances occur. This leadership style quickly evolves into a reactive or crisis approach to problem solving, in which one tolerates those disturbances that cannot be avoided or suppressed. For example, the administrator with the office space problem might be tempted to postpone the decision on new space, since the need to comply with the regulations for accessibility for the handicapped is more than a year away. By neglecting to set up a committee to study the problem or to present alternatives to the board of directors, managers with a tendency to flee from problems or to procrastinate soon find themselves faced with a crisis.

Even with the best of managerial intentions, however, crisis leadership orientation toward problem solving tends to be less a matter of personal choice than a realistic description of the present state of management. Future events are so uncertain, adequate information is so spotty, and each decision is so contingent on other circumstances that rational planning toward clear goals is practically impossible (Cyert and March, 1963). The administrator in our first case would have difficulty convincing the board directors of the need for new space if they view funding for the new program as problematic and the handicapped regulations as having "no teeth."

Each of these personal styles of leadership is, in turn, influenced by personal values and beliefs about organizations and services. One style is not necessarily better than another, although the participative style seems to be the most successful for getting decisions implemented. In fact, depending on the time available to solve the problem, the amount of information needed or at hand, the amount of resistance, and the relative importance of joint commitment, more than one style might prove helpful. The important point is that a manager's personal choice of leadership style influences the entire problem-solving process.

Equally important, managers must remember that, whatever leadership style is assumed, they are leading task-oriented groups and therefore need to recall what they learned as clinicians about group process: groups go through stages of development; norms for behavior will surface; informal alliances will form; roles will emerge to define the kinds of permissible interactions for the group; and conflict is important for creative interaction. When managers begin to apply group process information to the actual decision-making process, they will recognize, for example, that a group might not be ready to make a decision or that the stage of development still reflects a lack of trust. They should also note that nonverbal communication and environmental factors like room comfort are important to problem solving (Perrow, 1978).

Political Elements

Problem solving and decision making also involve consideration of political issues such as power, position, gain, loss, advantage, control, and survival (Miringoff, 1980). Who is going to give the agency trouble if we do this? What will we lose by moving? Can we afford to offend the United Way by taking these steps? Often political considerations will dominate decision making when a clear problem-solving process or strong personal convictions are lacking. Therefore, attention to the interplay of political and value considerations is crucial. For example, the program manager in our case study may be unable to promote a particularly well-qualified staff member to the position of day treatment manager because certain board members are personally opposed to the individual.

Analytical and Interactional Tasks of Problem Solving

The problem-solving process includes both analytical and interactional tasks (Perlman and Gurin, 1972). As Table 1 indicates, the analytical tasks engage the administrator in making cognitive choices among various data-gathering instruments, types of actions to be considered in the problem-solving process, limits of problem definition, types of committee structures used to involve others, key agents, and criteria for goal selection. The interactional tasks involve eliciting and receiving information from others, delegating responsibility, presenting alternatives to decision makers, and marshaling resources. Analytical tasks involve considerable thought and reflection; interactional tasks require such qualities as tact, sympathy, initiative, perseverance, and faith in self and others.

The process of thinking through all aspects of a perceived problem is traditionally approached by looking at the data and reaching a conclusion based on either deductive or inductive methods. However, complex problems sometimes defy all deductive and inductive attempts to solve them. In recent years, another method, trial-and-error thinking, has been applied to unblock the thought process. In early childhood, most learning occurs through feedback from trial-and-error behavior—making things move, fitting objects into corresponding spaces, attempting to control objects or persons. In play, trial-and-error behavior predominates, offering opportunities to experiment with novel situations (Maier, 1980). For example, Watson and Crick used the trial-and-error method in their search for the structure of DNA, playing with sticks for a whole night, until they happened on the idea that DNA consists of a double-helix structure (Watson, 1968). Play involves inventing, and inventing is a key to the learning-thinking process. For this reason, Boeing Aircraft Company executives go on retreats in which they play with ideas in the process of tackling a complex problem, and creative thinktanks are provided for planning staffs in other companies.

Facing a problem can be a grim experience, or it can be creative, and educators have long recognized that creative solutions to problems tend to emerge in the midst of perseverance, diligence, and hard work. Often, however, the solution does not come, and dullness, rather than brilliance, may characterize the enterprise. Recently, the introduction of the Japanese concept of *satori* to this process has provided a new understanding of the relationship between creativity and problem solving.

In expertness, the highest point attainable is satori, a sudden flash of enlightenment (Torrance, 1979). In addition to persistence and hard work, attainment of satori requires intensive absorption, practice, and minimizing outside distractions. The approach entails being immersed in the details of the problem and at the same time letting go of one's personal involvement. For example, in private industry, thinktank rooms are equipped with waterbeds and whirlpool baths for executives in the midst of creative planning. The executives are expected to dig as deep as possible, work on the problem until exhausted, and then let go of it as they lie in the waterbed or relax in the whirlpool. Often the "aha!" of creative solution appears as the subconscious works overtime. Similarly, Japanese trainees

Table 1. Analytical and Interactional Tasks of the Phases of Problem Solving.

	Analytical Tasks	*Interactional Tasks*
1. Defining the problem	Studying and describing the problematical aspects of a situation. Conceptualizing the system of relevant actors. Assessing what opportunities and limits are set by the organization employing the practitioner and by other actors.	Eliciting and receiving information, grievances, and preferences from those experiencing the problem and from other sources.
2. Building structure	Determining the nature of the practitioner's relationship to various actors. Deciding types of structures to be developed. Choosing persons as experts, communicators, influencers, and so on.	Establishing formal and informal lines of communication. Recruiting persons into the selected structures and roles and obtaining their commitment to address the problem.
3. Formulating policy	Analyzing past efforts to deal with the problem. Developing alternative goals and strategies, assessing their possible consequences and feasibility. Selecting one or more of those goals or strategies for recommendation to decision makers.	Communicating alternative goals and strategies to selected actors. Promoting their expression of preferences and testing acceptance of various alternatives. Assisting decision makers to choose.
4. Implementing plans	Specifying what tasks need to be performed by whom, when, and with what resources and procedures to achieve agreed-on goals.	Presenting requirements to decision makers, overcoming resistances, and obtaining commitments to the program. Marshaling resources and putting procedures into operation.
5. Monitoring	Designing system for collecting information on operations. Analyzing feedback data and specifying adjustments needed and new problems that require planning and action.	Obtaining information from relevant actors based on their experience. Communicating findings and recommendations and preparing actors for a new round of decisions to be made.

for new bank positions undertake painful endurance hikes as part of their orientation and experience flashes of exhilaration and creativity at that time and long afterward (Torrance, 1979). Often satori works best in group problem solving, either in dyads or in brainstorming groups. Although brainstorming—a technique in which only positive ideas, no matter how bizarre, are encouraged to flow unhindered without comment—is usually applied to seeking alternative solutions to problems, the same method can produce creative insights in the problem-definition phase, as well. Creative dramatics or sociodramas may also be applied to the problem. Excellent results from the use of satori techniques have encouraged managers to apply the so-called right, or creative, aspect of the brain to difficult problems and not just to assume that problem solving is a totally rational, left-brain process.

In summary, a manager's approach to problem solving includes: the choice and activation of a leadership communication style or pattern; the choice of key interactional tasks related to the process; analytical and interactional tasks centered on problem description, design of the system, and appropriate structure; attention to value issues, political considerations, and personal dispositions; and allowance for time to be creative. These activities might be described as the process of problem solving and decision making. These practices then are applied to each of the decision-making content areas—problem identification, formulation of action alternatives, and implementation of the solution—which will be described in detail later in this chapter. The interaction of process and content elements in the problem-solving framework is described in Table 2.

Problem-Solving Frameworks

In addition to identifying the numerous prejudgments, political concerns, personal values, leadership styles, and communication patterns that influence the problem-solving process, a manager must recognize that there are different content models for decision making. A composite model—including identifying the problem, determining available alternative solutions, selecting a strategy, and implementing the strategy—affords a middle ground between brief models and more complex presentations. The *S-T-P* model is an example of a shorthand approach (see Table 3): describe the *situation* as it is now and the conditions that are causing disturbance; identify the *target* or goal; and outline the *process* needed to reach the target (Manzell, 1965).

Pino, Jung, and Emory (1971) present a more complex model that includes: identification of the concern; diagnosis of the situation; formulating action alternatives; feasibility testing of selected alternatives (including training and evaluation); and adoption, implementation, and diffusion of good alternatives. This model includes a force field analysis that defines problem situations in terms of the driving forces, which push toward improvement, and the restraining forces, which resist improvement. According to the model, driving and restraining forces are identified, forces most easily and constructively acted on are selected, and action steps are identified and given priorities. Persons responsible for carrying out each action are then chosen. Such detailed models can be used as outlines for developing grant proposals or for solving more complex problems when sufficient time is available. For example, the Pino and others model might be useful for the agency problem related to adequate space but not for the problem of hiring the new day treatment manager.

Once managers are clear that they need to utilize interpersonal skills relating to leadership styles, values, and group process, they are ready to examine the steps of problem solving. The problem-solving model presented in this discussion, continuing aspects of the S-T-P model and the Pino and others model, involves:

Table 2. Problem-Solving Framework.

PROCESS ELEMENTS	CONTENT ELEMENTS		
	A. Problem Identification 1. Gathering data 2. Writing problem statement a. problem specification b. problem analysis	B. Formulation of Action Alternative	C. Implementation, Adoption, and Diffusion of Solution
A. Leadership Styles 1. Open, exploring, developmental 2. Authoritarian, controlling 3. Accommodating, compliant 4. Crisis-oriented 5. Defensive, hostile			
B. Group Process Skills Interactional Tasks 1. Eliciting and receiving information, grievances, and preferences 2. Reporting structures to be used 3. Communicating alternative goals 4. Presenting requirements to decision makers 5. Guiding the process			
C. Analytical Tasks 1. Studying and describing the problem 2. Researching and deciding on appropriate structure and rules 3. Reviewing past decisions and selecting alternatives 4. Designing the system for collecting information 5. Analyzing feedback			
D. Political Considerations E. Value-Screen and Personal Disposition 1. Personal preferences 2. Choices and personal judgments 3. Criteria for deciding 4. Training and educational influences			

Table 3. Problem Example—Using S-T-P Worksheet.

Situation	Target	Proposal/Plan
Starting point	Terminations	Path from S to T
Facts, opinions, explanations about the current conditions, predictions about efforts to change	Goals, aims, ends, values, purposes, objectives	Means, plan, strategy, implementation procedure
Environment as the group perceives it	Outcome desired by the group	The group's behavior
What is it now?	What do I want—now, soon, eventually?	What can I do now to get it—how, who, when, where?
• Not enough space in Center for staff; renovations are required. Question of whether it is more beneficial to renovate and stay or to move.	• Acquire some additional space in same building. • Renovate additional and present space to accommodate new computer and additional staff as well as renovate to meet handicapped requirements.	• Develop and implement fund-raising strategy including grants. • Approach real estate agents for acquiring new space. • Get bids on work to be done. • Assign project director.

1.   Problem identification.
     a. Data gathering
     b. Building consensus
     c. Drafting problem statement
        • Problem specification
        • Problem analysis
2.   Formulation of action alternatives.
3.   Feasibility testing.
4.   Selection of strategy for implementation.
5.   Implementation, adoption, and diffusion of solution.

Problem Identification

Problem identification is extremely important because the way in which a problem is formulated will strongly influence how it will be handled in succeeding phases of problem solving. Administrators often look at symptoms rather than at the problems themselves. Symptoms are messages, disturbances, or pieces of information that indicate that a problem exists. In one of our case examples, low staff morale expressed by increased absences and sick leaves following the resignation of the third day treatment manager demonstrated that a problem existed; the symptoms were not the problem, however. The problem was continuing unstable leadership in day treatment administration.

Problem identification is often hindered because information flowing to the manager is inaccurate or incomplete. Some staff members feel comfortable with the status quo and want someone in management to handle the crisis; others are reluctant to supply helpful information because they feel threatened by the administrator. "What if I tell him that the last manager was a controlling S.O.B. who did not understand clinical procedures, and then he uses that information against me?" Still others prefer to avoid conflict by calling in sick. Groupthink also prevents some staff members from sharing information with the manager. For all of these reasons, staff views are screened or blocked from reaching the administrator. The administrator must judge what is accurate, differentiate between symptoms and causes, and determine whether or not more information is needed to clarify the problem situation.

At this early stage of the problem-solving process, maximum openness to problem clarification is desirable. Too early closure on problem identification may bias the entire process. For example, the administrators with the space problem might bias the problem-solving process by stating at the outset that the agency needed to move.

Two steps comprise the problem-identification stage: gathering data and building a consensus, and writing a problem statement. In data gathering, the manager may tend to accept the general formulation of the problem as received and seek no further information—as when the problem appears to be clearly presented by a funding body or site-review team. However, because of political considerations, the manager should seek further views of the problem, both corroborative and contradictory. For example, an administrator might take under advisement a site-visit report stating that the agency is in trouble for allowing volunteers to vote on its board of directors until he or she determines whether such a conclusion is a matter of policy, has regulatory power, and can be appealed. In seeking information and building consensus about the state of the problem, the manager plays the crucial role of programmer of the problem-solving process, determining the type, amount, and quality of information needed and deciding when the search for information begins and ends.

Data Gathering and Consensus Building

Questionnaires, surveys, interviews, literature searches, and statistical computations are all tools the manager can use to gain further information for clarifying the problem. In the case relating to space requirements, for example, the manager might solicit the expression of staff needs, interview representatives of the handicapped accessibility office, and gather ideas from realtors about the office rental market. The search for relevant information helps to clarify and elaborate on one's definition of the problem. In other words, the information search helps both to narrow and to expand the problem by setting realistic boundaries (March and Simon, 1958). Search for information ceases when the problem appears to be defined adequately enough to enable problem solving to continue. The problem statement then provides a framework for the rest of the problem-solving process.

In a highly volatile situation, the problem might be clarified through a series of negotiations with consumers or dissident staff members as to their different perceptions of the problem. Again, political factors must be considered. In crisis situations, problem consensus might be reached through a meeting with representatives of different sides of the issue. In any case, consensus on problem definition is crucial, because, if the central problem is not specified and agreed on, rival explanations and proposals will compete for dominance and the real problem may be buried, only to reassert itself in the future. A participative leadership process can facilitate consensus building.

Repetition of the same problem occurs when administrators habitually offer last year's knowledge as a base for describing today's problems. Rather than using a more analytical or scholarly approach—for example, conducting marketing analysis or surveying the available literature on the problem—managers may apply old explanations to new problems. As a result, an agency can lose its momentum and bog down in an ever-growing mass of unresolved problems and tired, unsuccessful solutions. Creative thinking at this juncture is critical.

Problem Statement

The development of a problem statement involves two steps, problem specification and problem analysis. Whether a manager works alone or in groups, a problem statement must be written. One approach to writing a problem statement is the use of a force field analysis process (Eisen, 1967) to answer questions like the following:

1. I understand the problem specifically to be that. . .
2. The following people with whom I must deal are involved in the problem:
3. Their roles in this problem are. . .
4. They relate to me in the following manner:
5. I consider these other factors to be relevant to the problem:
6. If I could, I would change the following aspect of the problem:

This outline can be expanded by other questions, such as: What is the origin of the problem? Who is causing it? What kind of problem is it? What happens if you succeed or don't succeed in solving it?

If each member of the staff or committee answers such a survey prior to a problem-solving meeting, a comprehensive problem statement becomes more feasible. Further, the meeting itself could use a survey outline of this kind as an agenda and use brainstorming techniques to surface a variety of perspectives. Other cultures also yield ideas on how to approach problem identification. For example, in a creative approach used in some Japanese businesses, the newest and most junior staff member is assigned the task of developing a problem statement. Through trial and error, research, and questioning of associates, a statement is developed in concert with others that, though often incomplete and filled with errors, may contain novel approaches to the issue (Ouchi, 1981).

Problem analysis, like problem identification, takes various forms. One commonly used analytical tool begins with the premise that a problem is a temporary balance of opposing forces and has the administrator list driving and resisting forces and prioritize them according to intensity, or degree. Another approach is to use a means-ends analysis, which begins by seeking an understanding of the origin of the problem, examines the connections and relationships that cause the problem to continue, and then determines how the problem should be solved.

These kinds of analyses see problems as obstacles to accomplishing agency objectives and help reveal a clear picture of all the problem's ramifications so that the problem-solving process can proceed. One of the main reasons for involving program managers and board members in the problem-clarification stage is to build a consensus about the nature of the problem. All too often a manager who goes through the analytical process in isolation has a difficult time convincing others that certain aspects of a problem should be addressed and may even find it necessary to form a study committee to engender interest in the problem. On the other hand, managers frequently make the mistake of unnecessarily involving line staff members and board members in problem-solving exercises when their time could best be spent in more appropriate activities. The administrator's role is to be a problem analyst, the board's role is to address the problem with appropriate policy responses, and the staff's role is to implement that policy through program strategies. The manager might choose to involve some line staff members in information gathering or certain board committees in problem clarification, but ultimately it is the manager's responsibility to present a full description of the problem at hand.

Formulating Action Alternatives

If the manager uses the force field analysis process the formulation of action alternatives flows naturally from the diagnosis of the problem. For each driving and resisting force, any number of action alternatives might be applied either to increase the driving force or to decrease the resisting force. At this stage, the manager's success as a leader depends on the extent to which he or she can stimulate novel ideas. Since the tendency is to accept the most standard responses to the problem, a creative brainstorming process should be applied to engage the management team, the appropriate board committee, and, if necessary, the executive director in arriving at the most innovative and novel solutions possible. Multiple action plans might even be required (Mintzberg, 1973).

Then, as allocator of resources, the manager must assess the human and physical resources available to the agency and decide who might best carry out each alternative solution. Alternative solutions are then ranked in order of preference according to either implicit or explicit criteria—that is, managers may rank the alternatives and then decide what made them choose one alternative over another, or they may list the criteria to be used (such as costs, feasibility, or difficulty) and then apply them in setting priorities.

In the case study of the manager confronting the need for space, staff and board members could be provided with a broad array of alternative strategies, including special study committees for examination of housing issues, staff committees to study future program alternatives, development of questionnaires, and interviews with funding bodies. This listing of alternative solutions and strategies would then lead naturally into the next step in the decision-making process—feasibility assessment and implementation.

Feasibility Testing and Selecting a Strategy for Implementation

The next stage of decision making requires the manager to again address his or her values, beliefs, and preferences in order to make explicit the criteria according to which choices will be made. At this point, the administrator should be able to quantify the options by giving a numerical weight to each criterion selected. In the case of hiring a new day treatment manager, the criteria for selection—such as years of clinical experience, years of management experience, type of management experience, continuing education goals, particular skills exhibited, and personal strengths and weaknesses—would each receive a numerical value, and each candidate would be given a relative ranking for each criterion. The total score for each candidate would then produce a final ranking (Table 4).

Table 4. Hiring a New Manager on the Basis of Weighted Criteria.

	Clinical Experience	Management Experience	Continuing Education	Special Skills	Particular Strengths	Apparent Weaknesses[a]	Total
Candidate A	9	6	10	4	6	-4	31
Candidate B	10	10	10	10	10	-1	49
Candidate C	8	5	10	4	6	-7	26
Candidate D	1	10	10	10	10	-10	31

Note: Candidate scoring highest on the basis of weighted criteria is chosen (10 = highest rating; 1 = lowest rating).
[a] Weakness is weighted negatively (-10 = greatest amount of weakness; -1 = least amount of weakness).

The administrator might also use a means-ends analysis in assessing strategies, scanning relationships and values in order to project the chain of interactions likely to take place for each alternative. Or the manager might use a systems analysis, scanning political elements to determine what groups will be affected, what elements in the organization or other agencies will be disturbed, and what boundaries should be examined. In the case of seeking more office space, for example, the manager would analyze what a move might mean to other organizations in the services delivery system and whether a move might be coordinated with other agencies needing space. A resources analysis would include the examination of funding, staffing, and services delivery possibilities and an analysis of existing policies to assess the benefits afforded to the various parties by each alternative (Perlman and Gurin, 1972). Whatever method is chosen, the manager must be clear that his or her own values and preferences affect the choices made. For this reason, some managers may seek assistance from panels of experts functioning as preselection screening committees, with the manager making the final decision.

Often the decision can be made only on the basis of information controlled by the administrator. Since managers know the resources, needs, and capabilities of the organization, they function at the heart of the organization's strategy system (Mintzberg, 1973) and determine, by their ability to use resources appropriately, the administration's success. For example, assessing the right time for a move or selecting an appropriate staff person to fit into a particular mix of staff is a managerial skill. In addition, the manager has the ultimate responsibility for committing the agency's resources in accord with policy decisions of the board and direction from the executive director. In order to help the board make policy choices, the manager must identify policy options and make recommendations from among a variety of alternatives.

Administrators often hesitate in reaching a final decision because they are concerned about their choice of the best alternative. What if they are wrong? What if disappointing outcomes result from improper decision making or errors in their judgment? What about political fallout? Who sets standards for tolerable mistakes or a reasonable range of error? An administrator faces these questions with the realization that much uncertainty exists in managing human services but that this uncertainty can be minimized by not ignoring the evidence in problem-solving matters (Eaton, 1980). Administrators become aware that they are constantly making decisions based on insufficient information; nevertheless, wise managers move ahead in the decision-making process, using all information available and taking what they consider to be reasonable risks.

A clear statement of the solution—as important as a clear statement of the problem—should include a description of what is to be done, in what time period, and by whom. For instance, in the case of the agency space problem, the statement might include the following: 2,255 sq. ft. of new space shall be acquired by the executive director, with assistance from the board property committee, at a cost not to exceed $150 per month, and renovations on present space to prepare for handicap accessibility shall be accomplished within six months, not to exceed

$4,000. This description enables the manager to move on to the final step of adoption, implementation, and diffusion of the solution.

Adoption, Implementation, and Diffusion of Solution

The final step in the problem-solving process should not be difficult if the preceding steps were followed. Yet things tend to go wrong precisely at this point. Some managers do not like implementation and therefore do not function well as implementers. Their expertise may lie in clarifying the problem, and they find implementation difficult because it depends on so many unpredictable variables, including uncertain future events. For example, the manager who chooses an applicant he or she considers to be the most likely choice for a day treatment position may discover at the last minute that the person has accepted another offer or, once on the job, exhibits personality quirks not uncovered in the recruiting, interviewing, or selection processes. In the office space example, the board might decide to stay in present quarters, add some additional space, or renovate existing space. Staff might battle with each other over territory, a proposed grant for renovations might fall through, or inflation might strike a government funding body, causing reduction in allocations. The proposed solution may fall apart at any time in the implementation phase, to the consternation of managers and agency personnel alike.

The implementation process involves logistics, in which the resources of the agency are applied to various aspects of the problem-solving strategy. This process requires explicit work plans and procedures that the manager must monitor, since disturbances most often occur where procedures are vague, implicit, or nonexistent. The manager must schedule his or her own time and the time of associates around the implementation scheme and must establish a priority for the tasks to be implemented. Clear lines of authority and procedures for authorization, as in the hiring and firing of employees, must also be established, lest the smooth implementation of strategies be disrupted.

Problem Solving: A Cooperative Process

Even though administrators carefully follow a problem-solving model, they may still encounter difficulties in implementing decisions unless problem solving is considered a shared process. Board members, staff members, community advocates, clients, and volunteers should all participate in the process at one stage or another, with the administrator deciding who should be involved and at what point. A checklist is presented in Figure 1 to assist the manager in involving personnel from inside and outside the agency in the problem-solving process. Since administrators guide the process they need to seek answers to the following questions: What persons are most directly involved with the perceived problem and should be included in defining the problem? Does the agency have the talent or expertise to define all aspects of the problem, or are outside consultants required? At what point, if at all, will consultants be introduced, and what roles will

Figure 1. Problem-Solving Checklist.

Steps	Phase	Who is Involved?	Time Allowed	
☐	1. Identify problem	Manager and ☐ Board members ☐ Staff members ☐ Volunteers ☐ Community representatives ☐ Others (for example, consultants)	☐ Day or shorter ☐ Week	☐ Month ☐ More than a month
☐	2. Select from a range of alternatives	Manager and ☐ Board ☐ Staff ☐ Volunteers ☐ Community representatives ☐ Others	☐ Day or shorter ☐ Week	☐ Month ☐ More than a month
☐	3. Select goal statement	Manager and ☐ Board ☐ Staff ☐ Volunteers ☐ Community representatives ☐ Others	☐ Day or shorter ☐ Week	☐ Month ☐ More than a month
☐	4. Choose alternative solution should first approach not be feasible	Manager and ☐ Board ☐ Staff ☐ Volunteers ☐ Community representatives ☐ Others	☐ Day or shorter ☐ Week	☐ Month ☐ More than a month

☐ 5. Design plan of action
 ☐ Who _____
 ☐ What _____
 ☐ When _____
 ☐ Where _____
 ☐ How _____

☐ 6. First step—
 to be carried out immediately
  ☐ Who _____
  ☐ What _____
  ☐ When _____
  ☐ Where _____
  ☐ How _____

☐ 7. Additional—for which responsibility is to be assigned.

they play? Are role expectations for the board and staff clearly outlined in the process? The decision-making process often flounders because clear responsibilities are not defined for each phase of problem solving or because the organization focuses too much energy on the problem and too little on developing alternative solutions.

Conclusion

The ability to implement a problem-solving process provides a foundation for a full repertoire of administrative roles. The analytical tools of problem solving enable managers to clarify their values, develop criteria for decision making, choose appropriate leadership styles and allocate interactive as well as analytical tasks. Also, commanding a variety of problem-solving frameworks provides managers with flexibility in approaching problems. Therefore, skill in problem solving is recognized increasingly as a keystone in planning and directing programs.

References

Bennis, W. G., Benne, K., and Chin, R. *The Planning of Change.* New York; Holt, Rinehart and Winston, 1969.

Blake, R. R., and Mouton, J. S. *The New Managerial Grid.* Houston, Texas: Gulf, 1978.

Cyert, R. M., and March, J. G. *A Behavioral Theory of the Firm.* Englewood Cliffs, N.J.: Prentice-Hall, 1963.

Eaton, J. R. "Errors and Mistakes in Social Practice." *Administration in Social Work,* Spring 1980, *4* (1), 43–54.

Eisen, S. *Problem Solving—Program Learning Model.* Princeton, N.J.: Princeton University Press, 1967.

Goffman, E. *The Presentation of Self in Everyday Life.* New York: Doubleday, 1973.

Maier, H. W. "Play is More Than a Four-Letter Word: Play and Playfulness in Interaction with People." Paper presented at Second Social Work With Groups Symposium, University of Texas, Arlington, Tex., 1980.

Mannheim, K. *Ideology and Utopia.* New York: Harcourt Brace Jovanovich, 1952.

Manzell, R. *C.H.O.I.C.E. Problem Solving Models.* Parkland, Wash.: Pacific Lutheran University, 1965.

Maple, F. F. *Shared Decision Making.* Beverly Hills, Calif.: Sage Publications, 1977.

March, J. D., and Simon, H. A. *Organizations.* New York: Wiley, 1958.

Mintzberg, H. *The Nature of Managerial Work.* New York: Harper & Row, 1973.

Miringoff, M. L. *Management in Human Service Organizations.* New York: Macmillan, 1980.

National Family Planning Management Institute, Advanced Management Seminar. Westport, Conn.: Educational Systems and Designs, 1972.

Ouchi, W. *Theory Z.* Englewood Cliffs, New Jersey: Prentice-Hall, 1981.

Perlman, R., and Gurin, A. *Community Organization and Social Planning.* New York: Wiley, 1972.

Perrow, C. *Organizational Analysis: A Sociological View.* Belmont, Calif.: Wadsworth, 1978.

Pino, R., Jung, C., and Emory, R. *Research Using Problem Solving.* Portland, Ore.: Northwest Educational Laboratory, 1971.

Schutz, W. *FIRO-B.* Palo Alto, Calif.: Consulting Psychologists, 1977.

Torrance, E. P. *The Search for Satori and Creativity.* New York: Creative Education Foundation, 1979.

Watson, J. D. *The Double Helix.* New York: Signet Books, 1968.

☙ 12 ☙

Working with
Citizen Governing
and Advisory Boards

Nancy Peterfreund

With considerable federal attention in recent years focused on the involvement of citizen boards in community mental health programs, managers of mental health agencies need to support and encourage the contributions of concerned, committed, and informed community members to agency governance. Nancy Peterfreund discusses the key responsibilities of governing and advisory boards and presents current models of citizen participation and a sample agenda for model meetings. Detailed attention is given to committee formation, to board self-evaluation and evaluation of directors, to approaches for developing effective working relationships between board, administration, and staff, and to clarification of role boundaries and shared tasks and responsibilities.

Citizen participation in the mental health system has been an integral component of community mental health legislation since the inception of the community mental health movement in the mid sixties. What began as a generalized concept of community involvement in the planning, delivery, and evaluation of mental health services has evolved into a more specific mandate for citizen boards to ensure accountability to the community and to funding sources.

Today, every federally funded community mental health center (CMHC) is required to have a functioning citizen board. Mental health centers that do not receive federal funding but rely instead on state and local monies are also subject to requirements for citizen involvement issued by state or local authorities. Only in those states that do not have strict laws affecting private and public corporations can a mental health center operate without a board of some type.

Given this proliferation of citizen boards, mental health administrators must have a working knowledge of the major issues involving citizen participation, governance, and board development if their mental health agencies are to be managed effectively. For example, the following statistics emerged in a recent study of citizen mental health board members (Peterfreund, 1979):

- 45 percent of board members never received orientation or education concerning their roles and responsibilities; of those who did, 50 percent felt it was inadequate.
- On the average, it takes six months before board members feel they can contribute to the board.
- 89 percent of board presidents received no orientation or preparation for their position.
- Only 54 percent of board members are said to participate in discussions; only 57 percent do their homework to prepare for meetings and board activities.
- 58 percent of CMHC directors felt their boards did not understand their roles and responsibilities.
- 74 percent of the sixty-eight boards queried never took the time to evaluate their own performance; even fewer boards conducted a formal evaluation of the executive's performance.
- Over 50 percent of board members reported being less than sufficiently informed about areas critical to board functioning.
- Overall board performance was rated as less than adequate by 53 percent of center directors, 47 percent of board presidents, and 39 percent of board members themselves.

These findings bring to light some of the serious deficiencies in the current performance of citizen boards of mental health agencies. Board members feel that they have little impact on the center, that their relationship with the staff is poor, and that the information they receive from the director and staff is filled with jargon and professional biases. They have difficulty recruiting, motivating, and keeping members, receive inadequate clerical, financial, and general support from center staff, and have difficulty fulfilling requirements of representation, particularly concerning sufficient involvement of minority groups (Ruiz, 1973; Warden, 1978).

For their part, directors complain that the boards are more a headache and a burden than an asset to the agency. Boards are seen by directors as lacking sufficient knowledge or expertise to handle decision making in critical areas or as threatening if they have too much expertise. Often an agency director can be just as unclear as the board about the appropriate division of responsibilities between the board and administration (Senor, 1963; Stein, 1978).

Staff members often feel distant from the board. In many mental health agencies, the vast majority of staff members never have the opportunity to meet board members or to attend board meetings. They often see the board as having tremendous power over such areas as salaries, benefits, and long-range plans for the agency, yet board members are considered highly inaccessible (Hanson and Marmaduke, 1972; Robins and Blackburn, 1974). Some staff members view the lay board as an obstacle to professional goals and initiatives and resent its power to make decisions affecting clinical operations and client satisfaction.

This discussion of problems currently experienced by directors, staff members, and board members only touches the surface. With a view to helping resolve these problems, as well as to strengthening and clarifying governance functions in general, this chapter describes the following issues regarding CMHC boards: historical and legal perspectives on citizen participation in mental health programs, current models of citizen participation, the role of the governing board in relation to the director and the staff, and effective execution of shared and separate governance responsibilities by the board and the staff.

Historical and Legal Perspectives

Although the passage of the Community Mental Health Centers Act of 1963 marked the beginning of the national community mental health program, no formal requirements for local governance and control existed until the 1975 amendments to the act. The CMHC act originally intended that informal citizen participation in community mental health programs would result in programs that best served the particular mental health needs of each community while making the best use of available resources. In fact, however, professional service providers and agency administrators retained the majority of control over the individual mental health centers (Trecker, 1970).

The thrust of the 1975 legislation (PL 94-63) was to place the control of CMHCs in the hands of boards comprised of community leaders and to allow local citizens to determine community need and program services. The legislation stipulates that in order to receive federal funds centers must have citizen boards that will approve the center budget, establish general center policies, be comprised of no more than 50 percent providers, be comprised of citizens residing in the catchment area (where "practicable"), meet once a month, and be representative of the community served. Board responsibilities also include reviewing: the cost of center operations; the pattern of utilization of services; the availability, accessibility, and acceptability of services; the impact of services on the mental health of residents of the catchment area; and evidence of citizen involvement in assessing services, determining community needs, and assuring center responsiveness. The following excerpt from PL 94-63 (1975) outlines the provisions for governing bodies of CMHCs:

> (c) (1) (A) The governing body of a community mental health center (other than a center described in subparagraph [B]) shall (i) be composed where practicable of individuals who reside in the center's catchment area and who, as a group, represent the residents of that area, taking into consideration their employment, age, sex, place of residence, and other demographic characteristics of the area; and (ii) meet at least once a month, establish general policies for the center (including a schedule of hours during which services will be provided), approve the center's annual budget, and approve

the selection of a director for the center. At least one-half of the members of such body shall be individuals who are not providers of health care.

Since the provisions do not state clearly how board responsibilities are to be carried out, each center must work that out individually. This legislation goes a long way toward ensuring that the community residents have ultimate power over what takes place within the mental health center. It should be noted that federal guidelines and laws, although they apply only to those centers receiving federal funding, are designed to provide guidance to mental health centers relying on state or local funding, as well.

In most states, CMHCs that are private, nonprofit corporations also fall under the auspices of state laws for incorporating nonprofit organizations, which mandate that nonprofit agencies develop articles of incorporation in accord with state guidelines. These articles provide the legal framework for the board of directors and include a list of the officers of the corporation, who may make up all or part of the board of directors, and a description of the purpose for which the corporation has been formed.

Accompanying the articles of incorporation are the corporation's bylaws. Bylaws are the official rules enacted by the corporation to govern its actions, officers, and board members. One of the board's most important legal documents, bylaws typically contain the purpose of the center; qualifications for board membership; methods of admission to the board; rights and privileges of board members; rules for withdrawal, censure, suspension, or expulsion; officers' titles, terms of office, powers, duties, and compensations; time and manner of election or appointment of officers; procedures for filling board vacancies; voting rules, including the number of members constituting a quorum, the number of meetings to be held, and amendment methods; and the major board committees.

Beyond federal and state laws and guidelines, the county or other local jurisdiction may have its own set of rules and regulations for the mental health center's governance. In some counties, the county commissioners are the governing authority for a county-funded mental health center, with a resident citizen advisory board serving as advisors to the county and the director. In this situation, the county may have laws affecting methods of public input into the county decision-making process. In some cases, county officials have developed rules that delegate final decision-making authority to the agency governing board. In addition to federal laws and guidelines, then, state, county, and local laws and guidelines and funding source requirements may also mandate the existence of citizen boards at mental health centers.

Governing and Advisory Boards

The previous section established the historical and legal basis for the existence of governing and, in some cases, advisory boards. This section presents a comparison between governing and advisory boards, information on the relationship of governance concepts to agency management, and a description of a model CMHC board.

Citizens serving on the mental health center governing board exercise authority by influencing the actions of the director in carrying out agency policies and goals. As the controlling agents of the mental health center, governing boards have ultimate responsibility for the center's operations and the power to make final policy determinations (Robins, 1976). The boards are the employers of the executive directors serving their agencies.

The advisory board, on the other hand, does not have governing authority but does possess power and influence. The strength of the advisory board is determined by such factors as the energy and dedication of its members, the representativeness by its members of population groups in the catchment area, the receptivity of the center's director to suggestions and advice, and the advisory board's relationship to the parent organization. An advisory board's power is of a political, rather than a legal, nature, with authority delegated by the governing body (Ahmed and Harm, 1979; Brodsky, 1972).

Some of the factors contributing to differences in the roles and functions of governing boards nationwide are the following (Bertelsen and Harris, 1973; Hartogs and Weber, 1974; Rabiner, 1972).

1. Geographical location of the center (rural, urban, suburban).
2. Composition of the board (socioeconomic, political, racial, cultural, educational).
3. Size of the board and the mental health center.
4. Relationship between board and staff, between board and community, and between board members themselves.
5. Funding sources of the center and their requirements (federal, state, local).
6. Legal requirements for a corporate board of directors (differs in each state).
7. Relationship to county commissioners, state department of mental health, and other governing bodies.

Given this variability in the factors influencing board roles and functions, identification of an ideal board role is difficult. Since the changing circumstances of a mental health center also affect the type of role that the board must fulfill, what appears ideal at one point may become inappropriate at another. Boards will be asked to focus their energies on agency development, resource mobilization, political activities, or community relations, depending on the agency's developmental stage and current environment.

Despite the difficulty in describing an ideal board's role and structure, Table 1 attempts to provide an outline of those characteristics that seem to contribute to board effectiveness in the center and the community (Peterfreund, 1979). The model describes a governing board, but most of the items listed would be applicable to an advisory board as well, except perhaps legal liability, ultimate responsibility for financial management, policy determination, hiring and firing of the executive director, and personnel policy development. Although not every

Table 1. A Model CMHC Board.

The model CMHC board fulfills the following roles:

1. Advocates for clients, community, center, and mental health in general.
2. Serves as a communication link between center, community, legislature, and other agencies.
3. Promotes program and financial accountability.
4. Monitors effective and efficient services delivery.
5. Plans for the future of the agency.
6. Makes administrative policy.

To fulfill these roles, the board performs or ensures the performance of the following functions:

1. *Establishment of personnel policies:* staff personnel policies, as well as policies governing the hiring, evaluation, and termination of the director.
2. *Short- and long-range planning:* needs assessment, goal setting, development of mission and direction for agency.
3. *Evaluation and quality assurance:* program evaluation, evaluation of the board.
4. *Financial management:* budget review and approval, monitoring of center's financial status, financial planning, audit review, fee schedule approval, salary approval.
5. *Community relations:* community informational and educational services, assessing public opinion of the center, client advocacy system, coordination with other agencies and boards.
6. *Political action:* legislative and administrative advocacy, support of mental health action groups.
7. *Board training and management:* recruitment, orientation, motivation, and education of board members.

---

item will be relevant to the unique situation of each particular center, most boards will find much that is applicable.

All governing or advisory boards need an organized approach to carrying out board roles and functions. Organization and structure are most typically provided by means of an established schedule for conducting full board meetings and activities; an established set of board officers; an established committee system; a formal process for recruitment of board members; a plan of action; and an established communication system between board, director, and staff.

Full board meetings, a locus for the policy-making activities of the board, are typically held once each month at a location accessible to the center catchment area. The meetings often require an agenda planned by the chairperson with assistance from the center's executive director. To ensure that agendas and minutes are recorded, the director of the center has responsibility for providing clerical assistance to the board.

Board Committees

Through the use of committees, the board's responsibilities are divided among its members to facilitate the study and formulation of specific proposals. Boards typically use two types of committees: standing committees, which perform ongoing tasks of the board and are listed in the bylaws, and ad hoc committees, which are appointed to fulfill a particular mission (usually short-term) and then disbanded. The size of the board, the size of the center staff, and the time commitments of board members will determine the number of committees and the extent of their roles and responsibilities. The following committees, commonly found on large governing boards of over fifteen members, have overlapping functions and are usually combined by advisory boards and smaller governing boards into finance and planning, personnel, evaluation and quality assurance, community relations and legislative action, and board membership and education:

Executive Committee

1. Acting on pressing or emergency matters that must be dealt with between regular meetings of the full board.
2. Assisting the chairperson in developing an agenda for board meetings.
3. Giving preliminary consideration to important policy considerations.
4. Guiding and directing the executive director between meetings.
5. Evaluating the executive director (results shared with full board).
6. Executive committee membership options: all officers, all committee chairpersons, geographical representatives.

Program Review Committee

1. Participating in and reviewing planning, development, and evaluation of services offered by the center.
2. Reviewing community needs assessment.
3. Reviewing quality assurance processes and results.
4. Ensuring that processes for assessing client satisfaction exist; checking results.
5. Maintaining contact with program managers.
6. Providing reports to the board on service and program developments and issues.

Budget/Finance Committee

1. Developing criteria for budget approval.
2. Reviewing the annual budget of the center with respect to community need, existing services, and the availability of the center's resources.
3. Reviewing the center budget with regard to cost effectiveness.
4. Recommending acquisition of additional funds (for example, new grants, contracts, fund raising).
5. Projecting the financial needs of the center for future years of operation.
6. Preliminarily reviewing monthly and yearly financial statements and operating statistics, with summary of findings to full board.
7. Formally reviewing the center's financial management systems at least once annually.

8. Meeting with the center's financial manager on a regular basis.
9. Selecting and meeting with external auditors; following up on auditors' recommendations.

Long-Range Planning Committee

1. Overseeing board development of a mission statement.
2. Working with director and staff to establish a set of long-range goals for the center.
3. Ensuring preparation of long-range plan by center staff.
4. Initially reviewing long-range plan, with recommendations to full board for approval if acceptable.

Personnel Committee

1. Advising board on personnel standards, policies, and practices.
2. Making recommendations for personnel policies regarding the following areas:

   a. Conditions of employment; the period of contractual employment; the probationary period; written evaluations and their frequency.
   b. Job classifications and salary ranges for each class of position; increment policies.
   c. Working hours, the work week, overtime compensation; scheduling of hours and days.
   d. Vacations, methods of computing earned vacation; specified holiday leaves.
   e. Leaves of absence; sick leave; maternity leave; study of educational leave.
   f. Health and welfare; insurance coverages provided by the center, including health insurance, hospitalization, workmen's compensation, retirement.
   g. Promotion policies; considerations of merit and seniority.
   h. Termination of employment; notice of resignation; conditions of dismissal; retrenchment or reorganization; conditions under which severance pay may be granted.
   i. Hearing procedures; methods of handling staff grievances and appeals.

3. Acting for the board with regard to hiring an executive director, including:

   a. Preparing a job description.
   b. Establishing interviewing criteria and processes.
   c. Interviewing prospective candidates.
   d. Making recommendations to the full board.

4. Evaluating the executive director.
5. Maintaining knowledge of staff capabilities and achievements through the executive director and program managers.

Legislative / Legal Committee

1. Reviewing matters of a legal or contractual nature and interpreting them to the board.
2. Keeping up with issues in national, state, and local government pertinent to center operation.
3. Reporting to the board on current legislative and political issues related to mental health.
4. Legislative advocacy, including lobbying, letter writing, telephoning, and testifying.
5. Maintaining contact with other boards and local or national mental health associations.

Membership / Nomination Committee

1. Developing criteria for selecting candidates for board membership (job description).
2. Maintaining a board membership file.
3. Advertising for board members.
4. Examining the qualifications of each candidate with regard to interests, associations, and capability for making specific and needed contributions to the board and the center.
5. Processing the resignations and examinations of board members.
6. Reviewing and enforcing the section of bylaws dealing with vacancies.

Community Relations Committee

1. Defining the roles and responsibilities of community relations.
2. Setting goals and objectives at least once annually for the board's community relations program, with input from staff and director.
3. Recommending at least once annually a community relations program (goals, objectives, and specific activities) for board approval.
4. Developing community relations policies and guidelines.
5. Reviewing the organization's community relations program and activities at least once annually, in relation to approved goals and objectives. Future public relations plans are adjusted accordingly.
6. Helping to develop community relations budget with executive director or financial manager.

Board Education Committee

1. Preparing and conducting orientations for new board members.
2. Planning educational programming for the board, including:

    a.   Assessing educational needs of the board.

    b.   Obtaining and distributing educational materials.

    c.   Arranging for speakers.

    d.   Arranging for seminars, workshops, and continuing education opportunities.

    e.   Evaluating board response to educational programming.

Housing/Space/Facilities Committee

1. Reviewing the physical maintenance and upkeep of center facilities.
2. Planning substantial repairs, renovations, or additions, in consultation with staff.
3. Reviewing contractual bids and costs for submission to full board.

    Each committee should develop a clear statement of its role and functions and a set of goals for each year. Committee goals and accomplishments should be reviewed at least once annually to determine whether the committee is fulfilling its role and is still needed by the board.

Board Recruitment

    A strong recruitment program is essential to the effective functioning of a CMHC citizen board and helps deal with such common problems as high absenteeism, high vacancy rates, difficulty in obtaining a quorum, lack of expertise, and lack of adequate representation (Brieland, 1971). The recruitment process should be the responsibility of a committee of board members, with the assistance and advice of the center's director and staff. The recruitment committee must be aware of federal and other requirements for board composition.

    The number of board members is determined by the board and usually averages about fifteen. Leadership abilities, experience in the mental health field, and political connections are among the criteria that may be important in recruiting board members. Client representation on the board—by actual clients or by friends or relatives of clients—is helpful in dealing with issues of accessibility, acceptability, and availability and with other issues of mental health care related to client satisfaction.

    The committee, with the help of the center staff, should also prepare a set of orientation materials providing basic information about the center and the board to enable prospective members to make an informed decision about whether or not to join the board. During the recruitment process, the board should be provided with needed support from the center's director and staff in the form of clerical help, assistance in explaining the center's operations to prospective members, and orientation of new board members.

Board Plan of Action

    Finally, a plan of action for board activities is vital to effective execution of board responsibilities. Just as the staff plans for its activities, the board also requires a formalized approach to task accomplishment (Conrad and Glenn, 1976). At least once annually, the board should conduct a planning session in which board members set goals and objectives for the board's activities in the coming year. The director and staff members may offer their viewpoints on what the center needs from the board and may be involved in the actual goal setting, if the board wishes. Board goals should be concise, clear, feasible, and of high priority, since board member time is limited. Objectives should define ways in which the goals may be achieved, as well as setting timetables and committee or individual responsibilities for specific programs.

Board-Staff Relations

Effective governance requires the coordinated efforts of board members, the executive director, and key administrative, clerical, and clinical staff members. An established system of teamwork for governance, necessary to provide the cohesion, sense of direction, and operating framework needed by the mental health center, must be developed and nurtured by the center director and the board, since such a system does not often evolve without conscious effort on the part of all involved (Meisner, 1970; Price, 1977).

Conflict between board and executive or between board and staff often develops in the absence of any planned approach to the shared tasks of governance and may include the following types of problems (Holton, New, and Hessler, 1973):

1. Lack of understanding of the roles and responsibilities of the board, director, and staff.
2. Lack of clear definition of role boundaries.
3. Lack of training and education for board members in their responsibilities and tasks and for executive directors and staff members in how to work with a board.
4. Lack of opportunities for contact between the board and the staff.
5. Insufficient support for the board from the director and the staff.
6. Clash between board and staff in terms of ideology, values, socioeconomic status, race, culture, education, and experience.
7. Board activities seen by board and staff as a time-consuming burden, rather than an asset.
8. Board interference in day-to-day administration.
9. Director taking over board duties, including policy making.
10. Board being used as a rubber stamp for director's decisions.
11. Board reluctance or inability to evaluate director effectively.
12. Lack of sufficient reinforcement and recognition of board accomplishments.

Through a process of board and staff development aimed at increasing awareness of roles, responsibilities, and methods for improving communication, the mental health director can help cultivate more positive relations between board and staff, which in turn can lead to more effective management of the center. A good starting point in this process is an examination of the model of interrelationships among board, director, and staff shown in Figure 1.

Special attention should be given to the board's role in establishing a framework for center operations. In this capacity, the board operates as a responsible link to the community and clients, thus reducing pressure on the center director. As employer of the director, the board also constructively evaluates his or her performance. Finally, because the board represents the community, it should be recognized as a political body with center advocacy responsibilities when state and federal funding is needed.

Since a community board made up of lay persons of varying backgrounds, education, and experience relies heavily on the director and staff for professional expertise and data concerning administrative and clinical areas, the director must establish an ongoing communication system through individual, committee, and full board meetings to provide the board with the information it needs. This system should provide information in a form that is understandable to the board, relatively jargon-free, and to the point. As discussed earlier, the director is directly accountable to the board for program and financial operations and is also responsible for providing the board with training and recruitment, clerical assistance, and information regarding role and function. Most important, the director must develop procedures for carrying out the policies of the board and must communicate these policies to the center staff.

The director should also make certain that staff members have regular opportunities to meet the board and to contribute to its policy and personnel decisions. Contact between board and staff not only assists the board with its analysis of center programs but also helps to reduce staff resentment of the board as an arbitrary regulator of policy and salaries. Suggestions for improving board-staff relations might include:

1. Common orientation and educational sessions.
2. Exchange of minutes of board meetings and staff meetings (or summaries of meetings).
3. Informal social events.
4. Annual planning and evaluation conferences where all three groups get together to review goals and objectives, evaluate progress, and develop programs to meet goals.
5. Joint committee work on special problems.
6. Formal process for channeling staff concerns through director and board.
7. Formal process for staff and director to develop issue papers or problem statements on policy areas that the board is handling.
8. Access of all three groups to a manual containing center goals and objectives, long-range plans, policies, and center bylaws.
9. Annual meeting to establish in writing the roles and responsibilities of staff, director, and board in areas where there is disagreement or confusion, as well as in areas where no guidelines are already written.
10. Commitment of all parties to achieving center goals as a cooperative team.

Figure 1. Relationships Between Board, Director, and Staff: A Working Model.

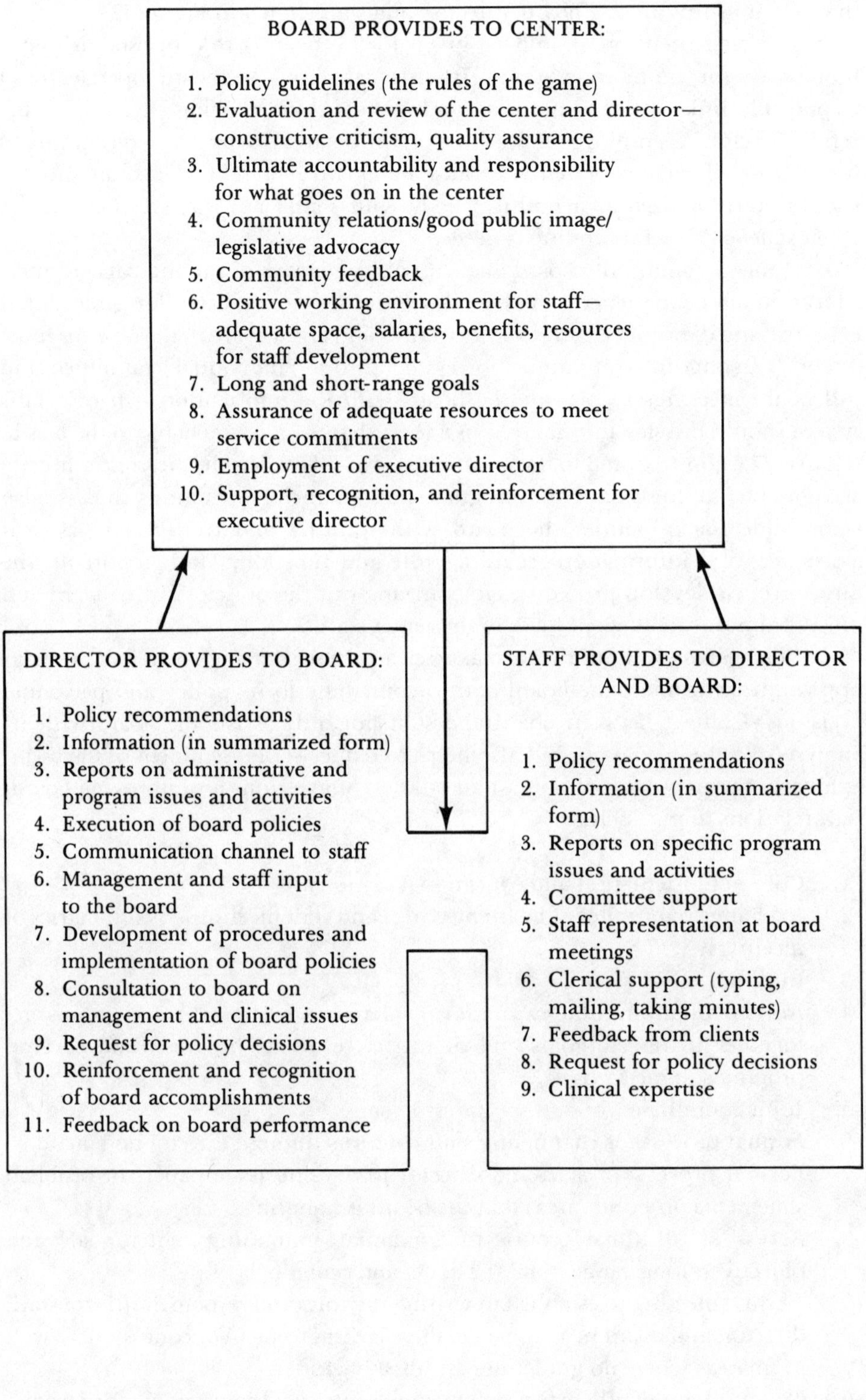

BOARD PROVIDES TO CENTER:

1. Policy guidelines (the rules of the game)
2. Evaluation and review of the center and director—
    constructive criticism, quality assurance
3. Ultimate accountability and responsibility
    for what goes on in the center
4. Community relations/good public image/
    legislative advocacy
5. Community feedback
6. Positive working environment for staff—
    adequate space, salaries, benefits, resources
    for staff development
7. Long and short-range goals
8. Assurance of adequate resources to meet
    service commitments
9. Employment of executive director
10. Support, recognition, and reinforcement for
    executive director

DIRECTOR PROVIDES TO BOARD:

1. Policy recommendations
2. Information (in summarized form)
3. Reports on administrative and
    program issues and activities
4. Execution of board policies
5. Communication channel to staff
6. Management and staff input
    to the board
7. Development of procedures and
    implementation of board policies
8. Consultation to board on
    management and clinical issues
9. Request for policy decisions
10. Reinforcement and recognition
    of board accomplishments
11. Feedback on board performance

STAFF PROVIDES TO DIRECTOR
AND BOARD:

1. Policy recommendations
2. Information (in summarized
    form)
3. Reports on specific program
    issues and activities
4. Committee support
5. Staff representation at board
    meetings
6. Clerical support (typing,
    mailing, taking minutes)
7. Feedback from clients
8. Request for policy decisions
9. Clinical expertise

11. Formal process for channeling board concerns through director to staff.
12. Board member representation at all staff meetings.
13. Board member volunteering a few hours per month at the mental health center.
14. Management and line staff representation on board committees.

Governance Responsibilities of Board, Director, and Staff

This final section provides a more detailed description of the roles of board, director, and staff in six key governance areas: policy making, long-range planning, financial management, program evaluation, evaluation of the executive, and evaluation of the board. The roles and responsibilities described here do not reflect the only way to divide the governing duties but are offered as guidelines and suggestions for boards and directors based on the experiences of mental health centers that have endeavored to establish clear lines of responsibility. Each center must engage in its own exploration of the optimal route to effective governance.

Common to each of these governance areas are several basic premises regarding the division of responsibility between board and staff. First, board members are part-time volunteers and should not be expected to perform tasks that would take more than an average of ten hours per month (or whatever is considered appropriate). Second, laypersons with no professional expertise in the mental health area should be able to handle board tasks with staff assistance. Third, a distinct line of demarcation should be drawn between policy and procedures; the board should set policy but should not interfere with the manner in which given policy is carried out. Fourth, the board should deal more with the broader and longer-range perspective than with the specific issues, which are the province of the director and staff. Fifth, the board must have enough data and information to feel comfortable in its role as policy maker.

Policy Making. The governing board, director, and staff must collaborate in the process of policy development, but only the governing board has the authority to give final approval for a given policy. The following is an overview of the roles of board, staff, and community members in the process of policy making. Who has authority for:

1. Policy development?   Board, director, staff, community
2. Policy determination?   Board alone
3. Policy implementation?   Director and staff alone
4. Policy review?   Board, director, staff, community

Policy development may involve board members, the director and staff, and community members. The director and staff should provide information to assist the board in identifying policy requirements for the center and should brief the board on such policy constraints as the requirements of funding sources or regulatory agencies and the limitations of center finances or service availability. Under certain circumstances, the board may want to delegate responsibility for the development of policy concerning day-to-day operations to the director and staff; however, the board should retain responsibility for resolving issues that are subjective or value-oriented. Regardless of who has the major involvement in the development phase, the authority for final policy determination rests with the full governing board alone; committee-level decisions are not valid for policy issues. The board will need to review the background information and the recommendations submitted by staff and board members before making final decisions.

Policy implementation is the responsibility of the director and staff and is the area in which board members are most likely to interfere inappropriately, since day-to-day administration is not a board responsibility. An important final step in the policy process is policy review. Policy requirements change as the center grows and changes, and policies should be kept up-to-date to reflect the actual practices and philosophy of the agency. At least once annually the board, director, and staff should meet together to review, modify, and add to center policies.

Long-Range Planning. Just as policy development is a shared responsibility of board, director, and staff, long-range planning requires the coordinated effort of all three parties. The process begins with a statement—to be developed by both board and staff, with final approval resting with the board—outlining the center's purpose, philosophy, and goals. Table 2 depicts the roles of board, director, and staff in the long-range planning process.

Financial Management. Although day-to-day management of the center's resources should be delegated to administration, the board retains authority over financial management, representing the community by directing the expenditure of public funds in the community's best interest (Metch and Veney, 1976; Mogulof, 1974). Management staff members carry out the board's directives, since they have the most knowledge of how the agency actually functions, as well as the technical financial skills needed to manage and provide mental health services. Responsibilities of the board in financial management include the following:

1. The board has the responsibility to make and approve policies on financial management and ensure that they are followed (see Appendix for a list of typical financial policy decisions the board needs to make).
2. The board must set center goals and priorities on which the budget is based.
3. The board must ensure the existence of financial planning for the center to meet short- and long-term goals and service commitments.
4. The board must approve the center's budget.
5. The board must become informed about basic financial terms and concepts and about how the center is funded.
6. The board must approve capital expenditures, grants, contracts, and other financial agreements.
7. The board should review selected financial reports and operating statistics on a regular basis to assess trends and ensure financial viability.
8. The board must ensure that the center is in compliance with requirements from funding sources.

Table 2. Who Does What in Long-Range Planning?

Board		*Director and Staff*
1.	Develops and approves the center's mission statement.	1. Develops the center's mission statement with the board.
2.	Establishes policy on planning: who should do it, what product should emerge and when.	2. Carries out the planning process according to board policy.
3.	Represents the community and clients in the planning process.	3. Represents management and line staff in the planning process.
4.	a) Develops criteria for approval of the plan. b) Oversees the needs assessment process; reviews results.	4. Obtains and disseminates data on internal organizational activities, on external forces influencing the center and its plan, and on community mental health needs.
5.	Determines goals for center activities.	5. Develops goals and objectives for center activities.
6.	Appoints a long-range planning committee.	6. Staffs the long-range planning committee.
7.	Reviews and approves the long-range plan.	7. Develops the long-range plan and submits it to the board for approval.
8.	Makes decisions for the center based on goals stated in the plan.	8. Suggests options to the board for achieving goals.
		9. Educates the board about planning.

9. The board has the responsibility to approve a salary scale for center personnel and to determine compensation for the executive director if an individual contract has been negotiated.

10. The board must review and approve the center's fee schedule developed by the executive director and staff.

11. The board should appoint the external auditor to conduct an annual audit of the center.

12. The board should ensure that the executive director formally evaluates the center's financial management system at least once annually.

The executive director and his or her management staff have the responsibility to:

1. Develop and implement plans for achieving financial and other goals set by the board.

2. Carry out financial policy developed by the board.

3. Conduct day-to-day business of the organization in the most effective and efficient manner possible.

4. Organize and adequately staff the financial management functions.

5. Regularly provide adequate and understandable financial and statistical information to the board and alert the board to trends in operations.

6. Make recommendations to the board regarding any major policies or contracts that affect the center's finances.

7.   Provide staff support to the board in financial matters.
8.   Prepare operational, cash, and capital budgets and present them to the board with adequate time for review and approval.
9.   Assist in educating the board as to the economics of the center's operations and general financial issues.
10. Establish and maintain a management information system to provide adequate data for internal control and management of the center resources.
11. Act as a liaison to governmental and other funding sources and maintain compliance with their regulations and requirements.
12. Evaluate the center's process of fiscal management at least once annually, with a report to the board on the results.

Program Evaluation. The board, director, and staff have significantly different roles in the area of program evaluation. The board represents the community's point of view, including the attitudes of consumers using the center's services (MacMurray and others, 1976; Mogulof, 1974). The director, as well as staff members delegated responsibility for program evaluation, contributes the professional expertise that allows for more technical and complex approaches to evaluation research. The role of the board in program evaluation is to:

1.   Become knowledgeable about basic concepts of evaluation.
2.   Develop policies on the level of evaluation to be done: how much, how often, and what types (within constraints of PL 94-63 requirement that 2 percent of the previous year's operating budget be devoted to program evaluation activities).
3.   Review evaluation studies conducted by the staff.
4.   Assure that program goals and structures are relevant to community service needs and amenable to evaluation.
5.   Review evaluation data related to the appropriateness, acceptability, availability, accessibility, and effectiveness of services.
6.   Act as a channel for citizen response (to programs, to services, to the center as as whole, to evaluation reports).
7.   Assure public dissemination of evaluation reports.
8.   Assure fulfillment of the evaluation requirements of funding sources— particularly federal, state, and local requirements.
9.   Advocate for different types of evaluation studies.
10. Keep professionals honest.
11. Review data requirements of program evaluation activities and determine the center's ability to obtain needed data.
12. Make policy decisions and set goals based on findings of evaluation.
13. Provide constructive criticism and suggestions for improvement in areas found deficient in evaluation studies.
14. Carry out evaluation studies in such areas as client satisfaction and nontechnical or community acceptance of the center.

The executive director and staff members have the responsibility to:

1. Carry out board policies on evaluation.
2. Advise the board on the types of evaluation studies that are needed and feasible.
3. Educate the board about basic concepts of evaluation.
4. Carry out evaluation studies as needed.
5. Hire staff members with capabilities for program evaluation.
6. Make regular reports to the board on evaluation findings in a form that is understandable to the board—often requiring a summary of findings and the interpretation of statistical information.
7. Set up annual review meetings and citizen forums, as needed.
8. Assist the board in carrying out its own evaluation studies, if desired.
9. Provide staffing for the board's evaluation committee.
10. Make available quality assurance information.
11. Make sure requirements for evaluation are carried out.
12. Keep the board aware of data and staff needs for evaluation.

Evaluation of the Director

As employers of the executive director, governing board members have primary responsibility for providing the director with timely performance feedback (Kahle, 1971; Ryan and Ullery, 1977). Yet this task of governance cannot be accomplished by the board alone; the full cooperation and involvement of the staff and the director are needed. Crucial to the evaluation process is the cooperative development of criteria for director performance and the determination of appropriate timing for formal evaluation by the board. The criteria used in evaluating the director should refer to the job description for the position of director typically developed during the recruitment process. In addition, the staff should be consulted on those areas of performance review that pertain to its particular needs and circumstances. Finally, the director should complete a self-evaluation using the criteria used by the board. Table 3 presents one example of an outline for an evaluation of the executive director (Kahle, 1971). The board and executive must determine the manner in which the executive's accomplishments will be measured. What will constitute adequate performance? Outstanding performance? Inadequate performance?

The final step is to set a process and timetable for review. Evaluation should be more frequent during periods of turmoil. The board should also try to avoid criticism after the fact by providing regular evaluations, which should prevent crises or dismissal of the director. At the time of the actual review, staff, board, and director should fill out the evaluation forms and submit them to a confidential committee, usually the executive committee, which should then review the evaluations and develop a summary report. The director should have the opportunity to meet and discuss evaluation findings with the committee

Table 3. Guide for Evaluating the Director.

I. *The purpose of the evaluation.* (This section should state briefly why the evaluation is being conducted, at whose instigation, what it proposes to accomplish, and the time interval since the last evaluation.)

II. *Responsibilities assigned and carried.* (This section should include a summary of the basic job description provided by the board at the time it was recruiting the director. The section should also indicate any new or additional responsibilities that have been added or have evolved since the beginning of his or her employment.)

III. *General aspects of practice.* (Strengths and weaknesses.)
   A. What is the extent of the director's professional expertise? Does the director attempt to increase his or her knowledge and keep informed of new developments?
   B. Does the director have an adequate working knowledge of the problems and structures and of key groups and individuals in the community?
   C. What are the quantitative aspects of his or her performance?
   D. How well does the director organize and prepare his other work?

IV. *Specific (qualitative) aspects of practice.* (Strengths and weaknesses.)
   A. Service to the board or governing body.
      1. Does the director relate well to board members?
      2. Does the director communicate ideas clearly? Is he or she receptive to communication from others?
      3. Does the director involve board members meaningfully in planning, policy making, and interpretation and in the overall operations of the agency?
      4. Does the director keep the board adequately informed of his or her activities and of the affairs of the agency?
      5. Is the director's general attitude acceptable to the board?
      6. Does the director provide leadership in board activities?
   B. Service to the staff.
      1. How well does the director relate to staff?
      2. Does the director understand their work and the problems that arise from their work?
      3. Does the director use personnel appropriately?
      4. Does the director delegate authority and responsibility appropriately?
      5. Does the director communicate well with the staff?
      6. Does the director encourage and use staff participation in planning, policy making, and operations?
      7. Does the director contribute to staff development?
      8. Is the director fair in his or her actions relating to personnel practices?
   C. Service to the community.
      1. How effective is the director in relations with funding bodies?
      2. How effective is the director in activities with planning bodies?
      3. How effective is the director in relations with other public voluntary organizations?
      4. How effective is the director in community and social action?
      5. Is the director effective in public relations and community education?
      6. How is the director viewed by his peers in other agencies?
   D. Service to the agency program.
      1. Does the director plan soundly?
      2. Is the director creative and innovative?
      3. Does the director assume the appropriate responsibility for making decisions?
      4. Does the director organize well?
      5. Does the director use agency resources well?
      6. Is the director effective in keeping the agency's program related to current community needs?
      7. Does the director demonstrate effective leadership of the agency staff?
      8. Does the director understand and use the budgeting process effectively?
      9. Does the director demonstrate ability in developing physical and financial resources?

Table 3, cont'd.

V. *Summary and recommendations.* (This section should provide a condensation of the total evaluation. It should indicate the director's progress toward achieving agency goals, his or her strengths, problem areas, and deficiencies. It should make recommendations for specific changes and indicate when they are expected to be accomplished. The summary should clearly state the board's satisfaction or dissatisfaction with the director's performance.)

before they are made public to the full board and staff. The meetings of the director and board should result in plans to resolve deficiencies.

Evaluation of the Board

Every CMHC board needs an established process for evaluating board functioning and accomplishments (Koontz, 1976; Lachner, 1977). A schedule of annual or semiannual evaluation sessions should be set, as the regular board meetings rarely allow time for such assessment. The evaluation process should include the director, appropriate staff members, and the board itself and may include federal, state, or local funding source representatives. Client or community residents may also offer their opinions, particularly in the area of board representation of community and client interests and values.

One useful framework for evaluation of the board uses questions categorized according to issues of structure, process, and outcome. Structural questions refer to the structural elements essential for effective functioning:

- Does the board have an adequate membership?
- Do members possess sufficient knowledge and skills to do the job?
- Does the board have an orientation manual?
- Does the board have a policy manual?
- Does the board have adequate resources (funding, staff support, and so on) to do its job?
- Does the board have a suitable place to meet?

Process questions deal with how well the board is carrying out its operations:

- Do most board members participate at board meetings?
- Do members do their homework to prepare for meetings?
- Do committees accomplish their tasks on time and with reports to the full board?
- Does the board use a process to facilitate decision making and information gathering beforehand?
- Is background material sent prior to board meetings?
- Does the board communicate regularly with the community?

Outcome questions relate to the actual effectiveness of the board in carrying out its duties and responsibilities:

• Did the board accomplish its stated goals and objectives?
• Did the board aid the center in accomplishing center goals and objectives?
• How many policy decisions did the board make during the current evaluation period?
• How many opportunities did the board create for communication with community residents? With clients?
• What changes in the center occurred as a result of board activities?
• What impact did the board have on the quality of care delivered by the center (in terms of availability, acceptability, accessibility, continuity)?
• How did the board help the director and staff to provide better quality care? More care? Different types of care?

These evaluation questions are just a beginning and serve as the basis for ongoing board development. To effectively accomplish the purposes for which it was established, the board develops its full potential as a working unit. An effective board is one that fulfills intended roles and accomplishes the objectives of the board, the center, and the community; it also takes the necessary time to prepare itself for its roles and responsibilities.

To prepare the board for its demanding and important roles, a comprehensive board development program is necessary. The board must develop an adequate and qualified membership, a firm philosophical and rational basis for its existence, an organizational framework from which to work, an understanding of the functions it is expected to perform, and the knowledge, skills, and assistance necessary to accomplish those functions. Board development programs may involve an initial orientation to the agency, the community, and board roles and relationships; subsequent training sessions can assist the board in improving skills and knowledge in key areas of board responsibility. A combination of readings and experiential learning situations, as well as opportunities for social interaction, enhances the board's ability to perform effectively as a group.

Conclusion

This chapter has focused primarily on the governing board of a community mental health center. The governing board—a critical element in the effective management of the CMHC—can provide leadership, community involvement and support, and political advocacy only if it has the resources and opportunities to develop its full potential. Assistance by the director and staff with membership recruitment and orientation of new members affords long-term payoffs in board efficiency. The board and staff must also work together to clarify their respective roles and responsibilities. This chapter presents an overview of such roles but does not provide a comprehensive solution—each center must develop its own system of cooperative and complementary functioning. Most crucial to the efficiency of the center is that role boundaries be defined as clearly as possible.

Finally, the board must evaluate both the director and the board itself. Assessment of the director should provide ways to improve the implementation of the center's policies. Evaluation of the board should identify areas for improvement in the center's governing authority and ways in which the director can be of greater help to the board. A director who assists the board in its development by increasing the availability of information and resources helps to ensure that the board will become an asset, rather than a burden. To ignore the enormous benefit provided by a board of concerned, committed, and informed community members is to ignore one of the richest resources of a community mental health center.

References

Ahmed, M. B., and Harm, C. S. "Developing a Community Board for a Mental Health Center." *Hospital and Community Psychiatry*, Apr. 1979, *30* (4), 256–258.

Bertelsen, K., and Harris, M. R. "Citizen Participation in the Development of a Community Mental Health Center." *Hospital and Community Psychiatry*, Aug. 1973, *24* (8), 553–556.

Brieland, D. "Community Advisory Boards and Maximum Feasible Participation." *American Journal of Public Health*, Feb. 1971, *61* (2), 292–296.

Brodsky, I. *Manual for Board Members: A Guide to Service.* New York: National Jewish Welfare Board, 1972.

Conrad, W. R., and Glenn, W. R. *The Effective Voluntary Board of Directors: What It Is and How It Works.* Chicago: Swallow Press, 1976.

Hanson, P., and Marmaduke, C. T. *The Board Member: Decision Maker for the Nonprofit Corporation.* Sacramento, Calif.: Han/Mar Publications, 1972.

Hartogs, N., and Weber, J. *Boards of Directors: A Study of Current Practices in Board Management and Board Operations in Voluntary Hospital, Health, and Welfare Organizations.* New York: Oceana Publications, 1974.

Holton, W., New, P., and Hessler, R. "Citizen Participation and Conflict." *Administration in Mental Health*, Fall 1973, pp. 96–103.

Kahle, J. H. "Assessing Executive Performance." *Social Casework*, 1971, *52* (2), 79–85.

Koontz, H. "Holding the CEO Accountable." *Hospital Progress*, Sept. 1976, pp. 68–74.

Lachner, B. J. "The Cost Accountability of the CEO and Board." *Hospital Progress*, Aug. 1977, *58* (8), 60–63.

MacMurray, V. D., and others. *Citizen Evaluation of Mental Health Services: A Guidebook for Accountability.* New York: Human Services Press, 1976.

Meisner, L. "A Training Program for Consumers in Policy Making Roles in Health Care Projects." Unpublished paper, Continuing Education in Health Sciences, School of Public Health, University of California, Berkeley, May 1970.

Metch, J. M., and Veney, J. E. "Consumer Participation and Social Accountability." *Medical Care*, Apr. 1976, *14* (4), 283–292.

Mogulof, M. B. "Advocates for Themselves: Citizen Participation in Federally Supported Community Organizations." *Community Mental Health Journal*, 1974, *10* (1), 66–76.

Peterfreund, N. *CMHC Board Development: A Manual for CMHC Boards, Staff, and Policy Makers*. Seattle: University of Washington School of Public Health, 1979.

Price, W. *Manual on Governance and Policy Planning for CMHC Board Members*. Silver Spring, Md.: Wolfgang Price Associates, 1977.

Rabiner, C. J. "Organizing a Community Advisory Board for a Mental Health Center." *Hospital and Community Psychiatry*, Apr. 1972, pp. 30–33.

Robins, A. "Governing Boards and Decision Making." *Administration in Mental Health*, Fall 1976, *4* (1), 18–25.

Robins, A., and Blackburn, C. "Governing Boards in Mental Health: Roles and Training Needs." *Administration in Mental Health*, Summer 1974, pp. 37–45.

Ruiz, P. "Consumer Participation in Mental Health Programs." *Hospital and Community Psychiatry*, Jan. 1973, *24* (1), 38–40.

Ryan, R., and Ullery, B. "Selecting an Executive Director." *Administration in Mental Health*, Spring 1977, pp. 66–77.

Senor, J. M. "Another Look at the Executive-Board Relationship." *Social Work*, Apr. 1963, *8* (2), 19–25.

Stein, H. "Board-Executive Relationships." In S. Slavin (Ed.), *Social Administration*. New York: Haworth Press, 1978.

Trecker, H. B. *Citizen Boards at Work: New Challenges to Effective Action*. New York: Association Press, 1970.

Warden, G. "Board Self-Assessment: Changing the Governing Structure to Meet Changing Times." *Trustee*, Mar. 1978, pp. 37–40.

ᎌ 13 ᎍ

Managing
Volunteer Programs
and Promoting
Self-Help Groups

William E. Hershey

In integrating volunteers into mental health programs, administrators often meet with staff or client resistance, as well as recruitment problems at a time when more and more women are pursuing careers. In establishing liaisons with or helping develop community self-help groups and resource networks, managers face community mistrust of professionals and a lack of training and organizational skills among agency staff members. In this chapter, William Hershey addresses these problems and suggests a model volunteer program that includes recruitment, screening, training, and supervising components. Volunteer job design, volunteer job satisfaction, and corporate involvement in volunteer programs are also discussed. The chapter concludes with a detailed description of self-help groups and community networks, additional volunteer resources for extending the services of a mental health program into the community.

Recent events have led mental health managers to examine once again the role and use of volunteers and community networks in planning and implementing comprehensive mental health services (President's Commission on Mental Health, 1978). The adequacy of treating the mentally ill in fifty-minute therapy sessions is being questioned, and the limitations and high cost of outpatient therapy and of inpatient services that isolate the resident from the community have been continuing problems for mental health services providers. In response, community involvement in treatment has increased through active follow-up programs, volunteer participation in agencies themselves, and community networks based in part on the participation of paraprofessionals and volunteers. This chapter will focus on ways in which planners and administrators can use self-help networks and volunteers to extend community mental health services.

Historical Perspective

Community networking and volunteer participation have long been a part of the treatment of the mentally ill. As early as the 1930s and 1940s, a positive alliance existed between psychiatrists and laypersons that fostered the development and expansion of moral treatment (that is, a combination of psychiatric and spiritual counseling), perhaps the first organized approach to the care of the mentally ill. A second by-product of this alliance was the increased acceptance of public responsibility for those who were unfortunate enough to become mentally ill. The psychiatrists of that period attempted to lower barriers between the mental hospital and the community by efforts to improve public attitudes toward insanity. They also sought to improve the treatment of those who were hospitalized for long periods of time by humanizing large institutions, thus facilitating their reentry into the community. At the same time, they proposed speeding up treatment of unhospitalized cases and encouraged early case finding in order to contribute to the highest possible rate of curability (Caplan, 1969).

Volunteers participated in hospital treatment by socializing with the patients and provided a link to the community by affording posthospitalization care in an effort to speed recovery. Dorothea Dix made considerable progress in her campaign to increase the number of public mental hospitals and almost achieved her goal of national legislation mandating public mental health services. Those who followed her were even more vociferous in their outcry against poor patient management, corruption, and the self-aggrandizement of professionals and superintendents. Among them were patient advocates who were able to ally themselves with liberal professionals who promoted new legislation for more humane treatment. These advocates of improved mental health services were the forerunners of today's participants in mental health associations, board members of mental health centers, fund raisers, and citizen advocates for improved legislation.

Many present-day activist volunteers differ from their predecessors in that they are more keenly interested in seeking changes in mental health policies affecting unserved and underserved ethnic minorities than in volunteering to assist in the delivery of treatment services. These new activists had experience in community organization in the late sixties and bring a desire to change programs in order to meet the needs of the communities they represent. Further, this activism is buttressed by recent federal legislation and regulations requiring citizen participation in programs where federal funds are used. The 1975 amendments to the Community Mental Health Center Act are very specific regarding the need for citizen involvement in all levels of mental health decision making: "Citizens shall be involved not only in planning and operation but also in review of services for the express purpose of ensuring that such services are developed in response to articulated needs" (Public Law 94–63, 1975).

Unfortunately professionals do not always welcome these new participants with open arms but meet them instead with token acceptance and even at times with resistance. Although professionals view volunteers as useful adjuncts to delivering mental health services, volunteers are frequently given work that is shunned or considered extraneous by other staff members. This tendency is decreasing as financial resources diminish and as mental health practitioners become increasingly aware of the rich and varied resources volunteer and community networks have to offer in such areas as community relations, preventive education services, self-help networks, and the organization and management of mental health associations.

If administrators are to make the best use of volunteer resources in improving services delivery, they must consider volunteers an integral part of the agency's services delivery system and must be creative in the recruiting, selecting, and developing of them. Competition for volunteers requires agencies to move volunteer programming to the forefront. Previously, volunteers were largely older women from middle- to upper-class social and economic backgrounds. Today's typical volunteer comes from a lower socioeconomic class, is young, employed, well educated, and expects a challenge; the agency needs to offer something in return for services rendered. Often these new volunteers are able to perform services in which agency staff members have little or no training, including legal advice, computer services, management consultation, financial investments, fund raising, and public relations; they may assist program managers by working with clients in providing transportation, home visit, case finding, home management, and housing relocation services.

Organizing a Volunteer Program

In order to involve the agency staff and board, mental health planners and administrators must be knowledgeable about, and committed to, the development and organization of a volunteer program. Administrators often encounter staff resistance caused by a lack of available training in how to work with volunteers and by staff fears that volunteers might not be competent to assist in the delivery of professional services. Clients themselves frequently feel reluctant to enter treatment with volunteer counselors whom they might know. These attitudes come from a lack of careful administrative planning regarding the development of a volunteer program and the integration of that program into the overall operation of the agency.

The volunteer program needs to be managed in the same manner as all other agency programs—volunteer programs do not run themselves (Schwartz, 1977). To prevent volunteers from experiencing a low-priority status, administration and supervising staff need to train staff to work effectively with volunteers. Such training may include instruction in supervision, performance evaluation, recognition and reward strategies, job clarification, and objective setting, as well as an evaluation of the entire volunteer program. Staff training should not proceed unless the administrator has appointed a coordinator for volunteers who is involved in administrative planning and programming.

Once the staff members of a mental health center recognize the potential benefits of a volunteer program, the agency's need for volunteers should be thoroughly examined, including an assessment of the overall goals of the agency and the potential role of volunteers, the number of persons needed to accomplish the tasks outlined, the community impact anticipated, and the agency programs needing support and expansion.

Administrators should involve interested staff and board members in the formulation or expansion of the volunteer program. The participation of board members is particularly important, for it elevates the administration of the program to the policy level, thereby institutionalizing the program and preventing it from changing at the whim of a new administrator. Volunteer program policies should include statements of purpose, direction, role expectations for both volunteers and staff, and the ways in which the program meets agency objectives, as well as attention to financing, staffing, training of volunteers, and program evaluation. For example, a volunteer personnel system, developed parallel to staff personnel procedures, might include individual volunteer files, work records, hour tabulations, a compensation system (recognition process), job descriptions, performance evaluations, personnel development and training programs, termination and exit interviews, and training reference materials.

Volunteer coordinators should be a part of the agency's management team. If a full-time or part-time volunteer coordinator cannot be justified on the basis of program needs and community liaison functions, then interested mental health staff can assume part-time responsibilities for the program, as long as the development of volunteer policies is not sacrificed. If, however, a mental health agency is committed to giving the volunteer program high priority, the volunteer program administrator must be a well-qualified person, particularly skilled in general management, decision making, and problem solving and knowledgeable in the problems and possibilities of the mental health system. The person should have a commitment to the concept of community change, both in the prevention and treatment of social problems, and should know the techniques for administering a volunteer program—recruitment, screening, selection, training, and evaluation (Wilson, 1976).

A key element in planning and developing volunteer programs, then, is organizational readiness, as reflected by board and staff commitment to a set of policies for the involvement of volunteers in the organization. A statement of purpose defines the volunteer program's role in helping the agency accomplish its mission, and major goals and procedures for assessment are defined and adopted by the board.

Roles Volunteers Can Play

Volunteers can work in behalf of a mental health agency in a number of ways. They can be members of governing boards or assist in resource development, organize guilds for fund raising and community relations, perform clerical or administrative tasks, help design a public relations campaign, or provide direct services to clients (Miller, 1979).

Volunteers on Governing Boards

The role of volunteers on policy making boards is the subject of another chapter. Since volunteer board members play such an active and authoritative role in agency functioning, the tendency is to forget that they are also volunteers. In fact, board members themselves often refer to volunteers who work with clients as "the volunteers," as if the board members were not a part of the volunteer resource themselves. Board training and development have not received the same attention as the training of direct service volunteers. Similarly, administrative staff lack training in facilitating board decision making. Tables 1 and 2 provide examples of board development goals, as well as components of a model board training program.

"Loaned Volunteers"—Corporate Interest in Volunteerism

In recent years, traditional recruitment devices like public service announcements, posters, and newspaper ads have not been sufficient to attract volunteers. With the large numbers of women having left the volunteer field to engage in salaried employment has come renewed effort to encourage corporations to promote volunteering as a community responsibility.

In response, some companies have placed key executives on loan to the agency for a month or more to assist in fund raising and to offer management consultation, keeping them on the company payroll during the period of the loan. Often companies allow agencies to come directly into plants or offices to inform

Table 1. Goals and Objectives of Board Development.

1. To assist board members in clarifying the board's role, purpose, functions, attitudes, relationships, structure, methods of operation, and legal requirements.
2. To improve recruitment practices of boards.
3. To ensure that board members have the opportunity to secure the knowledge and develop the skills to be effective in performing their tasks and functions.
4. To increase awareness of the need for ongoing board training and development within each mental health center.
5. To reinforce in-house capabilities for providing ongoing board orientation and education.
6. To reinforce board members' ability to seek out needed information from director, staff, community residents, clients, and other boards.
7. To reinforce the board's ability to initiate its own activities and work.
8. To keep board members up-to-date on policies, programs, issues, and regulations.
9. To reinforce the cohesiveness of the board as a group.
10. To give board members a common vocabulary of the language and concepts needed to communicate in the mental health system.
11. To ensure the board's development and utilization of its full potential.

Table 2. Components of a Model Board Development Program.

---

1.   **Philosophical and Organizational Framework**

Includes assistance with clarification of board roles, functions, legal requirements, attitudes, relationships (with director, staff, other agencies, community residents, and center clients), organization, structure, methods of operation, and goals for action.

2.   **Recruitment**

Includes assistance with development and implementation of a process for recruitment of qualified, representative, and committed board members.

3.   **Orientation**

Includes assistance with development and implementation of orientation plans, programs, and materials for new members.

4.   **Ongoing Education**

Includes provision of workshops, training sessions, and technical assistance in aspects of board functioning and in issues of mental health, the mental health center, or the community.

5.   **Assessment**

Includes ongoing assessment of board functioning and informational and membership needs to determine progress and areas needing improvement.

6.   **Access to Information**

Includes provision of access to needed information by means of a resource bank, board library, center director and staff, board member network, and so on.

7.   **Board Exchange**

Includes provision of opportunities for meetings, conferences, or visits to other board meetings to share experiences, problem-solving techniques, and information.

8.   **Support System**

Includes assistance with development of supportive relationships and structures for the board, including staff and clerical support, financial support (board budget), and educational support.

---

employees of services available and opportunities for volunteering. For example, the night shift of an aircraft plant is told through the company about the possibility of volunteering for several hours on an early morning crisis hot line following its shift. Stewardesses are advised of interesting opportunities to volunteer at an information and referral center on their time off. Volunteer bureaus in local United Way agencies or action centers in local government agencies can assist corporations in volunteer program development. At the request of the Xerox Corporation, for example, a mobile van staffed by Xerox volunteer personnel traveled around from neighborhood to neighborhood in New York, informing people about rape prevention, alcoholism, and consumer education and about volunteer opportunities in those areas (Raebel, 1980). Some corporations even have volunteer coordinators or employee management teams to match employee interests with agency needs. Offering released time for community service may attract some people to these companies in the first place, benefiting both the community and the corporation. Recently, labor unions have also encouraged their officers and members to volunteer in mental health agencies.

In a somewhat different approach to volunteering, well-informed members of labor and management can serve as informal, on-the-job, mental health information and referral specialists, thereby extending the agency's services into the work place itself. For example, members of the Barbers, Beauticians, and Allied Industries International Association, who deal with individuals on a one-to-one basis in their work, can attend an extensive array of courses covering such subjects as psychology, crisis intervention, leadership, and management. In one such course, members spend eight hours learning the effect of drugs on hair and the way to refer customers to drug treatment facilities (Raebel, 1980).

Another sign of growing corporate interest in volunteerism is the increasing number of volunteer management assistance programs (MAP) designed to improve management expertise in nonprofit agencies. Since the cost of management consultation is a growing concern, several United Way agencies across the country (in New York City, Cincinnati, and Seattle, for example) have created MAPs that help agencies solve their problems while maintaining their autonomy. Under these programs, volunteers are recruited from local corporations to assess problems and recommend changes and to provide seminars for agency personnel on management techniques. Generally, the program provides consultation in the following management areas: general administration, personnel management, accounting, finance, and public relations. Agencies are assured that information is held in strictest confidence. When an agency asks for assistance, management assistance committee members review the scope of the problem, determine the numbers and types of volunteers needed, and then recruit volunteer consultants from local corporations. A contractual agreement between the volunteer consultant and the agency, developed in order to eliminate possible misunderstandings about the scope of assistance, serves as a guide for gaining acceptance of the final recommendations.

Direct Service Volunteers

Direct service volunteers provide assistance that extends the agency's services. For example, they can enhance outpatient services by driving someone to a clinic, doing information and referral work, tutoring children in a day treatment program, or assisting as crisis counselors on a telephone hot line. By extending the range of agency services, volunteers allow staff to engage in a wider range of activities. For example, a volunteer crisis phone counselor can answer calls from clients after appropriate training in crisis intervention, enabling paid staff to develop in-depth treatment plans, supervise the more complex calls, and follow up on other clients.

Evidence does not indicate that volunteers are less reliable than paid staff in handling confidential information; in any event, the appropriate handling of information about clients can be a matter treated as a part of signed confidentiality agreements between the volunteer and the center. Volunteers often bring a kind of contagious enthusiasm and creativity to direct service work that is not generally found among professional staff members and may provide fresh insights into old problems. Because they are often closer to clients—ethnically, culturally, or socioeconomically—than their staff counterparts, they may provide an empathy that some staff have lost. In addition to volunteers who work with clients, administrative and clerical volunteers are also valuable additions to the staff of agencies, provided that their tasks are more than mere busy work. In general, volunteers need to feel they are making a significant contribution in order to maximize their benefit to the agency.

Volunteer Job Design

Even before taking the first step in recruitment, the volunteer program administrator must determine the extent of volunteer participation in the agency and develop a program plan for each area of volunteer activity. The plan should include objectives to be achieved, staff supervisory responsibilities, and a description of where and when service will take place. Program staff should have an opportunity to voice their concerns in the development of the plan. The plan should also specify who will recruit, select, assign, and train volunteers and who will do the consultation, supervision, and evaluation. In addition, since staff members are often not skilled in working with volunteers, the plan should include in-service staff training in the supervision of volunteers.

Volunteer job design also involves a detailed analysis of the tasks to be accomplished, as it does with job descriptions of paid staff. It should also include key responsibilities and related performance standards (see Table 3). Since volunteers get their primary rewards from the satisfaction of doing the job itself, care and attention should be paid to providing a sense of achievement, opportunities for some control and power, and ample opportunity for interaction between staff members and volunteers. To what extent is there challenge in the job? Is there an opportunity for clear feedback about volunteer performance? How much time is allowed for volunteer-to-volunteer interactions? A volunteer program administrator must ask such questions prior to recruitment. Because of the competition for volunteers, attention needs to be given to motivating volunteers through special recognition, challenging opportunities, increased responsibility, and opportunities for personal growth and development.

Components of a Volunteer Program

Recruitment

Volunteer recruitment involves more than posting notices on bulletin boards and sending public service announcements to the media. Like other aspects of volunteer management, it requires a plan. The recruitment plan can best be developed by consulting with public relations persons on the agency's board or staff or, if this assistance is not available, with a public relations firm. The public

Table 3. Sample Volunteer Job Description.

Position: *Volunteer Service Worker.*
Accountable to: Supervisor's name (trained professional).

Overall Responsibility

Community Information Line

Creative problem solving—facilitate caller's recognition and alleviation of problems; identify appropriate resources and assure linkage by doing follow-up calls.
Work extensively with clinic resource file of over 1,500 social, health, and welfare services in King County.
Crisis intervention (see below).
Advocacy—assist clients who have difficulty acquiring appropriate services.
Statistical recording of calls.

Crisis Line

Crisis intervention—identify and respond to feelings of clients; facilitate client's self-awareness; assist client in exploring personal problems, identifying resources, and developing action plans.
Psychiatric emergency service—refer emergency situations to community services providing outreach; schedule next-day appointments for people needing immediate help.
Advocacy—help client acquire appropriate services; occasionally do follow-up calls to clients.
Statistical recording of calls.

Qualifications

Time commitment of one four-and-one-half-hour shift per week for a minimum of six months after training.
Willingness to fill three holiday or other hard-to-fill phone shifts.
Punctuality, responsibility.
Legible handwriting for recordkeeping.
Completion of specialized training (approximately fifty hours).
    A. Twenty-four to thirty hours in classes taught by mental health professionals in:
       •crisis intervention skills
       •case files and logs
       •communication skills
       •community information and resource retrieval
       •suicide intervention
       •clinic personnel practices and administration
    B. Twenty hours of on-the-job training under experienced phone worker-trainer

Opportunities for Personal Growth

Promotion to trainer—train incoming volunteers.
Promotion to speakers bureau—represent clinic in community after training in public speaking.
Participation in in-services—attend presentation of specialized mental health community resource information by experts.
College credit—most area colleges grant credit for participation in the clinic's volunteer program.

---

relations effort must develop a good image for the agency program in order to market the product—the volunteer program and the agency's mission—and must make specific requests, such as asking for a certain number of persons to do specially designed volunteer jobs.

Job responsibilities should be honestly and accurately described. Volunteers will quickly discover if the agency is not being straightforward in its advertising for assistance, and mutually agreed-on expectations provide an important foundation for the volunteer experience. Human interest stories about the agency in brochures, public service announcements, and newspapers are typical approaches to letting the potential volunteer know what might expected. Rather than advertising generally for volunteers, an effective recruitment plan specifies the audience to be addressed and includes a speakers bureau of agency representatives sent to key professional, religious, and public service organizations to recruit volunteers. Since universities and community colleges are prime recruiting grounds, articles about the agency's services and volunteer opportunities in campus newspapers (or even paid advertisements) are often especially productive.

Senior citizens and retired employees have not traditionally been recruited but provide a particularly abundant source of volunteers. A number of companies prepare their employees for retirement through training institutes. One way to tap this service is to get on the agenda of retirement preparation seminars provided by some companies for their employees. It is also valuable to seek the assistance of other agencies concerned with volunteerism among senior citizens—for example, the Retired Senior Volunteer program reimburses senior volunteers to cover travel expenses, and retirement associations in some companies and unions have volunteer placement bureaus. Community volunteer action centers also have resource information for recruiting different types of volunteers.

Few organizations take youth volunteers seriously, yet they have proven themselves quite capable of rendering services in a variety of fields. Some mental health agencies have effectively employed youths as peer counselors, referral sources, and aides to professional staff. For example, youths have been trained in suicide prevention and successfully placed on youth suicide prevention telephone lines. Early fears and reservations about the use of youthful volunteers have diminished in recent years, and some states even have youth volunteer programs that partially subsidize youths to give a year of service in community agencies. Youths have also been used effectively as volunteers in children's treatment programs.

The agency's affirmative action program should actively recruit minority and handicapped persons as volunteers and should include representatives of minority and handicapped groups in the planning, development, and implementation of a volunteer program. Similarly, the affirmative action plan and personnel policies manual, which provide grievance procedures for paid and unpaid staff, might also cover the rights of volunteers. If it is necessary to fire a volunteer, what rights does he or she have? Is there due process? What is the appeal procedure? A number of agencies have developed a volunteer bill of rights. By whatever method, the potential volunteer should know what to expect in terms of rights to supervision, consultation, training, recognition, and due process.

Screening

The purpose of screening is to provide a process through which the volunteers and the agency staff have an opportunity to assess the suitability of the match between agency and volunteer interests. The self-selective process of volunteering should be designed to screen in, not screen out, capable individuals. As with the selection process for paid staff, volunteer screening should include such procedures as an application form, an orientation, and a personal interview. Screening for volunteers must be as careful as screening for paid staff because inappropriately placed volunteers can do equal harm—clients may be hurt, the agency reputation injured, and morale affected. In addition, screening should involve program supervisors, line staff, and the volunteer program coordinator so that the program staff assumes shared responsibility for volunteer programming.

The personal interview may take a variety of forms but should be limited to a set of important issues or questions. For example: Would the volunteer find it difficult to work with certain kinds of agency programs or clients? Is the volunteer biased toward any persons or groups, or does he or she hold a particular ideological or religious position that would prevent him or her from performing the work? Since the purpose of the interview is to probe for emotional stability and maturity of purpose, the interviewer should only ask questions related to the ability of the person to perform the task. Whether the person is married or single, heterosexual or homosexual, should not concern the agency unless these factors would affect work performance. Another approach is to use role playing to act out client problems or behaviors, asking the volunteer to respond. Other issues can be explored through a discussion of the volunteer's motivation in coming to the agency.

A second widely used screening tool is an application form designed to probe for maturity and emotional stability, frequently through some type of essay question, and to give the volunteer an idea of the agency's program. Some application forms include a contract between the volunteer and the agency that specifies the period or time of work and the working conditions (see Table 4).

The screening process continues through the probationary period of orientation and training, during which volunteers may discover that they are unable or unwilling to carry out the expected job, and concludes with an evaluation interview. The volunteer should be informed in the initial interview that training and evaluation are included in the selection process.

Training

The volunteer program administrator coordinates the training function and involves line staff, administrative representatives, and volunteers in designing a detailed training plan. The training plan should include the goals of training, learning objectives, specialized groups to be trained, an indication of who will do the training and how the training phases will be organized, analysis of the various training procedures and materials, and attention to evaluation. The goals and learning objectives may include specific knowledge to be learned, as well as self-concepts to be enhanced. Often the enhancement of self-concept is as important as the acquisition of knowledge, since self-confidence and commitment to the agency tend to carry the volunteer through difficult moments when principles or proce-

Table 4. Sample Volunteer Screening and Training Agreement.

As a phone worker trainee, I am aware that the training period, which encompasses both classroom and on-the-job training sessions, is a continuing screening process that allows me and the crisis clinic to evaluate one another, and that my acceptance as a phone worker is contingent on my successful completion of training and on the outcome of the final evaluation by my assigned supervisor. If, at any time prior to or during training, I decide not to participate further, I will notify the volunteer coordinator of my intention to terminate.

I will be on time for and participate in a minimum of four four-hour classroom training sessions, as scheduled by the volunteer coordinator.*

    * If extenuating circumstances prevent me from meeting this commitment, I will notify the volunteer coordinator and my supervisor prior to the session for which I will be late or absent.

As discussed with the volunteer coordinator or supervisor, I am willing, on my acceptance as a phone worker, to work a ____-hour shift weekly. Indicated below are times and days I will be available for shift assignment. I understand that my assigned supervisor and I will arrange mutually agreeable working times based on the information given below and on the current staffing needs of the agency.

SUNDAY	_____	_____	_____
MONDAY	_____	_____	_____
TUESDAY	_____	_____	_____
WEDNESDAY	_____	_____	_____
THURSDAY	_____	_____	_____
FRIDAY	_____	_____	_____
SATURDAY	_____	_____	_____

On receipt of my $20 deposit, I will be issued the agency training manual. At the end of classroom training, I will return the manual, and my deposit will be refunded.

_____   _____
    Phone Worker Trainee   Volunteer Coordinator or Supervisor

_____
    Date

dures do not come readily to mind. For example, a volunteer may remain calm while a client is expressing considerable emotional upset by remembering not to personalize such a situation and thereby maintain one's self-confidence.

In addition, the training plan should include a variety of teaching strategies to match the tasks for which the volunteers are being trained. For example, clerical trainees would need to be exposed to agency filing or telephone answering procedures, whereas prospective board members need training in agency policy development, legal responsibilities, board functioning, committee work, financial and resource management, decision making, planning, and general agency management.

Spreading the responsibility for training throughout the agency by including supervisors, line staff, and volunteers adds diversity to the training program. Some agencies have volunteer teams that specialize in writing and presenting simulated case studies for role playing throughout the various phases of training. Other agencies divide the training responsibility into teams of staff members and volunteers. Often agencies use outside groups as guest trainers to present specialty interests or skills, paying for these sessions by bartering or trading services. Another training possibility is to send volunteers to conferences or continuing education courses.

A typical training plan includes both orientation and ongoing in-service training. An orientation includes an overview of the mental health system; a description of the agency's mission and history and agency funding sources; a staff and volunteer organizational chart; and a discussion of the role of volunteers and of career development possibilities, including performance evaluation and recognition for work accomplished. The participation of administrators in the orientation phase lends a sense of cohesion and purpose to the volunteers' performance. The in-service phase of training addresses the different ways in which volunteers learn how to do the job. The nature of the client population is described; the specifics of job performance are outlined; the theory of various treatment modalities is explained; and the training manual, usually a regularly updated looseleaf notebook, is reviewed in terms of agency policies, standards, emergency procedures, and important reference material.

The methods available for training are varied, and trainers should not depend on lectures, except for brief talks preceding or following such exercises and presentations as role playing, videotapes, films, slides, games, and simulations—all of which can be used to transmit significant material. Since adult education sessions work best when there is participation, ample time should be allowed for feedback and questioning. Trainers need to realize that the ability to absorb a great deal of in-service training material is limited and content must therefore be repeated through on-the-job training.

Attention to the climate or setting of training is important, and space, decor, seating arrangements, room temperature, and even suitable refreshments should not be overlooked. Training sessions should be held to a reasonable time period. Since volunteers give freely of their time—and also since word of mouth is the most effective recruitment device—they should be made to feel welcome, comfortable, and respectfully treated.

Evaluation

Before the trainee enters the volunteer work force, she or he should be evaluated in an informal interview by the volunteer program supervisor or in a test administered to see what has been learned and where more work is needed. While the volunteer is carrying out tasks, continuous written feedback should be given. And an exit interview before the volunteer leaves the agency helps the center learn how to improve training or services delivery and gives the volunteer a sense of completion.

Mental health agency staff members might wonder whether the seemingly enormous task of volunteer programming is worth the undertaking—the dropout rate of volunteers is high, as is the cost of staff energy expended. For this reason the volunteer program should be evaluated as it evolves. Screening, training, and supervision should be examined in phases, along with the organizational climate and general attitude toward volunteers, and the impact of volunteer participation on the delivery of services should be assessed. This evaluation will assist the agency in keeping the volunteer program an asset in meeting the agency's goals.

Community Networks and Self-Help or Mutual Aid Groups

In exploring ways to extend the services of the mental health system into the community, the mental health administrator must pay particular attention to the informal community networks and self-help and mutual aid groups that serve as the voluntary counterparts to organized social services and, in many areas, carry the major share of the service load (Collins and Pancoast, 1976). Providing staff support and encouragement to the development of these community networks, often called natural or self-help networks, is a vital aspect of mental health services delivery that the staff members of mental health agencies are only beginning to appreciate. In this section, we make a distinction between *community networks* involving related agencies and self-help groups and *natural helping networks* that may provide informal support to an individual or family or formal support through an organized self-help group.

Types of Self-Help or Mutual Aid Groups

The terms *self-help, mutual aid, community,* and *natural* are used interchangeably to refer to groups or networks developed on a voluntary, self-help basis, usually without professional help, to provide mutual aid or to solve a common problem or need. They are usually initiated and organized at a peer level by neighbors, friends, relatives, and other persons to deal with some handicap, life transition, or life-disrupting problem. Emotional and material support comes with membership; expertise for solving the problem comes from the sharing of successful experiences in coping. The group is action-oriented and is characterized by short-lived personal participation involving empathetic, often spontaneous, face-to-face interaction (Katz and Bender, 1976). Such groups differ from other voluntary organizations—for example, the United Way or the Shriners—in that they often operate without social or political power and emerge because existing social institutions have failed to answer their needs or appropriately solve their problems. The kinds of groups vary and may be classified according to whether they focus attention on fund raising, political advocacy, consumer advocacy, or personal orientation (Silverman, 1978). Some of the best known groups related to consumer advocacy and personal orientation are Parents Anonymous, Recovery Incorporated, Advocates for the Mentally Ill, and Schizophrenics Anonymous.

Fund Raising for Survival. Groups that bring people together to raise funds on an ad hoc basis spring up wherever traditional community-fund organizations fail to respond to a felt need—for example, a group may organize a community food bank to supplement poverty-based government interventions, may provide emergency transportation for elderly persons, may develop a clothing exchange, or may establish a drop-in center for grief-stricken widows or survivors of suicide. Sometimes these fund raising drives become part of larger community drives organized by the United Way. More frequently, however, these fund raisers believe that their appeal for funds is best kept outside the domain of organized community fund raising.

Political Activism. Another type of self-help group is comprised of political activists who wish to change the way mental health services are being delivered by lobbying for changes in mental health legislation. Often mental health professionals assist these change agents by providing case examples and statistics to suggest points of view, although professional involvement may actually hinder legislative change because legislators tend to perceive mental health professionals as representing their own vested interests. Relatives of mental patients, patients themselves, and other concerned persons spend vast amounts of time writing legislation and lobbying for its approval, but simply getting an act passed is not enough. These activists have found that they need to follow their legislation through all stages of implementation, since attached regulations and interpretations of law nèed to be monitored to assure the implementation of legislative intent.

Consumer Advocacy. Clients of the mental health system or their relatives often become upset by the way they have been treated in the hospital or mental health agency and advocate for changes in operations or become a part of mental health advisory committees in local communities. Such consumer advocates can be both friend and gadfly to the mental health administrator and planner. They can help promote funding for improved or supplemental services by appealing to the media with an authenticity arising from their personal experiences. Some administrators, however, perceive advocacy as interference in the operation of the agency and do not recognize the need to provide adequate communication channels for consumer advocates.

Personal Help Groups. Another type of self-help group is the personal help group which provides its members with mutual aid in solving the problems involved in the transition from mental hospital or drug treatment facility to ordinary life. Self-help groups also offer assistance, skills, and emotional support for coping with a handicap or problem. When one first recognizes that one is different from others or faces a radically new position or role in life the feeling of isolation can be overwhelming; making the transition from isolation back to society often requires help. For example, a mother learns that her child is brain damaged and experiences feelings of anxiety, fear, self-doubt, and embarrassment. However, she soon discovers that other mothers with mentally handicapped children were devastated at first and that, over time, help from mothers in similar situations can assist mother and child in living a normal, happy life.

Members of these groups go through necessary life transitions, from first learning to recognize their difference from others through facing the impact of that recognition to learning how to cope (Silverman, 1978). These stages have been most clearly identified in the case of people coping with death and dying. Kübler-Ross describes the numbing effect of knowing that death is approaching, either for oneself or for a close relative—*denial* is followed by *rage* and finally by *acceptance* (Kübler-Ross, 1969). A similar process is at work when one faces a handicap and mutual aid groups offer hope as an alternative to despair; someone is there to say, "I know your feelings, I've been there. You can go on."

Another stage of transition is called recoil, in which a person regains his or her emotional strength to cope by using role models who offer a range of feelings and provide both perspective and information on the problem. Even when no cure and no end to the process of coping exist, the range of possible behaviors is explored. The alcoholic in a meeting of Alcoholics Anonymous points out that the problem is present daily and will not go away; yet, each day must be faced with the awareness that ways to accommodate to constant stress are also available. The self-help group provides anchors or waystations for persons learning to live these new roles. Often persons with the problem themselves become helpers of others.

Another key characteristic of self-help groups is the exchange of shared feelings and concern, which come from the reality of being "in it together" and which can often supplement or replace the worker-client relationship. Experience with the problem provides some of the knowledge and skill to help others. Therefore, the ability to listen and to learn is sharpened.

Most self-help groups organize regular meetings to exchange information, express feelings openly, and practice in learning new skills. At the meetings, those who were recipients of help are often shown how to be helpers themselves. Each group seems to have special requirements for members to become helpers, some being more formalized than others. For example, in Alcoholics Anonymous a person who has demonstrated the ability to stop drinking for at least a year is encouraged to become a sponsor or helper. Veteran sponsors teach others the sponsor role and sometimes provide training sessions for new helpers.

Mental health professionals need to understand that self-help groups and natural helping networks emerge to address an unmet need. Professionals have not provided all the assistance that alcoholics or chronic patients need, and, as a result, such disabled people have learned to help themselves. Mental health program managers need to learn how to help promote self-help groups and how to incorporate such community resources into intervention strategies and program development.

Community Service Networks

The first step in integrating formal and informal mental health resources into a community service network is to map the territory. At least two kinds of networks for providing mental services exist in most communities: the informal network, including self-help organizations, natural neighborhood helpers, relatives and friends, ethnic groups, social clubs, union halls, and various neighborhood organizations; and the formal helping network, consisting of mental health agencies, hospitals, religious organizations, crisis and emergency services, private and public schools, private and public social services agencies, and child guidance centers (Fields, 1980). It is surprising how frequently mental health professionals are unaware of the resources that these formal and informal networks provide.

The local information and referral services of United Ways or city or county human service offices have classified the services offered by formal networks into such groups as health, employment, and housing and actively engage in identifying gaps in services such as inadequate intermediate care facilities or community support systems. Such recognition has led to the development of human services coalitions of public and private agencies to meet specific needs. A similar effort should be made to map the territory of informal community networks. Sending staff into the field is a necessary first step that often discloses innumerable resources. For example, a summer intern at a Seattle mental health agency mapped the neighborhood resources of a small rural community in order to begin improving outreach services and discovered over 150 new, unlisted resources that were not contained in any local social services resource directory—groups that provided emergency food, transportation, and shelter for local residents in trouble.

Knowledge of such available resources provides mental health workers with new referral opportunities. The self-help group might be just what a client needs to cope with his or her condition. For example, a mental health counselor providing counseling to a widow could supplement and facilitate the counseling by referring the widow to membership in a widow-to-widow association. Possibilities are varied, and, if a resource does not appear to be available, the mental health professional may even assist in the development of a self-help group. For example, workers in a suicide-prevention center organized a group of suicide survivors in need of emotional support and coping skills into a self-help group. After a period of time, when peer leadership was established, the workers withdrew from involvement. On occasion, these groups may become more formalized and seek incorporation as social agencies themselves.

Other persons in the community can serve as informal helpers; for example, nurses, disc jockeys, clergymen, schoolteachers, and policemen have been trained to serve as crisis counselors, working as informal extensions of the emergency/crisis services of the mental health system. These persons are often called gatekeepers—available and accessible persons perceived by the community as resources in times of trouble. Yet they do not necessarily have the skills to handle crises or identify potentially suicidal behavior. Since mental health professionals may be requested to do this kind of training, mental health administrators need to ensure that staff members are trained in community organizing and group work skills. Staff members should not be surprised, however, if self-help groups are not especially impressed with the skills or motivations of mental health professionals, since such professionals have failed in the past to meet their needs. Nevertheless, if the professional does not compete with or undermine self-help groups, he or she might be able to make a valued contribution—for example, by serving on an advisory board, by assisting in training, or by acting as a consultant in organization and development. In a time of shrinking resources, imaginative and creative administration will be required to train mental health workers in the skills necessary for the support of self-help groups.

Some associations of self-help groups, individual helpers, and social service professionals are experimenting with linking and integrating services for persons in need. In Baltimore, for example, mental health agencies and neighborhood self-help groups use each other's buildings for meetings and have developed a cross-referenced informational system for the use of counselors and the provision of emergency services, as well as a hot line for communicating about unmet client needs within the network. Volunteers and professionals work together on developing common projects, and mutual support groups have been established to meet newly identified needs.

Another innovative approach to community networking involves the development of an extended support system of friends, relatives, and neighbors to assist families in crisis or in times of emotional stress. Therapists using this model convene an ad hoc support team, which consists of neighbors, relatives, and professionals and which may number as many as seventy persons, to provide information and physical and emotional support to meet the dysfunctional family's needs. Such an intervention team focuses considerable resources and energy on the problem—extending the capabilities of the therapist and, in most cases, providing help beyond the scope of any agency's services—in order to bring about constructive changes in a brief period of time, usually not more than several weeks (Rueveni, 1979).

Difficulties encountered by program administrators developing support networks include the following: (1) The process requires consent and cooperation from the family in trouble; (2) the public character of the intervention is difficult to accept, and the support system may be rejected; (3) the team needs to be gathered, trained, and guided through a fairly complex set of interventions; and (4) until the crisis abates, a high level of commitment is required. Nevertheless, the mobilization of family networks involving intense cooperation from a corps of volunteers and professionals has proven to be an effective technique for assisting families in crisis.

Conclusion

The community mental health system seeks to serve the person in his or her own environment. This chapter suggests ways in which volunteers can provide human resources to extend the services of the mental health center into the community. In addition, mental health workers can link their formal organizational and professional skills with informal community self-help networks. Both of these approaches to providing true community mental health services involve the integration of professional and lay skills and experiences in a partnership and collaboration that supports a new and healthy movement in community mental health.

References

Caplan, R. B. *Psychiatry and Community in Nineteenth Century America.* New York: Basic Books, 1969.

Collins, A., and Pancoast, D. *Natural Helping Networks.* Washington, D.C.: National Association of Social Workers, 1976.

Fields, S. "Mental Health Networks: Extending the Circuits of Community Care." *Innovations,* Spring 1980, 7 (1), 2–29.

Katz, A. H., and Bender, E. I. *The Strength in Us: Self-Help Groups in the Modern World.* New York: New Viewpoints, 1976.

Kübler-Ross, E. *On Death and Dying.* New York: Macmillan, 1969.

Miller, S. O. "Citizen Participation in Community Mental Health Programs." In Alfred Katz (Ed.), *Community Mental Health.* New York: Council on Social Work Education, 1979.

President's Commission on Mental Health. *Report of the President's Commission on Mental Health.* Vol. 1. Washington, D.C.: U.S. Government Printing Office, 1978.

Public Law 94–63, 1975 Amendments to the Community Mental Health Centers Act of 1963.

Raebel, J. "Volunteers From Business." *The Grantsmanship Center News,* May/June 1980, pp. 38–49.

Rueveni, U. *Networking Families in Crisis.* New York: Human Services Press, 1979.

Schwartz, I. *Volunteers in Juvenile Justice.* Washington, D.C.: National Institute of Law Enforcement and Criminal Justice, 1977.

Silverman, P. R. *Mutual Help Groups: A Guide for Mental Health Workers.* Rockville, Md.: Department of Health, Education, and Welfare, 1978.

Wilson, M. *The Effective Management of Volunteer Programs.* Boulder, Colo.: Johnson Publishing, 1976.

❧ 14 ❧

Dealing with Unionization and Collective Bargaining

William E. Hershey

Managers need to acquire the knowledge and skills of collective bargaining if they are to meet the challenge of unionization. This chapter first describes the history and process of unionization and then outlines the components of collective bargaining, including union security and management rights, the wage and effort bargain, individual employee security, and contract administration. The importance of determining appropriate bargaining units is stressed, selected National Labor Relations Board bargaining guidelines are presented, and relevant bargaining team strategies are described. Finally, union issues unique to mental health settings—professionalism, ethical codes, and public opinion—are explored.

Unionization in community mental health agencies is a comparatively new development for both administrators and clinicians, since nonprofit community human services agencies were exempt from the collective bargaining procedures of the Taft-Hartley Act until the 1974 amendments. In addition, the marked decrease in federal funding of community mental health centers in the 1970s led to the increased turnover of executive directors, which in turn contributed to staff unrest over inadequate recognition of personnel needs by local agency boards of directors. As a result, unionization became a viable option for expressing staff concerns about competitive salaries and job security.

Many mental health workers see unionization as a way of improving economic and working conditions and obtaining a voice in service planning. Traditionally, salary levels in mental health settings have been quite low—for example, a mental health worker with a bachelor's degree is often hired by a residential treatment center for minimum wage, and entry-level therapists often receive salaries far below comparable entry-level professional salaries in other fields. The surplus of mental health workers in some areas has made it an employers' market. Further, autocratic managers or boards of directors have at times set policies that fail to take employee needs into consideration. As a result, salaries and conditions have been arbitrarily determined, rather than negotiated. A desire to improve these economic and political conditions has made mental health workers increasingly receptive to unionization.

Managers in mental health agencies have also realized that they can address objectionable working conditions. Participatory management styles, career development programs, and attention to working conditions have precluded the need for unions in some cases. However, many of the conditions influencing the need or desire for unionization are beyond management control. Economic factors, such as inflation, and political factors, such as the election of conservative anti-mental health politicians, have affected employment conditions. Therefore, managers have begun to prepare themselves for collective bargaining by acquiring mediation and conflict resolution skills (Shaffer, 1979) and by employing management and legal consultants.

At least two major philosophical perspectives on the need for unions in mental health agencies have emerged. One perspective argues that good personnel management precludes the need for unions. The other view states that workers need a forum for expressing and acting on their organizational needs. This chapter will address these two perspectives by identifying the reasons mental health personnel seek unionization, the conditions that cause employees to join unions, and the labor-management strategies used in the collective bargaining process. The chapter also includes a description of the management skills required in mediation, contract negotiations, collective bargaining, and determination of the components of a labor-management agreement. Unionization will also be viewed in relationship to professional codes of ethics, public opinion, and bargaining unit development. As community mental health programs become increasingly unionized, both administrators and clinicians will need to acquire the knowledge and skills of collective bargaining.

Historical Perspective

Although a variety of laws have indirectly affected collective bargaining since colonial times, not until the Morris-LaGuardia Act of 1932 was a national labor relations law passed that directly related to the collective bargaining process. The Morris-LaGuardia Act became a cornerstone of American labor relations policy by making representation a private issue to be resolved among workers, employers, and unions; by eliminating so-called yellow dog contracts, which required employees to pledge that they were not and would not become union members so long as they were employed by that company; and by curtailing the use of injunctions by employers for the prevention of strikes (Beal and Wickersham, 1967).

Labor rights expanded in 1936 with the passage of the Wagner Act, which specifically protected employees from unfair labor practices by prohibiting employers from interfering with, restraining, or coercing employees in the exercise of their right to self-organization; dominating or interfering in the affairs of the union; discriminating in regard to hiring, tenure, or any other condition of employment for the purpose of encouraging or discouraging union membership; discriminating against or discharging an employee because he or she had filed charges or given testimony under the act; and refusing to bargain with chosen representatives of employees. An independent administrative agency, the National Labor Relations Board (NLRB), was established to hold hearings and to issue decisions and orders preventing unfair labor practices. NLRB orders and decisions—which are subject to court review for enforcement, although courts have been reluctant to intervene—have included cease-and-desist orders, court-ordered requirements to prevent labor law violations, and affirmative action requirements (Beal and Wickersham, 1967).

Although the Taft-Hartley Act of 1947 preserved the basic gains of unions, particularly the right to bargain and the prohibition of unfair practices that hinder the bargaining process, managers hailed it as a redress of the balance of power, perceived by them to be in the union's favor (Beal and Wickersham, 1967). The act spelled out unfair labor practices within unions, provided that employees be protected from union restraint and coercion just as the Wagner Act had protected them from employer coercion, and protected employees from union pressure exerted through employers, such as excessive or discriminating initiation dues and fees. In addition, the Taft-Hartley Act stripped unions of their power to induce employers to discharge persons who were antiunion, protected nonunion workers in nonunion firms from union pressure, provided a cooling-off period in the termination of collective bargaining agreements, and required the party intending to terminate or modify a collective agreement to serve a written notice of such intention on the other party to the agreement sixty days prior to the proposed date of termination. Finally, the Landrum-Griffin Act of 1959, another innovative piece of labor legislation, provided detailed regulation of the internal affairs of unions by the federal government.

All these acts attempted to protect the rights of the employer, the employee, and the union as they interacted in the collective bargaining process. The government thereby became the third agent in the labor-management relationship. Although the Taft-Hartley Act of 1947 and the Landrum-Griffin Act of 1959 added significantly to the regulations, most important for mental health program managers and employees were the 1974 Hartley amendments, which eliminated the exemption of employees of nonprofit hospitals (interpreted by the courts to include all nonprofit social agencies) from the collective bargaining process.

Pre-Collective Bargaining Period

The question of who in fact is covered by particular bargaining units must be answered before collective bargaining can begin. Several unions might be necessary to represent different bargaining units within a mental health center. Clerical workers might be represented by one union, and clinical staff members and program managers by another. No perfect solution is available, because what works for one institution may not work for another. Management, union officials, and professional associations need to determine the most appropriate bargaining units (Nigro, 1979).

The NLRB functions as a third party in collective bargaining by seeking answers to the following questions: What is an appropriate bargaining unit? What is the will of the majority in this unit? How can a change in the will of the majority be accommodated? These are difficult questions to answer, since mental health programs vary in size and complexity. Managers may prefer a single bargaining unit for all staff because many of the specific problem areas can be more easily controlled (Nigro, 1979). In contrast, professional associations have preferred more narrowly defined units in order to maximize attention to professional matters.

The collective bargaining process does not begin until a group of employees agrees to form a bargaining unit, secures union representation, and gains management recognition. This pre-collective bargaining period is important for both labor and management, since hostilities created at this time may linger into the collective bargaining process and hinder the negotiating relationship (Beal and Wickersham, 1967).

Employee Initiative

Either employees or union organizers usually take the initiative in organizing for agency unionization. Potential for dissatisfaction exists within any job, and typical complaints among mental health workers include low pay, insecure positions, short-term funding, long hours, bad working conditions, and chaotic or capricious management. Workers seeking a voice in shaping the issues that affect their lives meet with union representatives to assess interest in unionization and in the feasibility of organizing—and do so while maintaining secrecy in order to protect themselves from management retaliation.

The union has an easier time organizing when a group of dissatisfied employees forms a nucleus for recruiting new members. The workers can supply names, make personal contacts, give inside information on organizational problems, and generally establish a climate for organizing. Mental health professionals, however, are usually not motivated to explore or become knowledgeable about union issues. In fact, before the 1970s, mental health workers thought that their colleagues could not be organized, since mental health professionals work so closely with management and tend to share management viewpoints (Shaffer, 1979). Because of these factors, organizing has been slow in some parts of the country, although active in locales where other unions have been strong.

Occasionally, unions take the initiative in approaching an agency they believe should be unionized. Unions have ambitions for growth and a need to defend themselves from the competition of the unorganized. If nonunion workers in a field can display better wages and working conditions than unionized workers, unions have difficulty organizing. Therefore, unions frequently contact workers within organizations to assess the feasibility of organizing. In the mental health field, the union might point to low wages, poor benefits, and the union's ability to influence the passage of legislation providing higher allocations to mental health programs, and consequently higher wages. Organizing in this way, however, is more difficult than building on already existing interest in unionization.

Management Activity

Skillful managers who sense rising interest in unionization among staff members will review their management structure and processes with the following issues in mind: a fair and competitive wage structure with salary and career ladders; a clear, fair, open grievance procedure; a solid staff development program with staff access to training money; a good supervisory structure with emphasis on supervisory skills; an upward communication process; potential for flex-time and job-sharing; and clarity of agency mission in relationship to worker tasks and activities.

When employee or union initiative has led to union elections in an agency, managers and employees alike need to be aware of NLRB guidelines relating to unfair labor and management election practices. According to those guidelines, elections are overturned if conduct is detected that interferes with the employee's exercise of "a free and untrammeled choice." Examples of such conduct include misrepresentation of material facts or other similar agency trickery; presentation of threatening or misleading information by a person known by employees to have access to the information presented; presentation of information so close to the election that the other party or parties have no opportunity to make an effective reply; a reasonable probability that misrepresentation may have a significant effect upon the election; and lack of labor or management qualification to evaluate the statements of misrepresentation.

Some managers take an aggressive antiunion stance by showing antiunion films, sending letters to employees outlining the organization's opinion about union membership, and giving "captive audience" talks, which are prohibited, according to NLRB guidelines, twenty-four hours prior to an election. Workers are allowed to distribute leaflets to other employees, put up posters, or give talks. Such activities can create hostility among employees and management and can negatively influence negotiations and the work place environment following the campaign. For example, the very language of union organizers might not appeal to workers who are inexperienced in power struggles or conflict tactics. Such terms as *collective struggle, rights, enemies, demands,* and *arsenal of weapons* may be a natural deterrent for workers who have been accustomed to management-organized democratic problem-solving sessions (Alexander, 1980).

Rules and Scope of Collective Bargaining

Before becoming involved in negotiations, both the worker and the mental health program manager should have an understanding of the rules and the scope of collective bargaining. Collective bargaining usually includes four major issues: union security and management rights, including the manner in which both will be represented; the wage and effort bargain, including wages, production standards, and work objectives; individual security, including fair treatment, just cause, discharge, seniority provisions, grievance procedures, available work, and layoff provisions; and administration of on-the-job representation or union visitation; and arbitration issues. Actually, the issue of union security sets the groundwork for the other issues, since wages, working conditions, and individual security cannot be discussed until union security has been assured (Beal and Wickersham, 1967).

Union Security and Management Rights

Union security is a primary issue, since no effective independent employee representation can take place without it. Exclusive bargaining rights are gained by winning NLRB-authorized elections (Public Law 86–257, 1959). The specifying of management's rights is important because mental health agency directors receive authority and responsibility for management control from the agency board of directors, who need to be aware of all the issues reflected in a union contract. The agency director is the person in charge and functions as the personnel manager, the allocator of resources, and the human resources planner. Each step in the unionization process tends to erode this managerial power, with unions seeking to acquire whatever control they can negotiate from management.

Additional forms of security obtained only through the consent of management include the following (Cormick, 1977):

1. *Union shop,* under which all employees become members of one union after sixty days of employment.
2. *Agency shop,* which provides that all employees who choose not to join the union are required to pay the union a fee equal to membership dues to help defray bargaining costs.
3. *Modified union shop,* under which all employees hired on or after the effective date of the contract become union members for the duration of the agreement. Present employees who are not union members are not required to join.
4. *Open shop,* under which there are no union-protected positions and staff are free to join or not.

In addition to these options, union representatives in public service organizations have attempted to gain credibility by seeking dues checkoff clauses, whereby the employer withholds union dues from members' paychecks, with employee authorization, and transmits the money directly to the union; and maintenance of membership clauses, whereby all employees who are members of the union when an agreement is signed, and all who join later, must continue to pay dues to the union for the duration of the agreement. However, right-to-work states—that is, states that provide only for an open shop—do not allow such clauses (Shaffer, 1979).

Another important issue is the duration and renewal of the labor agreement. A notice of termination or negotiation must be given, as well as openers for wage adjustments during the contract period (Beal and Wickersham, 1967). In the case of mental health programs, where outside funding controls the revenue resources, a confused set of allocation schedules, ranging from biennial to annual, makes negotiation on this matter complex.

Management rights are not necessarily covered in union contract agreements on the theory that all rights not specifically bargained away belong to management. However, some agency managers feel it important to balance the union security issue with such management rights as the freedom to set goals of the organization, the freedom to determine the use of capital resources of the agency, and the power to discipline for cause. These management rights are particularly important in the mental health field, where limited resources can make the right to participate in setting agency directions even more important than wage issues. For example, in voluntary agencies, conflict may emerge between the board of directors and the professional staff over agency goals or services delivery approaches and may be more important to mental health workers than salary issues (Lightman, 1978). However, the trend seems to be to limit the scope of bargaining to wages, hours, and other terms and conditions of employment and to exclude from mental health agency union contracts such management rights as policy formulation, program planning and organization, budget development, and utilization of new technology. In some cases, contracts explicitly prohibit employers from bargaining on defined or implied management rights or state that employers are not required to bargain on management issues (Shaffer, 1979).

However, many of these same management issues—for example, caseload size, ethical practice, services delivery plans, and quality of service—are also of concern to professional staff members and might, in the future, become a part of the collective bargaining process, as is the case in the nursing and medical professions (Shaffer, 1979). Unions generally recognize management needs and therefore are sometimes willing to grant limited management rights clauses. Union concern is not so much to control the agency as to influence the form and content of management action.

Wage and Effort Bargain

Bargaining over wage and effort is the heart of the collective negotiation process and results in the major portion of a contract agreement. Since every wage and effort item can be translated into management time and costs and since higher wages, better hours, and better working conditions are still the primary goals of unions (Alexander, 1980), careful preparation for this aspect of the contract is crucial to both labor and management. The wage and effort portion of an agreement—the fundamental contract offer that new employees receive when they accept work—usually includes pay for time worked, the effort bargain, premium pay, pay for time not worked, and contingent health and welfare benefits (Beal and Wickersham, 1967).

Pay for Time Worked. Pay, of course, is geared to expected employee production; discussion in this area usually centers around job structure, wage and salary levels, and method of payment. Agencies should have carefully constructed job descriptions, performance standards, and work objectives in operation prior to negotiation on this item, and administrators who follow sound personnel management principles will argue for building wage negotiations on such job descriptions and performance standards, rather than opting for shortcuts—for example, a 5 to 10 percent increase for all employees. The wage bargain that includes the skills and knowledge required to perform an assigned task and the amount of work expected to be done by the worker ought to reflect consensus on what constitutes adequate worker performance.

In industry, managers and workers are familiar with the process of measuring worker outputs. Time studies help determine expected levels of production, and worker production rates can be compared to the rates of workers at other job sites. In professions such as social work or nursing, however, workers have, until quite recently, argued that such variables as task complexity, skill levels, and production objectives cannot be measured. On the other hand, managers and social agency boards of directors have argued that jobs in the nonprofit field involving the servicing of human needs should not be compensated at rates comparable to those in other service industry jobs because mental health workers are obviously working for more than just the money. In the light of current inflation rates, this argument has little, if any, merit. Performance in mental health services agencies can be measured, and persons deserve an adequate wage for effort expended, regardless of their motivation.

Salaries in the mental health field are difficult to determine due to the lack of salary surveys, job descriptions, and inadequate salary information, which is often hidden or kept as a professional secret. When classification schedules such as the annual United Way of America salary survey are published, they frequently do not relate levels of education and experience to job categories. State and federal civil service salary administration schedules present similar problems. Industry itself at times establishes rates within single industries or companies without regard for comparable rates in the community (Beal and Wickersham, 1967). Agencies might enhance their own personnel management system by engaging a personnel consultant to determine ratings, comparable work, and potential career ladders.

Management is not the only party that benefits from the availability of accurate job descriptions and performance standards. Often, worker dissatisfactions are directly related to impossible work expectations. Only after the key responsibilities of a particular job are spelled out can both manager and worker get a realistic picture of the work involved. However, overly specific contract language can lead to such narrow interpretations as, "I only do what the contract says." Since large wage increases are not likely to result from skillful negotiation because of external limitations on financial resources, negotiation on realistic job expectations and working conditions can prove especially critical to workers and managers alike. The freedom to paint one's own work space and a few dollars for the paint, for example, can contribute appreciably to improving worker morale and increasing efficiency. Flexible working hours, shared jobs, and job rotation are all issues that workers might negotiate in this portion of the process.

Premium Pay and Fringe Benefits. Premium pay is extra pay for work performed outside the normally contracted time or at unreasonable hours. Because of the nature of their work, mental health professionals have been traditionally expected to work until the task is completed with no extra compensation. However, mental health services managers know from experience that employees who work beyond a forty-hour week under stressful conditions are subject to burnout. This problem must be recognized and action taken, either by reevaluating the task or worker performance in each situation or by providing some extra compensation for overtime work. The U.S. Department of Labor requires such action for clerical workers, but mental health professionals have long suffered from a lack of attention in this matter, thereby increasing the appeal of unionization.

The use of fringe benefits such as vacation pay, holiday pay, paid rest periods, and special bonuses is one way in which management might provide time off with pay as a compensation for seniority or meritorious service (Beal and Wickersham, 1967). Some agencies have expanded fringe benefits, such as educational leave with pay, where salaries have not kept pace with inflation. Such benefits not only serve to improve morale and provide a release from work stress but also increase job competence. Other fringe benefit components of collective bargaining packages have expanded significantly in recent years and have included death benefits, pensions, supplementary employment benefits, severance pay, and health and welfare plans. Managers have learned to be careful in negotiating in this area, since health and welfare insurance rates continue to increase rapidly, and the perceived needs of employees for more or less benefits fluctuate and are difficult to anticipate.

Individual Security. The individual security component of a contract covers job rights and due process and is perhaps the most important contractual guarantee to the employee, since it ensures continuity of employment. Although management does not like to deal with an unstable work force or engage in layoffs, resources do fluctuate and political circumstances change. Guidelines should be developed with staff in order to accommodate both employee and management rights during periods of cutback management. Merit and ability, in contrast to seniority, are highly valued professional criteria that often conflict with seniority clauses in contracts. The mental health manager would like to have the freedom, in periods of cutback or expansion, to cut the least-able or promote the most-qualified staff members. High turnover rates in the mental health field have

diminished attention to the seniority issue, but recent funding cutbacks will probably lead to new demands for this aspect of individual security (Beal and Wickersham, 1967).

The grievance process is another common element of individual security in
union contracts. Almost every mental health program has some statement of fair
treatment conditions and grievance procedures designed to handle unfair job practices. The collective bargaining agreement may establish both the rules of employee conduct and the judicial review by which the disciplined employee is
judged—in other words, unions and management negotiate the procedures related
to "just cause" grievance procedures.

Management, traditionally responsible for maintaining good employee-
employer relationships under collective bargaining, also makes the initial accusa-
tion of employee failure to perform duties. If employees feel that they have been
unfairly treated, they may call upon the union to act as defense attorney. Usually
the labor agreement gives the worker and union a final recourse to arbitration to
guarantee the worker's right to fair treatment. Most mental health programs
should have detailed grievance procedures in place, even without unionization. If
situations do get to the hearing stage, the appointed judges usually are guided by
such principles as: policies must be known and reasonable; violation of policies
must be proven, and the burden of proof rests on the employer; the application of
principles must be consistent; where employees are held to a standard, that standard must be reasonable; the training provided employees must be adequate; the
job rights of employees must be protected from arbitrary, capricious, or discriminating action; actions must be impersonal and based on fact; and, where the
contract speaks, it must speak with authority (Holley and Jennings, 1980).

Administration

The final component of a collective bargaining agreement includes the
machinery for establishing due process and the delegation of authority to individuals responsible for the administration of the agreement. Some agreements include reimbursement procedures for time spent by stewards, appointment by the
union of representatives for handling grievances, and permission for stewards to
leave their work place to confer with employees and supervisors. Other elements
dealing with arbitration include opportunities for union officials to visit work
places during working hours,. under specified conditions; composition of an outside board of arbitrators; and a description of the duties, powers and limitations of
the arbitrator (Beal and Wickersham, 1967).

The stewards are usually elected by the union, and the number of stewards
is agreed upon by the union and the agency. The use of an outside mediator or
arbitrator usually involves authorizing the third party to rule on all disputes
pertaining to the interpretation or application of the agreement. Arbitrators are
generally selected by the parties from lists provided by the American Arbitration
Association.

Disputes or problems are usually resolved either by outside arbitration, mediation through a "friend of the family," or strikes. None of these devices need be applied if the parties first attempt to settle differences internally. No-strike and no-lockout clauses are usually included in contracts involving mental health agencies. Although mental health workers have engaged in strike activity in the past and will no doubt do so in the future, many are concluding that the alternative of binding and compulsory arbitration is preferable to strike action in the public service arena. Before the 1974 Taft-Hartley amendments, mental health center workers had the right to strike or picket if recognition was not forthcoming. Such striking or picketing is no longer possible, which means that management at mental health centers will most likely only recognize the need for an existence of unions by means of outside mediation and/or arbitration.

Appropriate Unit for Collective Bargaining

If the majority of employees at a mental health agency informally decide they want a certain union to represent them, and can convince the agency management that this is indeed the case—for example, by showing authorization cards or petitions signed by a majority of workers—then the management would simply recognize and bargain with the union. If the management of a mental health program refuses voluntary recognition of a union or if there is a question about the adequacy of worker interest in a union, government intervention may be needed and is initiated by filing a representation petition with the NLRB, which uses the guidelines noted in Table 1.

By law, an employer is required to bargain with representatives of his or her employees. In some cases, all of the employees of a mental health program may want to be in the same bargaining unit, feeling that, since their numbers are small, collective representation is more appropriate. On the other hand, clerical employees at a mental health agency may have interests substantially different from those of professional employees. In these situations, each group of employees, called a unit for collective bargaining purposes, is entitled to have a different union represent it in bargaining with the employer. Acting through its regional office, the NLRB determines which employees should be included in which appropriate unit. For example, in hospitals, the NLRB has recommended such units as professional employees, registered nurses, office and clerical employees, technical employees, and service and maintenance employees (Nash, 1978).

The bargaining unit is of considerable importance to employees, management, and the unions seeking representation rights. The wage concessions available to particular groups of employees can be influenced by the bargaining unit established. For example, a bargaining unit composed exclusively of professionals recently demanded that the scope of collective bargaining be expanded to include such issues as the size of caseloads, the course content for training programs, and the right to discuss professional issues on work time—prerogatives previously regarded as belonging to management (Alexander, 1980). The bargaining units of

Table 1. Selected Guidelines Used by the National Labor Relations Board (NLRB).

Groups Eligible to File Representation Petition

1. An employee or group of employees interested in unionization.
2. Any person or union acting on behalf of a substantial number of employees.
3. An employer who is presented by a union with a claim that it represents a majority of his or her employees.
4. An employer presented with a claim of representation from two or more unions (Title I, National Labor Relations Act, PL 86-257).

Contents of a Representation Petition

1. Description of the unit of employees in which the election is sought.
2. The approximate number of employees in the unit.
3. The names of all unions that claim to represent the employees in the unit.

NLRB Question of Fact

1. Are the employer's operations within NLRB jurisdictional standards?
2. Is the proposed unit appropriate for collective bargaining?
3. Is there a sufficient showing of employee interest?
4. Is the filing of the petition timely? (PL 86-257).

NLRB Criteria for Bargaining Unit Recognition

1. Demonstration of interest, signed worker authorization cards.
2. Submission with forty-eight hours of completion.
3. At least 30 percent of eligible workers represented on petition.

NLRB Criteria for Time Lines

1. No election can be conducted if a valid election has taken place during the preceding twelve months.
2. Representation elections are prohibited ("contract bar") for the life of a valid, signed collective bargaining agreement (usually three years or less).
3. A petition for elections may be filed at least sixty days but not more than ninety days before the expiration of a contract.
4. A formal hearing is held if there is no agreement on issues related to an election.

Components of an Election Agreement (Consent Agreement)

1. Description of the bargaining unit.
2. Time and place for holding elections.
3. Basis for determining who is eligible to vote.

Election Procedures Using Secret Ballots

1. Within seven days of NLRB ordering an election, the agency administrator must submit a list of names and addresses of all prospective bargaining unit members.
2. Names of prospective members are shared with the prospective union prior to posting election notices.
3. Secret balloting is usually monitored by NLRB staff.
4. Election speeches are prohibited by either party within twenty-four hours of the election.
5. Fraud, coercion, and injurious statements in election propaganda are prohibited.

Certification of Election Results

1. If a union receives support from a majority of workers, a certificate of official representation is issued.
2. If no union receives a majority, a twelve-month period of stability is guaranteed before the next election.
3. Within five days of counting the votes, either party can file objections alleging misconduct or challenging the ballots.

Table 1, cont'd.

Criteria for Union Recognition Without Secret Ballot Elections

1. Evidence reveals that a fair, impartial election would have been impossible at the time that the election was held.
2. Authorization cards were clear and unambiguous.
3. Employee signatures were obtained without threat or coercion.
4. A majority of employees in the bargaining unit have signed the cards (*NLRB v. Gissel,* 1969).

Decertification Procedures

1. A decertification petition requests an NLRB-supervised election to determine if the majority of workers no longer want union representation or representation by a particular union.
2. Procedures can be used by both management and labor.
3. Decertification elections follow the same procedures as certification elections.

---

highly skilled staff may negotiate higher salaries that may in turn penalize the less skilled. The argument for single bargaining units composed of professionals and paraprofessionals is that most mental health programs tend to be small and decentralized and that attempts to organize and bargain collectively on a professional or areawide basis—by doctors or lawyers, for example—do not appear to be especially successful. Alternative organizational forms, such as larger and more powerful bargaining units, may become increasingly attractive (Lightman, 1978).

The manager of the mental health program may favor small bargaining units in the hope of playing one unit off against the other. However, negotiating with larger, single bargaining units has the advantage to management of reducing costs related to multiple agreements and negotiations. Managers are also interested in ensuring that certain jobs reflecting significant management responsibilities should be excluded from the bargaining unit—for example, a line worker also carrying program management responsibilities for a small consultation and education unit or a psychiatrist who does medication but also supervises the screening program. Managers have considerable power in determining the composition of bargaining units in that they may legitimately withhold information on plans for developing new programs until after union representation elections or designate certain staff as a part of the management team.

Union management agreements excluding certain individuals from the unit have been set aside by the NLRB where it was believed that the persons involved should properly have been included in the unit. In exercising its power to determine appropriate units, the NLRB strives to determine the meaning of actual day-to-day relationships among workers. This aim is best served by seeking to determine the community of interest existing among employees (Beal and Wickersham, 1967)—a situation that prevails in mental health programs where professionals and paraprofessionals work daily in interdisciplinary teams in which roles are exchanged and interchanged. The community of interest criterion in such settings favors a single bargaining unit.

Managers and the Election Process

Typically, the time before an election is a troubling one for managers. The administrator tends to operate with a siege mentality, seeing formerly cooperative colleagues as the enemy now demanding the intrusion of outsiders into what once seemed a family operation. Managers report feeling hurt or at least severely limited in action and may, from that point on, feel restrained from even acting benevolently toward workers. Since most managers would probably prefer to operate without a union, some have launched successful campaigns against unionization by carefully following the rules and avoiding such behavior as the following just prior to the election: threatening behavior, such as eliminating certain services or programs; raising of wages or benefits prior to the election in order to influence the outcome of the election; promising to increase wages or benefits as a condition for voting against the union; and reducing the wages prior to the election in order to avoid the promotion of hostility among workers. If, however, the election announcement is sudden and unexpected, then management has little time for a campaign. In any case, the practices and policies of the agency will either help or hinder the campaign process. Some managers welcome the union as a method for establishing a worker organization that functions in a democratic fashion and as a countervailing force to the policies of the board of directors.

A union may also request recognition by proving that a majority of workers are interested in joining the union and by submitting signed authorization cards to an impartial mediator. If there is agreement on this procedure, a manager may save a considerable amount of time, money, and energy, to say nothing of the hostility that can develop during election campaigns, by assuming that recognition is a foregone conclusion. A research study has concluded that the cost for the employer of an NLRB election runs to approximately $126 per employee (Imberman, 1975).

Negotiation Process. If the workers win the union recognition election, preparations for negotiations begin immediately. Preparing for negotiations requires management and labor to specify their respective goals in order to reach a settlement. Each group enters the process with a different position regarding the maximums and minimums it would like to receive or be willing to relinquish (Stevens, 1963). These positions are ranked and become the basis for the collective bargaining process. For example, the mental health manager might determine that a top wage offer would be a 10 percent increase, which includes both 5 percent for merit and a new dental coverage plan in a package of benefits, and that a bottom-line offer would consist of a 3 percent increase with no merit or extra benefits. The union representatives, on the other hand, might propose a 20 percent increase in wages, a union shop, and four additional floating holidays. Negotiations then revolve around these positions. The union must be careful not to make unrealistically extensive demands, and management must take care not to make too limited an offer.

Part of the preparation process involves deciding whether to negotiate item by item or to work on a total package that includes several issues. The general preference seems to be toward packaging all items together, an approach that allows greater flexibility and a more realistic statement of positions than the item-by-item approach. The flexibility comes from each party raising several issues for discussion purposes—for example, "We might drop the items on floating holidays and voluntary overtime if you drop the items on extended retirement pay and union shop." This approach also indicates which issues are open for negotiation and which issues are firm (Holley and Jennings, 1980).

The two major aspects of collective bargaining are the economic wage and effort negotiations and the administrative communications and union security issues. Despite a certain amount of ritualistic game playing and posturing and the need to overstate positions, the key to successful negotiating is the maintenance of an atmosphere of respect and honesty that includes mutual trust; respect for technical competence, experience, and personal qualities; and the ability to admit mistakes, to keep one's word when a concrete position is taken, and to stick to issues, rather than focusing on personalities. Realizing that his or her counterpart on the opposing side needs to make a good impression on his or her team, the wise negotiator will recognize the need to save face and will give the other party room to move gracefully from a seemingly unyielding position (Holley and Jennings, 1980). Regardless of what is being communicated to the management or to union members, negotiators learn to hear what is being said beneath the actual words by asking: How final is the statement? How specific is the statement? and What are the consequences associated with the statement? (Holley and Jennings, 1980).

The Negotiating Team. The composition of the negotiating team is an important factor that varies from one organization to another. The union usually sends one of its principal officers as chief negotiator, along with several staff members, and may also want to include outside experts on its team. The mental health management team may be comprised of board members who have labor negotiation or legal experience, the executive director assisted by a labor relations consultant, and/or a third-party labor relations consultant who alone speaks for management. Whatever the pattern, each party should have a knowledgeable negotiator who can assume leadership in the bargaining process. An outside consultant may not have sufficient knowledge of internal issues, and a board representative might not be the best choice if he or she undermines the director's position as chief executive officer. No one solution is the best; however, the chief negotiator should possess full knowledge of labor-relations rules, negotiation strategies, legal issues, and agency operations and policies (Beal and Wickersham, 1967).

The Art of Negotiating. How issues are presented and the setting in which they are presented are also important factors. Special interest groups within bargaining units, for example, should make their wishes known by contacting union representatives prior to the negotiating session, rather than being represented on the bargaining team (Holley and Jennings, 1980); a unified approach is important once negotiations have begun. Conducting negotiations in private is also necessary, since real conflict may take place during negotiations, and the presence of an audience increases the likelihood of acting-out, namecalling, and even clowning. For progress to take place, a secluded, quiet, private environment is essential. Since personality conflicts may also emerge during negotiations, the negotiator needs to bring patience, basic intelligence, stamina, an open mind, and fairness to the bargaining table (Beal and Wickersham, 1967). The effective use of self and the use of various interpersonal strategies to modify attitudes are critical skills in the bargaining process (Spector, 1977).

Both union and management bargaining teams should be provided time to caucus in order to consider the financial and political implications of proposals and counterproposals. Both parties are politically motivated in their negotiations, assigning imprecise yet significant values to certain items that preserve their discretion and organizational strength or reward influential participants on their respective negotiating teams (Holley and Jennings, 1980). The management team should have financial advisers on hand for these caucuses, especially if they are not available at bargaining sessions, to assist negotiators in evaluating and prioritizing various nonwage proposals, particularly those numerous items that are not a part of the wage-effort bargain (Holley and Jennings, 1980).

Since most mental health agencies draw their revenue from direct federal grants or from public allocations, negotiators addressing the wage-effort bargain will often have minimal discretion. In fact, when public allocations are reduced, the union is placed in a difficult position. Having sold itself to the membership on the basis of improving wages, it finds itself in a position similar to management's—at the mercy of a changing political climate, reduced governmental spending for human services, or a general economic decline.

Bargaining in Good Faith. The NLRB requires the bargaining parties to negotiate in good faith by demonstrating a sincere and honest intention to consummate a labor agreement and by exhibiting reasonableness in their bargaining positions, tactics, and activities (Cox, 1958). Nevertheless, good faith is difficult to define precisely. The NLRB interpretation speaks of "meeting at reasonable times," of "not refusing to bargain collectively," of "incorporating any agreement reached if requested by either party." But this does not compel either party to make a concession. Violations of good faith take four forms: the nature of bargaining issues; specific bargaining actions—for example, announcing a wage increase without consulting the union; overall conduct—for example, going directly to employees instead of bargaining; and failure to recognize a successor's bargaining obligations. A major problem with bad faith bargaining is that the regulations are practically unenforceable. The NLRB can cite an agency for not bargaining in good faith and can order affirmative action, but failure to comply means appeal to the courts, which can take several years. As a result, unions feel that the lack of significant recourse has vitiated the regulations governing good faith bargaining.

Ratification. After a period of time with or without mediation, the negotiations should end with a tentative written agreement initialed by all parties, which must then be ratified by the union members and, in the case of nonprofit mental health agencies, reviewed and ratified by the board of directors. If union and board members ratify the agreement, the new labor contract becomes part of the agency's personnel policy.

The ratification process determines whether or not management and staff are willing to abide by the new policies. Since approximately 10 percent of such tentative agreements are rejected by workers because of misunderstandings, internal politics, or feelings of being shortchanged, the resolution of an impasse may require third-party mediation (Federal Mediation and Conciliation Service, 1977)—a voluntary process whose costs are borne by one or both parties. A professional mediator seeks to clarify positions and perceptions of the bargaining climate, assists in reaching agreement on financial data, and aids in estimating the costs of agreement (Holley and Jennings, 1980). Success depends on the mediator's skill and the capacity to develop trust (Cormick, 1977).

Contract Arbitration and Final-Offer Arbitration

Contract arbitration involves the selection of a neutral person or panel to hear the bargaining positions of the parties and make a final, binding decision on what should be included in the negotiated agreement. In final-offer arbitration, both parties present reasonable and hopefully acceptable proposals, and the arbitrator accepts just one, without compromise. The problem with final-offer arbitration is that the party whose proposal is not accepted may see the decision as undermining its interests or as not totally comprehending the issues or costs involved. This form of arbitration can be costly, and delays may be encountered in scheduling an arbitrator. However, the costs may prove worthwhile if an even costlier strike is averted (Beal and Wickersham, 1967).

A third type of third-party intervention is mediation arbitration, in which the parties agree in advance that contract language, whether reached by mediation or arbitration, will be final and binding. The process begins with mediating the issues to achieve some compromise and ends with arbitrating unresolved matters that have not been agreed on. The pressure of knowing that certain unresolved matters will be decided by arbitration often causes the parties to compromise on issues previously thought to be irreconcilable (Holley and Jennings, 1980).

Union and management may prefer not to involve a third party and thereby engage in a test of strength in terms of winning or losing the election. When economic conditions lead to reduced budgets for mental health services and staff members are unable to find work, a strike is not a strong weapon. Although strike activity is always possible, both union and management tend to see binding and compulsory arbitration as preferable and more productive (Shaffer, 1979).

Administering the Labor Agreement

Neither the contract agreement nor the settling of a strike is the final stage of the collective bargaining process; the process is actually ongoing. During the life of the wage-effort agreement and working conditions contract, issues or problems evolve that affect interpretation of the points of agreement and even the substance of the contract itself. Monitoring the results of the collective bargaining process is called agreement administration (Holley and Jennings, 1980).

The machinery usually established to handle agreement administration includes on-the-job representation and arbitration. The authority of union representatives derives from the labor agreement itself. Specifications related to shop stewards may include payment for time spent in handling grievances or authority to leave the work place to confer with employees or supervisors. The role of the steward is usually confined to helping settle grievances prior to the need for arbitration. The grievance procedure, which can be quite complex, generally includes the following steps: (1) an employee, with or without the steward, discusses a grievance with an immediate supervisor; (2) if the grievance is not resolved, a grievance committee, composed of managers and employees, seeks resolution; if still not resolved, the grievance is put in writing and sent to management for an answer within a specified time; (3) management responds in writing and, if the grievance is not resolved, allows time for appeal, again within a specified time; (4) a full grievance hearing is held with more management and union grievance committee members; and (5) if the grievance is still unresolved, the last step is arbitration through a neutral third party to reach a final decision.

Although most cases are settled by the employee or shop steward and the employee's immediate supervisor, all steps of the grievance process should be clearly outlined. For example, the grievance machinery enables the union steward to serve as an employee advocate when an employee needs to appeal a case to a supervisor at another level. The advocate role is missing from most nonunion personnel policies, a lack that could easily be rectified by staff election of an employee representative. In any event, good mental health agency management requires the careful and expeditious handling of complaints that affect worker performance.

The grievance procedures of most labor contracts also include the provision that specific problems or issues will not be eligible for arbitration. In these situations, management reserves the right to take action, and the union the right to strike, if not happy with the decision (Beal and Wickersham, 1967). A number of contracts also include in this section the limits of management liability if the decision goes against them—for example, up to $500 damages for any one decision.

The use of arbitration once all else has failed brings outsiders into the agency to assist in reaching an agreement. The contract agreement should therefore provide permission for union officials to visit work places during working hours under certain conditions; describe the composition of a board of arbitrators or a disciplinary board; and outline the duties, powers, and limitations of the arbitrator (Beal and Wickersham, 1967). Since arbitration is costly for both unions and management, grievances should be settled before they escalate into full-fledged arbitration. Such settlements depend on the skills and mutual trust of union stewards and supervisory management, as well as on their own assessment of their status in the organization (Holley and Jennings, 1980).

Union Issues Unique to Mental Health Settings

Professionalism. Some observers of mental health unionization see the union movement as a serious challenge to professionalism (Shaffer, 1979). From this point of view, unions are perceived as organizations of lower-class manual laborers antagonistic to the interests of middle-class professional workers. Although this image still persists, it is losing its force as more and more professionals become union members. Professionals working as a part of interdisciplinary teams recognize the importance of solidarity in the work place, and professionals are concerned as much with financial remuneration as with the public good. If professionals are to reconcile their union membership with professionalism, they may need to modify cherished beliefs about individual merit, consensus, and professional standards (Alexander, 1980).

The growth of white-collar unions indicates that beliefs are changing. As professionals change, they notice that the nature of unions and union bread-and-butter issues are changing also; establishing career ladders, creating innovative staff development programs, and designing flexible work-sharing jobs may be more significant than traditional wage-oriented collective bargaining agreements. When unions and professionals interact over time, unions become more professional, and professionals become more union-oriented (Alexander, 1980). For example, the American Nurses Association is a professional association that also functions as a union.

Ethical Codes. Professionals have also worried about unions undermining codes of ethics, overwhelming concern for the client with the self-interest of the group. For example, the adverse effect of strikes on delivery of services has deterred some professionals from joining unions. No-strike clauses and the guaranteed continuation of basic or emergency services during strikes are approaches that have been used to handle this problem. In some instances, in fact, worker self-interest may turn out to be highly congruent with concern for clients. For example, negotiating for a worker voice in mental health services planning or a position on the board of directors may provide workers with an opportunity to serve the broader needs of clients. The nursing and medical professions have been effective in incorporating such provisions into their contracts in order to improve services to clients, as well as to improve their own working conditions (Shaffer, 1979).

The National Association of Social Workers reaffirmed in 1975 that members may participate in the formulation of personnel policies and procedures through whatever means they may democratically choose, and collective bargaining was endorsed as one means of providing a rational and coherent method of solving problems (Lightman, 1978). One method of bringing together union and professional ethical interests might be inclusion of the professional code of ethics in the labor agreement as criteria for settling disputes. The Ohio State Nursing Association, for example, incorporated the American Nursing Association Code of Ethics into the collective bargaining agreement to ensure adherence to their point of view (Holley and Jennings, 1980).

Public Opinion. What will the public say, and will public and voluntarily supported services lose their funding, if strikes and other union activities increase? These kinds of questions have troubled professionals and paraprofessionals in other service-related fields, such as education and health care. But government, union, and research reports have generated a good deal of public awareness about teachers' salaries and hospital working conditions. As a result, public information may provide a base for public sympathy. For example, as the public has come to see hospitals as big business concerns, rather than charitable institutions, nurses have received a surprising amount of public support during their strikes (Holley and Jennings, 1980).

Conclusion

Whether unionization is an answer to wage and working condition problems is difficult to assess. Certainly, unionization will affect the personnel management system in mental health settings. Some employees are seeking for the first time to participate in determining salary and working conditions. In addition, even without unions, the conditions of employment are receiving increased management attention, and the traditional styles of management are being modified to allow for increased worker participation in decision making.

This chapter has described the formal process of collective bargaining, as well as informal activities that affect labor-management relations. Unionization is growing in mental health settings, and managers must prepare themselves for effective involvement in the unionization process by understanding the legal requirements that encompass labor-management relations; the formal, step-by-step process of collective bargaining; contract components, including the wage and effort bargain and fringe benefits; and the rights of unions and management.

The chapter has also described the art of negotiating a contract, including economic issues and the process of communication. Knowledgeable and skillful negotiation involves the effective use of self, individual and group interpersonal relations, and the development of political strategies. The contract agreement, however, is only the beginning of ongoing labor-management relations; agreement administration, the final phase of the bargaining or arbitration process, involves the monitoring of contract interpretation and implementation.

References

Alexander, L. B. "Professionalism and Unionization: Compatible After All?" *Social Work*, 1980, *25*, 476–483.

Beal, E., and Wickersham, E. D. *The Practice of Collective Bargaining.* Homewood, Ill.: Irwin, 1967.

Cormick, G. W. "The Ethics of Mediation: Some Unexplored Territory." Paper presented at 5th annual meeting of the Society of Professionals in Dispute Resolution, New York, 1977.

Cox, A. "The Duty to Bargain in Good Faith." *Harvard Law Review*, 1958, *71*, 1418.

Federal Mediation and Conciliation Service. *Thirtieth Annual Report*. Washington, D.C.: U.S. Government Printing Office, 1977.

Holley, W. H., and Jennings, K. *The Labor Relations Process*. Hinsdale, Ill.: Dryden Press, 1980.

Imberman, W. "How Expensive is an NLRB Election?" *MSU Business Topics*, 1975, *23*, 13–18.

Lightman, E. S. "An Imbalance of Power: Social Workers in Unions." *Administration in Social Work*, 1978, *2* (1), 75–85.

Nash, P. (Ed.). "Impact of the Amendments on the Law—NLRA and NLRB Changes in Berkeley." *Labor Relations in Hospitals*, 1978, *1*, 27.

Nigro, F. A. (Ed.). "Health Labor Relations: A Symposium." *Journal of Health and Human Resources Administration*, 1979, *2* (1), 6–87.

Sandover, M. "The Validity of Union Authorization Cards as a Predictor of Success in NLRB Certification Elections." *Labor Law Journal*, 1975, *28*, 698–701.

Shaffer, G. L. "Labor Relations and the Unionization of Professional Social Workers: A Neglected Area in Social Work Education." *Journal of Education for Social Work*, 1979, *15* (1), 80–86.

Spector, B. "Negotiation as a Psychological Process." *Journal of Conflict Resolution*, 1977, *21*, 607–618.

Stevens, C. *Strategy and Collective Bargaining Negotiations*. New York: McGraw-Hill, 1963.

๛ 15 ๛

Human Resource Planning

Mary Richardson

This chapter describes the effects of need and demand, labor supply, and productivity on human resources planning in the mental health field. After outlining the four major mental health disciplines—psychiatry, psychology, nursing, and social work—Mary Richardson explores the impact on services delivery of such factors as the utilization of paraprofessionals, labor mobility and career advancement, the shift to community settings, and third-party reimbursement mechanisms. She also considers a number of fundamental issues and trends in mental health human resources planning, including deinstitutionalization, treatment teams, and access to services.

Human resources planning in mental health care involves ensuring an adequate supply of personnel to match, but not exceed, future demands for services. In addition to the problems inherent in determining the numbers of persons and the skill levels necessary to meet service needs, geographical and demographic maldistribution of labor supply, rising labor costs, recruitment and training of future mental health care personnel, and increasingly complex governmental regulations are concerns and issues that make human resources planning difficult. This chapter discusses several important factors relevant to human resource planning in mental health: need and demand for services, productivity, the major mental health professions, utilization of paraprofessionals, labor mobility and career development, the shift to community-based services and its impact on staffing, and the influence of services reimbursement on staffing. The chapter concludes with a discussion of current human resource planning issues and trends.

Need and Demand for Services

In planning human resources, one must first assess the need for mental health care and the supply of resources available to provide that care (Warheit, Holzer, and Robbins, 1979). The need for mental health care services is often defined as the quantity of care that expert opinion considers necessary to keep a population healthy (Lave, Salve, and Leinhardt, 1975). Demand, a related concept, is a combination of the quantity of services used and public attitudes and preferences toward mental health care consumption.

Many factors influence demand for mental health care services. Access and availability of services are certainly influential factors (Neilsen, 1979; Rubin, 1978). Yet they are often viewed only in geographical or financial terms, whereas in fact the racial and sexual composition of staff also affects the access and availability of services. Knowledge about and attitudes toward mental illness and help among potential clients, as well as the attitudes of those who refer people for mental health services, may also influence demand for mental health services. All of these factors vary across geographic, social, and cultural divisions.

Four methods are suggested for determining the quantity of mental health services that will be demanded:

1. *Professional standards method.* Demand can be based on qualitative criteria related to expert opinion and available technology to provide a level of service that professionals believe will help ensure the maintenance of a mentally healthy population. Estimates are then translated into human resources requirements using staffing and productivity standards.
2. *Professional-population ratio.* The number of mental health professionals divided by the total population served produces a professional-population ratio. By multiplying this ratio times the estimated population for a targeted future year, human resources requirements may then be estimated. Despite its popularity, this method assumes that demand for mental health care and the mix of services delivered will remain unchanged over time and that efficiency and productivity in the delivery of services will not necessarily increase.
3. *Economic-demographic method.* Demand for services is related to selected economic and demographic variables, the magnitude of probable change is predicted, and calculations are then made of the impact on demand for services and on mental health care personnel requirements.
4. *Service target method.* Targets are determined for the kinds and levels of services required by a population, and then a task analysis is conducted to relate staffing and productivity factors to determine personnel needs.

Once the need for services and the anticipated demand are estimated, the current supply of available services can be measured. Estimates can then be made for changes in the labor market over time due to graduations, migration, retirement, and death. Techniques to increase the human resources pool include increasing wages, lowering educational or licensure requirements for entry into a job category, and increasing the capacity of training institutions. Taube (1978) suggests the importance of the following in assessing the supply of mental health care resources: specification of the geographical unit of analysis; specification of the units of supply; definition and classification of the units of supply; and measurement of the capacity to produce services.

Each state has a plan for the development of mental health services in which the availability of and need for mental health resources are analyzed by catchment areas. Such a plan must consider the supply of mental health services in each of three distinct organizational categories: mental health facilities; medical, social services, or educational facilities; and private practice settings (Taube, 1978). For each of these service settings, modalities of services should be specified. Taube (1978) recommends that the service modality categories include inpatient hospital or other residential care, outpatient care, and day treatment.

Productivity

Labor productivity plays an important role in the interaction between the demand for services and the supply of labor. Simply defined, productivity is the amount of a particular good or service produced over a specific period of time. Since mental health care does not produce a clearly defined product, productivity is generally expressed according to units of service. A unit of service in the mental health field is most often defined as the amount of time required to serve an individual—for example, one hour of individual therapy, three hours of day treatment, or a fifteen-minute medications evaluation. Productivity is measured, therefore, according to the number of units a particular service provider can produce in a given period of time, and determinations of staffing needs are then based on staff productivity. Productivity is also related to case mix; personnel serving a highly dysfunctional population, such as the chronically mentally ill, will likely produce fewer units of service in a work day than personnel serving less-disturbed, easier-to-serve clients. Often measures of productivity are not considered in relation to case mix, thereby leading to inaccurate estimates of staffing needs.

Productivity can significantly affect the cost of services, as well. Using an hour of individual therapy as a unit of service for illustration, the following calculations can be made:

- Assume a productivity rate of 60 percent (twenty-four hours out of a forty-hour work week spent in individual therapy). Twenty-four people will receive services from one therapist in a week's time.
- Assume the cost of one hour of individual therapy is $50. Over a forty-hour week, total costs of services provided will equal $1200.
- Assume the $1200 cost, which is composed primarily of personnel costs, will remain constant despite some fluctuation in productivity.

An increase or decrease in productivity will reflect the following change in costs per unit of service:

	Productivity		
	40 percent	*60 percent*	*80 percent*
Number of service hours per week	16	24	32
Cost per hour	$75	$50	$37.50
($1200 divided by the number of direct service hours)			

Therefore, a 20 percent reduction in productivity results in a 50 percent increase in cost per unit of service, whereas increased productivity clearly results in a decrease in the cost of services.

The Major Mental Health Professions

Although it is important to understand the concepts of supply, demand, and productivity in assessing human resources utilization, it is also important to take into account the four core mental health disciplines.

Psychiatry. Psychiatry, psychology, nursing, and social work emerged as professions over the past century as a result of a wide variety of social forces. Psychiatry became firmly established as a legitimate branch of medicine when Kraepelin, a German physician, developed a disease classification system for psychiatric disorders. As mental disorders came to be viewed as diseases that were organic in origin, psychiatrists became the acknowledged providers of services to those deemed mentally ill.

Today, psychiatrists are more clearly established in institutions than in community mental health services and often assume administrative roles in federal and state agencies, hospitals, and, to a lesser degree, in community facilities (Straker and Cummings, 1978; Winslow, 1979). Some psychiatrists work in both public and private settings, and the distribution of psychiatrists across public and private sectors is approximately equal. The geographical and demographic distribution of psychiatrists is also of concern—psychiatrists are frequently not available in rural areas, and the representation of women and minorities in psychiatry, although improving, is poor. In fact, many would argue that a shortage of psychiatrists exists (Koran, 1979; Pardes, 1979). The number of American medical school graduates entering psychiatric training dropped from 1,051 in 1970 to 842 in 1976, while the total number of medical school graduates in the same period rose 50 percent (Pardes, 1979). During the post–World War II period, the shortage of psychiatrists, particularly in state mental hospitals, was offset by the use of foreign medical school graduates. However, the enactment of federal legislation restricting immigration and student visas has drastically reduced the number of foreign doctors practicing in the United States. Consequently, the availability of psychiatrists is expected to continue to decline.

Psychology. As it emerged from a philosophy into a science, psychology was involved in identifying and describing normal behavior as a foundation for the detection of abnormal behavior. Until the middle of the twentieth century, most psychological activity was aimed at conducting tests and measurements under laboratory conditions. Gradually, a few psychologists began to work with psychiatrists, primarily in child guidance clinics. With America's concern during World War II for the psychological fitness of its soldiers, the Veterans Administration began to train psychologists to clinically apply their scientific knowledge, and over time, clinical psychologists moved into roles as direct care providers, frequently competing with psychiatrists.

Psychologists have come the farthest of the nonmedical health professions in developing regulations governing licensing or certification. Currently, psychologists are licensed or certified in all states and the District of Columbia, with almost all states requiring a doctoral degree for licensure. Limited licensure is available in a few states to graduates of master's degree programs, however, and some settings, such as public schools and community mental health facilities, do not require licensure at all. Psychology has few minority practitioners, but graduate programs have increased the number of minority and women students over the last several years. In 1976, 33 percent of psychology doctorates were awarded to women, and approximately 10 percent of psychology graduate students were minorities (President's Commission on Mental Health, 1978).

Nursing. Nurses began as assistants to physicians and have gained increasing autonomy over the years. Although the first psychiatric nurse training program was established in 1882, psychiatric hospitals were poorly funded and rarely could afford trained psychiatric nurses. Not until the development in the 1930s of somatic treatments for mental illness, such as insulin shock therapy, psychosurgery, and electroshock therapy, did a substantial need arise for trained psychiatric nurses. With the advent of the therapeutic milieu in psychiatric hospitals, the psychotherapeutic role of nurses increased. Maintenance of such a milieu requires twenty-four-hour care from a therapeutic team, and nurses, unlike psychiatrists, are available for all shifts. Although nurses on these teams are practicing as assistants to physicians, a shortage of psychiatrists in many hospitals means that nurses have increased authority and responsibility for psychotherapeutic care. In community settings, nursing does not yet have a clearly defined role; psychologists and social workers frequently view nurses as contenders for the same therapeutic territory.

Social Work. Social workers, unlike the other mental health professionals, have their roots in the social welfare system, having evolved from the volunteer charity workers of the early 1900s. As psychological theory came to include the social and cultural determinants of mental disorder, social work practice expanded into the mental health system, with social workers first assuming a therapeutic role with the families of children treated by psychiatrists in child guidance clinics. Gradually, with increased demands for services and the limited availability of psychiatrists, social workers began to practice psychotherapy. Like nurses, they continue to struggle to establish a distinct professional identity in the mental health setting. More than any other mental health care professionals, social workers reflect the merging of social welfare and health care ideologies and have contributed an increased awareness of the social and cultural implications of mental health services delivery for the population in need. Social work training includes a variety of levels, including bachelor's-, master's-, and doctoral-level programs. Currently, social workers are required to be licensed in twenty-three states, and efforts to establish social work licensing regulations are underway in many others.

Utilization of Paraprofessionals

As new levels of workers enter the system, little thought has been given to how best to integrate these roles with the existing professions, and many professionals have a limited understanding of the most effective way in which to utilize paraprofessional workers. As paraprofessional positions have been created, a job-factoring approach has often been taken, which factors out the simpler professional tasks and assigns them to new workers. This approach has resulted in a series of positions seen as special assistants to the professional and given such titles as psychiatric nurse aide, social work case aide, and psychology assistant. These positions, under direct supervision of the professional, have allowed for little independence of judgment or action.

Another method that has been used in creating jobs for different levels of workers has been the developmental approach, which focuses on what must be done to meet the needs of clients. According to this approach, work is defined according to roles and then clustered into jobs for individual professional and paraprofessional workers. Roles include (Southern Regional Education Board, 1979):

1. *Outreach*—reaching out to identify people with problems, referring them to appropriate services, and following up to make sure they achieve their maximum level of rehabilitation.
2. *Brokering*—helping people reach existing services and helping services relate more effectively to clients.
3. *Advocating*—pleading and fighting for services, policies, rules, regulations, and laws for clients.
4. *Evaluating*—assessing client and community needs and problems, whether medical, psychiatric, social, or educational; formulating plans and explaining them to all concerned.
5. *Education*—performing a range of instructional activities with individuals and groups, from simple coaching to teaching highly technical content.
6. *Behavior changing*—carrying out a range of activities planned primarily to change behavior, ranging from coaching and counseling to case work, psychotherapy, and behavioral therapy.
7. *Mobilizing*—helping to secure resources for clients and communities.
8. *Consulting*—working with other professions and agencies regarding their handling of problems, needs, and programs.
9. *Community planning*—working with community boards, committees, and other groups to assure that community developments enhance positive mental health.
10. *Care giving*—providing services for persons who need ongoing support of some kind, such as financial assistance, day care, social support, and twenty-four-hour care.
11. *Data managing*—performing all aspects of handling data: gathering, tabulating, analyzing, synthesizing, program evaluating, and planning.
12. *Administering*—carrying out activities that are primarily agency- or institution-oriented, rather than client- or community-oriented, such as budgeting, purchasing, and personnel activities.

The clustering of roles into jobs can occur around specific tasks or activities, major program functions, the need for assistance of specific professions, agency logistical problems (such as twenty-four-hour coverage), or the needs of groups of clients. Formulating jobs according to specific tasks or roles helps clarify workers' understanding of the job and helps specify the agency's expectations.

In actual practice, the ways in which workers are trained and integrated into the mental health system vary considerably. Response to specific needs is an important factor. Roles are often established and jobs created because personnel systems and funding agencies have certain requirements, because a strong individual in the system thinks it best, or simply because that is how it has always been done. Existing patterns of professional and paraprofessional utilization are identifiable with the following types of mental health settings (Southern Regional Education Board, 1979):

1. Hospital programs for the acute care of the mentally ill tend to use the medical model and make primary use of fully qualified professionals in traditional roles. Paraprofessionals tend to be present in custodial roles or as aides to one of the professions.
2. Specialized treatment units, such as children's, geriatric, mental retardation, and alcohol and drug abuse units, are more likely to use paraprofessionals and professionals according to a generic model. The overall treatment plan is determined by the full team, but the execution is assigned to individual members, including paraprofessionals.
3. Mental health programs in cities and prosperous suburbs use primarily professional workers, with a modicum of paraprofessionals who function as aides to professionals. In community mental health programs in poverty or ghetto areas of cities, however, paraprofessionals tend to function as generalists.
4. Mental health programs in rural areas are likely to make considerable use of paraprofessionals who, along with the professionals, function in generic roles. The relative shortage of staff requires everyone to work more collaboratively and relate to each other in more personal ways.
5. Mental health programs with a social-rehabilitation orientation make greater use of paraprofessionals than those with a heavy medical and psychiatric orientation. Social and rehabilitation programs are also more likely to work with chronically ill or mentally retarded persons than with the acutely ill. The job orientation of the paraprofessionals in such long-term care programs tends to be that of the generalist.
6. Programs that work with clients in their own homes, foster homes, group homes, and neighborhood settings make extensive use of paraprofessionals, since professionals are frequently not available for home visiting and neighborhood travel, both of which are time-consuming and expensive.
7. Large, bureaucratic agencies tend to use paraprofessionals as aides to professionals; smaller and more innovative agencies, using functional job titles and

organizational forms, seem to be able to use both professionals and paraprofessionals in more flexible ways.

Labor Mobility and Career Advancement

Labor mobility is an important factor in the mental health field. Professionals entering mental health facilities, confronted by few opportunities for advancement, make frequent job shifts within the mental health field and into and
out of other human services sectors. An advantage of such mobility is a broader
understanding on the part of the mental health professional for human services in
general and for the integration of human services and health care in particular.
Disadvantages include the unpredictability of the labor market and the loss of
trained personnel from one sector to another.

Career advancement systems for mental health professionals are generally limited. Some advancement within agencies and facilities may exist in the
form of small, incremental pay steps based on length of service; most often,
though, advancement means moving out of clinical roles and into supervisory or
management roles for which clinical practitioners find themselves ill prepared.
Furthermore, career ladders within the mental health professions are more often
based on academic training than on in-service training and experience. Persons
with considerable practical experience and expertise but a limited academic background are afforded little opportunity for advancement.

Shift to Community-Based Services and Its Impact on Staffing

The introduction of psychotropic medications (1950s) and the move toward
deinstitutionalization (1970s) necessitated the creation of a vast array of community-based services that have attempted to move from medical to behavioral,
social, and educational models of care. The rapid development of community
services in turn created an overwhelming demand for newly trained professionals,
as well as a need to retrain those who had moved from institutional to community
settings. Increased federal participation in the provision of mental health services
signaled increased federal support for training programs to staff those programs;
consequently, the number of persons in the core mental health disciplines grew
dramatically between 1950 and 1976, as noted in Table 1.

In addition, new levels of workers were trained in an effort to meet immediate demand (Alley and Blanton, 1976; Austin, 1978; Granet and Talbott, 1978).
For example, paraprofessionals offered a less-expensive, more rapidly trained substitute for professionals, were more readily available in small or rural communities, and were more often representative of the low-income and minority groups
frequently targeted in outreach efforts. Paraprofessionals are now employed in all
types of community and institutional programs, and in 1974 represented 33.6 percent of persons employed in mental health facilities (Taube, 1978). Beginning in
the late 1960s, paraprofessionals were frequently trained in community college

Table 1. Number of Mental Health Professionals by Discipline, United States, 1950–1976.

Year	Psychiatrists	Psychologists	Social Workers	Registered Nurses
1950	7,100	7,300	NA*	NA*
1955	10,600	13,000	20,000	NA*
1960	14,100	18,200	26,200	504,000
1965	18,500	23,600	41,000	600,000
1970	23,200	30,800	49,600	722,000
1975	25,700	39,400	64,500	906,000
1976	26,500	42,000	69,600	961,000

*Not Available
Source: President's Commission on Mental Health, 1978.

programs that reflected the philosophical and technical orientation of the psychologists, social workers, and nurses who developed them.

As the trend toward community-based services has grown, so have efforts to help clients live as independently as possible—efforts that have involved vocational rehabilitation workers, occupational therapists, educators, and recreation therapists, as well as mental health workers. Although often considered auxiliary, such social services and rehabilitation practitioners today comprise 12 percent of direct patient care staff (Vischi, 1980).

With the emergence of community awareness of mental health services needs and the inability of the community mental health system to meet all of those needs, alternative care sources have developed. These sources are often grassroots movements, funded on shoestring budgets and organized by people who are aware of unmet needs. In the 1960s, for example, services for runaway young people, generally started by community philanthropy, began to develop around the country. Other alternative programs, such as neighborhood drug and alcohol treatment centers, long-term residential programs, women's mental health services programs, rape/crisis centers, shelters for battered women, and service programs for the elderly, followed. Many of these alternative services utilize established mental health techniques but depend on paraprofessionals and volunteers to provide care (Richardson, 1980).

Influence of Services Reimbursement on Staffing

In 1975, patient fees accounted for 34 percent of total mental health center revenue, private insurance for 15 percent, and federal and state funds for 21 and 30 percent, respectively (Vischi, 1980). Most mental health services are purchased with tax revenues by governments. As the major purchaser of services, governments have considerable impact on the organization of services through the contractual arrangements whereby services are purchased through legislative and judicial action. This practice has led in turn to considerable regulation and demands for accountability—mandates that affect such matters as who is allowed to provide what services to whom, salary levels of staff, the facility or location in which an individual is allowed to practice, the types of services to be produced, and the population to be served.

Consumer interests have been introduced through some legislation but the greatest impact has come primarily through case law. The right of the mentally ill person to due process was first addressed in the 1966 case of *Rouse v. Cameron.* Subsequent case law has established the right to adequate treatment, the right to treatment in the least-restrictive environment, the right to informed consent, and the right to refuse treatment. The 1972 *Wyatt* v.*Stickney* decision, for instance, mandated specific staffing ratios in state hospitals (for example, for each 250 patients, the hospital shall have a minimum of two social workers with the master's of social work degree and five with the bachelor of arts degree).

Although all the mental health professions have assumed a broader therapeutic role as the locus of services has shifted from institutions to communities, considerable concern has been given to establishing a more equitable relationship among professional groups—a trend that has not been supported by academic training programs or third-party reimbursement schemes. Each profession has developed its own terminology to express technological perceptions and the concept of its role in the clinical process, based, in part, on an allegiance to the medical model or the psychosocial rehabilitation model. Despite the need for interdisciplinary and multidisciplinary practice, most academic training programs provide practitioners with more preparation for practicing independently than for practicing in groups. Once in an organizational setting, however, practitioners are often confronted with services organized into teams, with little formal definition given to the manner in which the professions are to relate to one another. Even when multidisciplinary decision making does occur, it is often described according to a medical model, with the psychiatrist or the licensed psychologist as primary provider, in order to withstand audits by third-party reimbursers.

Issues and Trends

Who should be doing what with whom is perhaps the major issue for human resources planners. Unfortunately, scant evidence is available for making such a determination. Decisions as to who provides services to what groups of people rest more often on professional lobbying and the resolution of turf battles than on any measure of client or patient outcome. Although the core mental health professions have their own clearly defined areas of expertise, much of their activity has begun to overlap, as each profession has developed its own approach to diagnostics, evaluation, intervention, and management. Further, issues of licensure and credentialing have importance in determining who has access to certain professional roles and what those roles will include. Human resources planners in mental health are therefore faced with difficult decisions about appropriate distribution and utilization of the core mental health disciplines.

Deinstitutionalization. The deinstitutionalization of patients in state hospitals has expanded the role of the service provider to include more rehabilitative and educational services and has therefore placed pressure on the administrator to meet changing staffing needs. Models of care used in community facilities are different from models applicable to institutional settings, and staff members from institutions are often not prepared to make the transition from inpatient to community services. In contrast, practitioners in community settings sometimes have difficulties working with deinstitutionalized patients. Less severely ill clients—often more verbal and motivated than their deinstitutionalized counterparts—are more appealing to these practitioners, who are usually trained heavily in verbal therapies and psychodynamics. Aftercare services for deinstitutionalized patients deemphasize verbalization and psychodynamics and emphasize instead the tasks of resocializing patients in basic living skills, motivating them to utilize services, and helping them secure housing and arrange finances—all of which resemble social services delivery more than mental health care. Questions have arisen as to the level of worker to deliver services to this population, as well as to the type of training necessary for those workers, and community service programs are being developed throughout the country that provide differing answers to those questions.

Mental Health Teams. Service trends in the mental health sector continue along team lines. Team models include (Southern Regional Education Board, 1979):

1. *The medical team.* In this model, a psychiatrist or another physician is the leader and directs the activities of all the other team members and the patient. This traditional model is used in mental hospitals and in the psychiatric units of general hospitals, is taught to physicians and nurses, and is expected by medical payment plans. Appropriate for acute inpatient care, it is less appropriate for other settings.

2. *The diagnostic team.* In this model, each of the professions does its unique assessment of the patient or client, all of the findings are brought together at a session, the diagnosis is decided, and a treatment plan established. This model usually includes inputs from professions other than the four core professions and often includes a vocational evaluation, an educational assessment, and laboratory or other special studies. As sometimes practiced, the diagnostic team approach may be inefficient because full batteries of tests and assessment studies are carried out for all clients when only a few of these tests may actually be necessary to establish a diagnosis and treatment plan.

3. *The coequal team model.* This model establishes all the professions involved as equals, with each having an equal vote in determining the client's treatment plan. This pattern may lead to a program in which each profession claims a segment of the services to be delivered to each client, even though that profession's expertise may be only marginally needed by some clients. In a variation of the coequal team, the overall team is assigned to a small group of patients or clients who in turn choose which of the team members they wish to have provide them with any or all of the services needed.

4. *The rehabilitation team.* In this model, sometimes used after the acute treatment phase is over, the various activities therapists (for example, occupational therapist, industrial therapist, special education teacher, social worker) are directed by a rehabilitation counselor, instructor, or other rehabilitational worker, who sets the plan and assigns the tasks.

5. *One-worker coordinated team (case manager).* In this model, one worker, either a professional or a paraprofessional, is responsible for coordinating all of the information and services on behalf of a client. Sometimes called the case manager model because the worker acts as the client's agent, personally delivering as many of the services as possible and calling for consultation or making referrals only when necessary, this model limits involvement to those specialists who are actually needed, rather than referring the client to an unnecessarily large number of specialists for services that may be only marginally helpful.

Increasing concern for comprehensive care has ensured continued growth in the use of the team approach, since teams are generally purported to provide especially comprehensive diagnoses, intervention, and follow-up. In addition, this trend has seen the introduction of other, related professions into the mental health team.

Integration of Medical and Mental Health Services. Increasingly, the integration of medical and mental health services is becoming an issue. Currently, it is estimated that 60 percent of those seeking mental health services do so in primary care physicians' offices (Regier, Goldberg, and Taube, 1978). The quality and type of response to these problems are unknown. Moreover, clients of community mental health facilities are likely to have had little or no physical diagnosis or evaluation, although evidence increasingly suggests that they may be at higher risk for physical disorders than other persons. Clearly, the mental health and medical care sectors have remained apart for too long, yet the cooperation of the two sectors will be important in the future staffing and organization of services.

Access to Services. Access to services remains a problem to many. Given the nature of mental disorder and the attitudes of society, the question of whether to channel an individual into the mental health services system or into one of the social welfare systems is often difficult to answer. Services for the developmentally disabled and the mentally retarded may be bureaucratically united with and closely parallel to mental health services but in practice remain functionally separate. Yet a chronically mentally ill person and a developmentally disabled or mentally retarded person may in fact be one and the same. Diagnosis and subsequent referral are highly dependent on when in the person's life the disorder is identified, who makes the diagnosis, and how available are resources within one system or the other. The legislation defining developmental disabilities has expanded to include certain mental disorders, and the mental health system is being increasingly looked to for services for the developmentally disabled or mentally retarded person who suffers from psychiatric or emotional disorders. Most mental health professionals, however, have little or no training or experience with the therapies appropriate to this population. Other access problems arise from people's poor understanding of mental health services and of what constitutes psychiatric or psychological disorders, from the stigma attached to mental illness, and from cultural differences.

Continuing Education. A major concern in human resources planning is continuing education. Academic and other training programs only begin to prepare people for roles in the mental health services system; once on the job, workers must adapt to unanticipated situations and learn many new skills. In addition, new ideas, techniques, and discoveries are appearing at an accelerated rate, making it impossible for any one person or profession to remain up-to-date at all times. Continuing education is therefore absolutely necessary to maintain competence, as well as to prepare people for change. Continuing education is often viewed as a luxury, however, and is poorly supported by training programs and mental health planning agencies alike.

Conclusion

The expansion of knowledge and theory beyond the early organic causation theory of mental illness, the introduction of psychotropic medication, and the subsequent shift in focus from institutional to community services have caused rapid changes in the organization and structure of mental health services over the past twenty-five years. These factors, along with the expansion of the knowledge and skills of each of the core mental health disciplines and the addition of new auxiliary and supplementary service providers, have made mental health human resources planning a complex, and, at times, frustrating task.

The use of supply, demand, and productivity concepts provides an important foundation for understanding mental health human resources planning. One must determine what jobs specifically need to be done and who, based on training and experience, is best qualified to do them. Allowances must also be made for the time it takes to train mental health workers before they enter the system and for the various pressures and influences affecting the way in which services are organized and delivered.

References

Alley, S., and Blanton, J. "A Study of Paraprofessionals in Mental Health." *Community Mental Health Journal*, 1976, 12 (2), 151–160.

Austin, M. J. *Professionals and Paraprofessionals.* New York: Human Sciences Press, 1978.

Dale, S. "School Mental Health Programs: A Challenge to the Health Professional." *Journal of School Health*, Nov. 1978, pp. 526–529.

Granet, R. B., and Talbott, J. A. "The Continuity Agent: Creating a New Role to Bridge the Gaps in the Mental Health System." *Hospital and Community Psychiatry*, 1978, *29* (2), 132–134.

Koran, L. "Psychiatric Manpower Ratios: A Beguiling Numbers Game." *Archives of General Psychiatry*, 1979, *36*, 1409-1419.

Lave, J. R., Salve, L. B., and Leinhardt, S. "Medical Manpower Models: Need, Demand, and Supply." *Inquiry*, 1975, *12*, 97-125.

Neilsen, E. D. "Community Mental Health Services in the Community Jail." *Community Mental Health Journal*, 1979, *15* (1), 27-32.

Pardes, H. "Future Needs for Psychiatrists and Other Mental Health Personnel." *Archives of General Psychiatry*, 1979, *36*, 1401-1408.

President's Commission on Mental Health. *Report to the President*. Vol. 2. Washington, D.C.: U.S. Government Printing Office, 1978.

Regier, P. A., Goldberg, I. D., and Taube, C. A. "The De Facto U.S. Mental Health Services System." *Archives of General Psychiatry*, 1978, *35*, 685-693.

Richardson, M. "Mental Health Services: Growth and Development of a System." In S. J. Williams and P. R. Torrens (Eds.), *Introduction to Health Services*. New York: Wiley, 1980.

Rubin, A. "Commitment to Community Mental Health Aftercare Services: Staffing and Structural Implications." *Community Mental Health Journal*, 1978, *14* (3), 199-208.

Ruiz, P., and Langrod, J. "The Role of Folk Healers in Community Mental Health Services." *Community Mental Health Journal*, 1976, *12* (4), 392-398.

Southern Regional Education Board. *Staff Roles for Mental Health Personnel: A History and Rationale*. Atlanta: Southern Regional Education Board, 1979.

Straker, M., and Cummings, J. "Staffing Patterns and Team Composition." *Hospital and Community Psychiatry*, 1978, *29* (4), 243-245.

Taube, C. A. "Assessing the Supply of Mental Health Resources." *Statistical Notes for Health Planners*, Apr. 1978, 7.

Vischi, T. R. *The Alcohol, Drug Abuse and Mental Health National Data Book*. Washington, D.C.: U.S. Department of Health, Education, and Welfare, 1980.

Warheit, G. J., Holzer, C. E., and Robbins, L. "Social Indicators and Mental Health Planning: An Empirical Case Study." *Community Mental Health Journal*, 1979, *15* (2), 94-103.

Winslow, W. W. "The Changing Role of Psychiatrists in Community Mental Health Centers." *American Journal of Psychiatry*, 1979, *136* (1), 24-27.

ॐ 16 ॐ

Financial
Management

Mary Davis Hall

Using a conceptual framework developed by Anthony (1965) to describe the relationship of finance and budgeting to the total management of not-for-profit organizations, Mary D. Hall presents principles to guide the manager in developing fiscal policy. She gives examples of fiscal procedures for operating an organization; discusses components of the program, planning, and budgeting (PPB) system that can be used in management control; and defines the roles of the manager, the clinical staff, and the board in the finance and budgeting process. One section of the chapter explores the differences between line-item, program, performance, and zero-based budgeting; another examines cost finding; and another briefly defines basic accounting methods. Although not intended to be a definitive treatise on financial management, the chapter does introduce the program manager to the basic concepts and language of fiscal management in not-for-profit organizations.

Financial management of mental health and other not-for-profit systems is a process of acquiring and using resources to meet the needs of the public and the goals of the organization. The process involves three interrelated management functions: planning, controlling, and operating. The primary tools of fiscal management are financial analysis, budgeting, and accounting. The basic skills needed to use these tools are conceptual rather than mathematical. To master the concepts and techniques discussed in this chapter, the manager need only be able to use basic arithmetic. Since most of the initial difficulties presented by the concepts of financial management are related to learning a new set of terms and relearning definitions for relatively common terms that are often misused in everyday conversation, technical terms will be defined.

Anthony (1965) proposed a framework for examining the planning and control systems of an organization that assumes that these systems have an underlying financial structure; that is, plans and results are expressed in monetary

units. He argues that "money is the only common denominator by which the
different elements, such as hours of labor, type of labor, quantity and quality of
material, amount and kinds of services produced, can be combined and compared" (Anthony, 1965, p. 4). His framework consists of the following three areas
(see Table 1):

1. *Strategic planning* is the process of deciding on objectives of the organiza-
    tion, on changes in these objectives, on the resources needed to attain these
    objectives, and on the policies that are to govern the acquisition, use, and
    disposition of these resources.
2. *Management control* is the process by which managers assure that resources
    are obtained and used effectively and efficiently in the accomplishment of the
    organization's objectives.
3. *Operational control* is the process of assuring that specific tasks are carried
    out effectively and efficiently.

Strategic Planning

The strategic planning functions described in Table 1 are primarily the
responsibility of a mental health agency's board of directors, with input from the
executive director and the staff. In general, the board is responsible for setting the
organization's fiscal policy and participating in the development and enactment
of a financial plan for the organization. Once the financial plan and fiscal policies
of the organization have been established, the role of the board is to monitor
management's implementation process, delegating day-to-day fiscal decision
making to management.

Financial Plans. Developing a financial plan for the not-for-profit organization is a critical part of the strategic planning process. Strategic planning refers
to the process—usually carried out by a task force made up of board members and
management—of identifying, analyzing, and selecting strategies to implement
policy. A financial plan facilitates management control and can, in most cases,
prevent management by crisis. Mental health agencies without financial plans are
managed by fiscal crisis, rather than controlled by management. One can recognize such an agency because it will frequently add new programs, expand services,
or make cutbacks in response to fund scarcity.

A strategic plan includes the goals of the organization as established in its
charter, objectives that are the basis for measuring the impact of services on client
and community problems, and a plan for meeting those objectives that specifies
and analyzes the activities to be carried out. If a major goal of the agency is, for
example, to reduce the rate of inappropriate institutionalization of the elderly,
then several alternative strategies may be used to attain that goal. The agency may
focus on providing services to aging centers and group homes (areas of least
restrictive care), or it may elect to use its resources to support staffs in nursing
homes. The point is that all strategies require financial resources, and the agency
must select among the alternatives and prioritize those selected. Once selected,

Table 1. Framework of Fiscal Management Activities.

Strategic Planning	Management Control	Operational Control
1. Setting fiscal policy.	1. Formulating budget guidelines.	1. Applying budget guidelines for hiring, promotion, and staff management.
2. Choosing funding sources.	2. Formulating allocation criteria.	2. Controlling expenditures.
3. Developing a fiscal plan.	3. Formulating the budget.	3. Identifying fiscal needs.
4. Deciding on nonroutine expenditures.	4. Planning of working capital.	4. Negotiating interagency contracts.
5. Appraising executive performance.	5. Deciding on routine capital expenditures.	5. Controlling the hiring and allocation of staff.
6. Choosing organizational goals.	6. Reporting to the board and others in the external environment.	6. Scheduling the production of services.
7. Setting program objectives.	7. Measuring, appraising, and improving management performance.	7. Conducting evaluations of programs and gathering data on client services.
8. Determining priorities for expansion or addition of new services.	8. Designing the structure of the organization.	8. Measuring, appraising, and improving worker performance.
9. Approving organizational structure.	9. Designing and using a management informational system.	9. Implementing policies and procedures.

they become the agency's service implementation plan and form the basis for the financial plan. A financial plan should have the following sections:

1. A section that establishes the basic revenue requirements of the organization, based on a projection of fiscal needs, to maintain the currently operating programs at a no-growth level for one year. The required level of funds should be tied to the organization's performance objectives for that year. This section provides management with a basis for monitoring income and evaluating the relationship of funding levels to performance.

2. A section that establishes target levels for funding any expansion of the existing system or the addition of new service programs. This section of the financial plan is usually a three- to five-year budget projection based on needs assessment data from the community, the region, and the state. For instance, it could take into account the mental health goals established in the county or regional health systems plan of the health systems agency. This part of the fiscal plan is used to guide management's monitoring of the environment for opportunities to acquire new sources of funds. It may also prevent management from acquiring funds if those funds are tied to the production of services not targeted in the agency's service and fiscal plan.

3. A section on capital investments for new space and major equipment purchases for the next three to five years. Included in this plan should be a standard that limits the level of capital expenditures or commitments that can

be made by management without prior board approval. Generally, expenditures for equipment over $1,000 are approved by the board or by a committee of the board, such as the finance or executive committee.

4. A section on cost containment that establishes a range within which service costs should be maintained by management. These figures are used by management as targets for monitoring expenditure levels and overall unit costs.

Financial Policy Statements. Financial policies are developed within the context of the overall administrative policies of an organization, but they are frequently developed without much care and concern. Who develops fiscal policy, and what are the content areas it should cover? In some cases, the administrative staff will develop a skeleton set of financial policies, with the details to be filled in by the board. In other cases, the board will have a finance committee with sufficient local expertise to develop its own financial policy statements. At a minimum, all mental health agencies should have financial policy statements on grants, contracts, cash management, credit and debt management, and auditing. Other fiscal policy issues, such as fringe benefits, wage and salary guidelines, and merit or performance pay policy, are usually included in personnel policy.

Grants. Grants are formal legal agreements between the agency and its funders that obligate the agency to invest resources to produce a prescribed set of services in order to attain some specific service objectives. Because most grants require matching funds in the form of hard dollars—that is, funds obtained from state or local governments or other nonfederal sources and not categorically earmarked or designated for a specific use by the organization—entering into a grant agreement is a fiscal investment decision. A common practice of most federal agencies, the matching grant typically requires an agency to provide one dollar of hard money for every two or three dollars of grant money it receives, as an expression of its commitment to the project or program.

Once priorities for the types of grant monies to be solicited have been established in the financial plan, the financial policy establishes a review structure to assure that the organization has sufficient hard dollars to match the requirements of those grants. Some grants include a long-term obligation for maintenance of effort and continued funding once the grant period is ended. Mental health staffing grants, for example, require agencies to maintain a level of financial effort: they decline on an annual schedule and obligate the agency, when the grant has expired, to pick up the costs previously funded by the grant. Since entering into such grant agreements may legally obligate the organization, all grant proposals should be reviewed through a formal management and board process.

Cash Management. The cash management policy of the agency defines how management shall assure that the organization maintains a positive cash-flow ratio, establishes the minimum cash-flow ratio to be maintained, and defines the constraints under which management can invest surplus cash in short-term investment accounts. A cash-flow ratio is the total amount of cash on hand divided by the total amount of expenditures expected for a specified period of time—for example, a cash-flow ratio of 1.2 would require $12,000 of cash in a checking account for every $10,000 in expected expenditures.

Cash management policies related to the banking and investments of the organization should address such questions as the following: Should the treasurer keep funds in interest-bearing accounts? Should the community mental health center maintain a cash-float or a continuous-loan account? What types of short- or long-term investments should be made by the treasurer? Most agencies use interest-bearing checking accounts and invest temporary funds surpluses in government securities, bank notes, certificates of deposit, or money market instruments. An agency that allows funds to remain in non- or minimum-interest-bearing checking accounts may lose several thousand dollars per year through poor cash management.

Some states will not permit the investment of public funds in interest-bearing accounts; however, this outdated approach to the management of public funds is rapidly disappearing. Most municipalities invest their taxes immediately on receipt. If the agency has a reasonably large sum—over $25,000—to invest, a special subcommittee of the board should probably oversee the investment and make separate financial policy statements dealing with the types and level of investments to be made.

Debt Management. At certain times and in certain circumstances, most not-for-profit organizations should borrow funds.When starting new programs, for instance, an agency may wish to borrow money to meet initial payrolls before grant funds arrive, enabling it to allocate and obligate monies that have not yet been received. The agency might also borrow funds during a period of negative cash flow, when monies from third-party reimbursements have not been paid on time. In such circumstances, the agency may borrow funds using as collateral its accounts receivable—fees already earned but not yet collected. In some instances, not-for-profit organizations should borrow money to make major capital investments in such items as furniture, typewriters, photocopiers, and clinic equipment, although the lease purchase arrangement, another form of short-term debt, is often a more economical way to acquire equipment than outright purchase. The debt management policy statement should establish limits on borrowing and board procedures for review of debt management activities.

As mentioned earlier, fiscal policies can also be included in personnel policy statements. Possibly the most legally complicated fiscal policy to be developed by the board is the organization's wage and salary administration policy. In that policy statement, the board usually determines the level and type of fringe benefits offered by the agency. If an agency is a not-for-profit corporation separate from state or municipal government, it can choose how to pay employees and in what form to give fringe benefits. If the employees of the organization are unionized, the fiscal wage and salary policies and fringe benefit packages are indicated in the organization's policy statement and the union contract. These policies must be reviewed at least once annually by the board's personnel subcommittee and legal counsel. As will become apparent when the structure of the budget is discussed, the form of the budget and the type of performance appraisal policy of the organization are interrelated. For example, if the mental health agency wants to use a behaviorally specific, performance-based job evaluation system with implications for merit pay increases, such changes need to be considered at the time the budget is prepared.

The financial plan and the financial policies of the organization are generally established by the board with input from management. They are written documents that should be dated and entered as official documents of the organization. Without such documents, the executive director and line management staff members will have difficulty maintaining management control of the organization.

Management Control

Management control is the responsibility of the executive director and administrative staff members such as the comptroller or business manager, the directors of clinical services, the personnel officer, and the planner/evaluator. The purpose of management control is to achieve organizational efficiency and effectiveness. Efficiency refers to attaining an optimum relationship between fiscal inputs (dollars and labor) and outputs (services); effectiveness refers to the accomplishment of stated objectives. Most fiscal management control activities (see Table 1) involve making resources acquisition and allocation decisions in the context of developing, implementing, and monitoring the budget. The major sources of data used to maintain management control come from management accounting records, the client informational system, strategic plans, and evaluation reports.

The major link between strategic planning and management control is the budgeting process. Ideally, an agency has assessed the service needs of its target populations; established program (service) goals and outcome objectives; determined the level of funds required to produce those services by developing a budgetary plan; acquired the necessary funds; and then allocated those funds in an operating budget. Actually, however, most agencies operate in an environment of fiscal instability and uncertainty, where the availability of categorical funds influences the choice of programs and service objectives.

Usually an agency is allocated a specific level of funds in state grant-in-aid, as well as some funding from federal grant programs (Feldman, 1973), and then determines its target population's service objectives based on that funding. For instance, an agency might have been allocated $100,000 of categorical funds to operate an outpatient treatment unit and have data indicating that the costs of the operation will be $25 per hour and an average of $750 per client per year. As a result, the agency would probably set its target output objectives at 4000 hours of service for 133 clients. Although oversimplified, this example should demonstrate what is meant by deductive budget decision making.

A deductive approach to budgeting does not present a problem if the agency is initiating or expanding programs that are needed by the client group it serves and are included in its strategic plan. Problems occur, however, when the agency adds programs that are not included in its strategic plan. Because agencies are so frequently faced with fixed-resource constraints and use deductive budgeting, the following discussion of the budgetary process assumes that management control in such organizations is based on producing the greatest level of services for a given level of funds. Such criteria are critical components of a fiscal policy and need to be determined prior to the budget development process.

The Budgeting Process

The budget of an organization is a dollars-and-cents plan of operation for a specific period of time. Most organizations have more than one budget—for example, a capital budget, a cash budget, and an operating budget. In this discussion, primary emphasis is given to the operating budget.

Budgeting is a political as well as a technical process. When the budget is in the developmental stage, consideration must be given to how the agency plans to use its resources to meet the social goals defined for it in federal and state statutes and guidelines, and those mandates must be balanced with the social goals of the community. Not uncommonly, federal or state goals may conflict with the needs of clients, and community mental health agency managers may need to redefine certain mandates in order to meet those needs in the allocation of state, local, and nonfederal funds. Although they seldom realize it, managers may use considerable discretion in determining the funding levels of different services. In addition, managers need to give due consideration to the social and political forces that influence the budget process. Because it is a plan, the budget can be constructed to reflect negotiations between the political priorities of local committees and the judgments of professionals and should remain sufficiently flexible to respond to the continuous demands of others in the organization's external environment.

Mental health agencies are frequently required by legal statute to be responsive to the needs of the community they serve and are encouraged by federal and state guidelines to form linkages with other human services agencies. Part of the political process of budget development includes the allocation of funds to develop those linkages. Although the fact is seldom mentioned in financial texts, the budget allocation process is in part a mechanism by which the organization attempts to gain political power or increase its service domain. For instance, a budget that allocates resources to other agencies in the form of contracts for services, shares staff across program boundaries, and uses multiple funding sources is a budget that indicates that the agency is aware of and responsive to the external economic and political environment.

The technical process of budgeting consists of establishing and implementing a set of policies, procedures, and rules (Hyde and Shafritz, 1978; Salmon and Pringle, 1977; Taylor, 1977). The structure of the budget constrains as well as facilitates the management of the organization. The three major types of budget formats are the line-item budget, the program budget, and the performance-based program budget. The budget format usually reflects the management style of the administration and the policies of the funding sources. Although some funding sources require the use of a specific budget form, such requirements should not dictate the development process or the agency's own budget format. Selecting the structural form of the budget is an internal, discretionary decision to be made by management with the board's concurrence.

Different Forms of Budgeting. The line-item budget was the first in a series of budget forms developed at the turn of the century. Sometimes referred to as the object-of-expenditure form of budgeting, line-item budgets are detailed tabulations of the myriad items required to operate a unit, including personnel, rent, office supplies, and other inputs (see Table 2).

In contrast to line-item budgeting, program budgeting seeks to identify all the costs associated with each mental health program. Many states and most federal funders of local mental health services require agencies to use some form of the PPB process in preparing requests for support. The primary function of PPB is to promote the development and analysis of alternative strategies by which an organization can achieve its organizational goals and implement public policy as expressed in statute. Briefly, the process of PPB involves:

1. *Program accounting*—allocating expenditures under output or service categories.
2. *Multiyear costing*—projecting costs on a three- to five-year time horizon (using the previous two years and the succeeding three to five years).
3. *Zero-based budgeting*—evaluating the base level of expenditures starting at zero dollars, rather than using the previous year's budget as the base.
4. *Quantitative evaluation of resources allocation alternatives*—using benefit-cost, cost-effectiveness, or cost-utility analysis.

In the following section, these components of the PPB process are examined in detail to provide some insights into the ways in which finance decision making, budgeting, and program evaluation are linked. Since absolute consensus on what makes up the PPB process does not exist, even among experts, this discussion should be supplemented with reading in other sources (Hatry and Cotton, 1967; Henrichs and Taylor, 1969; Lyden and Miller, 1978; Bierman and Smith, 1966).

Program Accounting

Program accounting is a way of organizing information to reveal how much is being spent for each purpose (Merewitz and Sosnick, 1971). The first step in the development of a program accounting system is to identify the programs. Defined as a cluster of activities functioning together to produce the same outputs, an agency program is frequently identified by its funding source, its target population, or the type of problem it addresses. If, for instance, the mental health agency receives funding from the National Institute of Alcohol Abuse and the National Institute of Drug Abuse, then both an alcohol program budget account and a drug abuse program budget account should be kept.

Table 2. General Form of the Line-Item Budget.

I. VARIABLE COSTS
  Personnel
    Salaries and Wages
      Physicians
      Psychiatrists
      Nurses
      Psychologists
      Social workers
      Clerical
      Administrative

      _____
      _____

    Employee Benefits
      Social security
      Life insurance
      Health insurance
      Retirement plan
      Workmen's compensation
      Unemployment compensation
    Professional Fees
                                Total Personnel   _____
  Operating Expenses
    Publications
    Subscriptions
    Dues
    Licenses
    Professional meetings
    Continuing education
    In-service training

    _____
    _____
                                Total Operating   _____
  Travel and Transportation Expenses
    Personal auto mileage, in state
    Personal auto mileage, out of state
    Public transportation
    Motels and hotels
    Meals
    Per diem
                    Total Travel and Transportation   _____
  Office Expenses
    Telephone
    Telephone, long distance
    Telephone, credit card
    Special telephone equipment
    Postage
    Air express
    Office supplies
    Photocopy supplies
    Office equipment and repairs
                            Total Office Expenses   _____
  Operating Supplies
    Drugs
    Medical supplies
    First aid supplies

Table 2, cont'd.

Operating Supplies (cont'd)
   Recreation supplies
   _____
   _____
                 Total Operating Expenses   _____
Contracts
   By name of vendor
            TOTAL VARIABLE COSTS   _____

II. FIXED COSTS
   Building Expenses
      Rent
      Electricity
      Gas/oil
      Water
      Waste disposal
      Sewage
      Insurance
      _____
      _____
                 Total Building   _____
   Equipment
      Renting/leasing
         Typewriters
         Furniture
         Photocopy machines
         Computer, time sharing
         Computer terminals
         Client van
         Automobile 1 (year)
         Automobile 2
         Laboratory equipment
               Total Equipment   _____
   Capital Outlay
      Laboratory equipment
      Office furniture
      Office equipment
      _____
      _____
             Total Capital Outlay   _____
   Other Expenses
      Prepaid leases, rents
      Depreciation
         Building (name)
      Equipment
      Public relations
      Credit losses
      _____
      _____
                 Total Other   _____
             TOTAL FIXED COSTS   _____

                 GRAND TOTAL   _____

Programs should not be defined by type of service mode, however. For instance, a halfway house for youthful offenders should actually be considered a youthful offenders program; the halfway house would be the program subcategory for budgetary purposes, even if the halfway house is the only program for youthful offenders. When other programs are then developed for this target group, they would also be included as program subcategories. Program subcategories in a mental health agency, which usually include such service modes as inpatient, outpatient, halfway house, crisis intervention, emergency, consultation education, and day treatment, are important accounting categories. When resources are scarce, a program subcategory can often be cut back without influencing the total program effectiveness.

At the basic level of program accounting, expenditures are assigned to program element. A program element, such as hours of outpatient service, is the unit of output produced and the base unit for measuring cost in a service organization. Since all agency program elements are services, they are best measured as service hours. Visits, although traditionally used as a unit in medical care, are not a program element that facilitates management control, because a visit in one program subcategory is seldom equivalent to a visit in another subcategory, and therefore the costs and benefits of subcategories cannot be compared. How can one compare a home visit with a medication review visit except in terms of cost per hour? Some may argue that in certain cases—inpatient services, for example—one should define the service day or the number of clients as the program element. The approach presents no problem as long as there is some way in which to compare inpatient and outpatient services.

The United Way has developed a system for categorizing programs that managers may wish to examine when they are establishing their program accounts (Sumariwalla, 1974). After identifying a number of programs, the next step in developing a program accounting system is to list the expenditures for each budget category by program subcategory and calculate the total expenditures for each program subcategory (see Table 3). Total expenditures per program are found by summing expenditures in the subcategories. One can then calculate the cost of a program element—that is, an hour of service—in each program subcategory by dividing the total expenditures in the program subcategory by the number of service hours.

The objects of expenditure included in the calculation of the cost of each program element should reflect total program costs and should be so constructed that management can calculate average costs and marginal costs. These and several other key terms are defined as follows:

1. *Total costs* are variable costs added to total fixed costs.
2. *Variable costs* are costs that vary with the quantity of service produced—for example, labor, fringe benefits, food costs, therapeutic supplies.
3. *Fixed costs* are costs that do not vary with production—for example, rent, utilities, equipment.
4. *Average costs* are total costs divided by the number of program elements produced in the same period of time—for example, service hours.

Table 3. Program Budget Summary: Sample for a Children's Program in a Community Mental Health Center.

	Program Subcategory									
	Adminis-tration	Salaries and Wages	Fringe Benefits	Profes-sional Fees	Contracts	Operating Supplies	Office Expense	Travel Transpor-tation	Building	Capital	TOTAL
Outpatient										
Day Care										
Twenty-four-Hour Care										
Inpatient										
Diagnostic Center										
Community Education										
Emergency										
Total Pro-gram Costs										

5. *Marginal cost* is the change in total cost resulting from changes in output, divided by the change in output for a specific period of time.

Fixed and variable costs, when clearly defined in the budget and expenditure reports, provide the basis for the agency to establish fee schedules and rates for third-party reimbursers. All too frequently, agency budgets do not specifically distinguish fixed costs from variable costs, or they omit from consideration critical elements of fixed costs such as depreciation and amortization allowances to maintain and replace buildings and equipment; cash-flow reserve allowances; and allowances for research, community education, and public relations.

Much controversy continues to exist among public sector accountants over the use of depreciation in not-for-profit organizations (National Committee on Governmental Accounting, 1968). Depreciation as an accounting procedure is defined as the process of recognizing a portion of the cost of an asset as an expense during each year of its estimated service life. For example, assume an agency purchases a piece of equipment that costs $16,000 and has a useful life of eight years. If the agency used a straight-line accounting method, the accountant would spread this expense over eight years by writing off $2,000 per year for eight years, rather than accounting for the full $16,000 in the year in which the equipment was purchased and delivered.

Depreciation of capital goods (known as fixed assets, such as buildings and equipment) is used to determine part of the cost of services for which the equipment is used. Therefore, depreciation influences the level of reimbursement the organization may obtain for those services. The generally accepted procedure for computing depreciation is to use the purchase price and standard life table that estimates the projected life of the equipment.

Variable costs, those costs that change as a function of the amount of services produced, include the cost of personnel, fringe benefits, the cost of supplies, office expenses, and travel and transportation expenses—in other words, all those costs that contribute to the production of a service or to the cost of supporting the personnel who provide that service (Horngren, 1967). Professional salaries are the major variable cost of most community mental health centers, and, if a staff member does work in several program categories, a portion of his or her salary should be allocated to each category (Feldman, 1973). Three techniques for allocating the costs of professional services are:

1. *Exact time approach* allocates professional personnel costs to various units on the basis of the exact amount of time spent by each professional in a program category. To use this method requires the worker to keep a time sheet on all activities each day.
2. *Estimated time approach* allocates personnel costs on the basis of estimated time spent by workers in a program category. The estimates are usually made by management with input from workers and are reviewed at least once quarterly.

3. *Periodic time study approach* allocates personnel costs on the basis of time studies. At least twice annually, and preferably quarterly, management will require all personnel to record the time spent in each task and program category for one randomly selected week.

Probably the most difficult costs to allocate are indirect costs—costs that are allocated from the organizational unit originally making the expenditure to another organizational unit benefiting from or influenced by the activity incurring the cost (Hagedorn, 1976). Central administrative services (including personnel, central records, accounting, and so on), utilities, repairs, and maintenance are examples of indirect costs (National Institute of Mental Health, 1977). Another form of indirect cost is costs incurred from interaction with another agency, such as the referral or placement of a client. The best source of information on how to calculate indirect cost is a set of rules and procedures developed by Sorensen (1976).

While confusion often exists with regard to accounting terms, the two major methods of accounting are enterprise accounting, used by organizations that produce goods or services for profit, and fund accounting, used by not-for-profit organizations such as mental health agencies. A fund is defined in the American Institute of Certified Public Accountants' *Audits of Voluntary Health and Welfare Organizations* (1974, p. 1) as "an asset or groups of assets, together with associated accountabilities (liabilities and equities), that are related as to activity or purpose and maintained as an accounting entity. Fund accounting is a double entry system for recording the transactions of each of several funds, which are separate accounting entities, with reciprocal entries for transactions between funds."

No general agreement exists among experts on what type of funds a mental health agency should establish. In many states, agencies are required to use the fund categories established for municipal governments, known as the general accepted accounting and financial information standards (American Institute of Certified Public Accountants, 1974). The advantage of using these or similar standards to guide the structure of the agency's accounting system is that it facilitates financial reporting to the funders, the board, and the general public. Fund accounting facilitates keeping track of the use of different sources of revenues on which the organization must prepare special financial reports. Most states, for instance, require fund accounting to account for the uses of state grant-in-aid.

Most managers of mental health agencies have little or no training in accounting and rely on accounting professionals to do the technical aspects of establishing program accounts. For those managers who would like to gain more expertise in program accounting, several excellent texts are available (Anthony, 1978; Gross, 1972; Hay and Mikesell, 1974; Lynn and Thompson, 1974; Matz and Curry, 1972; Neuner, 1974; Silvers and Prahalad, 1974).

Multiyear Costing

Multiyear costing requires the specification of standard rules for projecting costs into the future, necessary in determining whether programs can, over time, continue to meet projected client demand at a given cost. Multiyear costing is usually done by direct service staff members working with the fiscal officer. Anyone who has prepared a three- to five-year grant proposal has done multiyear costing, because such grants require a projected budget for each of the years for which funding is being requested. To do a reasonably good job of projecting costs into the future requires that the organization have some data on past years' costs for a program of similar type and scale of operation. Since such data are frequently not available to a local agency, management is often unwilling to risk making funding decisions based on projections. As only one component of PPB, multiyear costing is a planning process whose results should not be considered absolute and unchangeable. The critical part of the multiyear planning process is management documentation of the rules that are to be used in making the cost projections.

In addition to the projection of expenditures, six elements are to be described in the budget package, according to federal administrative guidelines for PPB: objectives that describe the benefits being sought, target levels of service effort, such as hours of outpatient service; choices made regarding alternative methods for obtaining the objectives; levels of service output expected; and the effectiveness with which target levels are obtained.

Zero-Based Budgeting

Zero-based budgeting (ZBB) is used in the strategic planning phase of budgeting. Frequently government funding agencies will request that the mental health agency prepare a budget that shows how various levels of funding will influence the level of services to be provided. For instance, the funder may suggest that the agency prepare budgets showing the impact of funding at 80 or 90 percent of last year's award (reduction due to inflation) and at a continuation level (last year's award plus adjustments for inflation). The agency might use ZBB to show that a 10 percent reduction from the current level would result in a 23 percent reduction in services but that the 10 percent cut could be absorbed with no loss in services if government reporting requirements were waived.

The key aspect of the ZBB process is the formation and selection of decision criteria. The zero-based budget documents show how the agency proposes to operate under different levels of funding. ZBB is a process that facilitates making decisions about what programs will be implemented at what level of activity, given a specified level of funding. The process is based on the assumption that resources are scarce and that to use available resources requires an annual review and evaluation of programs and activities comparing each program in terms of actual output, effectiveness, and costs (Pyhrr, 1973). The ZBB process forces management to organize information into decision packages. If the agency elects to prepare a ZBB decision package, it should obtain a manual or set of guidelines that specify each step (Anthony, 1978; Lynn and Thompson, 1974). If the request for a zero-based budget comes from a government agency, guidelines are usually provided, since the process is not standardized.

To formulate a zero-based budget, an organization is required to evaluate and review all programs and activities (current and new); review activities on a basis of outputs, effectiveness, and cost; and analyze all increases (Pyhrr, 1973). Six common components of the ZBB process are:

1. *Selection of the decision unit.* A decision unit is a program or other organizational entity for which alternatives in the scope of work and amount of resources allocated must be reviewed.

2. *Preparation of a decision package.* A decision package is a document that presents the information necessary to make resources allocation decisions. A decision package set is a group of decision packages representing the total budget for an organization or program.

3. *Preparation of consolidated decision packages.* A consolidated decision package set is prepared by top management for the board of directors and may include additional programs or delete original decision packages.

4. *Ranking of decisions.* Decisions are ranked in increasing order of priority by managers and board members.

5. *Documentation of the minimum level for program funding.* The minimum funding level for a program or a subprogram activity is the level below which continued operation of the program is not feasible because, in management's opinion, stated program objectives cannot be reached.

6. *Documentation of current levels of funding.* Current levels of funding represent a continuation budget level, without policy change but with increments representing only adjustments due to personnel salary change or changes in expenses due to inflation. Current level implies no growth in the product or services produced.

Quantitative Analysis of Alternatives

Benefit-cost analysis and cost-effectiveness analysis are the methods most commonly used for quantitative analysis in PPB. Benefit-cost analysis, a technique where the costs and benefits derived from agency activities are compared in monetary terms, is often used to compare alternative uses of capital (Layard, 1976). For instance, if the agency had funds to establish a new inpatient unit, management would examine the benefit-cost advantage of an agency-based inpatient unit over a subcontracted unit within a local hospital. Cost-effectiveness analysis is a technique whereby the costs of agency activities measured in dollars are compared with effects or benefits measured in nondollar terms. Cost-effectiveness is often used to measure the difference in cost per hour between two types of service modes against the difference in client behavior associated with each mode.

Agencies have traditionally used cost-effectiveness analysis as a management tool. With this method, programs are compared both on the basis of costs and on the basis of the amount, quality, or overall effect of the outputs. Cost-effectiveness analysis uses the same approach as benefit-cost analysis, except that the term *effectiveness* implies that the service benefits cannot be measured in dollars. As an approach to examining alternative resources allocation decisions, cost-effectiveness is seldom an appropriate technique to use by itself unless: costs of alternatives are identical, and therefore only benefits need be compared, eliminating the need to convert benefits to dollars; or benefits are identical, and only costs need be compared.

Cost-effectiveness analysis provides no direct guidance when one is unsure whether the total benefit from a program justifies the total cost or when one is trying to select the optimal budget level for a program—that is, the best possible budget level within agreed-on constraints (Stokey and Zeckhauser, 1978). Whenever possible, agency management should use both benefit-cost and cost-effectiveness analysis to compare alternative operating expenditure or capital expenditure decisions.

Despite some limitations, benefit-cost analysis is an extremely valuable tool for local agency managers to use to make strategic planning and management control decisions. In benefit-cost analysis, all program costs and all direct and indirect benefits are translated into monetary terms. Programs can then be compared to find the most efficient choices. The analysis can be used in the strategic planning process to analyze alternatives and make nonroutine capital expenditure decisions; to assist in choosing which programs to operate or expand; and to choose among new programs. Benefit-cost analysis can also be used in making routine management control decisions.

Using ZBB and benefit-cost analysis, a manager can also examine the operating efficiency of programs of different scales or levels of effort. For instance, "minimal desired" and "optimal" levels of an inpatient alcohol detoxification unit can both be subjected to benefit-cost analysis and then compared in terms of marginal cost alternatives to locate the optimally efficient programs or program scales. Marginal cost refers to the cost of adding the last additional unit of service or personnel. All too often agencies add a full-time staff member to take up cases on the waiting list, only to find that after a few months the capacity to deliver services exceeds the demand. The addition of one direct service worker may mean that the cost of a program will exceed its revenues.

Perhaps the greatest benefit of benefit-cost analysis is that management must choose criteria for making decisions prior to conducting the analysis. The three most common criteria used by human services managers are: maximizes services produced for a given level of funds or costs, maximizes net benefit, and minimizes cost while achieving a fixed level of benefit.

Capital Budgets and Cash Budgets

Although operating budgets have been the main focus of discussion, this chapter would not be complete without at least some mention of capital budgets and cash budgets. A capital budget is usually prepared annually but projects anticipated capital expenditures for buildings and equipment three to five years into the future. The cash budget is particularly important to mental health agencies, since it designates sources of funds and indicates projected revenues from each source. An agency that uses fund accounting usually maintains separate categories for each source of funds—each tax source; the federal funding source; state grant-in-aid; other state funding sources; and fees, reimbursements, contributions, and depreciation. All of these sources and their expected value should appear on the cash budget.

Throughout this chapter, it has been emphasized that a budget is a plan and should therefore be amenable to change during the year. One of the major sources of data used by management to monitor the need to change the budget is expenditure reports and other financial reports produced by the accountant for management. For every budget form, an associated quarterly expenditure report is prepared; in addition, cash-flow budgets may be prepared monthly. Accounting and management also prepare financial accounting reports to provide information on the fiscal status of the organization to board members and others external to the organization. Such reports, which include a balance sheet, a statement of sources and uses of funds, a cash budget report, and an annual audit statement, are not usually used as a basis for management control decisions.

Management control decisions are made by reviewing quarterly expenditure reports and client informational systems data, which may be part of an overall management informational system. Changes in the budget are usually made in response to exceptions in a line item or program category. If the level of projected revenues or expenditures is significantly different from that planned in the budget, the budget is changed to reflect exceptions to the plan. The original plan is not discarded but updated. The record of such budget changes gives management a source of data for retrospective analysis of management decisions and for the development of new budgets. Most exceptions occur in line items of program budgets, particularly personnel items, since costs vary from one year to the next. Variations in personnel costs are usually due to turnover and lags in hiring placement staff. In some state and many federal guidelines, agencies may not reallocate more than 10 percent of their total personnel budget line to any other budget line. Because of this restriction, start-up costs must be carefully projected; otherwise, money not expended for personnel will lapse and often must be returned to the funding source as unexpended revenue. An agency cannot absorb such a loss and expect to maximize benefits for a given level of revenue.

Monitoring the Financial Condition

Financial condition refers to the degree of financial stability or uncertainty. Because most mental health agencies have been adapting to funding cutbacks for the past five years at least, managers have some method for reviewing the impact of cutbacks on the financial condition of the agency. By looking at financial indicators, management can determine if trends related to the following financial problems may influence the financial condition: a declining revenue base, concurrent with an increase in service demand; an increase in the cost of services over and above what might be expected because of changes in the cost of living; dependence on external funding sources, decreasing the agency's flexibility to respond to changes in client needs; and inadequate fiscal policy or fiscal management practices.

Considerable progress has been made in the development of indicators to monitor financial condition (Hall, 1982). Such indicators are tools to assist management in examining financial trends over a three- to five-year period using information from financial statements, budgets, expenditure reports, audits, and annual reports. Indicators useful to mental health agency managers provide data that can inform managers whether the agency will be able to maintain programs in the future that are presently funded with resources scheduled to decline or be eliminated and maintain capital facilities and equipment in such a way as to protect the investment. Such indicators also help managers determine: what proportion of total revenues are restricted; what dollar commitments exist in the form of matching funds and unreimbursed overhead; to what extent increases in fringe benefits exceed those of other sectors; what agency cash management practices are used to produce revenues from current assets; and to what extent the agency uses short-term debt to even out cash flow (see Table 4). Answers to these and other questions based on an examination of financial trend information can assist management in strategic planning and in the review of fiscal policy and practices and can facilitate the development of an agency that is in sound financial condition.

Operational Control

Of the activities that comprise the operational control of an agency, which is in the hands of supervisors and directors of service units, only four specifically relate to fiscal matters (see Table 1). Nevertheless, fiscal crises are most often caused by laxity in the application of budget guidelines to staff management and by a lack of control of expenditures at the operational level.

Line items most frequently overspent are travel and consumable supplies. The control of travel cost has become a major management problem, given the cost of fuel and the capital investment individuals must make to own an automobile—no longer is the mere reporting of mileage an adequate management procedure. Workers should prepare travel plans, along with their weekly or monthly work plans, that justify their travel. Some agencies have worked out a travel reimbursement schedule for job class groups that sets limits on monthly travel and requires justification of exceptions and overuse. Not local travel but travel to professional meetings and out-of-state travel—frequently given to, and expected as a fringe benefit by, professional workers—put the biggest fiscal burden on agencies. In some agencies, travel to professional meetings is an earned, rather than an automatic, benefit. The control of non-service-related use of office supplies has always been a problem, and treatment supplies such as drugs also require inventory control, since costs of some items may increase by as much as 30 percent per year.

Funding Sources Now and in the Future

Large, usually urban, community mental health centers have been successful in tapping many funding sources, but some agencies have managed to

Table 4. Indicators to Measure the Financial Condition of Not-for-Profit Human Service Agencies by Type of Financial Problem.

Indicators of Declining Revenue Base

Increasing percent of revenues per client served
Increasing percent of one-time revenues
Stable percent of client fees
Decreasing percent of expenditures for repair and maintenance of fixed assets
Increasing percent of unfunded pension liabilities
Decreasing percent of unrestricted fund balance
Increasing percent of operating deficits

Indicators of Dependence on Unstable Revenue Sources

Increasing percent of revenues from government
Stable percent of revenues from memberships and contributions
Increasing percent of restricted operating revenues
Increasing percent of available sources of funds used
Increasing percent of unreimbursed overhead
Stable percent of revenues from client fees

Indicators of Increasing Costs of Services

Increasing percent of expenditures for support personnel
Increasing percent of personnel costs per client served
Increasing percent of expenditures for fixed costs
Increasing percent of fringe benefit liabilities
Increasing percent of nonlabor costs

Indicators of Inadequacies in Fiscal Policy and Management

Liquidity
Decreasing percent of interest earned from investments of current assets
Contract efficiency

Source; Hall, 1982, p. 28.

survive with only state grant-in-aid and a modicum of federal funds. In this concluding section, current sources for mental health funding are reviewed, and some attempt is made to look at the fiscal management implications of anticipated future state and federal policy changes.

Federal laws will have a major impact on the financing of mental health agencies, especially when certain population groups, such as the chronically mentally ill, children, the aged, and other underserved groups, are targeted for services. If federal policy mandates shift to these target groups, agencies will probably depend more on contracts from other human services agencies, such as Title XX social services, area agencies on aging, and youth services, for their funding. For example, few mental health agencies are not financially dependent to some extent on Medicaid. Reliance on contracts with other agencies usually involves some kind of fee-for-service arrangement.

Today, almost all mental health agencies obtain some form of state grant-in-aid, but the amount of that support and how the allocation is determined differ significantly from one state to another. In most cases, state funding is based on a capitation rate, with a base operational grant. For instance, a state may give a mental health agency 45 cents for each person living in the region served by the center and to that add $25,000 as a budgetary base. The capitation rate is usually calculated according to some complex formula that takes into account the demography of the population served. By using an adjusted capitation rate, states are attempting to redistribute resources by awarding more funds to those centers serving low-income and other underserved populations.

As federal funds begin to disappear, mental health managers are looking for other sources of funding. Some managers seek to shift services to different populations, others change their organizational structure, but all are attempting to tap private insurance payments as a source of funding. When agencies become reliant on insurance payments, they begin to serve increased numbers of working middle-class clients. Of those mental health agencies changing their structure, some became part of a community hospital or a health maintenance organization (HMO). A mental health unit in an HMO is financed by a fixed fee paid by the client, who has elected to participate in a prepaid group plan providing medical, dental, and mental health care.

Other innovative methods used to fund mental health care include contracts with public schools, nursing homes, and community hospitals; contributions from organizations like the United Way; and fund-raising efforts of local mental health associations. Some centers have received demonstration money from private foundations; others set up their own not-for-profit educational institutes and receive research and demonstration grants. In many states, mental health managers have been successful in getting contracts with local government under revenue-sharing block grants.

At the time this chapter is being written, no new sources of funds for mental health agencies exist—the financial future of mental health programs is hanging in the balance and will be influenced by new federal legislation. This chapter was written with the conviction that the concept of community mental health will survive, but the financial structure of the provider agencies will probably change drastically. Reimbursements and contracts seem to be the likely funding source of the future, particularly for services for the chronically mentally ill, who have needs far exceeding the traditional domain of community mental health agencies.

References

American Institute of Certified Public Accountants. *Audits of Voluntary Health and Welfare Organizations.* New York: American Institute of Certified Accountants, 1974.

Anthony, R. *Essentials of Accounting.* Reading, Mass.: Addison-Wesley, 1978.

Anthony, R. *Planning and Control Systems: A Framework for Analysis.* Boston: Harvard University Press, 1965.

Bierman, H. J., and Smith, S. *The Capital Budgeting Decision.* New York: Macmillan, 1966.

Feldman, S. *The Administration of Mental Health Services.* Springfield, Ill.: Thomas, 1973.

Gross, M. *Financial and Accounting Guide for Nonprofit Organizations.* Chicago: Ronald Press, 1972.

Hagedorn, H., and others. *A Working Manual and Simple Program Evaluation Technique for Community Mental Health Centers.* Rockville, Md.: National Institute of Mental Health, 1976.

Hall, M. D. "Financial Condition: A Measure of Human Organization Performance." *New England Journal of Human Services,* 1982, *2* (1), 25–35.

Hatry, H., and Cotton, J. F. *Program Budgeting for State, County, and City.* Washington, D.C.: George Washington University Press, 1967.

Hay, L., and Mikesell, R. M. *Government Accounting.* New York: Irwin, 1974.

Henrichs, H., and Taylor, G. *Program Budgeting and Benefit-Cost Analysis.* Santa Monica, Calif.: Goodyear, 1969.

Horngren, C. *Cost Accounting: A Managerial Emphasis.* Englewood Cliffs, N.J.: Prentice-Hall, 1967.

Hyde, A. C., and Shafritz, J. *Government Budgeting: Theory, Process and Politics.* Oak Park, Ill.: Moore, 1978.

Layard, R. (Ed.). *Cost-Benefit Analysis.* New York: Penguin, 1976.

Lyden, F., and Miller, E. *Public Budgeting: Program Planning and Evaluation.* Chicago: Rand McNally, 1978.

Lynn, E., and Thompson, J. *Introduction to Fund Accounting.* Reston, Va.: Reston, 1974.

Matz, A., and Curry, O. *Cost Accounting Planning and Control.* Minneapolis: South-Western Publishing, 1972.

Merewitz, L., and Sosnick, S. *The Budget's New Clothes: A Critique of Program Planning and Budgeting.* Chicago: Rand McNally, 1971.

National Committee on Governmental Accounting. *Government Accounting, Auditing, and Financial Reporting.* Chicago: Municipal Finance Officers Association of the U.S. and Canada, 1968.

National Institute of Mental Health. *Guidelines for a Minimum Statistical Accounting System for Community Mental Health Centers.* Rockville, Md.: National Institute of Mental Health, 1977.

Neuner, J. *Cost Accounting: Principles and Practice.* New York: Irwin, 1974.

Pyhrr, P. *Zero-Base Budgeting.* New York: Wiley, 1973.

Salmon, E., and Pringle, J. *An Introduction to Financial Management.* Santa Monica, Calif.: Goodyear, 1977.

Silvers, J. B., and Prahalad, C. K. *Financial Management of Health Institutions.* New York: Spectrum, 1974.

Sorensen, J. E. *Cost Finding and Rate Setting for Community Mental Health Centers.* Rockville, Md.: National Institute of Mental Health, 1976.

Stokey, E., and Zeckhauser, R. *A Primer for Policy Analysis.* New York: Norton, 1978.

Sumariwalla, R. D. *Accounting and Financial Reporting: A Guide for United Way and Not-for-Profit Human Service Organizations.* Alexandria, Va.: United Way of America, 1974.

Taylor, G. *Program Budgeting and Benefit-Cost Analysis.* Santa Monica, Calif.: Goodyear, 1977.

☙ 17 ❧

Management Information Systems

Linda Dreyer
Nancy Koroloff
Linda Bellerby

Designed for managers who do not have a background in systems analysis and who work in agencies without a sophisticated data processing unit, this chapter presents the basic components of information systems and describes techniques for identifying common problems that impede systems performance as well as a model for improving such performance. The mechanics of data processing are reviewed, commonly used terms are defined, and key questions are raised that need to be answered at each stage of a system's development and improvement. In addition, tables are provided for assisting managers in determining the data recorded by their current information systems and in deciding among equipment and software options.

Administrators have been under intense pressure from funders, legislative bodies, and other political constituencies to improve their agencies' information systems, and program managers are beginning to recognize the value of reliable information, especially when making difficult decisions related to declining resources. At the same time, rapid technological change in computer equipment is making it possible for even small agencies to manage their information resources at reasonable costs.

The process of implementing or improving an information system is complex and involves much more than technical analysis and design. System development or improvement creates changes in organizational structure and behavior and can consume scarce staff and fiscal resources. These technical, organizational, and managerial aspects must be carefully balanced if a management information system is to meet the agency's requirements. This chapter provides an overview of management information systems development, with special attention given to the program manager's tasks and responsibilities in that process. Portions of this chapter were adapted from a training project developed and published by the authors, in which more detailed information about management information system improvement can be found (Bellerby, Dreyer, and Koroloff, 1981).

Four Basic Components of Formal Information Systems

The term *information system* frequently conjures up images of computers. However, an information system is more than equipment—it is an integrated network of people, procedures, and equipment that systematically processes data about past and present events into information about the agency's internal operations and external reporting requirements. To be useful to decision makers, the information must be timely, accurate, uniform, and relevant. The four basic components of an information system are people, procedures, equipment, and the specific management informational content.

The keystone of any system is staff members who interact with the data from the point of collection to the point of utilization. Policies and procedures provide standards for ensuring that data are entered accurately and handled appropriately as they are processed into useful information. A wide range of equipment, including files, filing cabinets, typewriters, photocopy machines, calculators, and computers, may be involved in processing data into formation.

The mechanics of data processing include data handling, data conversion, and information presentation. The data-handling process includes the activities of generating and collecting data from staff members and routing data to a place where they can be stored and retrieved for later use. Data conversion involves sorting, summarizing, and analyzing the data in order to convert them into information. Information presentation includes interpreting and disseminating reports to the right people. Some common data-processing terms include:

- *Data*—specific, unrelated facts that have little value or interest by themselves.
- *Information*—data that have been aggregated or processed into an ordered and useful form.
- *Information processing*—cognitive activities that result in action, such as setting objectives, allocating resources, or making decisions.
- *User*—the person who processes information.
- *Data element*—a specific item of information—for example, a client identification number or date of birth.
- *Record*—a set of data elements usually related to a common subject—for example, a payroll record.
- *File*—a grouping of related records treated as a unit—for example, a file of client records.
- *Data base*—the composite of all the data systematically collected and stored for retrieval so that information can be generated to support decision making; a collection of files. An agency's usual data base components include client, staff, and fiscal data.

Most of an agency's data will be collected by clinical and support staff members and used primarily by administrators and board members. Users rarely concern themselves with data-processing activities unless these activities fail to produce information that is timely, accurate, uniform, and relevant. However, since signs of impending problems will surface in one or more of the data-processing components, the operation of the current information system should be assessed in order to correct problem situations before they cause a system failure. The results of an assessment can also provide the starting point for a major system improvement effort. Table 1 presents questions to be raised in a general assessment of a system's data-processing components.

The source of problems in the three data-processing components, data handling, data conversion, and information presentation, can be found in the people, the procedures, and the equipment network that supports the system. For example, if forms are not filled in accurately or completely (data-handling problem), the source of the problem may be poor instructions (procedures) or disagreement over data element definitions (people). The following questions related to people, procedures, and equipment are useful in assessing the operation of a managerial information system:

People

- Is there confusion about who has what responsibility for data-processing activities?
- Are bottlenecks created by staff members who do not have enough time to accomplish routine data-handling procedures?
- Do a small number of people make the majority of data collection errors?
- If a key staff member involved in data handling leaves the agency, does the information system continue to operate effectively?
- If the agency uses some type of computer support, is there a staff member with sufficient technical expertise to serve as a liaison with technical staff?

Procedures

- Do forms, reports and files get lost, go to the wrong people, or arrive late?
- Are procedures for completing forms, distributing reports, and filing records clearly documented?
- Do forms and reports have to stop at many different desks before they are completely processed?
- Do you have adequate procedures to control access to files and reports containing confidential data?
- Does the agency rely on one person's knowledge about how the information system works, instead of documenting these procedures in writing?
- Are procedures for correcting or updating forms and reports clearly specified?
- Are forms and reports checked for accuracy, completeness, and timeliness?

Equipment

- Is the equipment required for data-processing activities suitable and readily available?
- Are the costs of operating or maintaining equipment excessive?
- Would other types of equipment provide faster, easier, cheaper, or more efficient handling and processing of data?

Good information can reduce uncertainty in decision making and problem solving. Not only must the technical aspects of the system work smoothly to produce good information but the system must also collect the appropriate data to assist program managers. The content of an information system is best determined by a careful survey of the information the agency will need for internal purposes and external reporting requirements.

Broskowski and Attkisson (1982) suggest that a system's content should include reliable information on resources, effort, utilization, quality, outcome, effectiveness, cost, and efficiency, among other topics. The following examples provide common applications in these areas:

Resources, Effort, and Utilization

- Statistical reports on numbers and types of clients
- Service reports by program or staff
- Billing applications
- Staff assignments or productivity measures

Quality, Outcome, and Effectiveness

- Comparison of the type of service provided to a particular client group with some normative standard
- Comparison of a program's accomplishment in terms of effort, utilization, or outcomes with its original goals

Costs and Efficiency

- Determination of which of two programs is most effective at reaching the target group in the shortest time and at the lowest cost

Table 1. Components of an Information System.

---

1. Data-Handling Component

Description

This component includes activities like collecting data, routing data between work stations, and storing data in files and is the most labor intensive of the three components.

Common Problems

Staff members do not complete source documents accurately. The agency uses too many forms or collects the same data elements several times. Procedures for collecting, routing, and storing data are not documented. No one checks forms for completeness or accuracy. Responsibility for the system is vested in one person, usually a support staff member, with no authority to keep other people accountable.

In this agency:

1. Are some data not being used because staff do not trust their accuracy?
2. Do staff members disagree on standard data definitions?
3. Can records usually be found where they ought to be? Are files kept in a centralized place?
4. Do forms sit too long on someone's desk waiting to be processed?
5. Do staff complain about the amount of time they spend handling data?
6. Are the same data elements collected on several different forms (or collected more than once?
7. Do staff have trouble finding data in files?

2. Data Conversion Component

Description

This component includes activities, such as sorting, summarizing, and analyzing, that transform data into information. These activities can be completed by manual or automated methods and can result in simple head counts or elaborate statistical computations.

Common Problems

Staff spends too much time reclassifying data that were collected in one unit but must be reported in another. Data for one report exist in several places. Users need help in applying more or different data analyses to their decisions. Computer capability is underutilized.

In this agency:

1. Do staff need to spend too much time sorting or classifying data before those data can be used?
2. Do staff spend too much time pulling data together for reports?
3. Could more or different statistical analyses be done with existing data?

3. Information Presentation Component

Description

This component includes activities like preparing reports on time, formatting them appropriately, disseminating them to the right people, and insuring that they are interpreted correctly.

Common Problems

Good data never get used because of poor presentation. Data that could be useful are collected but never summarized and reported. Internal management informational needs are not linked to external reporting requirements. Users need help in interpreting report formats.

In this agency:

1. Are useful data collected that never get summarized or analyzed?
2. Are reports distributed to the right people at the right time?
3. Are reports tailored to meet different user groups' needs? Are reports easy to read and interpret?

Paton and D'huyvetter (1980) have observed that a system can produce information to facilitate management decisions if the data collected include answers to the following questions: Who delivered services? How much? What type? To whom? When? Under what program? At what location? With what results? At what cost? Reimbursable by what fee? Using what source of funds? In addition, agency personnel can derive their own list of data elements by identifying all of the agency's reporting requirements or by analyzing the decisions they themselves make.

Many agencies collect data just because the data may be needed some day, or the same data are collected on several different forms. Another common problem involves the use of different definitions by the agency and the funding source in presenting problems. In order to assist in determining if the system collects all the necessary data and is consistent with the definitions used by different agencies, Table 2 has been included as an assessment tool, incorporating the questions raised by Paton and D'huyvetter (1980) and the specific applications noted by Broskowski and Attkisson (1982).

Model for Improving an Information System

Almost everyone knows of an agency where the process of implementing or improving a management information system went badly. Complaints like the following, for example, are not uncommon:

> "We were unprepared for the behavioral side effects of automating the system. It wasn't that the computer dehumanized the staff, but that the staff humanized the computer."

> "We hired a programmer to design a client billing system for us, but we failed to cover ourselves in the contract. When it took him two months longer to complete the job, we were liable for the cost overrun."

> "We opted to go with the state information system six months ago because it looked like it would meet our needs. We have yet to get any reliable information back from it because of technical problems."

At least three major factors account for such problems and failures. First, the organizational characteristics of many human services agencies frequently come into conflict with information system ideology in such areas as ambiguous agency goals and objectives; diversity of staff, programs, and work technologies; unstable organizational structures; and conflicting values among staff members about the purpose and use of the information system (Weirich, 1980; Noah, 1978). Second, many agencies do not have optimal control over their information system environments due to the demands of state or federal systems or agencies, insufficient financial control over external data-processing contractors, or previous

Table 2. Determining the Data Recorded by an Information System.

You can do this exercise by yourself or with a few other people who are interested in working with you. Collect a copy of all the forms that are filled out in your agency. You may need to ask several staff members, including the person in charge of fiscal activities, to make sure you have a complete set.

Use this collection of forms to determine whether or not data are recorded that could be used to answer the following specific questions. Note that a continuum of responses has been provided: information is contained on a report; data are collected but not summarized; and data are not collected.

Some of the eleven general question categories will be more important to you as a manager than others. For example, if you supervise a clinical staff, you will probably be more interested in how much service is provided and who provides it. After determining which questions are of most interest to you, review the pattern of your responses to them. If you find many responses under "data are collected but not summarized," this indicates that you are collecting the right data, but other problems in the system are preventing those data from being summarized and reported in a way that makes them available to you when you need them. If you have many responses under "data are not collected," this suggests that all data elements should be reviewed, unnecessary elements deleted, and new ones added.

	information is contained on a report	data are collected but not summarized	data are not collected

1. How much service was delivered?

   How many clients were admitted during the month prior to this one?
   How many clients were terminated during the month prior to this one?
   What was the average number of contacts in the past month for each client receiving individual services?
   What was the average number of meetings attended in the past six months for each client involved in group services?
   In the past year, has the average number of contacts per client increased, decreased, or stayed the same?
   How many appointments were missed (and not cancelled) during the past full week?
   How many appointments were cancelled during the past full week?

2. What types of services were delivered?

   In the past full month:

   How many clients were screened for intake?
   How many clients received individual therapy?
   How many clients were involved in group therapy?
   How many persons received information and referral?
   How many contacts were made with collaterals?
   How many contacts were made with other agencies regarding clients?

3. To whom were services delivered?

   What percentage of the clients admitted in the past fiscal year were racial or ethnic minorities?

Table 2, cont'd.

	information is contained on a report	data are collected but not summarized	data are not collected

What percentage of the clients admitted in the past
fiscal year were younger than age eighteen?
What percentage of the clients admitted in the past
fiscal year were older than age sixty-five?
What was the most common presenting problem
(or diagnostic category) for clients admitted in the
past fiscal year?
What was the average income of clients admitted
in the past fiscal year?

4. When were the services delivered?

Can you identify the date each element of service
was delivered to each individual client?
Does service demand fluctuate during the year?
Does this fluctuation depend on the type of service?
Is there a month in the year when total service de-
mand is heaviest?

5. Which staff members delivered the services?

Can you identify which staff member delivered each
element of service to each individual client?
How many hours of direct service were delivered
by professional staff members in the past six
months?
How many hours of direct service were delivered
by social workers in the past six months?
How many hours of indirect services (consultation, education) were delivered by professional
staff members in the past six months?

6. Through what program were services delivered?

If your agency has more than one program, can
you identify which program delivered each element
of service to each client?
How many clients are served by each program?
How many hours (or units) of each type of service
were provided by each program in the past six
months?
How many hours of direct service were generated
by professional staff members in each program in
the past six months?

7. At what locations were services delivered?

If your agency delivers services from more than one
building or site, can you identify the site at which
each element of service was delivered to each client?
Are more services delivered at one location than
another?
Are requests for a particular type of service more
frequent at any one location?
Is a particular type of client more likely to come
to any one location?

Table 2, cont'd.

	information is contained on a report	data are collected but not summarized	data are not collected

8. What was the result or outcome of services?

What percentage of clients improved after receiving services?
What percentage of clients regressed after receiving services?
What percentage of clients stayed the same after receiving services?
How long did improvement last after the client terminated services?
Were certain types of clients more likely to improve than others?

9. What did it cost the agency to deliver the services?

How much does it cost the agency to deliver an hour of individual therapy (including administrative overhead and indirect cost)?
How much does it cost the agency to deliver an hour of group therapy?
How much does it cost the agency to deliver an hour of consultation?

10. What fee was charged or reimbursement claimed?

Can you identify who was charged how much for each element of service delivered to each client?
How much is a client charged for an hour of individual therapy?
How much is a third-party reimburser charged for an hour of individual therapy?
How much is a client charged for a group therapy session?
How much is a third-party reimburser charged for a group therapy session?

11. What sources of funds paid for the services?

What percentage of clients is eligible for third-party reimbursement?
How many third-party reimbursers does your agency currently bill?
What is the rate of nonpayment by third-party reimbursers?
What percentage of clients pays for their own services?
If your agency uses a sliding fee scale, what percentage of clients pays the lowest rate?
What percentage of client accounts is currently delinquent?

commitments in equipment, staff, and software. Finally, even when these constraints are not present, a system improvement that has too large a scope, is poorly managed, and is viewed only from the technical perspective is a candidate for failure (Ackoff, 1967; Cohen, Noah, and Pauley, 1979).

A system development and improvement model that minimizes the effects of these problems is built on the following premises: the technical work of improving a system progresses through planning, design, implementation, and maintenance phases, each of which necessitates that a number of key decisions must be made before the next phase of work can be started; incremental improvements to an existing system are preferable to an extensive overhaul whereby a sequence of small projects can reflect priority information needs and available resources; and the improvement projects should be managed by a staff member who can act as the liaison between the agency and the technical staff or vendors in order to ensure that the technical design reflects user requirements, that major impacts on organizational behavior are anticipated, and that cost and time overruns are avoided (Flengte, 1981; Lucas, 1974; Schoech and Arangio, 1979).

Phases of System Improvement

The process of improving a system parallels other program design models in which each phase varies according to what work must be accomplished and by whom. Both users and technical staff must be clear about their shared and separate responsibilities. This section briefly describes the planning, design, implementation, and maintenance phases and key decisions in the improvement process.

Planning. This phase begins with agreement among the agency administrator and other key staff members that something must be done about the existing data system. The organizational politics of system improvement may not be discernible until much later, but, in general, some person or event initiates the planning process. In the planning phase, agency personnel review the existing system's strengths and weaknesses and organize informational needs into a series of improvement projects, such as eliminating unnecessary data elements, improving data control procedures, automating the staff activity data base, and modifying existing report formats.

At the same time, staff motivation and morale and available staff and fiscal resources must be assessed in order to determine the agency's readiness to improve the system. Even at this early phase, key decisions must be made in order to integrate the technical, organizational, and managerial aspects of system improvement:

Technical

- Do we need to improve the existing system?
- What parts can be improved?
- What is the best sequence for proceeding with the improvements?

Organizational

- Who supports system improvement at this time?
- Where will we find barriers?

Managerial

- What resources are required and available?
- Who can assume the role of system advocate?

   Design. Agency personnel must investigate each improvement project thoroughly to define what the system improvement must accomplish and therefore what equipment and software options will be used. The description of the new system's desired characteristics is then turned over to technical staff members, who complete a detailed design of the improvement. Agencies can either use existing equipment, acquire new equipment, or use another organization's equipment. The software can be obtained by purchasing a package, developing it in-house, or contracting out to external technicians. A summary of the options available in making this critical decision is shown in Table 3.
   Writing a request for proposals (RFP) for equipment or software, negotiating contracts, working with technical staff, and anticipating the organizational impact of the improved system combine to make this a difficult phase for many agencies. Close attention must be paid to the following issues:

Technical

- What capabilities must the improved system have?
- What are the best equipment and software options for this agency?

Organizational

- Will staff members accept the changes in established work relationships and responsibilities created by the improvement?

Managerial

- How should the technical work be divided between agency and technical staff members?

   Implementation. After the technical staff has tested the system's design and resolved any problems, it shares the responsibility for the system implementation with agency personnel. The technical work in this phase focuses on preparing the system supports, such as documenting policies and procedures; orienting and training staff members; and installing equipment and supplies. Since the new system must demonstrate that it can operate in a "live" environment, some per-

Table 3. Summary of Equipment and Software Options.

Options	When Appropriate	Advantages/ Disadvantages	Approach
1. Purchase software package, use existing equipment	• Existing equipment is adequate. • Existing software is poorly designed or does not meet current informational needs.	• The number of packages feasible on existing equipment may be limited. • System may be operationalized easily and quickly. • Packaged system may require modification.	• Identify vendors selling packaged software. • Evaluate and compare various packages. • Negotiate contract.
2. Develop software in-house, use existing equipment	• Existing equipment is adequate. • In-house staff members have the time and expertise to do analysis and programming tasks. • Funding is available to hire new staff, if needed. • Ongoing system development efforts are anticipated.	• Existing staff members are familiar with the existing system and the center's operations. • Staff members may not have enough expertise to undertake the proposed system design.	• Prepare job descriptions if new data-processing personnel are to be hired. • Negotiate a work schedule with technical staff, outlining products, milestones, target dates, and job responsibilities.
3. Contract out software development, use existing equipment	• System requirements are too specialized to be met by packaged software. • Ongoing system development work is not anticipated. • Existing equipment is adequate.	• Center can acquire technically sophisticated personnel for a limited period of time. • Center is not responsible for day-to-day monitoring of design and programming tasks.	• Identify software vendors. • Prepare a request for proposal (RFP). • Negotiate contract.
4. Purchase software package, acquire new equipment	• Computer is not currently being used, or existing equipment is inadequate. • Existing software is inadequate or not available.	• Total system cost can be high. • System may be operationalized easily and quickly. • System may require modification. • Staff members need to learn simultaneously how to use the new system and how to operate the new equipment.	• Identify vendors. • Prepare RFP for equipment selection. • Evaluate vendor packages. • Negotiate contract.

Table 3, cont'd.

Options	When Appropriate	Advantages/ Disadvantages	Approach
5. Develop software in-house, acquire new equipment	• Equipment needs to be upgraded at same time as new applications are added. • In-house control over data-processing operations is desired.	• Converting existing applications to new equipment can be a time-consuming task, requiring large commitment of fiscal and staff resources. • New staff members need to be hired when a center converts to automation for the first time.	• Identify equipment vendors. • Prepare RFP for equipment selection. • Prepare job descriptions if new staff are to be hired. • Negotiate a work schedule with technical staff.
6. Contract out software development, acquire new equipment	• No in-house data processors are available. • System requirements are too specialized to be met by packaged software. • Computer is not currently being used, or existing equipment is inadequate.	• Contractor may not have prior experience using the type of equipment you select. • Total system cost can be high. • System will be customized to meet your particular needs.	• Identify software and equipment vendors. • Prepare RFP for both software development and equipment selection. • Negotiate contract.
7. Use an external computing facility	• Purchasing or leasing equipment is not feasible at this time. • Portions of the information system are being automated for the first time.	• This approach may provide access to larger equipment than the center could afford to buy, as well as to programming and other support services. • Price discounts may be available for processing not done during prime time.	• Contact local service bureaus or state and county computer facilities. • Obtain cost estimates and descriptions of available software and support services. • Negotiate contract or memorandum of agreement.

formance indicators must also be developed that will flag problem areas. Many agencies find this phase to be very hectic, but attending to the following key implementation decisions can avoid a premature conversion.

Technical

- Is the new system operating as intended?
- When can the old system be abandoned?

Organizational

- Have all staff members been oriented and trained in the operation of the system?

Managerial

- Have the staff and fiscal resources needed to operate the system been allocated?
- Are the system supports ready to convert from the old system to the new?

Maintenance. Even after the new system is operating under live conditions, it needs regular attention to keep its performance at acceptable levels. A system is not static for long and must respond to changes in organizational structure, reporting requirements, and personnel (Elpers and Chapman, 1973; Sorensen and Elpers, 1978). Periodic performance reviews can identify those areas needing modification in order to keep the system responsive to agency needs.

The extent to which staff members use the system's reports also deserves attention during the maintenance phase. That is, data-handling staff members have diminished incentive to provide accurate data for the system if they see that the resulting information has little value to users. Thus, data utilization becomes the ultimate performance test for many systems. Key questions for this last phase of the improvement process include:

Technical

- Is the system operating as intended?
- What minor modifications can improve its performance?

Organizational

- Are staff members using the system's output?
- Can data utilization be increased?

Managerial

- Are the staff and fiscal resources allocated to the system's operation adequate?

The System Advocate

The agency's control over the improvement process is best maintained by assigning as project manager a staff member who can organize, staff, direct, and monitor the activities associated with each phase. This person, called a system advocate, must often defend the improvement process against competing priorities and ensure that it is not jeopardized by inadequate resources.

The concept of a system advocate is new in human services agencies. Some system advocates have job positions linked directly to the system—for example, program evaluators or medical records clerks. Regardless of technical background, system advocates must have enough knowledge and interpersonal skills to relate effectively to the agency personnel who will use the improved system and to the technical staff who complete its detailed analysis and design. The critical elements of this liaison function include access to administration, linkage to staff and board members, and sufficient time to manage the improvement project.

Managing Organizational Change

The introduction of a new information system can create changes in organizational behavior whereby different work modes in the administrative and clinical domains of the agency can lead to friction (Kouzes and Mico, 1979). Failure to anticipate the impact of these changes has complicated the implementation of many new systems. Support and clinical staff members are often most affected by changes in procedures and equipment because they collect and process most of the agency's data and yet have very few specific uses for the information themselves.

As in any other planned change effort, all staff members must be able to identify benefits for themselves in the new system and must have the opportunity to voice their ideas or objections. If the information system is identified as an exclusive tool for program managers, then the improvement process may result in tension between clerical, clinical, and administrative staffs. Change strategies that emphasize staff participation should be built into the planning and design phases to ensure that staff needs are incorporated into the technical design. When the system is ready to be implemented, a sound orientation and training plan is needed to help staff members adjust to their new work relationships and responsibilities.

Current Issues in System Improvement

Several issues related to system improvement are currently being debated in the field of mental health. Particularly relevant to people in middle management positions are the issues of automation, core data sets, and data utilization.

Agencies are moving toward automation as the preferred way to improve a system. A recent survey of 343 community mental health centers showed that 79 percent had some level of computer support and 32 percent with computer support owned or leased their own in-house computer (Bellerby, Dreyer, and Koroloff, 1981). These figures will undoubtedly increase as the microcomputer and minicomputer marketplace expands and prices continue to decrease. Of the centers without computer support, 11 percent were planning to automate their manual systems within one year.

The shift to automated data systems contributes to a significant amount of agency stress. An automated system requires extensive staff and capital resources to develop and operate. Resources allocation decisions alone can set up a conflict between administrators who want to manage information more efficiently and clinical staff who want to increase services. Program managers, who may be ambivalent about automation themselves, are often the mediators in this conflict.

A second issue relates to the increasing demand on agencies to process a minimum data set that will meet external requirements. At the federal and state level, considerable interest and support exist for developing packaged systems that contain core sets of data to meet the agency's external and internal reporting requirements. These prototype systems, which reduce many of the costs associated with obtaining software, are developed on the assumption that agencies do not substantially differ in the way services are defined and delivered.

Agency staffs must clarify their informational needs and compare those needs with what a packaged system offers before a system is selected. Since problems in the content component of the system affect program managers more than other staff members, they should help identify what modifications a package may need to fit the agency's requirements or values. Otherwise, staff will resist implementing the system, and the needs of managers will not be met.

A third issue relates to data utilization by clinicians and the use of data in agency decision making. Many staff and board members need some initial assistance in learning how to use the system's output for decision making. In particular, clinicians and managers may need time to identify the system as a services delivery and management tool. Increasing people's skills in data utilization is important if we are to improve that decision making with the use of better information.

Conclusion

If agency staff members can determine the characteristics an improved system should have and can communicate those characteristics to the technical staff, then the probability of achieving a satisfactory system is high. Although difficult, these tasks can be completed using the phases and key questions presented earlier in this chapter to give structure to the work. Establishing staff participation and the system advocate function will also contribute direction to the process. Given the tendency for many administrators to rush the process, program managers may need to advocate a participatory approach to system improvement.

Benjamin (1971) provides a useful set of principles for carrying out the management system improvement process that serves to summarize the major points of this chapter:

Information Is a Resource
An information system is a tool for handling this resource. As such, it is a capital investment that should provide benefits that justify its costs and should be managed as carefully as other organizational resources.

People Are the Key

Although management information systems are usually thought of as controlled by the computer, involved staff members are the people who provide both the initiative and the barriers to system improvement.

Management Must Participate

To be effective, the system must relate to the purposes and activities of the organization as they are identified by administrative and clinical staff.

The System Is for the User

The end result of any system improvement is better information for use within the organization. Therefore, the different staff perspectives on improving the system need to be acknowledged.

References

Ackoff, R. L. "Management Misinformation Systems." *Management Science,* 1967, *14,* 147–156.

Bellerby, L., Dreyer, L., and Koroloff, N. *MIS Perspectives,* Vols. 1–5. Portland, Ore.: Portland State University Regional Research Institute for Human Services, 1981.

Benjamin, R. *Control of the Information System Development Cycle.* New York: Wiley, 1971.

Broskowski, A., and Attkisson, C. *Information Systems for Health and Human Services.* New York: Human Sciences Press, 1982.

Cohen, S., Noah, J., and Pauley, A. "New Ways of Looking at Management Information Systems in Human Service Delivery." *Evaluation and Program Planning,* 1979, *2,* 49–57.

Elpers, J., and Chapman, R. "Management Information for Mental Health Services." *Administration in Mental Health,* Fall 1973, pp. 12–25.

Flengte, D. "Building a New Management Information System in a Community Mental Health Center: A Case Study." Unpublished manuscript, University of Washington School of Social Work, 1981.

Kouzes, J. M., and Mico, P. R. "Domain Theory: An Introduction to Organizational Behavior in Human Service Organizations." *Journal of Applied Behavioral Science,* 1979, *15,* 449–469.

Lucas, H. *Toward Creative Systems Design.* New York: Columbia University Press, 1974.

Noah, J. C. "Information Systems in Human Services: Misconceptions, Deceptions, and Ethics." *Administration in Mental Health,* 1978, *5,* 99–111.

Paton, J., and D'huyvetter, P. *Management Information Systems for Mental Health Agencies: A Planning and Acquisition Guide.* Washington, D.C.: U.S. Government Printing Office, 1980.

Schoech, D., and Arangio, T. "Computers in Human Services." *Social Work,* 1979, *24,* 96–102.

Sorensen, J. E., and Elpers, R. "Developing Information Systems for Human Service Organizations." In C. C. Attkisson and others (Eds.), *Evaluation of Human Service Programs.* New York: Academic Press, 1978.

Weirich, T. "The Design of Information Systems." In F. Perlmutter and S. Slavin (Eds.), *Leadership in Social Administration for the 1980s.* Philadelphia: Temple University Press, 1980.

ৡ 18 ৡ

Program
Evaluation

Gary B. Cox

As defined in this chapter, program evaluation is a process for improving services delivery by providing information for decision making and planning. Although evaluation is often undertaken initially to meet external requirements, data can be of value for internal management purposes as well, and Gary B. Cox outlines an approach designed to maximize the agency's data utilization. Methods are also described for choosing relevant evaluation questions and for conducting the evaluation itself; program monitoring and special evaluation studies are distinguished, and basic resource needs are detailed.

This chapter provides an introduction to the use of program evaluation by mental health administrators. It emphasizes the broad issues and purposes of evaluation and addresses procedural details only from the perspective of the administrator's tasks. Hence, the actual processes of designing and managing evaluation projects will not be discussed. For interested administrators, evaluation design manuals are noted in the reference section (see, for example, Attkisson and others, 1978; Cook and Campbell, 1976; Fink and Kosecoff, 1978; Hagedorn and others, 1976; Isaac and Michael, 1972; Morris and Fitz-Gibbon 1978; Struening and Guttentag, 1975; Weiss, 1972.

Issues of Evaluation

Program evaluation can be defined as the activities of collecting, analyzing, and interpreting data for the purpose of providing program administrators and planners with information regarding the effectiveness of programs. This definition, covering a broad range of activities, emphasizes the support function of evaluation in relation to administration. Other definitions stress the research function of evaluation and often restrict the content focus of evaluation to program outcome. Elmore (1980, p. 2), for example, defines evaluation as "the application of social science methods to the discovery of program effects." Rutman (1977, p. 16) defines evaluation research as "a process of applying scientific procedures to accumulate reliable and valid evidence on the manner and extent to which specified activities produce particular effects or outcomes." Rutman and others emphasize the importance of rigorous scientific methodology. In this view, evaluation research strives to improve services by developing theory and an understanding of basic processes. As described in this chapter, however, program evaluation aims to improve services delivery by providing information for directly improving decision making and planning.

Two types of evaluation are usually distinguished: formative and summative. Summative evaluation assesses program outcomes—for example, whether treatment goals have been accomplished—to determine whether a program is worth continuing. The data go to a manager, planner, or funder and are used to decide whether to continue, change, or drop the program. Good summative evaluations are very difficult to conduct. Formative evaluations assess program operations to provide data to program implementers concerned with making the program more effective. In practice, while large numbers of ostensibly summative evaluations are done, particularly at the federal level, true summative decisions are rare. In this chapter, we will assume an explicitly formative stance.

A related issue concerns whether an evaluator should be employed directly from within the organization being evaluated or through some process outside the organization's control. The issue involved is credibility—an external evaluator presumably operates with a more objective viewpoint and hence produces more valid data. Credibility tends to be a problem in summative evaluation situations where program managers are trying to convince higher-level administrators and legislators that programs are efficacious and should be continued. In this chapter, however, credibility is not considered as a central problem, since the evaluations discussed are primarily for formative purposes internal to the agency. In such cases, since bias in the findings is counter to everyone's self-interest, a competent internal evaluator is acceptable.

Another important issue in evaluations is the method by which evaluations are conceived and questions selected. For a number of years, the preeminent conceptualization of the evaluation process has been the goal and indicator model, also known as management by objectives. This approach requires an organization to define its overall goals, to successively refine them until one or more measurable variables are identified for each goal, and to indicate desired levels of performance for each variable. Evaluation consists of comparing actual and desired performance levels.

This model of evaluation, although widely advocated over the past decade, has not proven very useful for internal agency management. Most agencies seem to use these evaluations for external documentation, because they are readily understood by outside funders and administrators. Finding productive ways to define and use goals in internal administrative functions, however, is much more difficult.

An alternative process for defining evaluation questions, the so-called utilization-focused approach to evaluation, has recently been promoted with the recognition that the utilization of evaluation data has always been a problem for administrators. An increasing body of research is making clear that utilization of evaluation data depends on such elements as timing, personal interests, and stage of organizational development. Utilization-focused evaluation, then, is based on the simple dictum that, in order for the data to be useful to an administrator, the program evaluation should address a question or problem that he or she perceives as important.

Why Conduct Program Evaluations?

Program evaluation may be done for two major reasons or purposes: to provide an answer or solution to an internal question or problem or to meet the requirements of an external funding source. Since external requirements are often general in nature, an administrator can choose to respond with either of two evaluation strategies. The first is to do a pro forma evaluation, designed primarily to meet the letter of the requirement; the second is to use the occasion of the requirement to identify an internal question that should be answered, design an evaluation project to answer that question, and package the results of the project to meet the external requirement. Depending on the flexibility of the requirements and the strength of the agency commitment to directing its own evaluation program, the project may vary significantly from the external guidelines. The pro forma project will nearly always be cheaper, especially in administrative and staff time, but the results will usually be less useful to internal operations. An aggressive evaluation effort, on the other hand, will usually satisfy external authorities and has the additional advantage of documenting rational, data-oriented management practice.

In the long run, it is argued, resources will be better spent if agencies develop evaluation programs around internal needs, use results from such projects for management and planning purposes, and then present the data, as well as evidence that the data have been used for management purposes, to meet external requirements. This approach assumes that an evaluation project will provide data that are useful enough to offset the additional costs of doing a complete evaluation.

Utilization of Evaluation Data

Evaluation has often been described as wasteful. Administrators have complained that evaluations are not completed in time for the results to be useful, that the results are often negative, that they do not answer relevant questions, and that they do not suggest ways to improve programs. Evaluators have replied that agency staff members do not know what questions they want answered, keep changing the question, do not understand the difficulties involved in doing research, and do not pay attention to the results.

The history of the utilization of evaluation data is somewhat akin to that of the efficacy of psychotherapy: early uncritical acceptance, followed by a period of vigorous criticism, and then a gradual emergence of supportive data. Recent experience indicates that evaluation data are being used, and we are beginning to understand some of the conditions that facilitate such use. For example, a considerable portion of the utilization problem has been attributed to differences between the perspectives of administrators and researchers. Differences in values, language, and rewards are so extensive, it has been suggested, that communication and cooperation are often difficult to establish. This two cultures notion, although especially relevant where large scale evaluation research projects are involved, may still be applicable to local agency situations, particularly where the evaluator lacks administrative experience or the administrator is untrained in research techniques. A major effort may be required to bridge this communication gap.

Another factor related to the utilization problem is that evaluation data are used by individuals to the extent that the data are important to them. Therefore, if the evaluation data are to be used internally, the users should define the important questions to be studied. Table 1 presents an outline of one evaluator's approach to conducting useful program evaluations (Patton, 1978).

Most of the other factors that influence utilization are more likely to be understood by administrators than by evaluators. Administrators know, for example, that utilization is often heavily political, that timely data are better than even the best data delivered too late, that evaluation is only one among many sources of information, and that programs cannot be frozen for the convenience of evaluators. A number of steps that can be taken to increase the use of evaluation data for internal purposes are presented in Table 2 (Rothman, 1980).

A useful program evaluation within an agency is a product of efforts by both the agency director and the evaluator. The initial question that any administrator must ask is whether he or she wants to commit the personnel and agency resources necessary for the project to be successful. If the evaluation is to flourish, the director must actively support it with an environment that makes use of evaluation data, provides the necessary resources, and involves the evaluator. For his or her part, the evaluator must view evaluation as a function useful to service planning, not as a weak form of social science research. At the local agency level, evaluation does not require a high level of technical research skill, although clinical or administrative experience is beneficial and prior successful evaluation experience is ideal. Above all, the evaluator should have a desire to involve administrators and staff in research processes and in the definition of issues.

In order for the evaluation results to be usable, a part-time or full-time evaluator must be thoroughly integrated into the administrative mainstream of the agency. For example, the evaluator should report directly to the agency director and should be thoroughly familiar with the agency's programs, policies, and problems. Two of the more obvious ways to facilitate this familiarity are to involve the evaluator on significant agency committees, such as the executive committee, the clinical services committee, and the quality assurance committee, and

Table 1. Outline of a Utilization-Focused Approach to Evaluation.

I. *Identification and Organization of Relevant Decision Makers and Information Users*

   A. Criteria for Identification: The Personal Factor
     1. People who can use information.
     2. People to whom information makes a difference.
     3. People who have questions they want to have answered.
     4. People who care about and are willing to share responsibility for the evaluation and its utilization.
   B. Criteria for Organization
     1. Provision can be made for continuous direct contact between evaluators and decision makers or information users.
     2. The organized group is small enough to be active, hardworking, and decision-oriented (my own preference is for a task force of fewer than five, and certainly fewer than ten, people).
     3. The members of the group are willing to make a heavy time commitment to the evaluation (the actual amount of time depends on the size of the group, the size and scope of the evaluation, and the members' ability to work together).

II. *The Relevant Evaluation Questions Are Identified and Focused*

   A. Criteria for Identification of Questions
     1. The members of the evaluation task force (that is, identified and organized decision makers, information users, and evaluators) agree on the purpose and emphasis of the evaluation.
       a. Information for program improvement (formative evaluation).
       b. Information about continuation of the program (summative evaluation).
       c. Both formative and summative evaluation, but with emphasis on one or the other (equality of emphasis is not likely in practice when a single evaluation is involved).
     2. The members of the task force agree on which components and basic activities of the program will be the subject of the evaluation (the point here is simply to delineate what aspects of the program are to be discussed in detail as specific evaluation questions are focused).
   B. Alternative Approaches for Focusing Evaluation Questions
     1. The evaluation question can be formed in terms of the program's mission statement, goals, and objectives.
       a. Evaluators must be active-reactive-adaptive in goals clarification exercises, realizing that the appropriateness of generating clear, specific, measurable goals varies depending on the nature of the organization and the purpose of the evaluation.
       b. Goals clarification provides direction in determining what information is needed and wanted, but goals do not automatically determine the content and focus of the evaluation, which depend on what task force members want to know.
       c. Goals are prioritized using the criterion of information needed, not just that of relative importance to the program.
     2. The evaluation question can be formed in terms of program implementation. Options here include:
       a. Effort evaluation.
       b. Process evaluation.
       c. Treatment identification approach.
     3. The evaluation question can be framed in terms of the program's theory of action.
       a. A hierarchy of objectives can be constructed to delineate the program's theory of action, wherein attainment of each lower-level objective is assumed necessary for attainment of each higher-level objective.
       b. The evaluation might focus on any two or more causal connections in a theory of action.

Table 1, cont'd.

---

    c. The theories or causal linkages tested in the evaluation are those believed relevant by evaluation task force members.

    d. The extent to which observed outcomes can be attributable to program activities.

  4. The evaluation question can be formed in terms of the point in the life of the program when the evaluation takes place. Different questions are relevant at different stages of program development.

  5. The evaluation question is formed in the context of the organizational dynamics of a program. Different types of organizations use different types of information and need different types of evaluation. Programs vary in organizational terms along the following dimensions:

    a. The degree to which the environment is certain and stable versus uncertain and dynamic.

    b. The degree to which the program can be characterized as an open or closed system.

    c. The degree to which a rational goal maximization model, an optimizing systems model, or an incremental, satisficing model best describes decision-making processes.

  6. The active-reactive-adaptive evaluator works with decision makers and information users to find the right evaluation question or questions. The right question from a utilization point of view has several characteristics.

    a. It can bring data to bear on the question.

    b. There is more than one possible answer to the question, that is, the answer is not predetermined or loaded by its phrasing.

    c. The identified decision makers want information to help answer the question.

    d. The identified decision makers feel they need information to help answer the question.

    e. The identified and organized decision makers and information users want to answer the question for themselves, not just for someone else.

    f. The decision makers can indicate how they would use the answer to the question, and they can specify the relevance of an answer for their program.

  7. As the evaluation question is focused, the fundamental question that underlies all the issues is: What difference would it make to have this information? How would the information be useful?

III. *Evaluation Methods Are Selected that Generate Useful Information for Identified and Organized Decision Makers and Information Users*

  A. Strengths and weaknesses of alternative paradigms are considered in the search for methods that are appropriate to the nature of the evaluation question. Options include quantitative and qualitative methods.

  B Design and measurement decisions are shared by evaluators and decision makers to increase information users' understanding of, belief in, and commitment to evaluation data.

    1. Variables are operationalized in ways that make sense to those who will use the data; face validity, as judged by decision makers and information users, is an important instrumentation criterion in evaluation measurement.

    2. Evaluation designs are selected that are credible to decision makers, information users, and evaluators.

    3. Major concepts and units of analysis are defined so as to be relevant to decision makers and information users.

    4. Multiple methods and measures are employed as much as possible to increase the credibility of findings.

    5. Decision makers and information users are involved in recurring decisions regarding methods, design, measurement, and basic data gathering, as changed circumstances, resources, and time constraints force changes in methods.

    6. Decision makers and evaluators weigh the methodological constraints intro-

Table 1, cont'd.

---

duced by limited resources, time deadlines, and data accessibility problems. All
task force members must be highly knowledgeable about the strengths and weaknesses of data collection procedures.
  7. It is better to have an approximate and highly probabilistic answer to the right
     question than a solid and relatively certain answer to the wrong question.

IV. *Decision Makers and Information Users Participate with Evaluators in Data Analysis
    and Data Interpretation*

  A. Data analysis is separated from data interpretation so that decision makers can
     work with the data without biases introduced by the evaluator's conclusions.
  B. Standards of desirability are established before data analysis to guide data interpre-
     tation; the nature of the standards of desirability will vary along a continuum from
     highly crystallized to highly ambiguous.
  C. Data analysis is presented in a form that makes sense to decision makers and infor-
     mation users. Decision makers are given an opportunity to struggle with the data
     as they become available so that surprises are avoided.
  D. Evaluators work with decision makers and information users to make full use of
     the data.
     1. Realizing that *positive* and *negative* are perceptual labels, the responsive evalu-
        ator avoids characterizing results in such monolithic terms. Most studies include
        both somewhat positive and somewhat negative findings, depending on one's
        point of view.
     2. Strengths and weaknesses of the data are made clear and explicit.
  E. Evaluation ultimately necessitates making leaps from data to judgment, from
     analysis to action. Utilization-focused data analysis and interpretation includes
     the judgments, conclusions, and recommendations of both evaluators and decision
     makers.

V. *Evaluators and Decision Makers Negotiate and Cooperate in Dissemination Efforts*

  A. Dissemination of findings is only one aspect of evaluation utilization, a minor
     aspect, in many cases. The primary utilization target consists of relevant decision
     makers and information users identified and organized during the first step in the
     evaluation process.
  B. Dissemination takes a variety of forms for different audiences and purposes.
  C. Throughout dissemination, both evaluators and decision makers take responsibility
     for the evaluation from initial conceptualization to final data analysis and inter-
     pretation. Options include:
     1. Both evaluators and decision makers are present at dissemination presentations.
     2. Both evaluators and those for whom the evaluation was conducted are identified
        in all reports and presentations.

  Source: Patton, 1978. Reprinted with permission of the publisher, Sage Publications, Beverly
Hills, California.

Table 2. Principles for Using Evaluation Research in Organizations.

Actions by Administrators

1. Demonstrate and communicate strong support for research within the organization.
2. Define research as clearly serving the planning and service functions of the organization
   [by the use of extensive] dialogue with researchers.
3. Establish structural linkage between researchers and planning and operational people.
   Locate the top research position at a high administrative level. If feasible, establish a
   high-level, specialized unit having joint research and planning functions.

Table 2, cont'd.

---

4. Establish special linking mechanisms such as development agents or development work groups.
5. Round out the competencies in the research staff through inclusion of people who have operational and organizational skills in addition to research capabilities.
6. Allow a sufficient allocation of time and people to carry out specific research utilization activities.
7. Be aware of and seek to improve the level of political and economic support in the external environment [for evaluative research].
8. Arrange for active participation of operational people with research staff in diverse aspects of the research process.
9. Define problems and identify research needs.
10. Carry out appropriate research tasks.
11. Develop conclusions, recommendations, and action plans.
12. Disseminate and interpret information.
13. Engage in developmental activities that concretize and operationalize action implications.
14. Establish appropriate mixed researcher-user task groups to carry out these functions.
15. Structure the use of time strategically and with parsimony for carrying out research process activities.
16. Arrange for a suitable mix of short-term and middle-range projects in order for the organization to be able to respond to different needs and pressures.
17. Create a climate of opinion that is supportive of research and its utilization; be an advocate for research in the organization.
18. Give moral and substantive support to researchers, recognizing that they are in an isolated position in most organizations.
19. Pave the way for participation of researchers in agency meetings and events. This entails encouraging researchers to take part and stimulating operational people to make them welcome.
20. Help researchers to understand key organizational problems and to focus their efforts on them.
21. Make friends for researchers within the organization.
22. Keep researcher-user relationships stable by providing for continuity of staff.
23. Take ample time to clarify with researchers the specific agency problems and concerns that particular reports should address.
24. Assist researchers in deriving appropriate action steps from the findings.
25. Review with researchers the resource situation of the agency and the resource implications of recommended actions. Look for positive resource implications in terms of conserving or expanding resources.
26. Help researchers to make their reports comprehensible and responsive to users in the agency. Review drafts with researchers in terms of brevity, attractiveness, simplicity of language, and self-contained coverage of the subject matter.
27. Assist researchers in analyzing psychological and organizational dynamics involved in a given report. Suggest ways of avoiding offending or threatening potential users.
28. Suggest different audiences that might be appropriately singled out to receive different forms of the report and how these different audiences might be addressed and reached.

Source: Rothman, 1980. Reprinted with permission of the publisher, Sage Publications, Beverly Hills, California.

---

to make him or her responsible for some other clinical or administrative role. If evaluation efforts are defined in collaboration with staff, results are more likely to be relevant, internally supported by agency personnel, and used when they become available.

Finally, the way in which the evaluator analyzes, interprets, and communicates data is important. Evaluation projects are not like academic research, where the investigator works primarily in seclusion and makes a public report as the final step. Evaluation data should be shared and interpreted as they are collected and analyzed. Further, evaluators should never let the results speak for themselves—every evaluation project should include recommendations that are developed in collaboration with the users.

Types of Evaluation Questions

In the mental health field, many questions can be raised about the types of clients being served and about the volume and effectiveness of services. Although manual systems can be devised to collect rudimentary data of this type, computer information systems provide greater flexibility and capacity.

How satisfied are clients with the services they receive? Client satisfaction data are easily collected and almost always gratifying to review. If little effort is made to get feedback, the proportion of clients responding may be unacceptably low, but questionnaire response rates above 60 percent are possible. Since they are usually positive, such responses are useful for external reporting purposes and may help uncover unanticipated internal problems experienced by clients in gaining adequate services.

How effective are the services being provided? For two major reasons, this type of question is the most difficult to answer. First, little consensus exists regarding the worth and utility of available outcome measures (see Chun, Cobb, and French, 1975; Comrey, Backer, and Glaser, 1973; Hargreaves, Attkisson, and Sorensen, 1976; Kiresuk and Sherman, 1968; Schainblatt, 1977; Waskow and Parloff, 1975 for outcome measures in current use). Second, the common use of pre-test/post-test designs often fails to provide needed information. For example, clients might be tested as they enter a program and again as, or at a fixed time after, they leave. Changes between pretreatment and posttreatment phases are noted. Again, such results are nearly always positive but do not necessarily indicate whether or not improvement was the result of treatment—untreated persons with similar problems may also show improvement—or whether or not a relationship exists between the amount of treatment and the degree of improvement.

Recent research provides fairly convincing, but not overwhelming, evidence that psychotherapy does have positive effects. Differences among therapies are not noted, however, nor are differences among therapists in type of professional training and amount of clinical experience—these factors remain to be sorted out in future research. In any case, highly reliable outcome data that unequivocally demonstrate treatment effectiveness or compare the treatment effectiveness of two programs are extremely difficult to obtain.

Despite problems, descriptive outcome data using client satisfaction questionnaires or pretest and posttest designs can be enormously useful for external and internal purposes. For example, a study of a day treatment program showed an unexpected sexual difference in the outcome of services to clients. Staff members questioned the result, since it violated their assumptions about the non-sexist nature of the program. The evaluator replicated the study, and the same pattern occurred. Further involvement in the analysis helped the staff realize that the content of its program was aimed primarily toward the male skid row inhabitants who made up the major portion of the program, and, consequently, the staff began considering ways to make the program more responsive to the needs of women.

Conducting a Program Evaluation

Starting a program evaluation involves defining the organizational context and planning strategies for initiating a particular project. After an evaluator has been chosen, the role of the evaluator and his or her relationship to the agency staff must be defined. Although staff involvement can be costly, its benefits include higher data quality, increased relevance of the evaluation, and greater potential for data utilization. The staff should also be involved in defining questions to be evaluated; whereas directors often propose projects oriented toward external funding agencies, clinical staff members are more likely to ask questions with implications for internal program management.

Clinical staff members are almost always involved in data collection. However, if this is their only role in the evaluation, they are less likely to be actively cooperative. No one is in a better position to identify certain problems in data collection procedures and program management than the front line staff, but this information is likely to be lost if persons in these positions are apathetic or neutral toward the project. Staff members should also be involved in directing the analysis of certain data—for example, to assist in interpreting results, clarifying the impact of certain client characteristics, and noting specific features of the program in relation to the results.

No evaluation should stop at simply reporting results. To facilitate utilization, the implications of the results should be outlined and recommendations made. Unless the evaluator is unusually well versed in the programs and the administrative, legislative, and political intricacies of the agency, he or she will benefit from staff ideas on the implications of the results and on steps that might be taken to implement any suggested organizational response. Finally, like most research, evaluation is more likely to raise questions than to answer them, and the evaluator will need staff help in prioritizing among the questions raised in order to begin new evaluation projects.

It may take a year or two for an administrator, an evaluator, and an advisory staff group to work smoothly and productively together. By that time, the evaluator would presumably be thoroughly familiar with the agency, several studies would have been completed and the results absorbed, and everyone would have developed reasonable expectations for the process.

Nevertheless, the overall process of defining questions, designing, implementing and monitoring projects, and analyzing and interpreting results is likely to produce friction at times. Such conflict tends to arise from miscommunication between the evaluator and the staff, frequently because of different bases of evaluation knowledge, different uses of terms, and different assumptions and values. Successful evaluations are usually characterized by the working through of conflict; the absence of conflict is more likely to indicate a lack of involvement and a low probability of data utilization.

Monitoring Agency Performance

Among general strategies for evaluation, distinctions must be made between the ongoing, continuous monitoring of some index of agency performance and occasional, possibly ad hoc, studies of currently salient issues. Characteristics that clearly lend themselves to monitoring include those client and service characteristics best handled by a good information system—for example, numbers of admissions, numbers of services provided, and numbers of clients served—and fiscal data returned regularly by an accounting office, such as billable services provided and revenues received.

The appropriateness of monitoring other kinds of data is less apparent. Some experts, for example, advocate the monitoring of outcome data, arguing that outcome is, after all, the single most important index of agency success. Inasmuch as agencies consume public resources for the purpose of providing for the public welfare, both ethics and reasonable accountability make ongoing, continuous monitoring necessary. The methods suggested for monitoring outcome data range from simple Global Assessment Scale ratings to mailed follow-up questionnaires or follow-up interviews.

The counter argument is that outcome data, although exceedingly valuable, are too expensive to collect continuously, especially since the validity of the collection procedure may be questionable. Adherents to this position are likely to suggest that outcome studies, perhaps of particular treatment components of larger programs, be performed periodically as needed and designed in collaboration with information consumers who participate in prioritizing the agency's informational needs. Studies are initiated and completed, and attention moves to new items. Priorities can change, and old results may lead to new studies, if consensus dictates.

Program evaluations are most successful when agencies are committed to continuous monitoring of service output. In general, monitoring works best if it is applied to indices identified as important. For example, there is no need to look at the volume of services unless it starts to drop or the no-show rate unless it gets too high. Key factors can be monitored over time using graphs and need only be noted in the event of significant change. Staff members will want to monitor the factors relevant to their needs.

Special Evaluation Studies

Beyond the regular monitoring of outputs, the value of the data system is its capacity to help improve the quality of special studies. The information system can help identify appropriate study populations and provide accurate demographic and service data on study subjects. In special studies involving clients, a reliable information system allows the casting of a much broader informational net and, because more data elements can be identified and collected, engenders results with broader meaning.

Many special studies can be treated either as retrospective or prospective projects. Retrospective studies rely on existing, generally archival data sources. Data may be extracted from old clinical records, existing data system files, or the memories of staff members. The advantages of this method are that studies can generally be done quickly and cheaply, with a minimum of intrusiveness. The disadvantage is that data quality is often not high. Existing data often do not precisely meet the study's requirements, and definitions of variables may vary, so that information collected by different investigators on the same variable may not mean the same thing.

Retrospective studies are a perfectly reasonable and acceptable strategy, provided the limitations are recognized, and are particularly useful for quick, preliminary, exploratory, or pilot work, where the results can help clarify unknown issues. More tightly controlled prospective studies, allowing for the collection of more reliable, complete, and meaningful information, frequently follow; however, they are usually more expensive and time-consuming to conduct.

Resource Needs

Ideally, an evaluator is familiar with computers and knows not only experimental design and statistics but also qualitative research techniques—technical training most commonly found in persons with doctoral degrees. He or she would also benefit from a range of administrative skills and a thorough knowledge of clinical programs. Even if additional resources and a specially trained person are not available, however, an agency can select a staff member who is interested in doing program evaluation, secure outside consultation, and then simply proceed. In any case, whoever is selected will need the strong support of the agency director, including additional staff and consultation support.

The potential resource needs of the evaluator fall into four categories that parallel the developmental stages of projects. The first type of resource need is assistance with defining projects, including eliciting questions suitable for study from the director or staff and gaining familiarity with techniques and studies conducted by other agencies. The most obvious sources for this assistance can be found at regional evaluation conferences and in direct contact with other evaluators, written evaluation materials, and newsletters or journals. The second resource need is consultation on research design. Ideally, evaluators will already have a good sense for research design, as well as an understanding of the implications of violating design principles. However, outside consultation can help to improve the evaluation design and thereby influence the way in which the data are analyzed and the results interpreted. The third type of resource need is assistance in implementing the study—a need usually filled by other staff members. Here again, knowledge of design principles will help an evaluator recognize and solve problems. Data analysis, the fourth resource need, would seem to be a prime candidate for the use of consultation resources, but, in fact, the level of sophistication required for most evaluations is low enough that help is often not needed. Most data analyses consist of extensive graphical presentations, such as histograms, frequency distributions, plots of variables over time, and scattergrams, along with a few descriptive statistics—for example, means, medians, standard deviations, and such basic inferential statistics as cross-tabulations, correlations, and T-tests. Projects requiring complex statistics like multiple regressions or analyses of variance or covariance may require further consultation. For interested administrators, several data analysis resource manuals are noted in the reference section (Bentler, Lettieri, and Austin, 1976; Bruning and Kintz, 1968; Campbell and Stanley, 1963; Linton and Gallo, 1975; Siegal, 1956).

A further question may arise as to whether the analysis should be done by computer or by hand. With increasingly inexpensive computers and the wider availability of packaged statistical programs, computer analysis is becoming more common. Manual analysis leaves all steps under staff control, but is usually restricted in the numbers of subjects and variables that can be managed and analyzed. Computers, on the other hand, although often unfamiliar and somewhat intimidating, have much greater flexibility and potential range of analysis than a manual system and can handle medium-sized data sets of up to several hundred subjects and fifty variables with little more difficulty than small sets.

If a computer is to be used, the three types of expense will be keypunching (usually minimal), computer time, and staff time for data entry and analysis. Computer time expense for most agency projects is low, under $100; staff time is usually higher, especially if beginners are used. Often local persons experienced in computer analysis can be hired on an hourly basis (expect to pay $6 to $10 per hour for students), with most straightforward data sets requiring not more than twenty to thirty hours.

Conclusion

Given the resource requirements and the inevitable time and energy commitments necessary, the agency must ask whether an evaluation will produce enough useful information to make it worth the investment of money and staff time. The answer to this question will depend in turn on whether the agency administrator and staff members have learned to value and use evaluation information in their decision making. Clearly, evaluation data need to be used if they are to be valued, and if initial evaluation experiences are positive, the likelihood of further evaluation efforts is increased. The natural strategy for increasing data utilization, then, is to start with a small, inexpensive project addressing a problem in which both the staff and the administrator are interested.

References

Attkisson, C. C., and others (Eds.). *Evaluation of Human Service Programs.* New York: Academic Press, 1978.

Bentler, P. M., Lettieri, D. J., and Austin, G. A. *Data Analysis Strategies and Designs for Substance Abuse.* Washington, D.C.: U.S. Government Printing Office, 1976.

Bruning, J. L., and Kintz, B. L. *Computational Handbook of Statistics.* Glenview, Ill.: Scott, Foresman, 1968.

Campbell, D. T., and Stanley, J. C. *Experimental and Quasi-Experimental Designs for Research.* Chicago: Rand McNally, 1963.

Chun, T., Cobb, S., and French, J.R.P. *Measures for Psychological Assessment: A Guide to 3,000 Original Sources and Their Applications.* Ann Arbor, Mich.: Survey Research Center, 1975.

Comrey, A. L., Backer, T. E., and Glaser, E. M. *A Source Book for Mental Health Measures.* Los Angeles: Human Interaction Research Institute, 1973.

Cook, T. D., and Campbell, D. T. *The Design and Conduct of Quasi-Experiments and True Experiments in Field Settings.* Chicago: Rand McNally, 1976.

Elmore, R. F. "Evaluation, Control and Learning in Organizations." Paper presented at annual meeting of the Western Political Science Association, San Francisco, Mar. 28, 1980.

Fink, A., and Kosecoff, J. *An Evaluation Primer.* Washington, D.C.: Capitol Publications, 1978.

Hagedorn, H. J., and others. *A Working Manual of Simple Program Evaluation Techniques for Community Mental Health Centers.* Washington, D.C.: U.S. Government Printing Office, 1976.

Hargreaves, W. A., Attkisson, C. C., and Sorensen, J. E. (Eds.). *Resource Materials for Community Mental Health Program Evaluation.* Rockville, Md.: National Institute of Mental Health, 1976.

Isaac, S., and Michael, W. B. *Handbook in Research and Evaluation.* San Diego: Knapp, 1972.

Kiresuk, T. O., and Sherman, R. E. "Goal Attainment Scaling: A General Method for Evaluating Community Mental Health Programs." *Community Mental Health Journal,* 1968, *4,* 443–453.

Linton, M., and Gallo, S. P. *The Practical Statistician: Simplified Handbook of Statistics.* Monterey, Calif.: Brooks/Cole, 1975.

Morris, L. L., and Fitz-Gibbon, C. T. *Evaluator's Handbook.* Beverly Hills, Calif.: Sage, 1978.

Patton, M. Q. *Utilization Focused Evaluation.* Beverly Hills, Calif.: Sage, 1978.

Rothman, J. *Using Research in Organizations.* Beverly Hills, Calif.: Sage, 1980.

Rutman, L. (Ed.). *Evaluation Research Methods: A Basic Guide.* Beverly Hills, Calif.: Sage, 1977.

Schainblatt, A. H. *Monitoring the Outcomes of State Mental Health Treatment Programs.* Washington, D.C.: The Urban Institute, 1977.

Siegal, S. *Nonparametric Statistics for the Behavioral Sciences.* New York: McGraw-Hill, 1956.

Struening, E. L., and Guttentag, M. *Handbook of Evaluation Research.* Beverly Hills, Calif.: Sage, 1975.

Waskow, I. E., and Parloff, M. B. *Psychotherapy Change Measures.* Washington, D.C.: U.S. Government Printing Office, 1975.

Weiss, C. H. *Evaluation Research.* Englewood Cliffs, N.J.: Prentice-Hall, 1972.

❧ 19 ❧

Quality
Assurance

Bernadette I. D. Lalonde

Mental health program managers are under increasing pressure to provide quality assurance to consumers, third-party insurance carriers, professional organizations, and the federal government. They must therefore be familiar with the various explicit quality assurance criteria. This chapter presents the context in which quality assurance developed, the means for distinguishing between program evaluation and quality assurance, and several model quality assurance programs. In addition, important conceptual issues in the definition of quality are discussed, including whether to select an input, process, or outcome approach; minimum or maximum levels of standards; a cost-containment or quality-of-care focus; implicit or explicit criteria; internal or external review; and peer or nonclinical reviewers.

The community mental health care system entered a new period of accountability with the passage of the Community Mental Health Act Amendments of 1975, known as Public Law 94-63. Federally funded community mental health centers (CMHCs) are now required by federal law to establish ongoing quality assurance programs employing utilization and peer review systems.

Quality assurance is important to clinical and administrative functioning because it is now mandated by federal laws, required by two important professional bodies—the Joint Commission on Accreditation of Hospitals and the Accreditation Council for Psychiatric Facilities—and expected by third-party insurance carriers. In the past ten years, quality assurance has evolved from being a worthwhile but little-talked-about voluntary self-assessment activity, entirely the domain of local service providers, to an important policy issue (Egdahl and Gertman, 1976), from being a vague, implicit, future-oriented concept (Riedel, Tischler, and Myers, 1974) to a structured explicit practice mandated by external agencies.

By definition, quality assurance is the promise or guarantee made by mental health care providers to funding sources, including third-party insurance carriers and consumers, that certain standards of excellence in mental health care are being met. It usually involves measuring the quality of care given to individual clients in order to improve the appropriateness, adequacy, and effectiveness of care (Brook, Williams, and Davies-Avery, 1976; Tischler and Riedel, 1973; Woy, Lund, and Attkisson, 1978). In addition, a quality assurance program is designed to detect deficiencies and errors in service and to control the costs of care by preventing overutilization of services (Woy, Lund, and Attkisson, 1978).

These objectives are met by conducting utilization and peer reviews. Utilization review is a case record review procedure evaluating the appropriateness and necessity of admissions, length of stay in treatment, services provided, and discharge practices. The purpose is to promote the most efficient use of mental health facilities and services. Peer review is a case review performed by clinical peers using predetermined sets of criteria outlining the norms of appropriate, adequate, and necessary care.

Evolution of Quality Assurance

With the growth of the health insurance industry and current professional and federal emphasis on accountability (the demand to justify health service practice and cost) has come a host of explicit quality assurance requirements from outside agencies. Of particular import to CMHCs are the requirements of the Professional Standards Review Organizations (PSROs), the Community Mental Health Act Amendments of 1975, the Joint Commission on Accreditation of Hospitals (JCAH), and the Accreditation Council for Psychiatric Facilities (AC/PF). Mental health agencies, depending on the services offered, may be subject to the quality assurance requirements of all these agencies.

Professional Standards Review Organizations. When the federal government took responsibility for providing financial coverage for the medical expenses of the poor and the elderly (Social Security Amendments of 1965, Public Law 89-97, Title XVIII), they initiated the national quality assessment trend that continues today. With Medicare and Medicaid came the federal government's insistence that each hospital and extended care facility institute a utilization review. Narrowly defined, utilization review is the study of the allocation of institutional resources to ensure their most efficient and economical use (Riedel and others, 1971). This review was and is intended to ensure that the medical services covered by Medicare, Medicaid, and Maternal and Child Health programs are necessary and that services are provided in the appropriate facility (Public Law 89-97, Section 1861k). Provision was made for a retrospective review of a sample of Medicare patients after hospital discharge to study the necessity for admission, length of stay, and services provided. A concurrent review, completed while a patient is receiving treatment, was also requested in order to study the necessity of long or extended hospital confinements. Participating hospitals were left with the responsibility for enacting and monitoring the utilization review.

In 1968, however, a Social Security survey found that almost half the hospitals were not reviewing admissions as required by statute (Stevens, 1971). With serious increases in federal health expenditures and the recognition that a significant proportion of the health services provided under Medicare and Medicaid were not medically necessary, Congress realized the need for a more effective cost-containment procedure and passed the Social Security Amendments of 1972 (Public Law 92-603, Title XI), which authorized the creation of PSROs. This law is an important milestone in the history of quality assurance for several reasons: it removed the primary responsibility for review of inpatient and extended care facilities from the hospitals and assigned it to local organizations of health care providers (Taft and Levine, 1976); it established the importance of concurrent review of admissions and length of stay to assure the prevention of unnecessary admissions and the necessity of all hospital days in both long- and short-term stays; it required the implementation of retrospective medical care evaluation studies; it marked the shift from implicit to explicit review criteria; and it introduced profile monitoring as a form of retrospective review.

Focusing attention on inpatient services, PSROs are involved in developing admission standards and length of treatment norms for the particular diagnoses or presenting problems handled by an institution. Patient records are systematically screened by trained medical records specialists or other reviewers to ensure that these standards are being met in practice. Records that do not conform to the criteria are assigned to practitioners for peer review. In the review, a clinician presents a case with his or her justification for admission, particular treatment, and length of stay. Peers assess the justification and suggest appropriate action—for example, the termination of the client from treatment, the removal of the client to another hospital, or an alternative, less-expensive treatment—when the clinician's justifications cannot be supported.

Both retrospective and concurrent review are mandated by PSRO law. In order to prevent unnecessary admissions and hospital days, concurrent review is required of all admissions and continued stays. Patient care evaluation studies and profile monitoring are aspects of retrospective review. Patient care evaluation studies are in-depth reviews of care and medical management practices intended to identify actual or potential service problems. Corrective action is then taken, and a reassessment is conducted to monitor the effects of the corrective action. Profile analysis is a technique for analyzing patterns of care.

PSROs, then, are responsible for ensuring that health care is medically necessary, consistent with professionally recognized standards of care, and provided in the least-costly setting possible. Whereas mental health services were not specifically mentioned in PSRO legislation, the law categorically states that reimbursement for services under Medicare, Medicaid, and Maternal and Child Health programs must have PSRO review. To the extent that inpatient mental health services are provided to such clients, they are subject to PSRO review. For a number of reasons, PSROs continue to focus their attention on inpatient services but will probably begin, in the near future, to focus attention on all services within mental health facilities. Facilities may therefore want to establish quality assurance programs that are compatible with PSRO requirements (see Office of

Professional Standards Review, 1974; Decker and Bonner, 1973; and National Institute of Mental Health, 1976).

Community Mental Health Centers Amendments. The national quality assurance trend continued in 1975 with the passage of the Community Mental Health Centers Amendments, which mandated that federally funded mental health centers establish, independent of PSRO activity, ongoing quality assurance programs that include utilization and peer review systems (Public Law 94-63, Title III, Section 201d). A quality assurance program is defined in the current guidelines as an approach for assessing and, when necessary, improving the quality of care. Peer review of clinical records and the development of written policies and procedures are not sufficient, according to these amendments; quality assurance requirements are fulfilled only when these activities contain effective mechanisms for implementing changes in substandard care and poorly utilized services.

CMHCs are required to establish a quality assurance committee composed of representatives from all the major relevant disciplines directly involved in the delivery of mental health services. Clinical staff may be joined by representatives from the program evaluation committee, medical records department, and agency administration. Such a committee might also include a PSRO liaison person to ensure that review procedures are consistent with PSRO requirements.

The guidelines indicate that the quality assurance committee should meet at least once per month and keep accurate records of all its activities, including times and dates of meetings, staff members present, number of cases reviewed by the committee, findings of the review, care evaluation studies performed, results of these studies, reports of all educational activities, and reports of all actions taken by the committee. A major responsibility of the committee is to develop a written policies and procedures statement (Joint Commission on Accreditation of Hospitals, 1979) that includes the objectives of the quality assurance program; the organization and composition of the committee; the functions, authority, and responsibilities of the committee; the relationship of the committee with other governance bodies; procedures for the development, adoption, adaptation, and continued refinement of criteria and standards; criteria for acceptance into treatment, length of treatment, validation of diagnosis, appropriate treatment modalities, discharge, and evaluation of treatment outcomes; procedures for screening and peer review; procedures for disseminating the results of the reviews; guidelines specific to the issues of confidentiality and disclosure; and procedures for implementing changes in patient care, should substandard practices or misuse of services be revealed.

The guidelines note that either concurrent or retrospective review of the care and services provided to clients may be conducted. The review must, however, be conducted using the written criteria, standards, and norms developed by the committee and peer reviewers. Concurrent review may be performed on all client records when the client enters treatment in order to assess the need for treatment and at periodic times during treatment to assess the quality of care provided and the necessity for continued therapy. Case records that do not conform to the committee's standards would then be selected for more intensive peer review.

A primary review function of the quality assurance committee is to conduct two retrospective clinical care evaluations per year. The topics of the studies are determined by the quality assurance committees, usually based on indications of possibly substandard patient care or on the potential for improving the general quality of care. Examples of clinical care evaluation studies might be a study of dropouts after first emergency contact or an investigation of consistently poor client outcomes for a specific treatment program. Criteria and standards are developed for study topics, information on the care given to a number of clients is gathered from case records, and the data are analyzed to identify deficiencies. An educational or administrative intervention plan is then developed and implemented to correct the deficiencies. A follow-up study is conducted later to assure that the recommendations have been implemented and the quality of care improved. Interested readers are referred to Goran (1975) for more detailed information on the specific steps involved in setting up clinical care evaluation studies.

The CMHC Amendments differ from the current PSRO requirements in that the amendments apply to all programs within the CMHC, not just inpatient services. The standards for appropriate, necessary care for outpatient and partial care services, however, are not nearly as well developed as those for inpatient services; mental health services have the task of developing those standards.

Joint Commission on Accreditation of Hospitals. To the extent that a mental health center operates an inpatient service in a general hospital, it may be subject to JCAH's quality assurance criteria, which were implemented in 1976 as part of patient care audit procedures. Regardless of the source of reimbursement for services, all programs seeking accreditation must comply with the principles found in JCAH's publication *Principles for Accreditation of Community Mental Health Service Programs* (1979). With respect to quality assurance, JCAH and the Accreditation Council for Psychiatric Facilities (AC/PF) require that the quality of services are evaluated by the staff members responsible for providing the services; the criteria represent the optimal level of service that can be achieved; the criteria are explicit and measurable; service variations from the norm are identified and justified; variations not justified to peer satisfaction are analyzed; corrective action is taken; follow-up studies are conducted to ensure that the corrective action was effective; the entire evaluation is documented and the results reported; provision is made for continuing staff development and training in areas found deficient; and provision is made for the reappointment of staff members, as appropriate (Richman, 1977b).

For example, the following list represents a selection of standards for treatment plans:

15.1 Each patient shall have an individualized, written treatment plan based on the assessments of that patient's fundamental needs.
15.1.1 The treatment plan shall be developed as soon after the patient's admission as possible.

15.1.2 Appropriate therapeutic efforts may begin before finalization of the treatment plan.

15.1.3 The treatment plan shall be a reflection of the program's philosophy of treatment and shall reflect appropriate multidisciplinary input by the staff.

15.1.4 The overall responsibility of the treatment plan shall be assigned to a member of the clinical staff.

15.1.5 The plan shall specify services required for meeting the patient's needs.

15.1.6 The plan shall include referral for needed services not provided directly by the program.

15.1.7 Speech, language, academic, and hearing services shall be available, when appropriate, either within the program or by written arrangement with a qualified clinician or facility, in order to meet the patient's needs.

15.1.8 The treatment plan shall include clinical consideration of the patient's fundamental needs.

15.1.9 Goals necessary for the patient to achieve, maintain, or reestablish emotional and/or physical health and maximum growth and adaptive capabilities shall be included in the treatment plan.

15.1.9.1 These goals shall be determined on the basis of the assessment of the patient and/or the patient's family.

15.1.9.2 Specific goals, with both long-term and short-term objectives, and the anticipated time expected to meet these goals shall be established.

15.1.9.3 Treatment plan goals shall be written in terms of measurable criteria.

15.1.10 The patient shall participate in the development of the treatment plan, and such participation shall be documented.

15.1.11 The treatment plan shall describe services, activities, programs, and anticipated patient actions and responses and shall specify the staff members assigned to work with the patient.

15.1.12 The treatment plan shall delineate the locations and frequency of treatment procedures.

15.1.13 The treatment plan shall designate the means for measuring the progress and/or outcome of treatment efforts.

15.1.14 The treatment plan shall delineate the specific criteria to be met for termination of treatment and aftercare services. Such criteria shall be a part of the initial treatment plan.

15.1.15 A specific plan for the involvement of the family or significant others shall be included in the treatment plan, when indicated [Joint Commission on Accreditation of Hospitals, 1979].

Clearly, the various quality assurance requirements of external agencies will create additional administrative demands on mental health agencies. While the quality assurance demands made by PSRO and the CMHC Amendments are similar in content, mental health agencies must ensure that their quality assurance program meets all applicable requirements.

Conceptual Issues in Defining Quality

The quality of mental health services appears to be a very complex and subjective issue, defying universal definition. The consumer, the clinician, the administrator, and the external funding and accreditation agencies might define and measure the concept in very different ways, depending on their stance on a number of important conceptual issues. At some point in the design and implementation of a quality assurance program, mental health administrators and clinicians will need to address the following definition and measurement issues.

Input, Process, or Outcome Approach. Quality can be defined and assessed from three different perspectives: structure or input, process, and outcome (Donabedian, 1966; De Geyndt, 1970). As the assessment of quality care varies by the method used, mental health administrators and clinicians are advised to select a particular approach or combination of approaches with care. Brook (1973) applied different methods of quality assessment to a group of medical patients and found that results differed by method. Many researchers advise an appropriate combination of all three components, viewing each as a necessary but not sufficient element of service quality (Donabedian, 1966; Thorne, 1977; Woy, Lund, and Attkisson, 1978).

The structural or input approach to defining and measuring quality of care refers to the description of a facility's characteristics. This approach assesses client characteristics, experience and qualifications of staff, condition of the physical plant (for example, safety features, adequacy of storage space for patients' personal effects, general condition of the building), equipment, and staff-patient ratios. A strict input approach to assessing service quality has several drawbacks, one of which is the assumption that high quality can be provided and maintained as long as input requirements are met. Whereas structural/input processes are considered necessary to the definition and measurement of quality care, many would hesitate to say that these processes are in themselves sufficient. For example, Linn, Gurel, and Linn (1977) found that over half of the input variables in their nursing home study were not correlated with outcome. Once minimum input standards are met, other factors influence outcome.

The process approach measures the quality of the interaction between client and provider, addressing the question, Did the client receive appropriate and effective service? This approach focuses on the overall service and assumes the existence of generally accepted methods of treatment for specific presenting problems. Individual cases are then compared with these normative standards to determine whether the treatment given was appropriate and adequate (Liptzin, 1974). Process analysis investigates such factors as admission criteria, length of stay in treatment, counseling methods, and management styles.

Although most of the procedures required in quality assurance reviews emphasize process issues, criteria defining appropriate, high-quality care are not always agreed upon by clinicians (Woy, Lund, and Attkisson, 1978). In medicine, these criteria are generally formulated on the basis of diagnosis; in community mental health services, however, the reliability of clinical diagnosis is open to question (Babigian and others, 1965), and the relationship between diagnosis and prescribed treatment is far from absolute (Tischler and Riedel, 1973). Over one hundred types of psychotherapy exist today, and, whereas most of them have been found to be more effective than no treatment at all (Parloff, 1980), the particular brand of psychotherapy that works best with different clients and problems has yet to be determined.

Outcome indicators of quality care reflect what happens to the client as a result of the services rendered. This approach refers to treatment outcome studies in which the effectiveness and quality of services are measured by the degree to which the client has improved as a function of therapeutic intervention. At first glance, outcome might seem to be the most scientific and objective indicator of quality care, but it too has its limitations. It is often difficult to set up highly controlled outcome evaluations that include comparable treatment groups and suitable control groups (Liptzin, 1974) and even more difficult to state with certainty that the treatment outcomes resulted only from the treatment interventions (Brook, 1977). Many factors beyond the evaluator's control, such as a sudden death in the client's family or a much-wanted job advancement, might have played a significant part in the treatment outcome.

In addition, the effects of treatment may vary at different points in time (Krubie, 1973; Donabedian, 1978). With those patients suffering from chronic mental illness, the time of discharge may not be useful in determining the effects of therapy, especially if quality is defined as the reduction or elimination of mental illness (Moorehead, 1976). Sometimes it takes years before the effects of therapy are seen. Assessment conducted months or years following termination of therapy is difficult, however, because clients are often impossible to track down.

The input, process, and outcome approaches to assessment have their respective strengths and limitations. Although some agencies may focus on the process approach, input and outcome dimensions are equally important. The 1975 CMHC Amendments acknowledge the value of outcome dimensions by stipulating two clinical care evaluation studies per year that address either process or outcome concerns. Beyond meeting the explicit demands made by these external sources, mental health agencies are free to decide how their quality assurance program will address input, process, and outcome concerns.

Minimum or Maximum Level Standards. How good is good enough? Quality is a relative concept that may be viewed, on the one hand, as the attainment of minimum acceptable standards or, on the other, as the attainment of optimally desired levels of care. Accreditation standards usually represent optimum levels of performance, whereas quality assurance standards appear to be more concerned with maintaining the minimum care acceptable. Agencies can choose to which level they will adhere, a choice determined in part by the views of clinicians and administrators. Standards that are too low may jeopardize the well-being of clients; standards that are too high may lower the staff's morale and contribute to unrealistic expectations on the part of consumers and funding sources.

Cost Containment or Quality of Care. The question of whether the cost of service figures in the definition and measurement of quality care is no longer open to debate. With the passage of the CMHC Amendments came the recognition that cost of service is a legitimate quality dimension and that utilization review can be a cost containment device. Agencies must, however, decide whether to focus their attention on cost containment or quality of care, since these two goals do not necessarily work in harmony (Luft, 1977). When the fiscal squeeze is not excessive and permits the preferred treatment to proceed, the two goals may harmoniously coexist. If, however, the preferred therapy cannot be supported financially, the two goals may come into conflict, and peer reviewers will need to decide whether to resolve the issue in favor of quality or of cost (Newman, 1974).

Implicit or Explicit Criteria. Another important issue in quality assessment is the decision to use implicit or explicit criteria for review. PSRO and CMHC legislation dictates the use of explicit criteria for selecting cases for peer review but does not favor a particular mode for the review itself. Implicit criteria, with their reliance on individual professional judgment, are subjective and arbitrary but also flexible, taking the client's unique problems and circumstances into account (Luft, 1977). Explicit review criteria, involving the application of sets of agreed-on formal criteria for assessing a client's diagnosis or level of functioning, are thought to be more consistent and objective (Noble, 1974), yet they provide many difficulties to clinicians and administrators. Some people question whether explicit mental health service criteria can ever be devised and whether objective criteria will lead to standardization of practices and the demise of innovation. The question is also raised as to what process should be used in selecting criteria (Luft, 1977). Should statistical norms on existing practices be used, and, if so, do these norms represent the highest quality care? What problems emerge when borrowing existing criteria from other institutions or from the literature? For example, highly developed quality assurance criteria and standards borrowed from inpatient services might be inappropriate for the ambulatory or partial-care services of mental health centers (Cohen and others, 1974; Richman, 1977b; Thorne, 1975).

The literature makes two suggestions regarding implicit and explicit criteria for review. The first is that the question Should implicit criteria be used? be changed to When should implicit criteria be used? The implicit criteria of clinical judgment continue to be important in community mental health decisions. The favored approach appears to be to use explicit criteria when selecting cases for review and implicit or a combination of implicit and explicit criteria for the peer review process itself. The second suggestion is that the professionals involved in the review also be involved in the design of the system and the establishing of criteria to ensure acceptability of the system (Luft, 1977; Luft and Newman, 1977). Any system, no matter how well designed, will fail unless it is accepted by the people who use it (Johnson, Kast, and Rosenzweig, 1973).

Internal or External Review. Review can be conceptualized and implemented as external or internal review. Whereas internal review is done by selected staff members within a particular agency, external review is conducted by a team of clinicians and administrators from other agencies who serve as consultants. Each approach has its advantages and disadvantages. External review may be more objective because external reviewers have less vested interest in the results of agency evaluation than internal reviewers, may carry more clout in suggesting and ensuring change, and may sidestep some of the sticky issues internal reviewers face when confronting coworkers with incidents of overutilization or substandard care. Staff members, however, may tend to consider external review more of an interference and a threat than internal review and may consequently become defensive, rejecting and undermining the review process. Some also argue that external review cannot adequately evaluate the process of care without lengthy and costly on-site visits.

The approach favored by Racusin and Krell (1980) is a combination external-internal review process. They consider external review to be the most effective way of initiating a quality assurance program if the review is restricted to the input dimensions, such as the adequacy of the record system, the quality of the professional staff, the adequacy of governance, and the adequacy of the physical facility. Mental health agencies that have not experienced a review may find an external review emphasizing input less threatening than an internal review that emphasizes process and thereby exposes individual clinical practice to colleagues on the review committee. External review also permits consistent application of the mental health laws and regulations to each agency. Typically, a multidisciplinary team of clinicians, administrators, and consultants would spend two to three days per year comparing an agency's structural dimensions against a set of standards such as those in the JCAH manual. The team might interview the agency director, the board of directors, a sample of the staff, and other agencies in the area for their opinions regarding the availability of the agency's services and might examine a random sample of case records to check the adequacy of record-keeping. A report of the findings and recommendations would follow the review, and subsequent annual reviews would monitor the degree to which the recommendations were addressed.

For evaluating process directly, Racusin and Krell (1980) consider internal review the most useful approach. Typically, the peer review committee, consisting of representatives from each of the major disciplines and programs within the agency, meets once or twice per month to review randomly selected case records. This random, retrospective chart audit does not guarantee that the cases exhibiting serious clinical management deficits will be reviewed, but it is considered the most efficient means available considering limited funds and personnel. In addition, all cases requiring more than six visits are usually brought to utilization review. In both chart audit review and utilization review, a record is kept of the review process, including the data of the review, the review members present and their professional degrees, a brief clinical description of the case, important points of discussion, a review of the treatment plan (including goals and modalities of treatment), and the length of treatment.

Educational or Punitive Approaches to Change. What should the review committee do when it is confronted with substandard practice? If the quality assurance program is viewed as a control mechanism, it may tend to be more punitive and focus on the competence of clinicians, rather than on the presentation of specific cases (Luft, 1977). If the program is viewed as an opportunity for self-improvement, the committee would tend to emphasize the presentation of specific cases for educational purposes. From the earliest days of utilization review, educational intervention was the preferred extension of review decisions, and this continues to be the intention of PSRO review and the CMHC Amendments. Good quality assurance systems should have timely feedback mechanisms to alert staff to gaps in knowledge and should provide for continuing education.

What should be done, however, when substandard practice continues and staff members refuse to seek continuing education? This issue is a difficult one because the review committee is dealing not with students but with professional peers. The danger, of course, is that a punitive atmosphere may lead to defensive behavior on the part of the clinicians and the ultimate destruction of the review process (Newman and Luft, 1974). Therefore, the quality assurance committee must first develop guidelines that clearly define job performance standards and staff development policies (Newman and Luft, 1974).

Quality of Care and Quality of Documentation. In the quality assessment process, data on client care must be compared to implicit or explicit criteria. Since such data are usually found within the original record or an abstract of the record prepared by record specialists or by the clinician, high-quality documentation is imperative. Some observers fear, however, that this emphasis on precise documentation lulls staff into defining and assessing quality in terms of high-quality documentation (Richman, 1977a). High-quality documentation does not guarantee high-quality treatment (Luft, 1977), nor does the review of documents without a mechanism for assuring high-quality care constitute a quality assurance program. A quality assurance program must have mechanisms for instituting changes to improve the quality of care when substandard practices or poor utilization of services is found.

Confidentiality. Confidentiality of records, always a sensitive issue in the mental health field, is also a major issue in quality assurance since the opening of a client's record for screening and peer review could violate the federal privacy act of 1974. Therefore, staff members must ensure that the documents used for quality assurance do not contain client identification.

And what of the confidentiality of staff? How much protection should the system afford professionals and staff members? The acceptability of a quality assurance program could be seriously undermined if individual clinical practices became common knowledge to other staff members (Luft, 1977). If a review system is established that emphasizes education rather than control, serious attention needs to be given to this issue.

Selection and Training of Peer Reviewers. In general, professionals resent review from nonprofessionals or professionals outside their realm of services, as they believe that quality service in a particular field demands an intimate knowledge of that field (Benveniste, 1977). The question of who is a peer becomes a major issue in a multidisciplinary mental health setting; many professionals, for example, argue that peers are only those persons who possess the same professional training. Each agency needs to work out its own answers to this sensitive question, recognizing that the assessment of quality care is affected by who is on the peer review committee—the review can only be as good as its reviewers (Luft and Newman, 1977). To promote an educational approach, peer reviewers should be good teachers, diagnosticians, therapists, and listeners, able to communicate suggestions for change in a tactful, nonthreatening manner (Luft and Newman, 1977). Special training sessions designed to enhance these reviewer skills might need to be developed in a way that does not antagonize clinicians who take pride in their communication skills.

In addition, if peer reviewers are not carefully selected, personality clashes may lead to one-upmanship, which can make a travesty of the peer review process. And means should be provided for identifying and dealing with reviewers who, once they have been chosen for a review committee, are found to lack the necessary skills. Luft and Newman (1977) suggest that, in order to avoid the delicate problem of incompetent reviewers, agencies move away from the notion that each professional must serve a term as a reviewer.

Use of Nonclinical Personnel. Another assessment issue relates to the use of nonclinical personnel in the review system. Clinicians may question the ability of persons without clinical training to interpret client records or understand the intricacies of a particular case in making a decision on quality care. Nevertheless, as a cost-saving device, records specialists, psychiatric technicians, and clerks are being trained for and included in the initial screening process of many review systems. The favored compromise between high cost and professional acceptance seems to be the utilization of specially trained staff for screening cases using clearly defined criteria and for preparing abstracts of the records for peer review.

In summary, a number of issues related to the definition and assessment of quality must be confronted before a quality assurance system can be planned and implemented. Although the literature presents helpful suggestions based on the experiences of existing mental health quality assurance programs, no hard-and-fast rules apply. Within the boundaries of the explicit criteria imposed by external agencies, mental health agencies must identify their own conceptions of quality and devise appropriate assessment procedures.

Quality Assurance and Program Evaluation

Quality assurance and program evaluation are the two primary mechanisms currently mandated by federal legislation for evaluating mental health services and used to meet the accountability demands of various external agencies. Woy, Lund, and Attkisson (1978) distinguish several dimensions of quality assurance and program evaluation: history and goals, degree of reliance on peer review, level of analysis, uses in decision making, technological requirements, and staffing requirements.

Major Differences. Quality assurance and program evaluation have developed independently of one another and stem from very different concerns. Since their inception in the 1960s, federally funded CMHCs were given the option of using some portion of their funds for research and evaluation. Numerous studies (Attkisson and others, 1974; McCullough, 1975) reveal, however, that many CMHCs chose not to take advantage of the offer—in 1974, program evaluation was still considered to be minimal or nonexistent among CMHCs (Comptroller General of the United States, 1974). To remedy this situation and to force CMHCs to face the concerns of program effectiveness and efficiency, the CMHC Amendments of 1975 required all federally funded CMHCs to continuously evaluate their programs and services. The impetus was not so much concern for quality of care or costs of services as it was the desire to improve the management and administration of CMHC programs by basing decisions on systematic and reliable information (Windle and Ochberg, 1975) and to assess the actual effects of services with outcome evaluation measures and client satisfaction surveys. Fiscal issues and quality of clinical care may have a place in program evaluation studies, but usually only to the extent that they relate to the program as a whole, to the particular service being provided, or to the treatment modalities being used.

Quality assurance programs are very much oriented toward the individual client, whereas program evaluation emphasizes data aggregation and statistical reduction to draw conclusions and make judgments about broad issues that affect the program as a whole or elements within it. Such issues as the effectiveness, acceptability, availability, and accessibility of the program, the level of staff effort, and the cost effectiveness of service modalities are central to program evaluation studies.

Quality assurance programs are intended to monitor and influence the process of service rendered to individual clients. Whereas outcome evaluation is always an important issue in clinical studies, quality assurance programs are mainly concerned with the process of care. In contrast, program evaluation studies are heavily outcome-oriented and are intended to provide information leading to program change as dictated through administrative action or policy change. Program evaluation relies more extensively on administrative review than on peer review. Program evaluation staff members tend to be managers, rather than clinicians, and to possess computer applications, accounting, and research design skills, rather than the clinical skills expected of the quality assurance staff.

Data from quality assurance review are used primarily by clinical staff in deciding issues related to the clinical care of the individual patient. Program evaluation data are intended for use in program operation, planning, management, and resources allocation.

Major Similarities. Program evaluation and quality assurance, traditionally connected to different areas of concern, have become more closely linked in federal legislation and are tending to converge. For example, program evaluation of outcome studies is now a quality assurance requirement. PSRO calls them medical care evaluation studies; the CMHC Amendments call them clinical care evaluation studies. Similarities are also found in the need of quality assurance programs to hire computer technologists to handle more highly developed quality assurance processes and management information systems. In addition, aggregation of patient-specific data, at one time thought to be a program evaluation device, is now being used in quality assurance studies called profile analyses that review patterns of practice. Woy, Lund, and Attkisson (1978) advocate a sharing of personnel and efforts to meet the demands for quality assurance and program evaluation as a way to help develop better evaluation systems and to solve the problem of allocating limited resources.

Model Quality Assurance Programs

Several mental health centers across the country have designed quality assurance programs that can serve as models for others interested in developing a system to meet both their own specific needs and external reporting requirements. The Connecticut Mental Health Center model (Riedel, Tischler, and Myers, 1974) is a comprehensive, computerized peer review system that meets the utilization and quality care demands made by the government and third-party reimbursers. In this system, the patient's record includes details of exactly what is being done for the patient and why. In the first step of the procedure, a computer is used to audit the adequacy and completeness of record content on all cases. The second step calls for peer review of data abstracted from the patient's record in comparison with locally established criteria and standards of excellence (Woy, Lund, and Attkisson, 1978). If the abstract reveals conformity with the standards and criteria, no further action is taken. If, however, deviations from the standards of excellence are revealed, the record is referred for a more detailed peer review process in which the record is examined in terms of the treatment plan and the actual service being delivered. The need for changes in intervention plans is communicated through a staff education and training program.

The model is very thorough and cuts down on staff time by having a computer do the initial screening, thereby maintaining confidentiality. The one drawback of the system is the high cost of computer use; some CMHCs cannot afford or do not have access to a computer.

The Peninsula Hospital CMHC model (Luft, Sampson, and Newman, 1976) represents a manual, or noncomputerized, peer review system. Initiated in 1971 as a cost-saving utilization review procedure, not as a quality assurance procedure, this system has had quality assurance as one of its welcome spinoffs. The program is now viewed by practitioners using it as an effective monitoring device of both cost of service and quality of care.

To maintain the delicate balance between increasing clinical needs and a limited budget, a peer review system was initiated that required every outpatient clinician seeing a client for more than six sessions to present the case to the outpatient peer review committee. The center has three quality assurance committees: an inpatient and partial care hospital committee, a child outpatient committee, and an adult outpatient committee.

The composition of the outpatient review committee, whose three members are selected by the chairperson of the department of psychiatry, reflects a high ratio of practicing professionals to administrative personnel in order to ensure that clinical, rather than fiscal, concerns will be emphasized by the committee and to ensure acceptability of the system by the center's staff. Another deliberate decision was to select committee members who favor long-term psychotherapies in order to counterbalance the predilection in utilization review for short-term treatment. The committee meets weekly for an hour and a half to review three cases that clinicians feel require more than six therapy sessions. The clinician presents the psychosexual history of the case, the diagnosis, the treatment goals, and, with input from the review committee, a proposed plan of treatment that authorizes a specific treatment modality, the frequency of sessions, and the maximum length of treatment. The patient's clinical record—containing admitting information, progress notes, the patient's ratings on the Global Assessment Scale, and prior peer review summaries—is usually present at each case review as a secondary source of information. A summary of the case review—including a synopsis of the clinician's oral presentation, a synopsis of the discussion in the review session, a termination date and, if applicable, a follow-up date—is always recorded after each committee meeting.

The deficiencies of this system are that it is not a comprehensive quality assurance program, since it only reviews cases that require more than six sessions of therapy; underutilization and the quality and appropriateness of care for patients in brief treatment are not reviewed; and the mechanisms for instituting change in the quality of care are not specifically noted. As mentioned before, a review system in and of itself does not constitute a quality assurance program; a quality assurance program must monitor the quality of service and, where appropriate, improve it.

Quality Assurance Procedures

Two important quality assurance procedures, admissions certification and continued-stay review, are described in this section. Admissions certification, a utilization procedure to ensure that all hospitalizations are necessary, is usually performed before admissions or within the first twenty-four to forty-eight hours after admission, and requires data collection, the application of admission criteria, and the application of length-of-stay norms. The data to be collected include: client identification; payment method; clinical identification; diagnosis or presenting problem; and selected signs, symptoms, and results of previous treatment. An example of a review chart is presented in Table 1.

Admission criteria specify whether admission is appropriate or inappropriate for the given diagnosis or problem. Typically, one of the following four criteria sets is used (National Institute of Mental Health, 1976).

1. *Diagnosis-specific criteria sets.* Diagnostic criteria from DSM-III are elaborated to specify the circumstances justifying hospitalization; to indicate the supporting documentation required; to establish the parameters governing the implementation of a treatment program; and to determine the circumstances warranting extended duration of stay, as well as the conditions for discharge.
2. *Clinical and social indications for hospitalization.* Separate clinical and social criteria are developed for all patients, regardless of diagnosis or problem (Paras, 1974). Social criteria are included in the belief that, in addition to the diagnosis or presenting problem, social variables may help account for the need for inpatient care in some clients.
3. *Symptom or behavior-specific criteria.* Specific behavioral criteria are developed for the hospitalization of patients exhibiting specific symptoms or

Table 1. Utilization Review Findings.

Client's Name: _____ Case Number: _____

	Initial	Change 1	Change 2
Primary therapist:	_____ :	_____ :	_____
Primary diagnosis:	_____ :	_____ :	_____
Primary treatment goal:	_____ :	_____ :	_____
Treatment program:	_____ :	_____ :	_____
Date admitted to program:	_____ :	_____ :	_____
Source of payment:	_____ :	_____ :	_____

Admission Review   Date: _____

Record entries complete: Yes____ No____
Certified by screening criteria: Yes____ No____
    Referred for peer review to: _____
Certified by peer review: Yes____ No____   ( ) Program change
Process of care (comment):   ( ) Termination
                                                             ( ) Notifications
                                                                 completed

Next Review Date: _____   Reviewer: _____

Treatment Review   Date: _____

Record entries complete: Yes____ No____
Certified by screening criteria: Yes____ No____
    Referred for peer review to: _____
Certified by peer review: Yes____ No____   ( ) Program change
Process of care (comment):   ( ) Termination
                                                             ( ) Notifications
                                                                 completed

Next Review Date: _____   Reviewer: _____

Extended-Stay Review   Date: _____

Record entries complete: Yes____ No____
Certified by screening criteria: Yes____ No____
    Referred for peer review to: _____
Certified by peer review: Yes____ No____   ( ) Program change
Process of care (comment):   ( ) Termination
                                                             ( ) Notifications
                                                                 completed

Next Review Date: _____   Reviewer: _____

Source: National Institute of Mental Health, 1976.

behaviors (for example, suicidal behavior). Such criteria can include a mix of clinical and social indications, rather than simply a diagnosis.

4. *A scaled judgment of the necessity for hospitalization.* The Connecticut Mental Health Center has also developed a general rating scale for appropriateness of hospitalization for all patients (Riedel and others, 1974). Questions about client behavior, mental status, physical condition, and clinician concern for client well-being are weighted on a scale of 1 to 4. Each prospective admission receives a score between 0 and 75 (see Table 2). In the Connecticut system, a score of 12 or more indicates definite need for hospitalization; a score under 12 requires review by a clinical consultant.

Continued-stay review, which assures that hospitalization for already hospitalized patients continues to be necessary and appropriate, has two components: length-of-stay review and quality care review. In most systems, a few days before a hospitalized client reaches the end of his or her initial number of approved hospital days, the case is reviewed by a review coordinator before the client is either discharged or granted further hospital days. The patient's chart is reviewed to ensure that the chart is complete, that the discharge or continued-stay criteria have been met, and that all appropriate, recommended medical examinations and laboratory work-ups have been completed and are documented in the chart. The chart's progress notes are examined for descriptions of the client's behavior and his or her response to treatment. The chart is also examined for evidence to determine whether the client requires further approved inpatient hospital days or is fit for discharge. In the Colorado system, continued-stay criteria are considered met when the chart indicates that psychosis is not in remission; client is suicidal or assaultive; physical complications exist; treatment of disruptive personality is in process; skill or role enhancement therapy is in process; similar services are still needed and unavailable in the community; client is awaiting economic support arrangements or transfer to another facility; or client has been rejected by family or community (Paras, 1974).

If the review coordinator finds the chart incomplete, the responsible clinician is contacted to provide the missing information. Once the missing information is provided, the chart is examined and a judgment made by the review coordinator on the appropriateness of the recommended discharge or continued inpatient stay. If the review coordinator is satisfied that the appropriate criteria have been met in support of the clinician's recommendation, the client is either discharged or granted additional approved hospital days. If additional days are granted, the review coordinator will assign another checkpoint when the review process will again be conducted.

If, however, the review coordinator judges the clinician's recommendations for discharge or continued stay to be inappropriate or unnecessary—for example, the clinician recommends continued stay, but the progress notes indicate a major improvement in the client's condition—the case is referred to the clinical adviser on the case for a final recommendation. The involved clinician is informed of the clinical adviser's recommendation and, in the event that the clinical adviser's

Table 2. General Criteria for Certifying Appropriateness of Hospitalization.

Instructions to Reviewers

1. Rate patient on each criterion as follows: none = 0, slight = 1, moderate = 2, and extensive = 3. Multiply the rating by the weight shown, and enter the score for each criterion. Sum the scores for all twelve criteria to obtain total score.
2. Ratings are to be based on the patient's condition during the seven days preceding evaluation for hospitalization.
3. In applying the criteria, an item of reported behavior should be employed to arrive at a rating on the first criterion on the list to which it applies. Do not use the same item of behavior to score a criterion that falls later in the list (for example, suicidal behavior should not be used again in rating criteria 4 and 5).

Criteria

1. Is there evidence of active suicidal preoccupations in the fantasy or thoughts of the patient? (Weight = 2)
2. Have there been suicidal attempts or active preparations to harm self (for example, buying a gun)? (Weight = 4)
3. Has the patient verbally threatened to hurt someone else physically? (Weight = 2)
4. Have aggressive outbursts occurred toward people? (Weight = 4)
5. Have aggressive outbursts occurred toward animals or objects? (Weight = 2)
6. Has antisocial behavior occurred? (Weight = 2)
7. Are there evidences of impairment of such functions as reality assessment, judgment, logical thinking, and planning? (Weight = 1)
8. Does the patient's condition seem to be deteriorating rapidly or failing to improve despite supportive measures? (Weight = 1)
9. Are there physical or neurological conditions or a psychotic, disorganized state that requires hospitalization to initiate the treatment process? (Weight = 2)
10. Does a pathological or noxious situation exist among patient's family or associates that makes initiation of treatment without hospitalization impossible? Or does the patient's disordered state create such difficulties for family or associates that he has to be removed and hospitalized for their sake? (Weight = 1)
11. Are emotional contacts of the patient so severely limited or the habitual patterns of behavior so pathologically ingrained that the use of a structured hospital program may be helpful? (This criterion should not be applied to acute patients, but only to those who are so limited as to be unable to establish and maintain emotional contacts.) (Weight = 1)
12. Does evaluation of the patient's condition require the twenty-four-hour observation and special evaluation (including stabilization or reevaluation of medication) that a hospital provides? Or has the patient been referred for treatment of drug or alcohol dependence? (Weight = 4)

Source: National Institute of Mental Health, 1976.

recommendation conflicts with the clinician's, the clinician is given the opportunity to appeal to a larger review committee. If the review committee upholds the decision that continued stay is not necessary, but the clinician continues to feel that it is, two choices exist: to discharge the client or to continue the stay even though reimbursement will not be received for noncertified days of care.

Chart review is not always necessary in length-of-stay review. Table 3 illustrates a method of continued-stay review that eliminates chart review by

Table 3. Certification of Need for Continued Stay.

Dr. _____ , on _____ , your patient _____ will have been hospitalized twenty-three days. If you anticipate that more than thirty days of inpatient care is needed, please complete and return this form before the twenty-third day. If discharge is anticipated before thirty days, check here ( ) and return.

1. What symptoms or behavior necessitated current admission?

2. Has patient been hospitalized before?
   ( ) No   ( ) Yes: ____ times; last hospitalization at _____ ; usual length of stay _____ .

3. Therapeutic goals for this admission:
   ( ) a. remission of symptoms
   ( ) b. evaluation of previous psychotherapy
   ( ) c. planning for psychotherapy
   ( ) d. planning for other care
   ( ) e. diagnostic evaluation
   ( ) f. other
   Elaborate briefly, making clear what is to be accomplished or what problems exist.

4. ( ) Discharge not possible because discharge plans not complete:
   ( ) a. planning not initiated promptly
   ( ) b. direction of planning had to be altered during hospitalization
   ( ) c. discharge difficulties related to:
       ( )(1) patient's motivation or acceptance of situation
       ( )(2) insufficiency of community resources
   ( ) d. physical illness of patient prevents completion of plans
   ( ) e. transfer pending
   Give specific details to illustrate the problem.

6. ( ) There was a relapse, but patient is now improving. Describe.

7. ( ) Type of therapy was changed during hospitalization. Specify.

8. ( ) Discharge within ____ days from now is anticipated.

9. Explain reasons for requesting further hospitalization beyond thirty days.

_____   _____
       Date   Review Coordinator

Action: ( ) Approved   ( ) Disapproved   ( ) More information needed

---

Source: Richman and Pinsker, 1973.

---

soliciting the required information directly from the clinician (Richman and Pinsker, 1973). In any case, a statistical record should be kept of the following continued-stay review activity: number of cases reviewed; number of extensions granted by the review coordinator; number of extensions referred to clinical advisers, with number granted and number denied (identifying client and clinician for each denial); and total number of inpatient days approved.

The procedures for quality care review are not as well defined as for length-of-stay review. Quality care review is usually conducted by a professional staff member and requires the continual monitoring of services and therapy to assure high-quality care. The review coordinator conducts quality assessment by studying the treatment plan to learn the initial diagnosis or diagnostic impression, the definition of the client's problems, planned interventions, and tentative release goals and plans; studying the rates of progress for descriptions of the client's behavior and responses to treatment; and reviewing the chart to ensure that physical findings are reported, all laboratory reports have been completed, and minimal lab workups have been performed. Inappropriate or inadequate care is usually brought to the attention of the clinical advisor, who is responsible for consulting with the involved clinician and, if necessary, initiating provisions for change.

Benefits of Quality Assurance Programs

The drawbacks of a quality assurance program include negative appraisals and sabotaging efforts by the professionals being reviewed, potential interference with the treatment process, compromising treatment modality and length of treatment in favor of budgetary concerns. Research by Block (1975), Newman (1974), and Luft (1977), however, has found that these shortcomings are not prevalent and that quality assurance has some very important secondary benefits.

The first benefit is that quality assurance tends to improve agency record systems (Block, 1975; Luft, 1977). Recordkeeping in clinical care is often quite poor because of the absence of explicit diagnosis and treatment criteria, the absence of explicitly defined treatment goals, and a general lack of clear and precise thinking on the part of clinicians (Liptzin, 1974). A peer review system aimed at monitoring and assuring high-quality care and efficient utilization of services forces clinicians to develop explicit criteria and standards, to clearly determine the goals of treatment and treatment methods, and to be more fastidious in their reports.

The second benefit is that quality assurance allows clinicians the opportunity to receive consultation on difficult cases. Although clinicians often feel anxious about presenting cases before a peer review committee, many consider it to be an educational process. Misgivings about the process seem to give way to positive, accepting feelings if the committee members are nonpunitive and tactful in their approach and remember that they are dealing with peers.

Initially, the implementation of a quality assurance program may prove to be something of a headache, as committee members struggle with the added financial burden of setting up a comprehensive program and with the reactions of staff members. However, an established quality assurance program has a positive influence on administrators, clinicians, clients, and mental health treatment programs.

Conclusion

Quality assurance has evolved from being a voluntary, somewhat vague and implicit concept primarily used by inpatient mental health services to being an explicit practice mandated by government agencies, accreditation bodies, and third-party insurance carriers. The mental health agency needs to monitor all external regulators to ensure that its quality assurance program meets the explicit requirements of all relevant review agencies. Each regulator has its own explicit quality assurance requirements, and, although the criteria may be similar, no one set of criteria is thought to supersede the others.

The quality of mental health care continues to be an underdeveloped concept needing further clarification. By definition, it refers to the appropriateness, adequacy, and effectiveness of care given to individual clients. When mental health care providers guarantee the quality of care, they are promising that certain standards of excellence are being met. In practice, the concept becomes complex and subjective, as agencies seek to define quality in terms of input, process, or outcome perspectives, to distinguish between qualitative and quantitative care, to employ implicit or explicit criteria, and to implement internal or external review. Unfortunately, no cookbook outlines what works best. Within the boundaries of the explicit requirements imposed by external review organizations, mental health agencies must develop their own definition of quality and devise appropriate assessment and change procedures.

References

Attkisson, C. C., and others. "A Working Model for Mental Health Program Evaluation." *American Journal of Orthopsychiatry*, 1974, *44*, 741–753.

Babigian, H. M., and others. "Diagnostic Consistency and Change in a Follow-up Study of 1215 Patients." *American Journal of Psychiatry*, 1965, *121*, 895–901.

Benveniste, G. *Bureaucracy*. San Francisco: Boyd and Fraser, 1977.

Block, W. E. "Applying Utilization Review Procedures in a Community Mental Health Center." *Hospital and Community Psychiatry*, 1975, *26*, 358–362.

Brook, R. H. *Quality of Care Assessment: A Comparison of Five Methods of Peer Review*. Washington, D.C.: National Center for Health Services Research and Development, 1973.

Brook, R. H., Williams, K. N., and Davies-Avery, A. "Quality Assurance Today and Tomorrow: Forecast for the Future." *Annals of Internal Medicine*, 1976, *85*, 809–817.

Brook, R. H., and others. *Assessing the Quality of Medical Care Using Outcome Measures: An Overview of the Method*. Philadelphia: Lippincott, 1977.

Cohen, G. D., and others. "PSROs: Problems and Potentials for Psychiatry." *American Journal of Psychiatry*, 1974, *131*, 1378–1381.

Comptroller General of the United States. *Need for More Effective Management of the Community Mental Health Centers Program*. Washington, D.C.: U.S. General Accounting Office, 1974.

Decker, B., and Bonner, P. (Eds.). *PSRO: Organization for Regional Peer Review*. Cambridge, Mass.: Ballinger, 1973.

De Geyndt, W. "Five Approaches for Assessing the Quality of Care." *Hospital Administration*, 1970, *15*, 21–42.

Donabedian, A. "Evaluating the Quality of Medical Care." *Milbank Memorial Fund Quarterly*, 1966, *44*, 166–206.

Donabedian, A. *Needed Research in the Assessment and Monitoring of the Quality of Medical Care.* Ann Arbor: University of Michigan, 1978.

Egdahl, R. H., and Gertman, P. M. *Quality Assurance in Health Care.* Germantown, Md.: Aspen, Systems, 1976.

Goran, M. J., and others. "The PSRO Hospital Review System." *Medical Care*, 1975, *13*, Supplement 1–33.

Johnson, R. A., Kast, F. E., and Rosenzweig, J. E. *The Theory and Management of Systems.* New York: McGraw-Hill, 1973.

Joint Commission on Accreditation of Hospitals. *Principles of Accreditation of Community Mental Health Service Programs.* Chicago: Accreditation Council for Psychiatric Facilities, 1979.

Krubie, L. S. "The Process of Evaluation of Therapy in Psychiatry." *Archives of General Psychiatry*, 1973, *28*, 880–884.

Linn, M. W., Gurel, L., and Linn, B. S. "Patient Outcome as a Measure of Quality of Nursing Home Care." *American Journal of Public Health*, 1977, *67*, 337–344.

Liptzin, B. "Quality Assurance and Psychiatric Practice: A Review." *American Journal of Psychiatry*, 1974, *131*, 1374–1377.

Lorei, T. W., and Schroeder, N. H. "Integrating Program Evaluation and Medical Audit." *Hospital and Community Psychiatry*, 1975, *26*, 733–735.

Luft, L. L. "Vital Issues in the Design of Quality Assurance Systems." In R. S. Kessler (Ed.), *Quality Assurance in the Ambulatory Setting: Nine Papers.* St. Albans: State of Vermont, Institutional Industries Press, 1977.

Luft, L. L., and Newman, D. E. "Therapists' Acceptance of Peer Review in a Community Mental Health Center." *Hospital and Community Psychiatry*, 1977, *28*, 889–894.

Luft, L. L., Sampson, L. M., and Newman, D. E. "Effects of Peer Review on Outpatient Psychotherapy: Therapist and Patient Follow-Up Survey." *American Journal of Psychiatry*, 1976, *133*, 891–895.

McCullough, P. "Training for Evaluators." In J. Zusman and C. R. Wurster (Eds.), *Program Evaluation: Alcohol, Drug Abuse, and Mental Health Services.* Lexington, Mass.: Lexington Books, 1975.

Moorehead, M. A. "Ambulatory Care Review: A Neglected Priority." *Bulletin of the New York Academy of Medicine*, 1976, *52*, 60–69.

National Institute of Mental Health. *Assessing and Assuring Quality in Community Mental Health.* (Contract report prepared by C. Windle and the A. D. Little Company). Washington, D.C.: U.S. Department of Health, Education, and Welfare, 1976.

Newman, D. E. "Peer Review: A California Model." *Psychiatric Annals*, 1974, *4*, 75–85.

Newman, D. E., and Luft, L. L. "The Peer Review Process: Education Versus Control." *American Journal of Psychiatry*, 1974, *131*, 1363–1366.

Noble, J. H. "Peer Review: Quality Control of Applied Social Research." *Science*,

1974, *185*, 916-921.

Northwest Federation for Human Services. *Microdata Sampling Systems: A Proposed Measurement Design.* Boise, Idaho: Northwest Federation for Human Services, 1976.

Office of Professional Standards Review. *PSRO Program Manual.* Washington, D.C.: U.S. Department of Health, Education and Welfare, 1974.

Paras, J. L. *A Guide for Development and Implementation of a Utilization Review and Medical Care Assessment Program.* Denver: Fort Logan Mental Health Center, Colorado State Hospital Project, 1974.

Parloff, M. B. "Psychotherapy and Research: An Anaclitic Depression." *Psychiatry*, 1980, *43*, 279-293.

Racusin, R., and Krell, H. "Quality Assurance in Community Mental Health Centers." *Administration in Mental Health*, 1980, *7*, 292-303.

Rapp, M. "Federally Imposed Self-Regulation of Medical Practice: A Critique of the Professional Standards Review Organization." *George Washington Law Review*, 1974, *42*, 823-843.

Richman, A. "The Differences Between Quality Assurance, Records Committee Review, Program Evaluation, and Clinical Supervision." In R. S. Kessler (Ed.), *Quality Assurance in the Ambulatory Setting: Nine Papers.* St. Albans: State of Vermont, Institutional Industries Press, 1977a.

Richman, A. "Developing Screening Criteria for a Patient Care Evaluation Study, PSRO/JCAH Type: Hints, Suggestions and a Checklist." In R. S. Kessler (Ed.), *Quality Assurance in the Ambulatory Setting: Nine Papers.* St. Albans: State of Vermont, Institutional Industries Press, 1977b.

Richman, A., and Pinsker, H. "Utilization Review of Psychiatric Inpatient Care." *American Journal of Psychiatry*, 1973, *130*, 900-903.

Riedel, D. C., Tischler, G. T., and Myers, J. K. (Eds.). *Patient Care Evaluation in Mental Health Programs.* Cambridge, Mass.: Ballinger, 1974.

Riedel, D. C., and others. "Developing a System for Utilization Review and Evaluation in Community Mental Health Centers." *Hospital and Community Psychiatry*, 1971, *22*, 229-232.

Stevens, R. *American Medicine and the Public Interest.* New Haven: Yale University Press, 1971.

Taft, C., and Levine, S. "Problems of Federal Policies and Strategies to Influence the Quality of Health Care." In R. H. Egdahl and P. M. Gertman (Eds.), *Quality Assurance in Health Care.* Rockville, Md.: Aspen Systems, 1976.

Thorne, M. Q. "PSRO: Future Impact on Community Mental Health Centers." *Community Mental Health Journal*, 1975, *11*, 389-393.

Thorne, M. Q. "Models of Quality Assurance Programs in Rural Community Mental Health Centers." In R. S. Kessler (Ed.), *Quality Assurance in the Ambulatory Setting: Nine Papers.* St. Albans: State of Vermont, Institutional Industries Press, 1977.

Tischler, G. T., and Riedel, D. C. "A Criterion Approach to Patient Care Evaluation." *American Journal of Psychiatry*, 1973, *130*, 913-916.

Windle, C., and Ochberg, F. M. "Enhancing Program Evaluation in the Community Mental Health Centers Program." *Evaluation,* 1975, *2,* 31-36.

Woy, J. R., Lund, D. A., and Attkisson, C. C. "Quality Assurance in Human Service Program Evaluation." In C. C. Attkisson and others (Eds.), *Evaluation of Human Service Programs.* New York: Academic Press, 1978.

❦ 20 ❦

Assessing Community
Mental Health Needs

Benson Jaffee

In presenting basic concepts and principles of community needs assessment, Benson Jaffee distinguishes among normative, perceived, expressed, and relative needs, then details such needs assessment methods as surveys, social indicators, selective community opinions, service statistics, and secondary analysis of existing data. In addition, he describes steps for conducting an agency-focused needs assessment, including selection of the appropriate type of questionnaire or interview; sampling of the target population; and collection, analysis, and utilization of data.

In recent years, interest has increased in conducting needs assessments designed to provide data about the mental health needs of actual or potential agency clientele and about the population in agency catchment areas, data to be used in the administration and planning of new or modified services. This trend has been related to the increasing demand for mental health services agency accountability—due in part to the passage of the Community Mental Health Centers Amendments of 1975—and to the burgeoning literature on how to conduct needs assessments. The purposes of this chapter are to specify and illustrate the basic concepts and principles involved in mental health needs assessment and to describe and discuss the major steps in conducting such an assessment.

Definition of Basic Concepts

Clearly and explicitly defining such terms as *needs, needs assessment,* and *mental health problems* is not merely an academic exercise undertaken for heuristic purposes. Rather, unless there is clarity about what the mental health staff wishes to measure and what is actually measured, the data that are gathered and the findings derived from those data will, at best, be confusing—and, at worst, meaningless and perhaps misleading—to the administrator, to agency board members, and to other relevant policy and decision makers, who may well have differing views of the true needs of the agency's target populations, the types of services that should be provided to meet those needs, and the degree to which current services are actually meeting those needs.

At the outset, the concepts of unmet needs and social problems need to be distinguished. A social problem has been defined as "a problem in living, a dysfunctional somatic or psychological state, or an undesirable social process . . . for which a satisfactory solution requires a major mobilization of additional resources or a major reallocation of existing resources" (Attkisson and others, 1978).

Thus, an unmet need is related to the recognition of a problem in living, which in turn involves an accurate perception of the dysfunctional psychological or somatic state or undesirable social process; a comparison level, standard, or norm; and an evaluation of the extent and seriousness of the disparity between what is and what should be. Furthermore, that the need is unmet implies that satisfactory solutions to the problem in the form of programs, personnel, or funding do not currently exist in the community or, if they do exist, that they are not adequate or are not readily accessible. Finally, unmet need involves a situation in which the problem in living can be remedied only by a mobilization of new resources or a reallocation of existing resources.

Unmet need, then, is a normative concept (Moroney, 1977), defined in a social context and involving a judgment and a value position. At a given point in time, an individual or a group of individuals is assessed as experiencing a problem in living that requires either the creation of new resources or the reallocation of existing ones, be those resources better housing, better health care, employment, more recreational services for the aged, jobs for the handicapped, diversionary services for acting-out youth, or one of a myriad of other resources. In other words, "needs do not show themselves. Someone must establish what constitutes a need" (Kimmel, 1977). Furthermore, since the concept of unmet need is elastic, not absolute (Moroney, 1977), what constitutes need changes over time. As a result, the assessment of unmet mental health needs would seem to be an ongoing or at least recurring process in any mental health agency committed to relating its services to the actual needs of its target population (Bell and others, 1976; Shapek, 1975).

In addition, the definition of the problems involved and the choice of resources required to satisfactorily solve those problems may differ widely, depending on who makes those judgments. The definition of problem or need can be viewed from four perspectives—normative, perceived, expressed, and relative—as shown in Table 1 (Bradshaw, 1977; Moroney, 1977). Each type of need concerns only one facet of the concept of unmet need, and consequently each has specific implications for what is being measured and for what information can be garnered in the needs assessment process. Thus, for example, if a mental health center were to measure the extent of need as established by professional judgment—that is, normative need—the administrator and board would obtain data that are considerably different from the data they would obtain if they were to measure need as perceived by the client. Similarly, expressed need as measured by waiting lists and

Table 1. Multiple Definitions of Need.

Normative Need

Determined by professional or other expert judgment, normative need may or may not be based on an objective, systematic study of the target population. The experts identify a desirable standard based on their experience, often expressed as a ratio, and compare this standard with the actually existing need. If the group or population falls short of this standard, its members are considered to be in need.

The obvious strength of this concept of need is that it makes possible the clear identification of individuals or groups in need of services by using highly knowledgeable persons to judge the nature and extent of need. However, this concept of need tends to be paternalistic or elitist, in that this need is determined by someone from outside the community. Furthermore, individually applied normative standards may reflect the personal biases of the judges and may not accurately account for the changes in both values and knowledge in a given community. Finally, assessments of normative need by experts using different standards can differ widely.

Perceived (Felt) Need

This type of need measures what people perceive to be their problems and the resources or services they desire. The principal advantage of this type of need is that the target population itself, rather than some intermediary expert, defines the problems and the resources required to deal with those problems, thereby contributing to the design of more directly responsive services.

However, a limitation of perceived need is that some people may not distinguish between problems they themselves are experiencing and problems experienced by others. In addition, experience has demonstrated an ofttimes marked disparity between what people say they need or want and their subsequent utilization of these needed services when in fact they are provided. As a result, statements of perceived need provide a somewhat tenuous basis for decisions concerning the creation of new or reallocation of existing resources. Finally, tapping perceived need may raise expectations for relevant services, expectations that may lead to the frustration and alienation of the target population if they are not subsequently met.

Expressed Need

This type of need is synonymous with demand for services and is indicated by the number of persons who actually seek specific types of services, as measured by intake statistics and waiting lists. The strength of this concept of need is that it offers a measure of truly experienced need reflected in people actually seeking specific services or resources for problems they are facing. A mental health agency measuring this type of need would thus have a sound basis for concluding that the problems presented by its current and potential (waiting list) clientele really exist and that services addressed to those problems are needed and would be utilized. If the measurement of expressed need is expanded to include a count of waiting lists in other agencies in the community serving similar clients, the basis for planning and offering similar services would be enhanced.

On the other hand, expressed need does not reflect the need of target population members who have not taken the step of applying for services, and waiting lists do not constitute an adequate definition of presymptomatic or latent need in a community.

Relative (Comparative) Need

This type of need measures the gap between those utilizing existing services in one geographical area and those with similar needs in another area who are not receiving similar services. Those failing to receive services are considered to be in need.

This concept of need addresses the issue of equity among areas and groups and can be used to attempt to standardize the provision of services to such areas and groups. One limitation is the great difficulty in defining and taking into account the significant differences in population characteristics and pathology—and therefore in specific kinds and levels of services needed—between two areas. Moreover, the more adequately serviced areas may themselves still be in need in more absolute terms.

---

intake statistics would provide the administrator and board with still different information. Obviously, such differing types of data could lead to very different conclusions about the changes in services delivery patterns that should be considered by the agency. For this reason, it is important to measure two or more types of needs whose strengths and shortcomings are complementary in order to get a more complete understanding of the range of needs in the target population (Mustian and See, 1973).

Needs Assessment Methods

Thus far, attention has been focused on the classification of unmet needs. Now the methods for assessing such needs must be identified. Attkisson and others (1978) distinguish between needs identification, which describes the nature and extent of mental health services problems in a given geographical or social area, and needs assessment, which estimates the relative importance of those needs in order to determine priorities for service planning and development. The distinction is between fact gathering and decision making, two complementary and indispensable but different processes that are based on different objectives and frames of reference and yield different types of data.

The needs assessment literature is replete with descriptions and discussions of an array of methods and techniques, including surveys, social indicators, selective community opinions (for example, key informants and community forums), service statistics, and analysis of existing data (Bureau of Research and Evaluation, 1975; Center for Social Research and Development, 1974; Project Share, 1976). Tables 2 through 6 present condensed summaries of these major needs assessment approaches and a description of their major characteristics, adapted from the most widely cited texts on the subject. Each of the major approaches has clearly identified limitations, in addition to its undisputed assets; therefore, no one approach can provide the mental health administrator or planner with a totally adequate or comprehensive picture of the unmet needs experienced by the target population served by his or her agency. For this reason, the guiding principle found throughout the needs assessment literature is that, to the extent that time and budget permit, combinations of complementary approaches should be used, either simultaneously or in tandem, with the various methods selected so that strengths and weaknesses compensate for one another (Minnesota State Planning Agency, 1977; National Institute of Mental Health, 1976).

For example, a survey of the general population of the catchment area of a mental health center could be conducted at the same time that utilization and waiting list data or management information system data were being gathered by systematically organizing and aggregating information already routinely compiled by the agency. Similarly, an optimal treatment approach could be developed and an adequate sampling of cases gathered while the mental health center was undertaking a key informant study, assembling social indicator data, or preparing for or conducting a community forum.

In determining which of the above methods to use, the mental health administrator needs first to assess the cost and time involved in the various ap-

Table 2. Surveys.

The survey approach involves the collection of data regarding the health or social well-being of a target population or the patterns of care or services it receives. Data are gathered from: a sample or an entire population of community residents; specific target populations within the community; service providers, both agencies and individual practitioners; or experts in specific social problem or services delivery areas.

A. *Major Data-Gathering Techniques*

The mailed questionnaire, the in-person interview, and the telephone interview.

B. *Major Advantages*

1. If properly gathered, the resulting data are the most scientifically valid and reliable.
2. Surveys yield specific information about the needs and service utilization patterns of individuals who are directly aware of or are experiencing the problems or needs.
3. Where units of analysis are households, data are available from various family members.

C. *Major Disadvantages*

1. Survey methods—for example, probability sampling and interviewing—are expensive.
2. Respondents may be reluctant to divulge sensitive information about themselves or family members.
3. Refusal to participate and nonreturn rates of questionnaires may make validity and reliability of findings questionable.
4. Survey methods may raise consumer expectations that desired services will in fact be provided. Failure to provide these services may result in frustration and anger in the target population, as well as cynicism about and alienation from the agency.
5. Respondents may indicate their intentions to utilize specific services if these are provided, but such intentions may not be translated into actual usage once services are established.

Source: Warheit, Bell, and Schwab, 1976; Research Group, Inc., 1976.

Table 3. Social Indicators.

The social indicators approach infers need from descriptive statistics found in public records and reports, especially those statistics found to be closely correlated with persons in need (Schneider, 1975). Examples of the statistics most commonly used as social indicators are housing patterns and population density; income, age, race, and sex; crime and substance abuse; housing conditions, such as overcrowding and substandard housing; family patterns; morbidity and mortality rates; accessibility to services.

A. *Major Data-Gathering Techniques*

Use of worksheets to gather data from public reports; reports of national, regional, state and local health, education, and welfare agencies; crime statistics; court records; health and welfare planning council reports; and records of vital statistics.

B. *Major Advantages*

1. Required data often already exist in organized form; thus, social indicators are usually inexpensive to develop by persons with limited research training.
2. Data can be developed with only limited amounts of information about the local community.
3. Data can be compared with data from other communities.
4. Wide range of data from many sources is valuable and can be incorporated in an index of need.

Table 3, cont'd.

C. *Major Disadvantages*

1. Social indicators claim to represent only indirect, correlational measures of needs; no causal relationship exists between social indicators and incidence of problems.
2. Data may be used to reinforce personal, class, or ethnic biases regarding social problems and patterns of social functioning.
3. Danger that the characteristics of a community, as measured by rates, averages, and so on, will be used fallaciously to stereotype all the individuals in that community. This is called the fallacy of ecological correlations.

Source: Warheit, Bell, and Schwab, 1976; Research Group, Inc., 1976.

Table 4. Selective Community Opinions.

I. *Key Informant Study*

Key informants are persons knowledgeable about the community's needs and service utilization patterns. Thus, typical key informants are public officials, administrative and program personnel in health and welfare organizations, physicians and nurses from both the private and public sectors, and clinical staff members of community mental health centers, vocational rehabilitation agencies, and health programs (League of California Cities, 1975; Warren, 1977).

Key informants are selected after the objectives of the assessment are defined. Then a data-gathering instrument is administered to each key informant, usually in a personal interview that permits face-to-face contact, a free exchange of ideas, and a high response rate.

A. *Major Data-Gathering Techniques*

Usually in-person interview; telephone interviews and mailed questionnaires may also be used, although they yield less-adequate data.

B. *Major Advantages*

1. Is relatively simple and inexpensive.
2. Permits input from many different perspectives.
3. Helps open and strengthen lines of communication among human services agencies.
4. Fosters more community involvement in setting priorities and allocating resources.

C. *Major Disadvantages*

1. May suffer from the built-in biases of informants based on individual or organizational perspectives not representing total community needs.
2. Tends to reflect personal opinions or experience only; thus, may omit important needs not known to informants; may lack hard objective data.

II. *The Optimal Treatment Approach*

This approach, appropriate primarily for local direct service agencies, involves the development of an optimal plan or case disposition for individual clients as part of the regular, ongoing procedure for creating an actual treatment plan. The optimal and actual plans are compared, and discrepancies due to missing resources or programs are noted. These are aggregated across cases, and the results, indicating needs, are fed into planning and management functions.

Table 4, cont'd.

A. *Major Data-Gathering Techniques*

The production of an actual and an optimal treatment plan for each active case; a formal comparison of any disparities in these plans concerning desired and actual treatment resources or programs; and the aggregation and organization of such disparity data for all cases served during a given period of time.

B. *Major Advantages*

1. Any data desired are gathered prospectively; thus, data quality can be monitored and weaknesses remedied before serious flaws develop.
2. Data should have generally high relevance to unmet needs (validity), depending on the legitimacy and knowledgeability of the person or persons determining optimal client need for and accessibility of services.
3. Costs of generating and analyzing data tend to be low.
4. Data can be highly relevant to agency decision making.
5. More-informal, less-systematic applications of this needs assessment approach are probably in use in many agencies.

C. *Major Disadvantages*

1. Conceptual confusion between needs and services may result from treatment plans phrased in terms of services, rather than in terms of meeting client needs.
2. This approach is subject to two types of bias: sampling bias, where the client sample used to generate the data is not representative of the agency's entire target population; and perspective bias, where the perspectives of those making the optimal treatment decisions are not congruent with the perspectives of those responsible for program and planning decisions.
3. The approach may involve an unacceptably long lead time for the accrual of a sufficient number of cases to generate adequate needs data.

III. *Community Forum*

This approach involves a group of persons, most often members of the general population but also frequently specially invited key informants, who attend a series of public community meetings. Here they express their ideas and beliefs about the needs and service patterns of the community.

A. *Major Data-Gathering Techniques*

A series of public meetings located strategically throughout the community, using small groups to aid and encourage individual participation. Ideas, attitudes, and perceptions expressed are recorded and a summary of suggested needs and services prepared according to priorities developed by forum attendees through the completion of a brief, structured questionnaire.

B. *Major Advantages*

1. Is relatively easy to arrange and relatively inexpensive to conduct.
2. Provides input from individuals from varied segments of the community.
3. Identifies persons interested in future involvement.

C. *Major Disadvantages*

1. May involve difficulties in gaining representative attendance at meetings and in finding sufficient strategically located meeting sites.
2. May become a grievance session dominated by one group that focuses on problems beyond the scope or control of the agency.
3. May raise unrealistic expectations for new services.
4. Results in difficult-to-analyze, impressionistic data, not necessarily accurate or representative of the community.

Table 4, cont'd.

IV. *Nominal Group*

This approach consists of a workshop in which selected individuals are asked to share their views on community needs and service patterns by means of a specific process (Delbecq, Van de Ven, and Gustafson, 1975). Group members write answers to predetermined questions without group interaction. Then each person's ideas are shared with the group without comment or discussion from other group members. All ideas are then discussed, and each group member selects and ranks five or ten ideas he or she deems most important. Individual rankings are tallied, resulting in a group ranking of all the ideas regarding needs and community services.

A. *Major Data-Gathering Techniques*

Silent, individual identification of needs and services, followed by group discussion and individual and group ranking of these needs and services.

B. *Major Advantages*

1. Allows for group decision making or idea sharing while avoiding the major drawbacks of an interacting group.
2. Allows participants to reflect and think individually, thus fostering minority opinions, avoiding hidden agendas, stimulating individual responsibility for the group's success, encouraging creativity, and preventing the domination of any one person or point of view.
3. Ensures that each person's views are heard during the sharing, nondiscussion period.
4. Promotes richer, more creative, and more acceptable solutions, especially for heterogeneous or tension-laden groups.

C. *Major Disadvantages*

1. Tends to lack precision in the voting and ranking.
2. May cause some participants to feel manipulated because they are not familiar with the process.

V. *Community Impressions*

This is a method of collecting and combining impressions about community needs and service patterns from key individuals, verifying this information with the community groups identified as having the greatest needs, and then involving those groups in acting to reduce their needs. In essence, this approach combines the key informant study with the community forum.

A. *Major Data-Gathering Techniques*

In-person interviews with key community persons; analysis of the resulting data to identify and locate geographically those groups with the greatest need; and community forums among the identified groups in need.

B. *Major Advantages*

1. Generally involves minimal expenditure of time and resources.
2. Permits consideration of a variety of often unpredictable responses to community needs, including both facts and impressions.
3. Involves those groups with greatest identified needs in determining whether or not they have such needs and in becoming actively involved in meeting the needs they think they have.

C. *Major Disadvantages*

1. Lacks the validity and reliability of the more formal needs assessment surveys.
2. Does not ensure that every community group with needs will be identified or that the needs of those identified will be recorded.

Table 4, cont'd.

Source: Warheit, Bell, and Schwab, 1976; Research Group, Inc., 1976; Siegel, Attkisson, and Cohn, 1976.

Table 5. Service Statistics.

I. *Utilization and Waiting List Data and Rates*

This approach, used widely to estimate the mental health needs and service patterns in general populations, involves descriptions of persons who have utilized, are currently utilizing, or who are waiting to utilize mental health services in a community (Epstein and Tripodi, 1977; Scheff, 1976).

A. *Major Data-Gathering Techniques*

Analysis of agency records for such client data as sociodemographic characteristics, presenting problems, characteristics of services provided, frequency and duration of services, referral sources, and treatment outcomes; then, with these data as a baseline, gathering and analyzing comparable data from other agencies and persons in the community.

B. *Major Advantages*

1. Uses usually readily available data, generally securable at low cost.
2. Helps increase communication among the community's service providers.
3. Tends to promote sensitivity to community needs.
4. Helps foster better integration of services.

C. *Major Disadvantages*

1. Involves problems in guaranteeing anonymity and confidentiality of data, particularly data from other agencies.
2. Involves the difficulty of determining whether data in the sample receiving services are representative of the population.
3. Involves the difficulty of projecting the number of unserved persons in the population.

II. *Review of Management Information System (MIS) Data*

This approach consists of the review of information collected by human service agencies, primarily for management or administrative purposes, related to demands for service; trends in services delivered, including distribution of service usage among services delivery areas; target populations or areas requiring special study; and comparisons of cost of services delivery in various services delivery areas.

A. *Major Data-Gathering Techniques*

Review of MIS data gathered routinely by the agency and comparison of such data with other secondary data and survey information regarding human services needs; analysis may reveal great barriers to services or limited information on the availability of services.

B. *Major Advantages*

1. Uses other existing methodologies to gather needed information.
2. Generally complements other sources of data.
3. Is relatively inexpensive because the information has already been gathered for other purposes.

C. *Major Disadvantages*

1. Current data have only limited applicability to needs assessment.

Table 5, cont'd.

2. Information is available only regarding persons who have participated in the formal service system.
3. Information may not be available in appropriate form for needs assessment.
4. Management information gathered by different agencies may well not be comparable, making it difficult to track clients or service patterns across agencies.

Source: Warheit, Bell, and Schwab, 1976; Research Group, Inc., 1976.

Table 6. Secondary Analysis of Existing Data.

I. *Analysis of Previous Studies*

This approach involves the analysis of previously gathered research data and data collected for other purposes by other sources, such as unemployment, crime, and juvenile delinquency statistics, to shed light on human services needs. These data can be used to determine the location and severity of various types of problems and the location and concentration of services designed to address those problems; assess the context in which problems occur; and identify possible target areas for service development or expansion.

A. *Major Data-Gathering Techniques*

Already existing social data gathered from a variety of relevant sources, organized, aggregated, disaggregated, and analyzed; such data assessed to determine if they are the most reliable and valid available; available across the geographical units being analyzed; available on an ongoing basis; related to the needs of the decision makers in regard to human services needs, rather than being utilized only because they are available; and combined on the basis of a common unit of analysis—for example, city or county.

B. *Major Advantages*

1. Uses already existing data and existing methodologies and therefore tends to be a flexible and low-cost technique that can gather data quickly in many situations.
2. Complements other needs assessment techniques.

C. *Major Disadvantages*

1. Data are often incomplete and thus unsatisfactory because they were gathered before the needs assessment study was conceived and designed.
2. Not all the necessary data may be available in usable form to assess all the needs of the population under study.
3. Problems with disaggregating data may preclude the use of some secondary data in assessing individual needs or in identifying individuals with more than one problem.

II. *Review of the Needs Information of Other Human Services Systems*

This approach involves a systematic review of the needs information gathered by other human services planning and delivery systems by means of meeting with other agencies (usually on a state level) and informally requesting their needs statements; reviewing the functional plans of other agencies, especially sections on the needs that those agencies are to address; and conducting program coordination surveys to identify duplication and gaps in provided services.

Table 6, cont'd.

A. *Major Data-Gathering Techniques*

Development and use, with other agencies, of an interview guide for gathering the following types of information: definitions of the services offered; the activities necessary to perform each of those services; eligibility criteria for service recipients; definitions of units of service; descriptions of services delivery areas; numbers of units of service currently being delivered; documented need, if available, for service by geographical unit; numbers of clients at risk, by type of service; and numbers of unserved persons in need of each type of service.

B. *Major Advantages*

1. Helps meet needs by reducing duplication and gaps in service.
2. Is a relatively inexpensive and flexible approach applicable to as few or as many ·other agencies as necessary.
3. Complements other needs assessment approaches.

C. *Major Disadvantages*

1. This approach requires considerable staff and time, if done correctly.
2. Data for ascertaining needs in an easily usable format may not be available in many agencies.
3. Compilation of the information required in this approach may be time-consuming.
4. Analysis of the resulting data may tend to be controversial and may require much discussion and reconciliation among agencies.

Source: Warheit, Bell, and Schwab, 1976; Research Group, Inc., 1976.

---

proaches under consideration. In addition, the administrator must evaluate the extent of the agency's commitment to change—its readiness to undertake major or minor reallocations of agency resources or reformulations of service priorities in the light of the findings of a needs assessment. Assessment approaches differ in their potential for producing data that could lead to recommendations for far-reaching changes in the agency's services delivery patterns or service priorities. Those approaches, for example, that directly query actual or potential recipients of the agency's services or those that utilize experts to report on the needs of the agency's clientele are more likely to result in findings with implications for radical modifications or alterations in services delivery patterns than indirect approaches such as social indicators and service statistics. The knowledgeable mental health administrator needs to keep these diverse potential consequences in mind in choosing needs assessment approaches from among the alternatives described in Tables 2 through 6.

Moreover, the assessment of the needs of a mental health center's target population should be the foundation for the planning and delivery of relevant and meaningful mental health services at the community, county, and state levels. Needs assessment should not be a process sporadically undertaken in isolation from the overall services delivery program; rather, it should be an integral and ongoing element of the center's service planning, development, and delivery process.

Conducting a Needs Assessment

Statement of Purpose. As with any research undertaking, if the results of the needs assessment are to ameliorate the problem that has occasioned the assessment, the entire undertaking must be based on clearly articulated questions, formulated in advance, that the assessment is to answer. The problem stimulating the research is found in the statement of the assessment's purpose and should be phrased as an assertion, not as a question. Once formulated, this statement of purpose should act as the source of the study's research questions. Data gathered by the assessment to answer those questions would then suggest approaches to remedying the problem.

Clear specification of the problem and the research questions in concrete operational terms is an essential precondition for gathering valid and meaningful data about the needs of the target population. Failure to be specific can result in unfocused data, at best, and in worthless findings not amenable to implementation, at worst. Moreover, an unclear statement of the problem and of the questions to be answered makes it difficult to determine whether or not a needs assessment is appropriate in the first place.

One constructive method for identifying and describing the main characteristics of a problem is to develop an issue paper, which is based on what is already known or what can easily be learned from existing sources and which includes the following topics (Kimmel, 1977):

1. The structure and likely causes and sources of the problem.
2. Known groups in the population that may be affected by the problem.
3. Objectives that might be met by agency action geared to remedying the problem.
4. Criteria that might be used to indicate progress toward resolving the problem.
5. An overview of both public and private programs already addressing the problem.
6. Estimated costs and impacts of efforts already underway and of other possible approaches to attacking the problem.
7. An identification of significant constraints on the reduction of the problem.
8. Major analytical or data problems that would have to be handled before further analysis can proceed.
9. A description of the additional study and analysis that must be undertaken and an estimate of the cost and duration.

A well-developed issue paper addressing these concerns totally or even partially would provide a firm foundation for determining whether a needs assessment or some other type of study should be undertaken. If the decision is to proceed with a needs assessment, the questions to be answered by that assessment must then be developed in a form that will assure that the resulting answers, in the form of needs assessment data, will illuminate ways of addressing the problem. A set of research questions might resemble the following:

- What are the social, emotional, and maintenance problems perceived by local citizens? How severe are these problems perceived to be?
- To what extent are citizens aware of the existence of services available to help them cope with or overcome these problems?
- Specifically, which services do they know to be available?
- If citizens are unaware of existing services designed to address those problems, to what extent do they believe that such services should be provided? If, on the other hand, they are aware of the existence of such services, to what extent do they believe that additional services should be developed to address those problems?
- Assuming that additional services were to be developed to address such problems, to what extent do the citizens believe that local tax dollars should be used to support such services?

All the major concepts appearing in the research questions should be defined concretely so that they can be measured and translated into unambiguous items in the data-collecting instrument.

Organizational Structure. Once the above considerations are confronted and resolved to the satisfaction of all the decision makers in the agency, an appropriate organizational structure should be established within the agency to legitimize the needs assessment, take responsibility for conducting it, and, on its completion, take steps to implement its findings. This structure should be a task force or steering committee with broad representation from all relevant segments of the agency, including board, administration, and clinical staff; the research personnel who will be involved in the assessment; the actual or potential client population; and the community at large.

A project director, who will take immediate responsibility for the day-to-day conduct of the needs assessment, must be selected. In doing so, the steering committee will have to confront the question of whether to choose someone from within the CMHC or someone brought in especially for this purpose. Both options have their advantages and disadvantages, but perhaps the most important factor is the size of the budget available for the needs assessment. If funding is limited, the agency may have no alternative but to assign to the project director's role the administrator or staff person thought to possess the most skills necessary for the task. However, if the CMHC has an adequate budget, a competent non-agency researcher could be engaged.

Review of Previous Studies. Starting from scratch in a needs assessment is both time-consuming and expensive; therefore, before any data-gathering work is begun, a thorough search for and examination of all available past and ongoing needs assessment studies and other pertinent information collection efforts should be undertaken. Such studies or data compilations might address some of the CMHC's current research questions underlying the proposed needs assessment, thereby reducing the scope, complexity, and expense of that study. In some instances, the location of an adequate range of pertinent data may even obviate entirely the need for a new assessment.

Many sources are available for already existing data, which usually can be obtained at minimal cost. One such resource is federal agencies that issue publications containing normative data potentially useful in interpreting local indicators of need. For example, the Biometry Division of NIMH publishes reports covering a wide range of topics relevant to local mental health programs, including data derived from an analysis of the annual *Inventory of Federally Funded Mental Health Centers*. In addition, the National Clearing House for Mental Health Information, the National Clearing House for Drug Abuse Information, and the National Clearing House for Alcohol Information all provide free computer literature searches in their areas of specialization and disseminate a broad range of information (Siegel, Attkisson, and Cohn, 1976).

Another especially valuable source of data particularly pertinent to the use of the social indicator method of needs assessment is the mental health demographic profile system (MHDPS), described in Attkisson and others (1978, p. 270):

> This data resource provides computer-stored demographic profiles on the standard community mental health catchment areas in the United States. These profiles contain data specific to individual catchment areas; they also present comparable data for the United States as a whole and for the state and county (counties) in which the catchment area is located. In addition, it is possible to integrate MHDPS data with the other data from the catchment area, such as service utilization statistics, public health statistics, vital statistics, and crime statistics. The flexibility of MHDPS has special value to a need study. The MHDPS output can be expanded or reduced in keeping with the specific interests of individual agencies. The availability of this extensive and useful demographic profile system allows human services agencies to have census data as a core building block for a broader social indicator analysis. The MHDPS tapes are available from state departments or divisions of mental health.

Developing Reliable and Valid Data-Gathering Instruments. After the planning and organizing phase has been completed, the next step is to select the specific types of instruments required to gather the data necessary to answer the needs assessment research questions. The principal task will be to locate already existing instruments or to develop new instruments that will yield the most reliable and valid data possible. Reliability refers to the consistency of measurement over time or of different measurements of the same phenomenon at the same time. To the extent that repeated measurements of the opinions or attitudes of people about their human services needs yield highly comparable results over a period too brief to have permitted real changes in those opinions or attitudes, the measurements are considered to be reliable. Validity, on the other hand, concerns the extent to which reality, or the true state of affairs, is being measured. Measurements are valid to the degree that they are actually measuring the phenomenon they purport to be measuring.

Although a variety of data-gathering instruments are used in various needs assessment approaches, by far the most common are the interview and the self-assessment questionnaire. An interview involves a direct interaction between the interviewer and the interviewee. Either in person or by telephone, the interviewer asks a list of questions called an interview schedule, which he or she fills out during the course of the interview. By contrast, a questionnaire is an instrument that is completed by a respondent or informant without the presence of an interviewer and is then either mailed back to the agency or collected. Table 7 specifies the principal types of questionnaires and interviews and describes the criteria for selecting among them.

Field testing the questionnaire or interview on a sample of the target population prior to its final administration is an essential step in developing a reliable and valid data-gathering instrument. Field testing is the only way to determine whether the instrument as a whole is intelligible to the population the agency wishes to sample and whether the instrument items convey to that population their intended meaning and are capable of eliciting a full range of responses. The penalty for not field testing an instrument is that the final data may prove meaningless or irrelevant with respect to the survey's research questions and the problem prompting the needs assessment.

The survey instrument should be field tested on a group of subjects who are as much as possible like the subjects to whom the finalized instrument will be administered—if at all possible, members of exactly the same population. Thus, if the CMHC's target population is the past and current recipients of any one or all of its programs, the questionnaire or interview should be field tested on a group of past and current recipients of the same services.

The field test subjects can, but need not, be a random sample from the population. Although the number of persons used for field testing an instrument is not fixed, the group should be large enough—minimally fifteen to twenty-five, optimally thirty to forty—to allow for the widest possible distribution of responses. The format for the field testing—that is, the conditions under which the instrument is administered, the length of the interview or questionnaire, the manner in which the interview is conducted, and the training of the interviewers—should be as identical as possible to the format envisioned for the final administration of the instrument to the target population. Because the field test is an essential troubleshooting procedure and not a mere formality, the data gathered from field test subjects should be carefully analyzed for inadequacies in the wording, sequencing, or content of one or more of the items.

Sampling the Population to Be Surveyed. Before any data-gathering instrument can be administered to collect needs assessment information, two important steps must be taken: first, the population to be surveyed must be identified; and, second, a plan must be designed to sample that population.

For purposes of the needs survey, a population, or universe, is the total group of cases with specified characteristics to which the study's findings are to be generalized. This may include all the clients that a mental health agency is currently serving, all the individuals or households residing in its catchment area, or, more narrowly, all persons admitted to the inpatient unit of the agency during a given period of time, all the case records closed during the past five years, or all

Table 7. Criteria for Selecting the Appropriate Type of Questionnaire or Interview.

I. *Mailed Versus Group-Administered Questionnaires*

   A. *Group-Administered Questionnaire*

      1. Use if and when the agency's entire target population or a representative sample of that population can be gathered in a natural way in one spot—as, for example, at a well-publicized community meeting sponsored by the agency, at an annual meeting, or at a meeting called to consider a situation or an issue of great concern to most of the target population.

      2. Advantages are low cost (elimination of postage expenses) and high response rate, particularly if respondents are given enough time to complete the questionnaire and are asked to deposit it in a prominent place as they leave the room or the building. These assets outweigh the liabilities of less time and lack of total privacy in the completion of the questionnaire.

   B. *Mailed Questionnaire*

      1. Use when a group-administered situation is not possible or desirable; where the nature of the instrument items indicates the need for privacy and for sufficient time to formulate considered answers; and where sample representation is of paramount importance.

      2. Advantages are that the questionnaire can be distributed at any time, rather than at an infrequent, appropriate gathering or meeting of the target population, that the mailed questionnaire may give the appearance of being more professional, and that it may permit greater anonymity of responses.

      3. Disadvantages are low response rates, additional cost for postage and follow-up reminders, and delay in the beginning of data analysis as questionnaires trickle in.

II. *In-Person Versus Telephone Interviews*

   A. *In-Person Interviews*

      1. Use when interview topics require good rapport to deal with sensitive material; when the purposes of the study must be explained in detail to elicit cooperation and the meaning of specific items must be interpreted; where extensive probing of interviewee responses is desirable; and where the schedule and the coverage of content areas are comprehensive.

      2. Other advantages are the ability to legitimate the interview through the presentation of visible credentials, which may be of importance to many interviewees; the opportunity to ask a broader range of questions due to such legitimation; the ability to visually monitor respondent nonverbal behavior, thereby reducing subjective impressions and enhancing data validity; and increased representativeness of the sample, which can be chosen to reflect all relevant strata of the population.

      3. Disadvantages are the high cost of callbacks, monitoring of field operations, and interviewer training and travel time; turnover of interviewers who may weary of or find arduous the interviewing process, thereby necessitating the recruitment and training of additional interviewers at additional cost; and the possibility of personal danger to interviewers traveling through or working in areas of the city experiencing social tension and high crime rates, which may require costly safeguards or insurance protection.

   B. *Telephone Interviews*

      1. Use when the agency or the needs assessment process is well known and legitimated to the target population; when the interview topics are relatively noncontroversial or nonsensitive; and when adequate data can be gathered in a relatively short time.

      2. Advantages are the low cost of less-trained interviewers, no travel allowances,

Table 7, cont'd.

and lower cost of callbacks; more comprehensive coverage due to shorter interview schedule; and some increased validity due to the anonymity of the telephone
conversation context.

3. Disadvantages are the limited amount of time possible for telephone interview;
   suspicion or wariness on the part of potential interviewees due to the lack of opportunity for full legitimation of the interviewer or the study and, consequently,
   a higher refusal rate; the greater ease with which an interviewee can break off
   contact before the interview is completed, thereby resulting in less usable information; and reduced representation of the target population due to nonowner-
   ship of telephones or to unlisted telephone numbers, which introduces systematic
   biases into the final data.

incidents of drug overdose coming to the agency's attention during a given six-
month period.

Any segment of the population specified by certain criteria constitutes a
stratum, or subpopulation, of the total population. Thus, the male members of all
families seen in counseling, all clients age sixty-five or older, all cases with a
designated presenting problem, or all census tracts with an ethnic minority population of more than 25 percent may be considered strata, or subpopulations, of
their respective populations. However, if it is more congruent with the purpose of
the needs assessment to do so, each of these specified aggregates of cases may be
considered to be the total population to which the findings are to be generalized,
rather than only a stratum of a larger population.

A sample is a segment of a total population selected in such a way as to
represent the characteristics of the population from which it is drawn. The purpose of sampling is to enable administrators or planners to make generalizations
about the total population; the characteristics of the sample itself are not the main
concern.

All the considerations involved in sampling cannot be considered in this
chapter. However, the needs assessment steering committee and the project director must be aware of the crucial nature not only of the type of sampling design
selected for a given needs assessment approach but also of the sampling process
itself and of the need to safeguard sample integrity throughout the assessment.
Since these factors directly affect the validity of the data and its generalizability to
the population, even a small investment in a research consultant early in the
undertaking will yield valuable payoffs, considering the time, energy, and money
being invested in the needs assessment. An expert methodologist can help to
ensure optimal sampling design, sample size, maintenance of sample integrity,
data analysis of sample findings, and generalizability to the population.

Conducting Field Operations. As in sampling, all the considerations involved in the gathering of needs assessment data cannot be discussed in detail in this chapter. However, it is important to note that field operations for the needs assessment must be carefully organized and supervised if sample integrity is to be maintained and if the final data are to be complete, valid, and reliable. The two principal data-gathering methods, self-administered questionnaires and face-to-face interviews, have essentially similar field requirements, although they do differ in some respects. For a more detailed consideration of research field operations, the steering committee and the project director should consult experts in survey research in private research firms or at the universities or colleges in their communities. In addition, certain published references provide step-by-step instruction in field operations (Warheit, Bell, and Schwab, 1976; Goode and Hatt, 1952; Selltiz and others, 1976).

Analyzing the Needs Assessment Data. Data analysis is the crucial phase of eliciting from the raw data the findings that will identify the target population's problems and service needs and will help the mental health center to better address those needs and problems. The data analysis phase of the needs assessment process should include a written plan for data analysis prior to the start of the study, a plan for computer use, and specification of the audience for the final report.

Since these and related tasks demand specialized expertise, sufficient funds should be included in the needs assessment budget for purchasing the necessary statistical and data analysis consultation from a research or statistical specialist at a local college or research-oriented corporation. Such consultation may sometimes be contributed without charge by a faculty member or corporate specialist.

Utilizing Needs Assessment Data. As the proof of the pudding is in the eating, the principal test and value of all the work that has gone into a needs assessment is in the utilization of its findings to inform services delivery policies and resources allocation decisions. As noted earlier, a commitment to implementing the results of a needs assessment should be a precondition for undertaking it in the first place.

However, even with the best of intentions, implementation may prove to be difficult or even impossible. An explanation of why agencies sometimes do not use the findings of competently executed agency research—program evaluation as well as needs assessment—to modify agency practice and policy is beyond the scope of this chapter. Nevertheless, an emerging literature does exist that analyzes the barriers to the utilization of research findings and identifies possible ways of overcoming those barriers (Patton, 1978; Warheit, Bell, and Schwab, 1976; Weiss, 1972).

The CMHC steering committee, project director, and administrator should attempt at the outset of the assessment to identify the major forces in their agency and community that would hinder or actively oppose the utilization of the assessment findings. Tables 8 and 9 present some of those principal barriers, as well as the steps that may be taken to overcome them and promote the implementation of the needs assessment findings.

Implementation is a difficult and often frustrating process requiring per-

Table 8. Barriers to the Utilization of Needs Assessment Findings.

I. *Staff Member Resistance to Change*

    A. Staff members, including the agency administrator, may have a strong commitment to the CMHC's current pattern of services.

    B. Staff members may be anxious about possible termination, major redeployment, or changes in staff responsibilities due to needs assessment findings.

    C. Some staff members may be concerned that such changes in assignments or responsibilities may have been motivated by inadequate performance on their part.

    D Some staff members may be suspicious of and resistant to the research process and the scientific method as a way of determining the problems and needs of the agency's target population.

    E. Some staff members may have a strong sense of being left out of the needs assessment process.

II. *Organizational Resistance to Change*

    A. Established patterns of interaction among board, staff, and administration may be strongly rooted in the organization's history and provide organizational stability.

    B. All organizations have functions and purposes other than goal achievement that tend to resist change.

III. *Communitywide Resistance to Change*

    A. Program territory or turf considerations among human services agencies may exist.

    B. In most communities, long-established and complex interorganizational relationships and interactional patterns exist that have been difficult to achieve and therefore resist major changes.

Table 9. Conditions for and Steps to Promoting Utilization of Needs Assessment Findings.

I. *Overcoming Staff Resistance to Change*

    A. Genuine staff involvement in all phases of the planning and execution of the needs assessment. Such involvement should begin with the onset of the assessment, continue through its conclusion, and involve at least the following steps:

        1. Explaining the rationale and purpose of the assessment, including the fact that it is not prompted by individual staff member performance, but rather by the need of the entire agency to appraise its services delivery policies and practices.

        2. Presenting realistic expectations for the assessment and providing an opportunity for staff input, both of ideas and of specific research tasks.

        3. Presenting to the staff periodic progress reports about, as well as the final results of, the assessment, prior to releasing that information to other agencies and to the community.

        4. Involving the staff in drawing recommendations from the findings for changes in agency policy, programs, and services delivery patterns.

    B. Realistic assurances to staff members that assessment findings will not result in staff layoff and that, if redeployment becomes necessary, the agency will help retrain them.

    C. Development of an interorganizational mechanism or structure for involving all staff members in translating assessment recommendations into clear, specific changes in ongoing policies, organizational practices, and job tasks.

    D. Clear documentation by study findings of the need for specific changes in the agency's services delivery system.

II. *Overcoming Organizational Resistance to Change*

    A. A strong, clearly enunciated commitment on the part of the CMHC board and

Table 9, cont'd.

---

administration to support and implement any changes deemed necessary by the assessment.

  B. Development of a mechanism or structure for translating the assessment recommendations into clear, specific changes in ongoing organizational policies, practices, and job tasks.

III. *Overcoming Communitywide Resistance to Change*

  A. Unequivocal documentation by the assessment findings of the need for changes in community agencies.
  B. Development of a coalition of agencies to sponsor and conduct the needs assessment.
  C. Development of an interagency change process for translating needs assessment recommendations into changes in communitywide service patterns.

---

sistence, careful planning, and a clear focus. However, as Warheit, Bell, and Schwab (1976, p. 62) have noted, "change is a process and, once that process is put in motion, it generates 'a life of its own.' Any change in the program structures of our organization, however small, may be sufficient to generate other changes of a more profound nature. Therefore, changes based on needs assessment do not have to be radical, highly visible, or dramatic. It may be that a few small changes can be seized for further modifications of greater scope. Thus, it is important to implement the most modest of recommendations for change, even when the immediate outcome seems inconsequential."

Conclusion

This chapter began with a discussion of the basic concepts and principles of needs assessment, followed by a description of the most common assessment methods. Attention was then devoted to the process of conducting a mental health agency needs assessment: getting organized and getting started; developing reliable and valid data-gathering instruments; sampling; and gathering and analyzing data. Finally, the difficulty of implementing study results in policy and resources allocation decisions was addressed, and the major barriers to the utilization of needs assessment findings and of the conditions and steps that can be taken to promote such utilization were summarized.

References

Attkisson, C. C., and others (Eds.). *Evaluation of Human Service Programs.* New York: Academic Press, 1978.

Bell, R. A., and others (Eds.). *Need Assessment in Health and Human Services: Proceedings of the Louisville National Conference.* Louisville, Ky.: International City Managers Association, 1976.

Bradshaw, J. "The Concept of Need." In N. Gilbert and H. Specht (Eds.), *Planning for Social Welfare.* Englewood Cliffs, N.J.: Prentice-Hall, 1977.

Bureau of Research and Evaluation, Division of Planning and Evaluation. *Annotated Bibliography of Needs Assessment*. Gainesville, Fla.: State Department of Health and Rehabilitative Services, 1975.

Center for Social Research and Development. *Analysis and Synthesis of Needs Assessment Research in the Field of Human Services*. Denver: Denver Research Institute, University of Denver, 1974.

Cox, G. B., Carmichael, S. J., and Dightman, C. R. "The Optimal Treatment Approach to Needs Assessment." *Evaluation and Program Planning*, 1979, *2*, 269–275.

Delbecq, A. L., Van de Ven, A. H., and Gustafson, D. H. *Group Techniques for Program Planning: A Guide to Nominal Group and Delphi Processes*. Glenview, Ill.: Scott, Foresman, 1975.

Epstein, I., and Tripodi, T. *Research Techniques for Program Planning, Monitoring and Evaluation*. New York: Columbia University Press, 1977.

Goode, W. J., and Hatt, P. K. *Methods in Social Reseach*. New York: McGraw-Hill, 1952.

Kimmel, W. A. *Needs Assessment: A Critical Perspective*. Washington, D.C.: U.S. Government Printing Office, 1977.

League of California Cities. *Handbook: Assessing Human Needs*. Sacramento: League of California Cities, 1975.

Minnesota State Planning Agency. *Needs Assessment: A Guide for Human Service Agencies*. St. Paul: Minnesota State Planning Agency, 1977.

Moroney, R. "Needs Assessment: Concepts, Issues and Methods." In Institute for Social Service Planning, *Problem Analysis and Needs Assessment: An Expanding Role for the Local Human Services Administration*. Chapel Hill: University of North Carolina Press, 1977.

Mustian, D. R., and See, J. J. "Indicators of Mental Health Needs: An Empirical and Pragmatic Evaluation." *Journal of Health and Social Behavior*, 1973, *14*, (1), 23–27.

National Institute of Mental Health. *A Working Manual of Simple Program Evaluation Techniques for Mental Health Centers*. Washington, D.C.: National Institute of Mental Health, 1976.

Patton, M. Q. *Utilization-Focused Evaluation*. Beverly Hills, Calif.: Sage, 1978.

Project Share. *Human Services Bibliography Series: Needs Assessment*. Rockville, Md.: Aspen Systems, 1976.

Research Group, Inc. *Techniques for Needs Assessment in Social Services Planning*. Atlanta: Research Group, Inc., 1976.

Scheff, J. "The Use of Client Utilization Data to Determine Social Planning Needs." In R. A. Bell and others (Eds.), *Need Assessment in Health and Human Services: Proceedings of the Louisville National Conference*. Louisville, Ky.: International City Managers Association, 1976.

Schneider, M. "The 'Quality of Life' and Social Indicators Research." *Public Administration Review*, 1976, *36*, 296–305.

Selltiz, C., and others. *Research Methods in Social Relations*. (3rd ed.) New York: Holt, Rinehart and Winston, 1976.

Shapek, R. A. "Problems and Deficiencies in the Needs Assessment Process." *Public Administration Review*, 1975, *35,* 754–758.

Siegel, L. M., Attkisson, C. C., and Cohn, A. H. "Mental Health Needs Assessment: Strategies and Techniques." In W. A. Hargreaves, C. C. Attkisson, and J. E. Sorensen (Eds.), *Resource Materials for Community Mental Health Program Evaluation.* Rockville, Md.: National Institute of Mental Health, 1976.

Warheit, G. J., Bell, R. A., and Schwab, J. J. *Needs Assessment Approaches: Concepts and Methods.* Washington, D.C.: National Institute of Mental Health, 1976.

Warren, R. "Community Needs: How to Identify and Understand Them." In F. Cox and others (Eds.), *Tactics and Techniques of Community Practice.* Itasca, Ill.: Peacock, 1977.

Weiss, C. H. *Evaluation Research.* Englewood Cliffs, N.J.: Prentice-Hall, 1972.

❧ 21 ❧

Residential
Facilities and
Programs

Barbara J. Friesen

*Managers of residential programs are often faced with a variety of compet-
ing demands from staff and clients, and it is difficult to separate clinical
from administrative decisions. This chapter addresses the problems of administering twenty-four-hour residential mental health facilities and introduces some of the issues and common tasks involved in developing and
managing them. Principles and methods of residential care are examined,
with specific reference to inpatient services, psychiatric halfway houses,
state hospital wards, and owner-operated group homes. The chapter presents a number of management approaches to assist administrators in meeting the requirements of physical, social, and treatment needs. Friesen favors
creating a treatment milieu that maximizes the health and the capability of
residents and staff.*

All residential programs must provide for clients' physical, social, and
treatment needs. The maintenance and survival of the organization require
attention to staff needs and to the expectations of funding sources and community. Residential programs struggle with a fundamental dilemma: The ability to
structure and organize the resident's experience up to twenty-four hours each day
can maximize the impact of the services provided, but accompanying this opportunity is the danger of contributing to the resident's disability by creating dependency and constricting social roles.

Clinical and Administrative Issues

Managing a residential mental health facility is something like learning to
juggle. The manager must simultaneously consider a variety of demands that may

be contradictory. Choices made in response to one set of needs may restrict the alternatives available to solve other problems. The separation of clinical from administrative issues is difficult, and few managerial decisions may be considered routine. I shall begin with breakfast at four residential settings, looking at the common tasks, demands, and problems the manager faces.

Ridgeville State Hospital

6:00 A.M. Mrs. Bleeker, psychiatric aide on nights, finishes waking the patients on Ward A. There is a lot to be done before the day shift at 7:00 A.M. The residents need to be up, dressed, medicated, and breakfasted. The beds must be made, the ward tidied. Mrs. Bleeker takes pride in her ability to get forty people organized and her work done by change of shift time.

Things have changed a lot in the last ten years. Before, the patients ate in a central dining room in the basement of the building, but now meals are served "family style" in the ward dining area as part of the new "normalization" program. The meals arrive in hot carts, and the patients take turns serving the food and clearing the dishes. The dining area has new curtains and bright plastic tablecloths.

6:25 A.M. Oatmeal, scrambled eggs, toast, and peaches this morning—a good breakfast. You can't expect them to cook pancakes or fried eggs for the 200 people in this building.

This normalization program is OK, but people hardly stay long enough to forget their table manners anymore. And it does make it harder to do a good job sometimes. Take the beds, for instance. Before, Mrs. Bleeker and two or three patient helpers could get them all done in a half hour and get them made right. Now patients are supposed to do their own. It's really hard to motivate some of the patients to do a good job, and it really does take longer. And men and women in the same ward can be a problem.

6:45 A.M. We need to get these dishes cleared up. No sense being bothered by all the changes. It's much worse during the day, they say. Lots of new people with lots of bright ideas, and the doctors seem to go along with it.

6:55 A.M. Here comes the day shift. They usually don't care what went on during the night shift. "How is everything?" "Just fine—it was a quiet night."

Mattox Community Psychiatric Unit

6:30 A.M. Scott, the psychiatric technician on the night shift, finishes his notes for the day shift. It was quite a night: two patients in seclusion and an admission at 3:00 A.M. He wasn't much trouble—appears to be senile or pretty confused, anyway. The police found him downtown and brought him in for his own good. Mrs. Ferguson in seclusion was pretty noisy for a while, but she went to sleep after the night nurse gave her some Thorazine, I.M. She's quite an interesting case. The diagnostic team is still doing their workup, but she'll probably settle down and be in group therapy in a few days.

6:45 A.M. Breakfast has started for those who are up and eat hospital food. Some of the patients just want coffee or fix Instant Breakfast in the kitchen. You can't blame people for not wanting oatmeal. Hope they don't leave a mess again.

The night shift isn't so bad, really. You get a chance to read the patients' files, and it's always interesting to talk to them and see how they really are. They say we're all a part of the treatment team, but you don't really get much chance to do anything when everybody's asleep. Harry C. had trouble sleeping last night, and he really opened up with me—talked about his army days, his wife, and his drinking problem. He called it a problem! That's really the first step. Hope a vacancy comes up on the day shift, though. Most of the therapy goes on during the day, and that's what I really want to do. Patients come and go pretty fast here. You see some of them every few months or so, but you really have to wonder what happens to the rest of them.

Lincoln Halfway House

6:00 A.M. Jim A. fixes himself eggs, toast, and coffee before he catches the bus to work. He used the last of the eggs, so he adds eggs to the grocery list on the kitchen blackboard. He's been on his job for three months and is beginning to enjoy the early morning routine of getting off to work. At first it was pretty frightening, and he was glad that Sue, one of the managers, had breakfast with him and rode the bus with him during the first week. Jim liked the idea of having a job for pay but was unsure about whether he could work well enough to please his boss. At a meeting last week, the job supervisor said that Jim was doing very well.

8:00 A.M. Mary and Stewart, the residents who are in charge of planning and cooking meals for the week, have a hasty conference about the breakfast menu. Jim ate all the eggs, so they can't have French toast, as planned. Maybe they didn't order enough eggs, but it makes it hard to plan when people just come in the kitchen and eat what they please. *And* he didn't do his dishes. He'll hear about that at the house meeting tonight.

Mary and Stewart settle on oatmeal, fruit, and toast, even though someone is sure to complain about the oatmeal. Maybe people should just get their own breakfast, anyway. Sharon comes into the kitchen, adds laundry soap to the grocery list, and says she just wants coffee. She has a dentist appointment this morning and doesn't feel like eating much.

8:45 A.M. Sue comes in and suggests that if Stewart and Mary ride along to Sharon's appointment, they can pick up some groceries.

9:00 A.M. Charles, the social worker, and Bill, the vocational counselor, arrive and stop in to see the director, Alice. They point to this morning as an example of the coordination problems in the program. They are trying to get a "prejob" group going, but three of the members have gone off with Sue in the car. They don't know if Sue is deliberately sabotaging the treatment program they're trying to start, but in any case, she "forgot" that a meeting was scheduled.

Mrs. Anderson's Group Home

7:00 A.M. Mrs. Anderson starts fixing breakfast. She puts on the coffee first because Joe, Martha, and Rose will be down soon, wanting coffee to drink on the porch while they smoke. Sometimes Mrs. Anderson feels a little sorry for them, especially when it's cold outside. But it's her house, the state doesn't pay her to take the risk of somebody starting a fire, and she doesn't like smoking. With these kinds of people, you just have to have some rules. They can't help being the way they are, and if they were able to take more responsibility, they wouldn't be here, would they?

Sometimes it seems like the state people don't understand the residents, and it puts Mrs. Anderson in a bind. Like the medication thing—the residents are supposed to take their own. The social worker explained the rules—that Mrs. Anderson is not a nurse, so she can't give out drugs. If the people really could be trusted with their meds, it would be OK, but she's not going to take the chance of somebody taking too much, or worse yet, not taking any at all. The social worker didn't really like the way she keeps the meds locked up and then watches to be sure each person takes the right things and the right amount. But they *do* need supervision.

A quick breakfast this morning because today is grocery shopping day. *That's* something nobody can complain about. Mrs. Anderson is a good cook, but can't stand to have anybody else messing around in the kitchen when she's trying to work. Residents do clear up their own dishes, but nobody, including Mr. Anderson, ever puts them into the dishwasher correctly.

Mrs. Anderson thinks she will ask Martha and Carol if they want to go along to the grocery store. It will do them good to get out, and they did clean their rooms nicely. Wish you could say the same for Joe. He just doesn't seem to care if things are messy, but you can't let things go forever. Mrs. Anderson will probably have to clean his room again today.

The social worker was concerned that people sat around a lot. They sure do, but what can you expect? You can't spend all day driving people around. There's enough of that, anyway, what with taking Rose and Joe to the mental health clinic for their treatments.

Some of them used to walk down to the shopping center. When Rose got caught with some cologne she hadn't paid for, Mrs. Anderson had to put a stop to that. Just as well that they stay home. She used to worry about where they were and what they were doing. And the traffic is so heavy where they crossed York Avenue.

7:30 A.M. "Good morning, all. Pour yourselves some coffee and come back inside in fifteen minutes. I'll have breakfast ready by then."

These glimpses of residential settings suggest some of the ways daily life can be organized. Differences between settings emerge as decisions are made about how to meet common requirements: provision for the physical and daily living needs of residents, development and implementation of a treatment or rehabilitation program, and organizational maintenance and survival.

Physical/Daily Living Needs

Daily living needs include the provision of food, shelter, clothing, laundry, and housekeeping. Residents' physical health and safety must also be ensured. At a minimum, meals must be nourishing, of sufficient quantity, and served on a fairly regular basis. Someone must plan, purchase, prepare, and serve the food and clear up after meals. One important decision is whether or how residents will be involved in this process and in other tasks, such as laundry and housekeeping.

The physical structures within which residents are housed can vary widely. Beyond basic shelter, questions of safety, maintenance, adequate space, and architectural arrangements that support the goals and purposes of the organization must be considered. Concerns for security and economy are reflected in the architecture of many older state hospital buildings. Arrangements such as the glass-enclosed nursing station placed to allow surveillance over many patients in a large area, toilet stalls without doors, and common bathing and sleeping areas were typical. Recent efforts to improve living conditions and treatment include provisions for privacy and structural arrangements that allow and encourage socialization.

Community residential programs often do not have such a legacy of architectural anachronisms. Many are fairly recent and relatively small; so appropriate facilities can be sought and remodeled without prohibitive cost. Decisions about space must be connected to the program purpose and function. For example, a halfway house where most residents are working or involved in community activities during the day requires much less space than a setting where the treatment program is primarily in-house.

Providing for the safety and security of residents is one of the knottiest problems in residential facilities. Two major considerations are involved: cost and the trade-offs between security concerns and the degree of autonomy and freedom desirable for residents. The cost of residential programs is high partly because of the need for twenty-four-hour staffing, sprinkling and alarm systems, adequate maintenance, and other precautions to ensure the safety of staff and residents. Security concerns include management of residents who may be a threat to themselves or others and protection of residents from outsiders who may harm or victimize them.

Concern for residents' safety is often at odds with encouraging increased participation in community life. Mrs. Anderson was concerned about physical safety (crossing a busy street) and about a resident's shoplifting. Although her response could be interpreted as maternalistic and overprotective, the issues that worried her are common to all residential programs.

Treatment Program

An emphasis on the treatment and rehabilitation of residents is what distinguishes a mental health treatment facility from a residence, a hotel, or other place where people might live. The extent to which treatment goals are central varies widely from one setting to another.

Putting together a treatment program requires attention to two major areas: identification and choice of methods for assisting clients to resolve problems and increase skills and definition of social arrangements and roles of staff and residents around treatment goals.

All residential programs are challenged with creating what Wolins and Wozner (1977) call a "reclaiming milieu." This is an environment that promotes independence and health rather than dependence and disability. Management decisions about the design and continuing operation of the residential facility are pivotal in creating and maintaining such an environment. The manager in this sense may be described as a "social engineer."

Current practice in residential mental health settings is influenced by the disabling effects of the "total institution." Goffman (1961) describes lessons from the state hospital experience. Locked into the social role of "patient," residents become dependent and institutionalized and their social and self-care skills atrophy. Goffman (1961) also describes a "binary system" of extreme separation of staff and resident roles and values. Staff members are the caretakers for the incompetent residents.

The limitations of the total institution are not confined to large state hospitals. When the same attitudes and restrictive practices occur in community residential facilities, the residents' experience may be very much the same. (See, for example, Bassuk and Gerson, 1978; Jones, 1975.) The development of a "reclaiming milieu" in residential mental health settings may be supported by the following propositions:

1. *No residential environment is neutral.* Except for those who stay very briefly, the residential setting becomes a socializing agent for staff and residents alike.
2. *"Overprovision" may be as harmful as neglect.* When the organization does for residents what they could do for themselves, their opportunities to behave responsibly and independently are diminished.
3. *Efficiency may contribute to disability.* A predictable, stable environment is a positive experience for many residents. To the extent that the residential experience becomes routine, requiring a minimum of effort and few decisions, it may also be stultifying.
4. *"Big is bad."* Increased size of wards and, in some cases, total organizations is negatively associated with individualized care, expectations for client independence, and discharge rates. Large size has been found to be positively associated with degree of disturbed behavior and cost of care. (See Holland, 1973; Hrebiniak and Alutto, 1973; Linn, 1970; Martin and Segal, 1977; Moos, 1972.) Although the manager may have no control over the total size of the organization, methods for reducing the size of living groups and administrative units should be considered.
5. *More staff is usually better.* Higher staff/resident ratios are associated with higher staff expectations for resident independence (Martin and Segal, 1977), treatment progress (Becker, 1969), and higher discharge rates (Linn, 1970).
6. *Decision making by lower staff levels tends to improve care.* Individualized

patient care (Holland, 1973) and expectations for resident autonomy (Moos, 1972) were higher when line staff members were involved in decisions about treatment planning and the organization of life on the living unit. In order for staff members to expect independent, responsible behavior from residents, they must also feel competent and responsible.

7. *The physical environment is important.* There is increasing awareness that the setting of mental health organizations reflects society's estimation of the inhabitants and may contribute to treatment progress or lack thereof. Holahan and Saegert (1973) describe a successful remodeling project that was undertaken with specific social goals in mind.

8. *Administrative and clinical issues often overlap.* Because of the powerful and constant effect of the organizational environment on residents, the manager should be alert to the impact of even everyday decisions.

Organizational Maintenance and Survival

Organizational maintenance and survival includes all those activities that do not directly address the residents' daily living and treatment needs. These activities include securing adequate funding, staffing, and obtaining clients. Effective mechanisms for coordinating services, staying in touch with the community, and making policy decisions must be created. Assuring compliance with health, safety, licensing, and accreditation standards has required increased attention in recent years.

Goals, Treatment Philosophy, and Organizational Structure

Goals, philosophy, and structure are abstract and do not beg for attention in the same way as a kitchen fire or a staff rebellion. It is easy for the manager to become involved in the business of running an organization with little time to reflect on how it got the way it is or how it might be better. My interest is in how the manager combines the goals, treatment philosophy, and structure of the organization to form what must be our ultimate concern, the resident's experience.

Some forces that affect the residential setting are external requirements and are not under the manager's control. Many internal decisions, however, also determine the direction and environment of the organization. As I review these "organization shapers," think about a residential setting with which you are familiar. Where does that facility stand in relation to these areas? To what extent is each factor amenable to intervention by the manager?

Although each residential organization may develop other objectives, three overall goals are common to any residential mental health facility:

1. *Treatment or rehabilitation* of residents.
2. *Social control* (protection of society from persons who are dangerous to themselves or others or whose lives must be managed or regulated in some way).
3. *Care and custody* of persons who are unable to provide their own needs, who need protection and a sheltered environment.

The degree to which any of these overall purposes is dominant varies with the type of residential settings. The emphasis on particular goals may also shift over time, either because of changes in client needs or because of changing priorities external to the organization. Differences between residential programs may be related to the following factors:

1. *Auspices.* Publicly funded and mandated programs usually have a greater responsibility for social control functions than privately funded and controlled programs. Responsibility for persons who are involuntarily committed, including those whose commitment results from criminal acts, rests with the public system. The state hospital has historically been assigned this function. As persons who are involuntarily committed are included in community facilities, emphasis on social control will increase in these programs.

2. *Degree of control over intake.* Residential programs that can screen and select residents also have greater control over the shape and direction of their programs. Residential facilities vary widely in the extent to which they are selective about the types and numbers of clients they serve.

3. *Type of client served.* Community residential programs are often developed around the needs of a specific population. Dimensions that shape programs may include age, sex, degree of supervision or physical care required, and the treatment and rehabilitation needs of each client. Thus, nursing homes may serve the elderly mentally disabled who are also physically infirm, and a halfway house program may be designed for ex-patients for whom partial or full employment is a goal.

    Community hospitals may have limitations on the length of stay that reflect financial considerations (the patient's insurance limit has been reached) and/or prognosis. Because the state hospital may place no restriction on admission or length of stay based on the patient's lack of money or degree of impairment, it has often become a repository for the poorest and most severely disabled persons.

4. *Recent incidents.* Residential programs may experience fluctuations in the degree to which certain goals are emphasized. A common phenomenon is pressure to increase the social control function of the program because of an incident involving a resident or even an incident "somewhere" involving an "ex-mental patient" that receives unfavorable publicity.

Goals concerning treatment, social control, and care and custody are not entirely compatible, and the emergence of one mandate may diminish the organization's capacity to respond fully to another. Social control concerns, for example, may impose restrictions on clients' movement and autonomy that contradict treatment aims. Resources devoted to ensuring minimum fire safety standards are then not available for transportation or other needs.

Two other goal-related issues complicate the manager's life. The first is that goals are often not explicitly stated. When formal goal statements do exist, social control is often not described as a goal, even though it may be of great importance to funding sources or to the community at large. Sometimes the residential facility manager may discover the real community norms only when they are violated. A second problem is that various sources of goals, such as funding sources, licensing bodies, the public, and staff, may disagree about which goals should be emphasized. It is important for the manager of a residential program to be clear about the extent to which overall goals influence the program shape. Reflect on your residential program or one with which you are familiar. What emphasis is placed on each major goal? What are the sources of these goals? What implications does this goal emphasis have for the management of this particular program? Where are there conflicts?

Each residential setting is characterized by a belief system about the nature of mental illness and about the appropriate responses to residents' needs and problems. When the philosophy and related goals are expressed in a formal statement, decisions about the numbers and kinds of staff members needed, the roles they assume, and how they should be organized may be made in relation to such a statement. Frequently, however, the philosophy is not formalized or coherent, reflecting the mix of training and socialization of the staff members. Many mental health setting employees have different and sometimes conflicting philosophies.

Organizational structures may be either carefully designed to support treatment philosophy and methods or may evolve piecemeal in response to demands and problems. Residential facilities will be most effective when the philosophy and treatment methods are clearly stated and organizational structure is developed to support the treatment approaches and methods used.

I shall examine two contrasting treatment approaches and complementary organizational structures. The illness/medical model is often combined with the hierarchical approach to organizational structure. The social treatment approach is supported by a horizontal, more democratic structure. These treatment approaches and structures are summarized in Table 1.

Illness/Medical Approach

Client problems represent an illness to be cured in the illness/medical approach. People are "patients" who place themselves in the hands of experts who administer the appropriate treatments, which usually occur at a specified time and place. The patient role is fairly passive. Patients are expected to cooperate with treatment and to supply information upon which diagnosis and treatment are based. The role is seen as temporary; patients are relieved of usual responsibilities until they are "better."

Staff roles and duties are clearly delineated. The physician is charged with overall responsibility for the patient. Other treatment providers may include social workers, psychologists, nurses, and occupational therapists. Supportive personnel provide housekeeping, cooking, maintenance, transportation, and other functions that keep the organization running.

Therapeutic functions are seen as largely separate from daily living activities. The organization is the "context" or place where treatment occurs. The

Table 1. Treatment Approaches and Structures.

Dimensions	Illness/Medical Approach	Social Treatment Approach
Problem cause	May be genetic, chemical, result of early experiences	More emphasis on social and environmental factors
Location of problem	Within client	Client/social environment
Definition of problem	Illness	Problems in living, need for interpersonal and social skills
Major treatment approaches	Medications, individual and group therapy	Teaching skills to live successfully in social environment. Community *is* treatment.
Emphasis on organizational environment	*Low-medium* (should be safe, pleasant context for treatment; daily living/treatment largely separate)	*High* (social and physical environment *is* treatment; daily living/treatment inseparable)
Role of resident	"Patient" (passive but cooperative)	"Community member" (active participant in own and others' development)
Staff roles	Expert, specialist (roles fairly distinct)	Catalyst, role model, resource person (roles blurred)
Administrative implications	Administrative and clinical functions often distinct	Administrative and clinical functions often mixed
Organizational structure	Hierarchical and bureaucratic	Flat and democratic

relationship between the institution and the community is often distant. The community is the place to which patients are discharged when they are well and a source of referrals and placements. Good community relations depend on preserving an image of good care and the avoidance of unfavorable incidents.

A bureaucratic structure complements the illness view of treatment. Advantages of this form of organization include the ability to maximize the use of technical knowledge through specialization. Thus, a treatment approach that includes specific therapies applied to particular diagnostic categories or types of patients can be efficiently delivered within this type of organization. Various specialties and/or departments can be organized to provide for clients' daily living needs. Efficiency is increased through centralized operations, such as planning, preparation, and service of meals. Supplies may be purchased more cheaply in bulk. Rules and procedures that guide the conduct and operation of various parts of the organization increase coordination and predictability.

Organizational hierarchy serves as a means of coordination through a supervisory structure that assures that tasks and treatment will be implemented as planned. Responsibility for goal setting and decisions about unforeseen events is invested with a few people at the top of the organization. Thus, decisions are made by those with the widest perspective about program needs.

Advantages of this form of organization include (1) efficient means of organizing and coordinating routine tasks, particularly for populations of severely disturbed patients requiring structured treatment environments; (2) centralized decision-making coordination between organizational departments, also providing a way of dealing with nonroutine events; and (3) continuity enhanced by attaching specific rights and duties to positions so that staff members can be hired on the basis of specific skills and abilities.

Possible disadvantages of this model include (1) the formalized structure may increase the extent to which staff members perceive human problems as routine and (2) reliance on bureaucratic organizational forms when many tasks and events are nonroutine may result in inappropriate application of existing rules and/or excessive dependence on top decision makers.

Social Treatment Approach

Within the social treatment approach residents' problems are seen as largely social and environmental, rather than as residing solely within the person. Treatment approaches involve all aspects of the person's life, with an emphasis on increasing his or her ability to assume responsibility for personal needs, and the development of necessary social and daily living skills.

Residents are active participants in their own treatment and development, as well as in that of other residents. Staff members serve as resource persons, role models, catalysts, and such. Professional boundaries are deemphasized and much role blurring occurs. Responsibilities are organized around the talents and skills of individual staff members rather than around specific positions or professions. The contributions of persons not usually considered treatment staff are also important. The social distance between staff and clients is smaller than in the medical model, although the line between the two groups is preserved.

The activities of living and the relationships and interactions of the staff and client group are the treatment. Preparing a meal, resolving conflicts over differing standards for neatness, or establishing rules of living are activities through which clients learn social and basic living skills. Thus, daily living and therapeutic functions are inseparable. The relationship with the community external to the residential facility is viewed as interdependent. The boundaries between the therapeutic community and the larger community are more fluid than in the medical facility. The community (internal and external) *is* treatment.

An emphasis on resident involvement in decision making calls for a more democratic form of organization, which Litwak (1978) has described as the professional or human relations model. Proponents of this model point out its appropriateness for human service organizations. Because client problems are complex, many tasks are not routine and cannot be specified in advance.

Generalists, rather than highly specialized staff, and warm personal ties, rather than the impersonal relations, are preferred. Involvement of all levels of staff in shaping organization policies characterizes this form. Rather than rules that guide the conduct of personnel, internalization of shared norms, values, and goals aids progress toward organizational goals. Hierarchy and status differences are deemphasized.

Many features of this model are appealing and may have advantages over the hierarchical form. However, there are also some disadvantages: (1) Reliance on the internalized norms to guide behavior often leads to conflict—although people may agree about general goals and philosophy, individual interpretations of general guidelines may produce disparate results. (2) The presence of few formalized rules may produce anxiety and insecurity for both residents and staff. (3) Decision making at the lowest possible level multiplies the need for frequent meetings and other coordinating mechanisms. (4) Decision making may be slow, tedious, and inefficient. (5) The absence of highly specific job descriptions may lead to territorial disputes.

Comparing Approaches

Neither the medical bureaucracy nor the social treatment approach is complete or ideal. The medical/illness approach works fairly well when the "sick role" is temporary. Hospitalization achieves its purpose: The patient and family each has respite from a stressful situation, and twenty-four-hour care and supervision are provided in times of crisis. The ex-patient, once recovered, returns home to resume normal roles. The use of psychotropic medications has greatly increased the number of people who can use hospitalization in this way. For those who do not recover quickly, the patient role and extended hospitalization can become a "Catch 22": Relieved of responsibility because they are "sick," patients find that lack of responsible behavior becomes defined as a part of their illness. The hospital environment often cannot develop enough flexibility to allow for gradual resumption of roles and responsibilities.

The social treatment approach is more widely used in small, transitional residential programs. It is more compatible with community mental health ideology and more easily accommodates the principles of residential care presented earlier. This approach is probably not sufficient for people who are acutely disturbed and disorganized. Attempts to include such residents may be disruptive to an open, less highly structured program and may require placing more restrictions than are desirable on all residents.

Managers who wish to build and manage a social treatment facility should consider the following requirements:

1. A very clear understanding of the limitations and advantages of this approach and a strong commitment to this philosophy and the complementary structure.
2. Willingness to delegate both responsibility and authority and the ability to live with less-than-perfect decisions.
3. Willingness to make unpopular decisions, to be authoritative when necessary in order to assure organizational survival.

4.   Flexibility. (A system of general rather than specific rules to guide day-to-day operations may result in more nonroutine events or crises).
5.   Ability to choose, hire, and train staff. (These tasks are somewhat more difficult than in a system where staff can be hired largely on the basis of professional training. Because some degree of uncertainty and less social distance between residents and staff are built into staff roles, jobs can be stressful.)

The illness/medical approach and the social treatment model are commonly used, and the relationships between these treatment approaches and organizational structures are fairly clear. Managers who understand the requirements and limitations of each approach and the possible conflicts between them may also successfully mix philosophical and organizational models. Awareness of the impact of the goals, treatment philosophy, and program structure on the environment of the organization allows the manager to make informed choices. Decisions such as the kind of treatment program desired, whether staff members with specialized skills or generalists are needed, and what to do about the laundry can all be considered within this framework.

With this general framework in mind, look again at the four residential programs. As each facility is reviewed, keep the following questions in mind: What problems does the manager face? What would it be like to be a resident in this facility? What are the limitations to change? What is the predominant treatment approach? What about the structure—does the tail wag the dog?

Ridgeville State Hospital

Ridgeville State Hospital was the prototype of the large, bureaucratic medical model organization. Several years ago, a task force studied problems within the organization and proposed the following changes in its report.

Size and Organization. With over 1,000 patients, and almost as many staff members, Ridgeville is too large to be managed effectively. The present system of moving patients through admission, treatment, and continuing treatment wards leaves no one except the hospital superintendent with continuous responsibility for the patient from admission to discharge. The current structure makes it impossible to coordinate effectively with the community because the hospital catchment area contains twenty counties, each with different resources and ways of doing things. Each ward may have patients from all twenty counties, and adequate discharge planning for each patient is difficult.

The system of separate professional departments for nursing, social service, psychology, and occupational therapy makes the team concept very difficult to develop at the ward level. Each line staff member has two supervisors, the ward physician and a supervisor from the department.

Recommendations. The hospital should be decentralized into semiautonomous units. Patients should be assigned to wards on the basis of their county of origin. Each unit director should be given the authority to assign and schedule staff and set unit policy. The heads of the professional departments should retain their titles and serve a staff rather than a line function. They would be responsible for maintaining professional standards and providing consultation to unit directors.

Anticipated Problems. Assigning patients to wards on the basis of geographic origin will necessitate converting to coeducational wards, with a mixture of chronic and acute patients on each ward. This will require remodeling on the wards to provide separate bathroom facilities. There may be some community reaction to this plan and some staff resistance.

Treatment Program. Except for medications, many patients are not actively involved in treatment programs. In order to seek accreditation by the Joint Commission on Accreditation of Hospitals (JCAH) and to meet the standards for Medicare and Medicaid, each patient must have a treatment plan that is reviewed quarterly. Current professional staffing levels cannot provide individual or group therapy for every patient, and many patients would not benefit from such an approach.

Many patients are idle for most of the day, and some are unable to care for their own personal needs adequately. The organization at the ward level appears to foster this problem because ward staff members assume responsibility for many tasks the patients could do for themselves. Staff members work while the patients watch.

Recommendations. A normalization program should be instituted throughout the hospital to encourage independence and self-care. Each unit director should survey practices on the unit and identify what can be done to increase patients' abilities to care for themselves and to upgrade the physical environment.

Specific hospital-wide actions should include the following:

1. Serving meals on the wards rather than in cafeterias.
2. Installing washers and dryers on each ward for patients to do personal laundry.
3. Coed wards.
4. Changes in current admission routines that may be humiliating or frightening to newly admitted patients.
5. Redecorating to make the wards more livable and attractive.
6. Activities and field trips outside the hospital.
7. Allowing patients to handle their own money.
8. Providing lockers with locks for patients' personal possessions.

Anticipated Problems. Encouraging patients to assume more responsibility for themselves will require a shift in the roles of nursing staff. Many of the psychiatric aides have served in their caring roles for many years and may find it difficult to change. An intensive training program may be necessary to support the recommended changes.

Administrative support is crucial. Patient involvement in caring for themselves may mean that the wards are less tidy and some jobs may take longer to get done. With the support of supervisory personnel, the ward staff will find it easier to assume new roles and responsibilities.

The task force report contained many other suggestions for improving conditions at Ridgeville. Many of the proposed changes were implemented, and the hospital is today a more humane, physically attractive place. Decentralization into geographic units did improve coordination with the various communities the hospital serves. Some wards developed a team approach to treatment planning that appears to work well. Where nurses have been given increased recognition for their contributions to the team effort, patients assume more responsibility for their daily chores, and staff members try hard not to "help" so much.

But Ridgeville is still a large, bureaucratic, medically oriented facility. A number of things make it very difficult to reform Ridgeville in any major way. The mission of the hospital is set by the state legislature, which also authorizes the funds for its operation. Of all residential settings, the state hospital has the greatest responsibility for social control and for care and custody of those who cannot care for themselves. The hospital has no control over involuntary admissions and can select only voluntary applicants who are incompetent and very sick. Although this procedure is desirable for the prospective patient, it results in a mixture of severely disabled patients with a wide variety of needs. Flexible programming is very difficult to achieve.

In any attempt to change its treatment philosophy, Ridgeville faces the problem that hospital accreditation and licensing standards require that certain levels of staffing and service from each of the disciplines be maintained. Physicians' responsibilities are prescribed and supported by law, so the team approach is built around the focal role of the psychiatrist. Integration of daily living activities and the treatment program has been attempted through the normalization approach, but many daily living tasks, such as meal planning and preparation, remain centralized.

When the normalization program was adopted, a comprehensive training program was developed, but staff shortages prevented the release of psychiatric aides and nurses for more than a few hours at a time. It appeared that some staff members did not change their behavior much after training.

In addition to dilemmas about treatment philosophy, Ridgeville faces some severe funding problems. Reasons for rising costs include inflation; increase in admissions and discharges, which requires more paperwork and more professional and secretarial time; unionization, which has resulted in higher wages; changes in commitment laws, which require that patients be paid for work they do; and remodeling projects to meet accreditation, fire, and safety standards.

Staffing is a headache. It is very difficult to find certified psychiatrists who are willing to work at the hospital for the wages that are offered. There is high turnover in the most junior psychiatric aide positions, and the directors of the departments of social service, psychology, and nursing have also changed frequently.

Mattox Community Psychiatric Unit

Mattox Community Psychiatric Unit is a thirty-bed mental health unit that is part of a private, nonprofit general hospital. It also provides inpatient services for the catchment area through a contract with the community mental health center. The average length of stay for patients is slightly less than two weeks.

The treatment program at Mattox primarily reflects the medical/illness philosophy, although attempts are made to promote a concept of community and to involve patients and their families in treatment planning. Most patients receive psychotropic medications and are involved in one or more groups while they are hospitalized. A wide range of group approaches is used, depending on patients' needs. The nurses and psychiatric technicians on the day shift rotate through these groups monthly. Psychologists and social workers serve as the permanent group leaders to provide continuity. Occupational therapy and recreational activities are also provided.

The unit medical director, who is the only psychiatrist employed directly by the hospital, serves as the physician for patients who do not have a private psychiatrist. He is often responsible for half the patients on the unit, as well as for his administrative duties. The psychiatrists in private practice are reluctant to assume medical responsibility for patients they do not know; they have limited time to make hospital visits, and they must accept less than their regular fees for public patients.

The physical environment of the unit is attractive, almost plush. Each patient has a private room or shares a room with one other patient. The doors are unlocked from 8 A.M. to 8 P.M. every day. When a patient is extremely agitated, seclusion rooms are used or a staff member is assigned to the patient. All patients are voluntary, except for those brought on twenty-four-hour police holds. Staff do not like to have to deal with involuntary patients. They believe that patients should go to the state hospital if they need that kind of supervision.

This situation has created considerable conflict with the staff of the mental health center, who charge that the unit wants to be a private, middle-class hospital on public money. The unit director has been meeting with the mental health center director to try to work out mutually acceptable policies.

The unit struggles with problems of money and staff morale. In order to run in the black, the unit must average a population of twenty-two patients. There is considerable pressure from the hospital administration to reduce costs and to keep the census up. Wild fluctuations occur in a short period of time; the population has been as low as eight patients and as high as thirty-two patients in a two-week period. The unit seems to operate best with about fifteen patients.

When the population is low, there are not enough patients to form reasonable groups, everything seems dead, and staff members worry about layoffs. When the unit is full, life seems very hectic and chaotic. During peak periods, nurses spend much of their time with newly admitted patients and often have to forgo their involvement in therapy groups, which many nurses see as the most rewarding aspect of their jobs.

The short length of stay and the constant flow of seriously disturbed patients also contribute to staff morale problems. Some of the groups never get off the ground because patients are discharged after one or two sessions. Staff members wonder whether they really contribute anything to patients' improvement. Although a community meeting is held every morning, the patients often do not appear to feel responsible for what goes on in the unit. The same topics come up time after time; new issues for the patients are ancient history for the staff. The medical director is concerned about the attitude and morale of all the nursing staff. There is high turnover among the psychiatric technicians, especially on the afternoon and evening shifts.

The director of the Mattox Psychiatric Unit faces several problems: defining the overall goals of the psychiatric inpatient unit; developing strategies for implementing a therapeutic community treatment environment; defining the relationship of the unit to the larger hospital, as well as to the local mental health center; and improving staff morale.

Lincoln Halfway House

Lincoln Halfway House was established in 1978, as a private nonprofit corporation. Interested citizens and mental health professionals serve as officers for the halfway house. The initial funds for planning and purchase of a building were provided by a local foundation, and most of the operating expenses are covered by rent paid by the residents. Sue and Tony, the resident managers, receive free rent, food, and a small salary. The local mental health program pays the salary of the half-time director and provides the services of a part-time social worker. A vocational counselor is available one day each week. The house has room for twenty-three residents.

The program goals are described in the institution's Articles of Incorporation: "Lincoln Halfway House is established for the purpose of providing a temporary home for persons between the ages of 18 and 65 who are released from psychiatric hospitals. The program is intended to provide a normal living situation, an environment in which residents can gain independence, increase self-esteem, and prepare themselves to fully return to community life, including employment. It is the belief of the undersigned officers that these goals are best accomplished through residents' taking charge of their own lives, and by learning social responsibility toward other people. To this end, we seek to promote a spirit of community, of sharing, and a sense of the positive contribution of all members at Lincoln Halfway House."

When Lincoln House opened with eight residents, there were some shaky times for a few months. When the director who had been hired decided at the last minute to accept a full-time job, two board members volunteered to work with the resident managers to build the new program. Initially, they had hoped that residents could have some experience with shopping, cooking, and using public transportation before they were released. Members of the board who approached the superintendent of the state hospital about developing a prerelease ward were told that funding limitations did not allow for such a special program.

Some of the first residents who came to Lincoln House said they knew how to cook, but they required considerable supervision, even when the ingredients for the meal were all assembled. After serving dinner at 10:00 P.M. two nights in a row, Sue and Tony decided that they should prepare the evening meal temporarily until the residents gained more skills.

The philosophy of the board members, which was shared by Sue and Tony, was that there should be no more restrictions on the residents than necessary. Part of the treatment for residents was in learning to make their own rules for living and working out their problems with each other. What was not very clear was who was responsible if the residents got into trouble in the community or if things did not go well in the house. Sue and Tony agreed with the idea that people should be responsible for themselves but were uneasy about their own responsibilities.

Slowly, things at Lincoln began to get organized. Rules were agreed on by the residents with Sue and Tony about smoking areas; a work schedule was developed, along with penalties for not doing an assigned chore; and many other house procedures were outlined.

Sue and Tony worked very hard during the first few months. They were relieved when a director, Alice Jonesburg, was appointed, but were also apprehensive about what she would think of the program. As it turned out, Alice was very complimentary about what had been accomplished. After meeting with the board, Alice began to put together a work plan. It was clear that Lincoln faced several immediate problems:

1. There were only eleven residents, and about eighteen were needed to cover expenses. The board had decided to slow down admissions until things got organized.
2. Lincoln had only the barest outline of a budget and no bookkeeping or accounting system.
3. Some of the current residents were quite limited in their social and self-care skills. The current residents needed more skill training. Some halfway houses include "normal" residents as catalysts and role models.
4. Job descriptions needed to be developed as more staff were added. So far, Sue and Tony had done everything.
5. A neighbor had telephoned to report that one of the residents was walking around and around the block. The neighbor asked if the resident should be out after dark.
6. Some of the board members appeared to be very imbued with the work ethic. The current residents were a long way from being self-supporting. The six-month limit on length of stay seemed to be too short.
7. A van was needed to transport residents.

If you were Alice, how would you rank the items on her work list in order of importance? What are some suggestions for approaching each problem? If

Lincoln Halfway House could be started all over again, what suggestions would
you make to the planners?

Mrs. Anderson's Group Home

Mrs. Anderson's group home does not really meet the definition of a formal organization because she *is* the organization. Her facility has been included
because it is a widely used placement for persons who leave state mental hospitals.

Mrs. Anderson had a crisis this year when the mental health division
proposed standards to license group homes. Her facility would have needed a
license because she has six or more residents. The standards would have required
fire and safety codes that her home could not meet without extensive remodeling
and considerable cost. They also would have required her to hire additional staff.
Mrs. Anderson has had seven people in her home for many years. She decided that
if the standards were passed, she would just have to send two people back to the
hospital. Nothing has happened so far.

Mrs. Anderson provides shelter, small-group living, good food, and "benevolent custody." She does for residents what they could do for themselves, and
the rules in her home are more restrictive than in many other settings. In a study of
community living situations, Hewitt, Ryan, and Wing (1975) found eight restrictive practices; no choice of main dishes at mealtimes; residents have no say in
planning menus, although personal preferences are taken into account; residents'
rooms can be entered at any time; residents do not have keys to their bedrooms;
residents may not smoke in their bedrooms; staff members wake residents or
check that they are up in the morning; staff members retain control of medicines,
although this may be varied to suit individual residents; there is no regular
meeting of residents and staff. Mrs. Anderson employs all these practices and adds
two of her own: Residents may not smoke in the house and residents may not go to
the local shopping center without supervision.

Mrs. Anderson does not have an explicit treatment philosophy. She takes
her responsibility for residents very seriously. The residents are well cared for
physically and do not complain about their situation. Mrs. Anderson would be
shocked at the suggestion that her home is similar to the state hospital in many
ways. Yet she does run an almost total institution. There is little stimulation;
expectations of the residents are very low and they are viewed as incompetent and
childlike.

Mrs. Anderson's home is typical of many such facilities, but it should not
be considered representative. In some other homes, residents are encouraged to
help with meals, to do their own laundry, and to become involved in community
activities. Some group home providers help residents learn basic living skills and
are pleased when they graduate to more independent living situations.

Before writing Mrs. Anderson off as hopeless, consider her problem:

1. She, too, is isolated. She has little time to see other people and knows no one
    else who runs a similar facility.

2. Beyond her common sense and experience raising three children, Mrs. Anderson has no particular skills and no training in dealing with the residents she serves. She has never been to a workshop and has never been invited to one.

3. Mrs. Anderson has no source of support or consultation about how to meet crises. The social worker from the local social service department is not seen as a resource because Mrs. Anderson feels that she is critical of the way things are done.

If Mrs. Anderson had access to some consultation and training from someone who knows something about the principles of residential care and could help her clarify her own responsibility, she might become more flexible. For example, Test and Stein (1976) report that their approach to dealing with minor criminal activities, such as shoplifting, might be to allow the client to be arrested and perhaps to spend a night or two in jail, depending on the needs and condition of the client. Mrs. Anderson would probably have needed a great deal of support and reassurance to make such a decision when Rose was caught with the cologne she had stolen.

The extent to which small group home providers such as Mrs. Anderson can be expected to provide more than custodial care is open to question. As licensing of group homes is accomplished, and as staff members are added and formal programs introduced, these facilities will become "organizations." Many providers may decide, with Mrs. Anderson, to reduce the number of residents in their homes in order to avoid such regulation.

Conclusion

Recently, there has been a shift in the mental health field toward avoiding hasty and totally unrestricted residential placement. Although the goal of helping clients remain in their own homes should be pursued, many people will continue to need a sheltered environment, at least temporarily. Unfortunately, the nature of these sheltered environments is often defined by our habits and assumptions about residential program development and by management practices.

Mental health facilities are built around the common requirements of meeting residents' physical, social, and treatment needs. Overall goals and choices about treatment philosophy and structure affect the residential experience. Whatever form the residential facility may take, the manager's central task is clear. Taking into account the needs of clients, the expectations of society, and the requirements of the organization, managers are challenged to create a "reclaiming milieu," an environment that emphasizes the health and capability of residents and staff members who live and work within the organization.

References

Bassuk, E. L., and Gerson, S. "Deinstitutionalization and Mental Health Services." *Scientific American*, 1978, *238* (2), 46–53.

Becker, R. E. "Staffing Level and Treatment Effectiveness." *International Journal of Psychiatry*, 1969, *115*, 481–482.

Goffman, E. *Asylums*. New York: Doubleday, 1961.

Hewitt, S., Ryan, P., and Wing, J. "Living Without the Mental Hospitals." *Journal of Social Policy*, 1975, *4* (4), 391–404.

Holahan, C. J., and Saegert, S. "Behavioral and Attitudinal Effects of Large-Scale Variation in the Physical Environment of Psychiatric Wards." *Journal of Abnormal Psychology*, 1973, *82* (3), 454–462.

Holland, T. P. "Organizational Structure and Institutional Care." *Journal of Health and Social Behavior*, 1973, *14*, 241–251.

Hrebiniak, L. G., and Alutto, J. A. "A Comparative Organizational Study of Performance and Size Correlates in Inpatient Psychiatric Departments." *Administrative Science Quarterly*, 1973, *18* (3), 365–382.

Jones, M. "Community Care for Chronic Mental Patients: The Need for Reassessment." *Hospital and Community Psychiatry*, 1975, *26* (2), 94–98.

Linn, L. S. "State Hospital Environment and Rates of Patient Discharge." *Archives of General Psychiatry*, 1970, *23*, 346–351.

Litwak, E. "Organizational Constructs and Mega Bureaucracy." In R. Sarri and Y. Hasenfeld (Eds.), *The Management of Human Services*. New York: Columbia University Press, 1978.

Martin, P. Y., and Segal, B. "Bureaucracy, Size, and Staff Expectations for Client Independence in Halfway Houses." *Journal of Health and Social Behavior*, 1977, *18*, 376–390.

Moos, R. "Size, Staffing, and Psychiatric Ward Treatment Environments." *Archives of General Psychiatry*, 1972, *26*, 414–418.

Test, M. A., and Stein, L. "Practical Guidelines for the Community Treatment of Markedly Impaired Patients." *Community Mental Health Journal*, 1976, *12* (1), 72–82.

Wolins, M., and Wozner, Y. "Deinstitutionalization and the Benevolent Asylum." *Social Service Review*, 1977, *51* (4), 604–623.

22

Community Support and Rehabilitation Programs for the Chronically Mentally Ill

Anne Strode Nelson

The adoption of a deinstitutionalization policy in many states across the country has focused increasing attention on the community support needs of the chronically mentally ill. This chapter describes a community support model and gives examples of support services for assisting consumers in securing government benefits, providing crisis stabilization support or medical services, and implementing a case management system. The development of a community support program requires a commitment to the task of building a community network of mental health and social services.

Mental health services have undergone tremendous changes in the last century. Early care focused on the removal of the psychiatric pathology using medical treatment modalities, such as rest and chemotherapy. Few if any rehabilitative and daily living skills were taught to clients. Patients became essentially captives of the institution to which they were admitted, due as much to an acquired dependency on the institution as to their illness.

Subsequent nationwide adoption of deinstitutionalization policy necessitated change of many beliefs, practices, and programs designed to serve psychiatrically disabled people. Both consumers of services and mental health workers suddenly were faced with new kinds of coping problems in the community, and the first two decades of the deinstitutionalization movement were characterized by inadequate and poorly integrated services.

The consequences of massive release practices prompted the National Institute of Mental Health (NIMH) to initiate actions for developing a range of services to meet the needs of severely mentally ill persons residing in the community. This chapter provides the mental health administrator with an overview of community care in general and specifically in the Community Support Program (CSP) initiated by NIMH in 1978. By way of introduction, a case example may shed some light on the consequences of inappropriate institutionalization.

> Janet is a fifty-five-year-old widow. She was hospitalized for depression after the death of her only child, who died in a car accident at age ten. Janet's husband visited her often during the first few years of confinement, but eventually he stopped seeing her. He gave up when he saw no hope for cure. He died ten years after Janet's hospitalization.

> Prior to the death of her son, Janet had a full-time job at the public library. She was active in civic organizations and was considered attractive and well-balanced. Following the death of her son, Janet sought help for severe depression. She enlisted a reputable psychiatrist. When the medications he prescribed failed to alleviate the depression, brief psychiatric hospitalization was recommended.

> Janet found it extremely difficult to adjust to hospital life. She was from a small, independent-minded family and found communal living unbearable. The people in her ward were unstimulating and bizarre. There was nothing to do on the ward but watch television. There were no opportunities to make decisions of any kind. When Janet complained about life on the ward, she was either ignored or the doctor changed her medication. Such complaints were considered a manifestation of her depression.

> After a few weeks of resisting authority and complaining, Janet realized that it was useless. She then concentrated on getting out. These efforts proved to be even more frustrating. After many attempts, she gave up, feeling defeated and hopeless. Even the daily news lost meaning. Janet finally learned how to be a patient! She learned always to obey and agree with staff. She took her medications, got up with the others, went to bed on time, and participated in group therapy as prescribed.

> After eight months, Janet lost any desire to leave the hospital. She was afraid. Even on excursions to movies and concerts, she felt insecure and uncomfortable until she was back within the protective walls of the hospital. Janet did not feel better about herself in the institution; she felt "sick" and incapable of living on the outside. She forgot what it was like to work, to shop, to keep house, or, for that matter, to do anything that would be considered normal in the community. She did, however, learn how to behave as a patient, to "fool" staff, and to beg for cigarettes.

> Janet is typical of many ex-mental patients who are now being placed in the community because the hospital is recognized as an inappropriate placement. Although an intensive psychiatric placement is inappropriate for Janet, she no longer can cope in the community without assistance. She, like many other institutionalized people, is in need of community support services. Awareness of cases like Janet's, as well as numerous class action suits and dissent decrees that further illustrated the debilitative results of long-term hospitalization, has contributed to the deinstitutionalization movement.

Historical Perspectives

To appreciate fully the issues that led to the Community Support Program, it is important to explore the characteristics of early institutionalization. Dorothea Lynde Dix led a social movement in the late nineteenth century that instigated the development of state asylums for the mentally ill. Her efforts, and those of Horace Mann, culminated in the Dix-Mann doctrine, which sought to make poor mentally ill people wards of the state so they would not be placed in prisons and almshouses or sold as slaves. The New York Care Act of 1890 was the first legislation establishing state "lunatic" asylums. Other states followed.

The asylums began as relatively small, isolated retreats where the clients' most pressing needs were met. The New York Lunatic Asylum, later renamed the Utica Psychiatric Center to improve its image, serves as a typical example of a traditional state hospital. In January 1843, it opened its doors to 276 patients. A century later the inpatient census had grown to 2,044 (State of New York, *History of Utica*, n.d.). The center, like most state psychiatric institutions, became overcrowded and understaffed. Mixing patients with acute problems with chronic patients and insane criminals led to severe problems and isolated facilities. Poor transportation systems made it difficult to reintegrate the mentally ill into the community. Few patients were able to maintain ties with family or friends. Within the institution, a whole new set of norms and roles evolved for the patients. The survival skills needed in the hospital were the antithesis of the skills needed to maintain oneself in the community. Patients rapidly lost community survival skills. Behavior became structured around minor privileges. If patients were not good (as demonstrated by obeying orders and recognizing their problems), they were punished and rewards were taken away. Changes in drugs or increased dosages were used to control behavior further. Every action was monitored. People were deprived of making decisions that affected their lives. In order to survive within a psychiatric center, a patient learned passive and dependent behavior. A sense of depersonalization gripped the client, which was seen as a manifestation of mental illness.

The Deinstitutionalization Movement

The recruitment and discharge of World War II soldiers increased the demand for psychiatric services. This demand was met in part by the Veterans Administration, which built new hospitals with psychiatric units to serve those affected by war. Shortly thereafter, in 1947, the National Institute of Mental Health was created to oversee mental health care. These events marked the beginning of federal involvement with mental health policy. It was not until 1961 that this involvement increased significantly.

In 1955, state psychiatric centers were serving 558,000 inpatients (Bachrach, 1976). At this time, failures of institutionalization were recognized, and a series of innovations was changing the focus of mental health services. Seven factors that contributed to the discharge of many patients and subsequently to alternative treatment modalities coalesced in the late fifties and early sixties: invention of

psychotropic medications, reduced number of admissions and readmissions, reduced length of stay, development of community mental health care centers, expansion of nursing home care, more mental health personnel, and civil rights and
class action suits.

The invention of psychotropic medications was probably the most significant factor in revolutionizing mental health treatment. Neuroleptics, antidepressants, and tranquilizers enabled many disturbed people who would have been
institutionalized to remain in the community. These drugs, particularly phenothiazine, decreased the number of institutional readmissions and significantly
reduced the average length of stay. Basic goals for a national policy on community
mental health care were set forth in the 1961 report of the Joint Commission on
Mental Illness and Health (quoted in Rose, 1979, p. 434): "The objective of modern treatment of persons with major illness is to enable the patient to maintain
himself in the community in a normal manner. To do so, it is necessary: (1) to save
the patient from the debilitating effects of institutionalization as much as possible; (2) if the patient requires hospitalization, to return him to home and community life as soon as possible; and (3) thereafter, aftercare and rehabilitation are
essential parts of all services to mental patients."

The commission's recommendations regarding long-term hospitalization
were bolstered by the new drugs. Many people felt that the psychotropic medications enabled professionals to seek alternative forms of treatment for the mentally
ill. However, others like Scull (1976) and Mechanic (1969) argued that medications were a poor rationale for deinstitutionalization since they reinforced the
medical view of insanity as an illness. Bellach (1964) argued that the drugs merely
made mental health care a "practical" policy. Certainly, the advent of psychotropic medications met the needs of financially desperate state hospitals, which
were overcrowded, poorly staffed, and in physical disrepair. It appeared cheaper
to discharge clients than to upgrade conditions on the wards. Thus, deinstitutionalization became the convenient solution to many financial, legal, and moral
problems.

Community Support Programs

The community mental health centers (CMHCs), developed through the
Mental Retardation and Community Mental Health Centers Construction Act of
1963, were designed to alleviate some of the problems manifested in the state
hospitals by providing aftercare and prevention services. While a burgeoning
array of community mental health services emerged, the centers, in general, failed
to address adequately the comprehensive and special needs of deinstitutionalized
persons. These circumstances led to the development of the Community Support
Program (CSP).

The CSP, initiated by NIMH in 1978, was a significant nationwide pilot
program designed to promote the establishment of community-based services for
the severely psychiatrically disabled adult population. The original CSP entailed

contracts between NIMH and state mental health agencies. States subcontracted with local service providers for the model demonstration projects, which included such specialized services as housing, transportation, teaching daily living skills, medications management, resocialization therapy, and other related services (Turner and TenHoor, 1978). NIMH hoped the original program funds would serve as catalysts for development of projects in other states and expansion in states with federal contracts. The CSP was based on the following ideas (National Institute of Mental Health, 1977, pp. 1–2):

> Mentally disabled people are now living outside of mental hospitals in increasing numbers. Reliance on hospitals for long-term care of such persons will continue to diminish. The costs of hospitalization are too high, the human and civil rights issues too complex, and the negative side effects too great to maintain the old pattern of institutional care.
> Deinstitutionalization of severely mentally disabled patients, on the other hand, may solve nothing. Simply moving patients out of one setting into another provides no guarantee that their lives or ability to function will improve.
> For severely emotionally disabled persons to benefit by release from mental institutions, they must have long-term access to rehabilitative and supportive services in the community. They need help, for example, with living arrangements, jobs, and other problems of everyday life . . . .
> At present, thousands of mentally disabled persons remain in institutions or continue to enter and reenter them primarily because few community programs are available. Many thousands more have been (and continue to be) released with inadequate provision for their care in the community. In light of these inadequacies, the need for constructive action is clearly urgent.

In order to receive CSP funds, states were asked to design a system of services that would alleviate, or at least reduce, three fundamental problems of providing community-based mental health care: (1) financing and interagency coordination, (2) client organizing and advocacy, and (3) accountability for case management and follow-up.

Although it seems natural that the CMHCs would take the lead role in serving chronically mentally ill people, this has not been the case. Deinstitutionalization progressed largely without their participation. Although the NIMH initiatives have facilitated the development of appropriate services for the severely disabled, many problems, such as community and staff attitudes, funding obstacles, and treatment modalities, must be overcome before adequate treatment occurs by and in the community.

Stern and Minkoff (1979, pp. 613–616) describe six paradoxes that shed light on the problems experienced by CMHCs in serving the CSP target population. They found that the problems of serving the severely mentally ill arose not from lack of staff commitment, but from too much commitment, as reflected in the following contrast of old and new values.

Old Values	*New Values*
1. Being a good community mental health professional means focusing on primary prevention and consultation with community caregivers who take direct responsibility for patient care.	1. Being a good community mental health professional for chronic patients means focusing on tertiary prevention and taking responsibility for the patients myself.
2. The goal of the clinic is to serve psychiatrically disabled patients and to serve as many people as humanly possible.	2. The goal of the clinic is to serve those most in need and least able to pay.
3. I am valued professionally for my academic training and for treating "good" patients.	3. Anyone can treat "easy patients." I am valued as a specialist, providing services to patients who are most difficult to treat.
4. I am a fully trained professional who needs to utilize my talents with those patients who can benefit from my skills.	4. My training, though thorough in other areas, did not prepare me to treat chronic patients. However, I am flexible enough to learn new skills for chronic patients in order to become fully trained.
5. A good therapist makes patients well.	5. A good therapist helps patients to attain and maintain their best level of functioning. A good therapist provides what a patient needs and knows that some patients need lifetime care.
6. If chronic patients do not do well in the community, life in the state hospital may be better for them.	6. If chronic patients do not do well in the community, new resources and approaches must be found to address their needs in the community.

The changes in values illustrate why the CMHCs may not be meeting the needs of the chronically mentally ill. Many staff members may experience difficulty in making the attitude and skill changes necessary to serve the CSP target population. In order to meet the CSP needs, staff members must adapt to these changes, face uncomfortable working conditions, or move on to different settings. These are challenging tasks.

The problems facing mentally ill persons are complex and require intervention from formal and informal resource networks. Many localities and states have developed formal interagency agreements on shared responsibilities and methods of coordination. For example, an agreement between the New York State Office of Mental Health, the Department of Social Services, and the Department of Health stipulates that mental health clientele, whose care will be reimbursed by Medicaid, will be given appropriate and rightful access to generic skilled nursing and health-related facilities. An agreement between Westchester County Mental Health Association and Harlem Valley Psychiatric Center calls for the psychiatric center to provide staff support to the association for intervention, advocacy, and case finding. Informal resource networks include such natural supports as family, friends, neighbors, landlords, and the community at large (Rabkin, 1974).

Community support services (CSS) are designed for severely mentally disabled adults whose primary disability is emotional, rather than developmental or organic, and for whom twenty-four-hour nursing is inappropriate. Individuals who display the following characteristics are eligible for services (National Institute of Mental Health, 1978b, p. 3).

1. *Severe mental disability* often results in hospitalization and is manifested in the following symptoms: thought disorders, hallucinations, inappropriate affect, severely disturbed interpersonal relationships, delusions, disorientation.
2. *Impaired role functioning* can be manifested by unemployment, needs for sheltered living arrangements, public assistance, and assistance in daily living.
3. *Social support* systems may be *absent* in the natural environment (close friends or group affiliations may be lacking or the person may live alone or be highly transient).
4. *Inappropriate social behavior,* which results in demand for intervention by the mental health and/or judicial/legal system, may be exhibited.

My first case example, Janet, clearly meets the criteria for a CSS participant because of her long-term hospitalization. The following example illustrates one type of severely disabled person who also needs supportive care:

> John (twenty-eight years old) has been living in the community, but he is severely mentally ill. He has been hospitalized for brief periods of time since his first admission at age twenty. As a youth, he lived with four foster families and had one six-month stay at a juvenile correctional center.
> John tried suicide numerous times as a child. After each incident, he was hospitalized briefly. After two attempts at suicide, a social worker recommended foster care. Unfortunately, the first foster care placement began a series of failures and subsequent shuffling from one home to another.
> John's self-esteem is low. He is grossly overweight and is frightened by people. He distrusts almost everyone. Mental health

professionals have almost given up on John. He has "burned out" the staff at the local mental health center, at the general hospital, and at the state hospital. They cannot find any method to "cure" him. He drifts in and out of the facilities.

Numerous attempts have been made to get John into a school or vocational program. Staff believe that if he could gain some job skills, it would enhance his abilities to cope on his own. Unfortunately, John's life-style does not lend itself to school or agency time schedules.

John is depressed and suicidal, estranged from his family, and currently lives alone. Although long-term institutionalization is not appropriate for John, he does need some structure and assistance in daily living, vocational, and social skills. He is typical of many younger severely mentally ill adults who need some kind of support services. The CSP is designed to provide services that meet the various needs of people like John.

The Community Support Model

NIMH stresses that a number of components of the human service system must coordinate activities and services with one another before a community support system exists. Natural helping networks and government and voluntary agencies must work together to provide the services essential for a CSP to work. At the beginning of the national CSP effort, NIMH stipulated that staff and resources should be available to perform these services (Turner and TenHoor, 1978, p. 329):

1. Identification of the target population.
2. Assistance in applying for entitlements.
3. Crisis stabilization services in the least restrictive setting possible.
4. Psychosocial rehabilitation services, including but not limited to
   • Goal-oriented rehabilitation evaluation.
   • Training in community living skills in the natural setting wherever possible.
   • Appropriate living arrangements in an atmosphere that encourages improvements in functioning.
   • Opportunities to develop social skills, interest, and leisure time activities, to provide a sense of participation and worth.
5. Supportive services of indefinite duration, including supportive living arrangements and other such services as long as they are needed.
6. Medical and mental health services.
7. Backup support for families, friends, and community members.
8. Involvement of concerned community members in planning and offering housing and working opportunities.
9. Protection of client rights, both in the hospital and in the community.
10. Case management, to ensure continuous availability of appropriate forms of assistance.

An additional component, which was not included in the original model, is transportation. Community support services are especially critical in rural areas. Without adequate transportation, neither the clients nor the staffs can fully participate in community support activities. In addition to the eleven essential service components, five elements are critical for linking the components of the service system together: state and local financial incentives, a coordinating and monitoring agency, discharge planning processes and procedures, a case manager for each client, and community resource development.

The following sections briefly describe some of the innovative community mental health and human services programs that have been designed to serve the severely mentally ill. The brief descriptions guide the program manager by suggesting alternative approaches to programming.

Identifying the Target Population. Methods of identifying the target population vary, depending upon the service delivery system. Where discharge from a psychiatric hospital is planned, clients can be assessed by mental health center staff prior to release and then followed in the community. But if the clients are at large in the community, using a variety of providers or none at all, then identification becomes difficult and time-consuming. In urban areas, where the severely mentally ill tend to frequent common establishments or the streets, identification may be easy, but getting the client into care may be impossible. Here, aggressive outreach is necessary, but the worker must recognize the client's right to refuse treatment. Workers must balance their efforts between the client's civil rights and the moral obligation to provide treatment.

Assisting Consumers in Securing Benefits. To assist consumers in obtaining benefits, workers must be knowledgeable about the range of possibilities and the eligibility criteria for financial, medical, and other benefits. These benefits cross numerous service boundaries, for instance, veterans associations; insurance entitlements; social security; supplemental security income (SSI); welfare; food stamps; Medicare (Title XVIII), Medicaid (XIX), and Social Service (Title XX) benefits; and local general assistance. In most states, the case manager is responsible for assisting clients in securing benefits they are entitled to.

Crisis Stabilization. Severely mentally ill persons suffering from psychotic episodes often are inappropriately placed in psychiatric centers or jails. The CSP strives to develop a range of admission diversion services, such as twenty-four-hour on-call mechanisms, crisis intervention, diagnosis, and acute care, and admission diversion programs, such as emergency houses (similar to halfway houses), special family-care homes, and acute psychiatric wards in general hospitals. In southwest Denver, the mental health center reduced admissions to psychiatric hospitals substantially by providing consumers in crisis with family-care services. Family caretakers have been trained to provide short-term care until clients stabilize. Of course, caretakers have access to support services themselves. In Albany, New York, there is an emergency house, owned by the state and located in the center of the city near a psychiatric center. This house serves as a halfway house for those coming out of the institution and as an admission diversion program for those who are in danger of being hospitalized.

Psychosocial Rehabilitation Services. Rehabilitation services were practically nonexistent in most institutions. Many innovative programs that enhance residential, vocational, and social and recreational opportunities for clients have evolved in the last few years. These services have become available both in the community and in institutions in some states.

Residential Alternatives. The CSP stresses placing individuals in least-restrictive settings, which calls for a range of residential environments. At minimum, people discharged from psychiatric centers need assistance in locating suitable and affordable housing. Some may benefit from housing in the community with twenty-four-hour supervision, but others need intensive inpatient care. Residential alternatives in the form of supervised apartments, group homes, and halfway houses have emerged across the country. Nursing homes, private proprietary homes for adults, and single-room occupancy hotels continue to house a large number of ex-patients living independently. Federal Housing and Urban Development funds (Section 202 loans for residential units and rent subsidies) have enabled states to contract for the development and renovation of living units. In some states, private, nonprofit agencies have been established to develop less restrictive housing for clients discharged from hospitals or otherwise in need of supervision. Search for Change in Westchester County, New York, operates sheltered cooperative apartments for clients released from Harlem Valley Psychiatric Center. Some of these have staff living in; in others, the staff supervise on an on-call basis.

Places for People in St. Louis, Missouri, is another private, not-for-profit agency. It was established in 1972 to assist persons being discharged from St. Louis State Hospital to obtain housing in the community (National Institute of Mental Health, 1978a). Fairweather Lodge model has been used by a number of communities. This model concentrates on using lodge members (ex-patients) to provide the support and care needed to maintain other members in the community. There are no live-in staff, and professionals are used only for technical consultation. Lodge members' group decisions are the basis for both community residence and business transactions (Fairweather and Sander, 1969). The lodges operate at an extremely low cost because clients pay for room and board out of wages and SSI payments.

Vocational Programs. A range of alternative work-related opportunities is necessary. These might include job referral and placement, skill training, skill assessment, sheltered workshops, and transitional employment programs. Fountain House, in New York City, is one of the best known psychosocial rehabilitation centers. The clubhouse, as it is called, is based on a work-oriented model stemming from a philosophy that work gives life meaning. Fountain House was established in the 1940s to support discharged patients from state psychiatric institutions. The clubhouse members use the club as a drop-in center, as a place to eat, and as a place to work. From three to four hundred members use the club daily. Some come just to hang around, but a large number go to Fountain House to work, either in the cafeteria, the cafe, or on various clerical and administrative jobs. Some members work as tour guides, taking hundreds of people through the clubhouse annually. There is a Fountain House thrift shop, located a few blocks away, that serves as a transitional employment site.

The Fountain House transitional employment program features jobs in a variety of private businesses. Members are often employed in placing tags on merchandise, working on assembly lines, and doing janitorial work. Staff members arrange the initial job interviews. After the member secures a position, a staff person accompanies him or her to the job. For the first few days, the staff person works alongside the member to ensure that he or she learns the job and is comfortable with it. Once the member feels okay about the work and the sur-roundings, the staff person discontinues working alongside. However, should the member fail to appear on the job, someone from Fountain House covers the position until the worker or someone else can come in. This is the key to the success of this program. The employer never is inconvenienced. The Fountain House model is being replicated across the country.

Although sheltered workshops have been in operation for mentally retarded individuals for some time, only recently have severely mentally ill people been able to take advantage of these opportunities. For example, Fernald State School in Massachusetts operates a series of graduated workshops within the institution boundaries. Clients are assigned to different levels based on the work and their behavioral skills. Conbela, a rehabilitation facility in Seattle, Washing-ton, operates a large, successful paper recycling plant by collecting and sorting large quantitites of paper, which are sold for processing. Consolidated Industries in Syracuse, New York, employs over 100 disabled persons from packaging items for a medical supply company to wrapping automotive parts in plastic using heavy and expensive equipment.

Social and Recreational Programs. Drop-in centers, clubhouses, and social centers are described as places where clients can go to socialize, play games, watch TV, or just hang out. Fellowship House in Florida is a community center with evening, weekend, and weekday activities, including a Saturday night coffee-house, potluck dinners, and trips to community events (National Institute of Mental Health, 1978a).

Westcott Cafe in Syracuse, New York, began as a renovated storefront de-signed to serve the social and economic needs of residents of the Westcott Street neighborhood by providing a place where people could meet, exchange ideas, and share information to help solve their common problems (Hutchings Psychiatric Center, 1978). The cafe serves low-income elderly, young working people, stu-dents, and numerous individuals with psychiatric symptoms. Many of the clients live in nearby halfway houses and come to the volunteer-managed cafe for an inexpensive meal and to mingle in an atmosphere of acceptance.

Medical and Mental Health Services. Most communities now provide tradi-tional health, dental, and mental health services to a major proportion of the less chronically disabled persons. However, staff members are discovering that they have to be more assertive or creative in getting the severely disabled to utilize services, especially those providing medication review. At Capital District Psychiatric Center in Schenectady, New York, staff members were spending an exorbitant amount of time trying to get clients to come in for their medication reviews. A volunteer working for the center came up with an idea for getting clients to come in every week for their prolixin shots. She suggested they offer incentives to the clients, such as cookies and punch. On the prolixin clinic day, there is a "party" at the clinic. Clients come to listen to music, drink punch, socialize, and have their medications reviewed. A simple, rather inexpensive idea has led to successful compliance with treatment.

Backup Support. When promoting treatment *in* the community and *by* the community, it is important that the people involved with the clients get the backup support services they need. Families, landlords, and employers especially need someone they can call upon to help them work out difficulties that arise because of interactions with the client. The police also must be considered. Police often come into contact with clients on the street and need to know how to treat these people and to prevent inappropriate placement in jail. Training workshops, seminars, conferences, and the provision of written materials can provide backup support to community helpers.

Administrators should recognize the importance of technical assistance, not only in programs within their own centers, but in other facilities used by their clients. Staff members should be encouraged to intervene in places of employment, residences, and in other community settings, as needed, so that problems can be solved as quickly as possible.

Involving the Concerned Community. A wide range of people should be included in the CSP. One way to include those who normally would not be active is to solicit volunteers. Volunteers can assume roles as board and advisory committee members and as direct service providers. Students from local community colleges and universities make excellent volunteers. Sometimes the business community is forgotten when trying to serve clients. For instance, in some small communities, staff often see little opportunity for transitional employment positions. After all, there may be no large department stores or office buildings. However, schools, grocery stores, and gas stations may provide entry-level jobs. In one eastern city, a concerned citizen happened to be in the same hospital room as the owner of a grocery store chain. After talking for a while about what each man did, they arranged for the placement of an ex-hospital client in the store as a transitional job. This brief interaction was the beginning of a transitional employment program. Small interventions such as these can lead to innovative programs. The same is true for residential units, where landlords may be willing to take clients if they are guaranteed backup support and technical assistance. If landlords are included in the planning for these programs, they are more likely to cooperate.

Protecting Client Rights. In 1973, Priscilla Allen, a noted advocate and ex-hospital patient, testified to the California Senate Select Committee on Proposed Phaseout of State Hospital Services. She stressed that "living in the community can hardly be said to be living in the community at all, that community facilities, such as board and care homes, are often as effective, if not more effective, in institutionalizing patients as a state hospital; that in my opinion, for specific types of patients, state mental hospitals will be for the foreseeable future a necessary treatment resource" (Allen, 1976, p. 147). In discussing patients' rights, Ms. Allen addressed not only the right to treatment but the right to refuse treatment, as well as confidentiality of records, economic protection, civil rights, and right to information about one's own well-being. In 1974, Ms. Allen wrote a bill of consumer, tenant, and human rights for citizens using outpatient mental health services. This bill is a thorough guide to the rights of consumers. It serves as a good orientation to staff who should be ensuring that clients' rights are upheld.

Case Management. The roles assumed by case managers are sometimes overwhelming, such as counselor, linker, supporter, broker, monitor, catalyst, and advocate. The proper support services mentioned previously are critical if the case manager's goal of providing continuity of care is to be realized. Models of case management include a team of workers specializing in one or more of the community support functions or one individual who is responsible for all activities. Case management services can be administered through a mental health center, a county office, or a private agency. For example, in Hennepin County, Minnesota, an independent living program is operated by a private, nonprofit, psychosocial rehabilitation agency designed to equip clients with the skills needed to achieve and maintain independent living (National Institute of Mental Health, 1978a). A case manager works closely with a primary counselor to evaluate the clients' needs and establish service goals related to continuity of care and the provision of such services as training in practical living skills, budgeting, housekeeping, consumerism, grooming, nutrition, medical consultation, social skills training, self-advocacy training, leisure time and recreational activities, housing arrangements, basic education, training in use of community resources, and vocational development.

In Madison, Wisconsin, an interdisciplinary team model has been demonstrated and replicated successfully in communities with fewer resources, carrying out five major tasks: assessment of clients' level of functioning, individual planning for unmet needs, resource development or creative use of existing resources, implementation of the service plan, and review and updating of the plan (Test, 1979, p. 18). Case managers do not provide therapy; rather, they plan for client needs and see that the individual acquires needed services. The team is ultimately responsible for referring clients to services and subsequently monitoring their progress.

Managing and Evaluating a Community Support Program

Program managers who must develop a new program should first examine their philosophy and attitudes toward mental health services. Unless they believe in the inherent dignity and worth of severely mentally ill persons, they will not foster an environment that aims to serve this population in the most appropriate, least restrictive setting.

They should also assess the services currently available and the number of clients utilizing them. The convergence of the data from the client needs assessment and the survey of existing services will show gaps in the current delivery system and thus supply information about service needs. In addition to identifying program needs in terms of the eleven community support system components listed earlier, it is important to contact staff members in other communities who have gone through the same planning process and can suggest program alternatives, additional funding, and procedures for creating new programs. For example, there are step-by-step procedures for establishing a group residence in the community related to zoning, community opposition, methods for analyzing the community, and identifying obstacles to developing a residence (Stickney, 1976).

Community support programs should begin on a small scale because they can always be expanded once all the start-up problems have been resolved. It is important to explore all possible funding avenues, including federal, state, local, and private foundations, and to monitor federal and state priorities, not only in mental health, but in other human service areas as well. By working closely with the state officials and gaining their respect, you have a better chance of resolving fiscal and administrative obstacles efficiently and effectively.

In addition to developing and managing a community support program, it is important to build an evaluation component early in the planning process. The evaluation efforts can be overwhelming unless the planning process is divided into manageable pieces, with priorities assigned to each phase. I suggest the following general strategies for engaging staff in community support program evaluation activities:

1. Determine your audience for the evaluation reports. This task is critical in order to avoid designing evaluation outputs that do not meet the needs of your audience. It is possible that different outcome components may be geared toward different audiences.
2. Identify questions to explore. Organize questions in order of priority and select the top priority questions as a starting point for evaluation. It is important to take into account the program legal and financial obligations.
3. Start small and keep it simple. When establishing priorities, think in terms of the relationship of staff time and agency resources to the benefit gained. Is it worth all that effort to answer certain questions?
4. Identify alternative methods for answering the top priority questions. Can the information be extracted from state or county information systems? Can the information be extracted from agency records? Are there any community-wide studies that address the same issues? Generate new data only when necessary.
5. Engage all levels of staff in designing and implementing the evaluation activities. Their acceptance of the evaluation process is directly related to the reliability and validity of the data. Their cooperation is essential.

The goal of the CSP is to assist chronically mentally ill persons to reside in the community with a reasonably high quality of life. The extent to which this occurs is difficult to assess because of the complexity of chronic mental illness and the problem of defining successful treatment. At minimum, clients should remain in the community longer with support services than without them. Mentally ill persons may need occasional hospitalization, but merely recording the number of times a person is hospitalized does not provide adequate evaluative information. One must also look at the length of time the person is retained and the reasons the person stayed as long as he or she did. The improvement of community living skills may not be possible for some chronically mentally ill persons, due to their illness. Therefore, maintaining clients at their current level of functioning may prove to be a valid evaluation standard. For evaluative purposes, one might aim to achieve progress in a certain proportion of the target population. Many CSP projects focus on one or more of the following baseline measures to begin their evaluative endeavors: description of the target populations, description of the service delivery network, documentation of systems change.

To the extent possible, CSP evaluators should use instruments that have been tested for reliability and validity to ensure valid data and save the staff much time. Schulberg (1979) suggests a number of ways to use existing data, such as incidence and prevalence studies, in an evaluation design. He suggests examining the following statistics:

1. The number of discharged mental patients living in the community.
2. The number of people living in identified community residences for mentally ill (that is, boarding homes and group homes).
3. The number of people who have a psychiatric diagnosis receiving supplemental security income (SSI) benefits.
4. The number of people receiving medication or other treatment at aftercare clinics.
5. The number of people found through community surveys to have low levels of social and vocational functioning.

Although these measures do not provide specific information on needs, they can give estimates of the demand for services. Such measures are useful for beginning the planning process and are much less expensive to obtain than community surveys.

The description of the service delivery network may be easy or difficult, depending on the size and complexity of the service delivery system. An inventory of services can begin with the local phone book, agency resource files, and local referral sources. These materials can be compiled to provide an overview of the system, although it will not provide information regarding the adequacy of services. If agencies are autonomous and isolated, an inventory of services made by the core service agency is an excellent means for beginning to establish interagency liaison.

The documentation of change in the community support system can occur at many levels, but the most common is the individual case. The evaluation of the service delivery system through the use of the case is feasible because the services intersect across agency boundaries. Although the examination of the case management process does not explain the entire delivery network, it is a good beginning point. More detailed studies focusing on interagency dependency, cooperation, and coalition are often needed, but are extremely complicated and expensive. The utility of this detailed information is questionable unless it is used to identify barriers and gaps in the system. Other evaluation activities might include cost studies, analysis of the effectiveness of the service system, and in-depth evaluation of such services as residential programs and sheltered work environments. Successful evaluations are based on identifying the audience for program evaluation, specifying the key questions, keeping the evaluation process small and simple, identifying methods for answering top priority questions with existing data, and involving all staff members in the design and implementation process.

Conclusion

A community support system program is an exciting and complex endeavor. It requires the dedication and cooperation of many individuals from government, the community, and service agencies. It requires a change of philosophy and rethinking on the part of many individuals. It also requires many resources, both fiscal and personal. Even with the complexity and the expense, the goals of such a program are both valid and attainable. The chronically mentally ill people in this country have a right to live in the most appropriate and least restrictive setting. With assistance, many mentally ill persons can become contributing members of society. Community support services can assist mentally ill consumers to lead more complete and productive lives.

References

Allen, P. "A Bill of Rights for Citizens Using Outpatient Mental Health Services." In H. R. Lamb and Associates, *Community Survival for Long-Term Patients*. San Francisco: Jossey-Bass, 1976.

Bachrach, L. *Deinstitutionalization: An Analytical Review and Sociological Perspective*. Rockville, Md.: National Institute of Mental Health, 1976.

Bellach, L. *Handbook on Community Psychiatry and Community Mental Health*. New York: Grune & Stratton, 1964.

Fairweather, G., and Sander, D. *Manual for Developing a Community Treatment Program*. Rockville, Md.: National Institute of Mental Health, 1969.

General Accounting Office. *Returning Mentally Disturbed to the Community: Government Needs to Do More*. Washington, D.C.: U.S . Government Printing Office, 1977.

Hutchings Psychiatric Center. *Description of Westcott Cafe*. Syracuse, N.Y.: Hutchings Psychiatric Center, 1978.

Mechanic, D. *Mental Health and Social Policy.* Englewood Cliffs, N.J.: Prentice-Hall, 1969.

National Institute of Mental Health. *Request for Proposal.* Rockville, Md.: National Institute of Mental Health, 1977.

National Institute of Mental Health. *CSP Project Summaries.* Rockville, Md.: National Institute of Mental Health, 1978a.

National Institute of Mental Health. "Operational Definition of Target Population for Community Support Program." Unpublished guidelines, Washington, D.C., 1978b.

National Institute of Mental Health. *Administration in Mental Health Services.* Rockville, Md.: National Institute of Mental Health, 1979.

Rabkin, J. "Public Attitudes Toward Mental Illness: A Review of the Literature." *Schizophrenia Bulletin,* 1974, *10,* 26–33.

Rose, S. "Deciphering Deinstitutionalization Complexities in Policy: Program Analysis." *Milbank Memorial Fund Quarterly, Health and Society,* Fall 1979, pp. 429–460.

Schulberg, H. C. "Community Support Program: Program Evaluation and Public Policy." *American Journal of Psychiatry,* 1979, *136* (11), 43–51.

Scull, A. T. "Decarceration of the Mentally Ill: A Critical View." *Politics and Society,* 1976, *6* (2), 173–212.

State of New York. *Appropriate Community Placement and Support, Phase One, Mental Health Five Year Plan.* Albany: Office of the Deputy Commissioner, 1977.

State of New York. *Case Management Services in Community Support Systems, A Training Manual.* Albany: Office of Mental Health, n.d.

State of New York. *History of Utica.* Utica: Utica State Hospital, n.d.

Stern, R., and Minkoff, D. "Paradoxes in Programming for Chronic Patients in a Community Clinic." *Hospital and Community Psychiatry,* 1979, *30* (9), 613–617.

Stickney, P. *Gaining Community Acceptance: A Handbook for Community Residence Planners.* White Plains, N.Y.: Westchester Community Services Council, 1976.

Test, M. A. "Continuity of Care in Community Treatment." In L. I. Stein (Ed.), *New Directions for Mental Health: Community Support Systems for the Long-Term Patient,* no. 2. San Francisco: Jossey-Bass, 1979.

Turner, J., and TenHoor, W. "The NIMH Community Support Program: Pilot Approach to a Needed Social Reform." *Schizophrenia Bulletin,* 1978, *4* (3), 319–348.

ॐ 23 ॐ

Services
for Mentally Ill
Offenders

Jean Marie Kruzich

Mental health managers need to understand the criminal justice process in order to identify decision points in the system where mental health professionals can play a part in making the criminal justice system responsive to the needs of the mentally ill. This chapter presents an overview of the administrative and clinical issues in serving the mentally ill offender, the range of clients' needs, the potential roles for mental health workers, the impact of deinstitutionalization, and the need for improved coordination between the mental health and criminal justice systems. If these issues are not understood, jails may become similar to the back wards of state mental hospitals.

Societies have always had a need to control the behavior of individuals who come into conflict with societal norms. In modern times, the issue of criminal deviance, its understanding and control, has been relegated to the criminal justice system (Cohn, 1978). The purpose of criminal law is to preserve social order by confining, punishing, and treating culpable offenders in the hope of deterring future antisocial conduct. However, a countervailing tradition in jurisprudence prohibits punishment when an offender is mentally disabled or acted without criminal intent (Keilitz, 1980).

Although no reliable figures on the number of mentally ill offenders in jails and prisons or on probation and parole are available, a few scattered studies indicate the size of the problem. A 1976 study of five county jail populations reported in *Corrections* magazine found 37 percent of the inmates suffering from a treatable mental disorder (Wilson, 1980). Another study based on interviews with 10 percent of the jail population found 57 of the 428 inmates interviewed (13.3 percent) were diagnosed with primary mental health disabilities (King County

Jail Services Project, 1978). There is little doubt that these figures reflect the results of deinstitutionalization policies, which moved to empty out state hospitals before the necessary community services were in place. Whitmer (1980), in a study of 500 defendants in need of psychiatric care, found that despite long histories of hospital treatment, almost 60 percent had no history of outpatient treatment. Thus, we find evidence that a significant number of chronically mentally ill individuals, who ten years ago would have been long-term residents in a state hospital, are now finding their way into the criminal justice system. Although estimates of the magnitude of the problem of the mentally ill in the criminal justice system vary, there is a growing recognition of the seriousness of the problem.

The Criminal Justice Process

The criminal justice system operates by apprehending, prosecuting, convicting, and sentencing to punishment those who violate the law. It addresses three needs beyond the punitive: removing dangerous people from the community, deterring others from criminal behavior, and giving society an opportunity to attempt to transform lawbreakers into law-abiding citizens (President's Commission on Law Enforcement, 1967). The criminal justice process for any given crime involves some or all of the following steps (Kerper, 1979, pp. 176–200):

1. Commission of crime	10. Preliminary hearing
2. Prearrest investigation	11. Filing indictment information
3. Arrest	12. Arraignment
4. Booking	13. Pretrial procedures
5. Postarrest investigation	14. The trial
6. Decision to charge	15. Sentencing
7. Filing complaint	16. Appeals, collateral attacks
8. Magistrate review of complaint	17. Probation and parole
9. First appearance	18. Final release

Before considering mentally ill offenders in the criminal justice process, it may be useful to define and clarify some terms and concepts as they pertain to the system in general.

Criminal offenses are categorized either as felonies or as misdemeanors and can be distinguished by the maximum punishment provided for the crime; if the offense is punishable by capital punishment or imprisonment for more than one year, it is considered a felony. If it is punishable by less than a year in prison or by a fine alone, it is a misdemeanor. Felony sentences are served in prison and misdemeanor sentences are served in jail. Many felons and the vast majority of misdemeanants do not go through all the steps.

The prearrest investigation (step 2) is carried out by police when they receive information relating to a possible crime. Its purpose is to determine if a crime actually was committed, and if it was, whether there is sufficient information to justify making an arrest. Arrest (step 3) can be defined as the taking of a person into custody for the purpose of charging him or her with a crime. The person is searched and taken to a holding facility, usually a jail. (In the case of some misdemeanors, the police may not transport the person to jail, but will issue a field citation ordering the person to appear in court on a certain day.) At the holding facility, the arrestee is booked (step 4), a process whereby an administrative record is made of the arrest. Usually the arrestee is fingerprinted, photographed, and searched again. Often there is a brief screening to assess physical and mental health. A postarrest investigation by police (step 5) is conducted only when necessary. It might involve putting the arrestee in a lineup or obtaining handwriting or voice samples or other kinds of information from him or her.

The decision to file charges (step 6) is based on the arrest report completed by a law enforcement officer. A high-ranking police officer reviews the report to determine whether the case should be approved for prosecution or whether the arrestee should be released. If higher ranking officers approve the charge, the case goes to the prosecutor's office. The prosecuting attorney must decide if the arrestee should be charged and, if so, whether the charge should be that recommended by the police. If the prosecutor decides to proceed in filing charges, a complaint is filed with the court (step 7). The complaint is reviewed by a judge (step 8) whose role is to assess the judgment of the police and prosecutor to assure that the accused was properly arrested and charged. The first appearance (step 9) usually occurs the day following the arrest. The judge informs the defendant of the charge and bail is set. The first appearance is the only court screening of a misdemeanor and is held in conjunction with step 13.

The preliminary hearing (step 10) is held before the judge whose task it is to determine if there is sufficient supporting evidence to send the charges forward to the grand jury (where the grand jury is used) or to the trial court. If evidence is deemed insufficient, the charges are dismissed and the defendant is released from jail. The judge also may release the defendant from jail under a personal recognizance program. The preliminary hearing is a public advisory hearing with both sides represented. By contrast, the grand jury, in those jurisdictions that have one, reviews cases in secret. Additionally, it hears evidence only from the prosecution; the defendant is not present. The job of the grand jury is to screen out cases where there is insufficient evidence to prosecute. If the majority concludes that there is sufficient evidence for the prosecution to proceed, the indictment is approved (step 11), which signals that the case is ready for presentation before the trial court.

At the arraignment (step 12), the defendant is informed of the specific charge against him or her and can plead guilty, not guilty, or nolo contendere (no contest). If the defendant pleads not guilty, a date will be set for the trial (step 14). Pretrial or discovery procedures (step 13) provide each side with the evidence to be presented. If the defendant pleads guilty or no contest, the case is set for sentencing. At sentencing (step 15) the judge determines the length of the sentence within the guidelines provided by the statute under which the defendant was convicted. Sentencing of felons usually takes place a week or more after the trial to allow for the collection and presentation of relevant information by a probation officer.

After the sentence is handed down, the defendant may appeal the conviction (step 16). If the appeals process fails, the defendant may make a collateral attack, the most common and most famous being the writ of habeas corpus—a directive to the court to bring the accused forward to consider the validity of continued detention.

Police

> On a call from a veterinarian, police picked up Emma, a forty-five-year-old woman, claiming her home was in the doctor's parking lot and therefore refusing to leave. The doctor had called after several customers had been frightened by Emma's angry demands that they remove their cars from her property.
> Brad, a fifty-five-year-old man with organic brain damage, is picked up by police at the bus depot. Witnesses say that a fifteen-year-old boy walked into the bathroom, where Brad, who had taken off all his clothes, assaulted him.

In most cases, the police or law enforcement officers make the initial contact with the accused. Their responsibility is for detecting crime, investigating after it comes to their attention, apprehending offenders, and gathering evidence to be used in the prosecution of the accused. Law enforcement officers cannot and will not arrest all the offenders they encounter. They in effect make law enforcement policy by the way in which they use discretion (President's Commission on Law Enforcement, 1967). A major factor in decision making will be the interpretation of the norms of the local citizens and community.

Montilla (1977), in looking at environmental factors that influence the criminal justice system, suggests three levels of decision making that influence whether an individual moves into the criminal justice system. The first and most significant is the tolerance of the citizens, family, and community agencies for deviant behavior. As in the cases of Emma and Brad, most crime reports, and therefore most arrests, are directly related to a citizen complaint. Clearly, citizens' attitudes are crucial determinants of police, court, and correctional work loads. The second most significant decision influencing entry into the criminal justice system is the kinds of services the community has developed to make it possible to keep and treat offenders in the community. As Montilla (1977, p. 528) notes, "treatment and services available in the community are measureable expressions of a community attitude about people who need the services." The third most significant level of decision making involves the formal agencies of the criminal justice system—the police, the courts, probation and parole, and other correctional agencies. The alternatives available to law enforcement people dealing with misdemeanants and felons can be illustrated by further description of the cases of Emma and Brad. Upon arriving at the veterinarian's parking lot, the law enforcement officer finds Emma demanding that the veterinarian get off her property. In this case, the prearrest investigation involves no more than the observation that a misdemeanor, trespassing, is being committed. Trespassing, breach of peace, and defrauding are the most frequent misdemeanors committed by the chronically mentally ill. The police officer has at least three options: call a mental health professional or crisis intervention team to intervene and refer, take the person to the emergency room of a hospital, or arrest. If an individual is drunk and acting in this manner, an alternative to an emergency room would be a detoxification center.

Community norms are not the only influence that will play a role in the police officer's decision to arrest or not. Other factors include the legal strength of the available evidence, the victim's willingness to press charges, the presence of witnesses, the number of prior arrests, the time and information at the police officer's disposal, and the officer's prior experience with the alternative services available. If a police officer has had the experience of taking an actively psychotic individual to an emergency room, only to wait for two hours and then be told they cannot treat the person because he or she is refusing medication, the choice will probably be jail. Virtually no systematic data exist on the number of mentally ill diverted from the criminal justice system at different points. However, Borgman's (1975) study of fifty adults accused of violating criminal laws who were directed to community mental health systems revealed that only 12 percent were diverted in lieu of arrest. In Brad's case, because of the evidence suggesting a serious felony charge, diversion away from the criminal justice system is not an available alternative.

The Prosecutor and the Court

> Fred was picked up by the police as a result of a phone call from a motel keeper who found Fred sleeping in one of the motel rooms after breaking the lock.
>
> Jack is arrested by police for a series of felonies stemming from his stealing a shotgun and holding his wife and girlfriend at gunpoint. A twenty-one-year-old, Jack has a history of assaultive behavior when he stops taking his lithium.

After Fred's arrest, the prosecution has a wide range of discretion. The first decision is whether the arrestee should be charged and, if so, whether the charge should be the one recommended by the police. The prosecutor could decide to divert Fred to a community support program for the chronically mentally ill, charge him with second-degree burglary, or release him. Numerous factors may come into play in the prosecutor's decision: the weight of the evidence, such as the amount of harm caused by the crime; the criminal record of the arrestee; assessment information gathered during booking; and the adequacy of any alternative remedies that may be utilized without involving the criminal process. In Jack's case, as was true of the earlier case of a felony charge, there is less discretion. However, because there would be a question of competence to stand trial, the prosecutor would most likely get a court order to send Jack to the state hospital for a pretrial competency hearing.

The next point at which a mentally ill individual may be diverted from the criminal justice system is the pretrial arraignment appearance. Assuming Fred was still in the system, he would have been booked and would have spent at least one night in jail before being brought before the judge. Jail conditions may have exacerbated his condition. If there were mental health consultants or screeners in the jail identifying Fred as needing inpatient treatment, an effort might be made to get him voluntarily committed and, by negotiating with prosecutor and defense attorneys, to get the charges dropped. If Fred refused, a mental health professional might be called to determine if he met the state involuntary commitment law criteria.

The availability of alternative community resources is a critical factor in determining whether a person can be diverted from the criminal justice system. For example, if the city or county has a supervised personal recognizance program that can provide case management and placement services, people like Fred or Emma may be able to stay in the community without continual involvement in the criminal justice system. Borgman (1975, p. 420) found that 55 percent of diversions of offenders to the mental health center occurred after the filing of charges but before the trial, the point at which the community, including the legal system, must begin coping with the defendant. The prosecutor, possibly faced with an overcrowded docket or lack of evidence, may find it expedient to dispense with the case by referral. If, instead, the prosecution decides to proceed, the next step is the filing of the complaint, which is followed by the first appearance or arraignment on the warrant. At this point, the court begins to be more heavily involved in the defendant's fate. Both the prosecutor and the judge are faced with some issues that are particularly significant for the mentally ill defendant. These include the issue of dangerousness and the use of an insanity plea as part of the defense strategy.

Dangerousness. "Dangerousness" refers to a propensity (that is, an increased likelihood when compared with others) to engage in dangerous behavior. Dangerous behavior refers to those acts that are characterized by the application or the overt threat of force that is likely to result in injury to other persons. The issue of dangerousness is important in the case of the mentally ill because they are feared whether or not they are in fact dangerous. Thus, to most people, the unpredictability or bizarre behavior of some of the mentally ill suggests the possibility of imminent violence (Jacoby, 1978).

There are many points in the criminal justice and mental health systems at which questions regarding an individual's dangerousness are raised—for example, in the granting of bail; at sentencing; at setting conditions of probation, work release, furlough; and in case of emergency involuntary commitment. In almost every instance, judgments about the person's future dangerousness must be made. The impact of assessment of dangerousness on an individual's future makes it important to examine continuously our ability to predict dangerousness.

Studies before 1970 indicated that people hospitalized for psychiatric reasons and released did not, as a group, constitute a greater risk for behaving in a criminal or violent way than did people who had not been hospitalized for psychiatric reasons. Studies done after 1970 have come to a different conclusion, indicating that the mentally ill discharged from state hospitals, clearly a subset of the mentally ill population, do have a somewhat higher rate of arrests for violent offenses. For example, Sosowsky (1978) found that the mentally ill had significantly higher arrest rates for violent crimes, especially twenty- to twenty-nine-year-old males, who had the highest arrest rates, approximately ten times more frequent than the males in the general population.

Thus, the latest studies do suggest that in some absolute sense the mentally ill who have been hospitalized are more prone to criminal activity. It is interesting to note that this change comes at a time when there are more mentally ill in the community. There is also the possibility that more people are being diverted from the criminal justice system to the mental health system. This in turn raises another issue, our ability to predict dangerousness. Clearly, people fear the mentally ill as dangerous. Not surprisingly, numerous studies have been done attempting to predict dangerousness of various groups of mentally ill. One of the most studied groups regarding this question are the "Baxstrom" patients, 967 criminally insane patients who were considered to be some of the most dangerous in New York State. Based on the *Baxstrom* v. *Harold* decision of the U.S. Supreme Court, they were transferred from a maximum security correctional mental hospital to a traditional state mental hospital. Only 20 percent were assaultive in any way during the following four and a half years. This group of patients had been detained an average of fourteen years in prison and hospitals for the criminally insane. Also, only 24 of the 967 patients were returned to correctional security hospitals between 1966 and 1970.

Monahan (1976), reviewing all the studies on predicting dangerousness, notes that the most striking conclusion is the degree to which violence is overpredicted. In these studies, 54–99 percent were false positive, that is, people who will not in fact commit a violent act are labeled as dangerous. Thus, he notes, the question we are left with is essentially a moral one: How many harmless men and women are we willing to sacrifice?

The Insanity Defense. The insanity plea, recently used in only rare instances, is important as it relates to the nature of dangerousness. Insanity is often confused with dangerousness. In common law, the restraining of insane persons without the usual legal process can be justified only when the use of the restraint is limited to situations that involve imminent danger to persons or property. Persons who are seriously disturbed may or may not be insane for legal purposes, and they may or may not be any less dangerous than persons not so diagnosed. Many criminal offenders, ex-felons, and persons convicted of drunk driving are likely to be equally if not more dangerous than persons who are mentally ill (Shah, 1978).

There is an inherent dilemma in the area of insanity between a deterministic modern theory of the causes of action, which recognizes the role of an individual's past in his or her behavior, and an enduring free will theory of the morality of actions and the responsibility of one's behavior. From a psychiatrist's view, if guilt is based on free choice, then no one is guilty for behavior that is predetermined (Brooks, 1974). If guilt is based on intention, then everyone is guilty, for every action is intended—if not consciously, then unconsciously, and the borders between the two are not clear.

For years, McNaghten rules have been the basis throughout most of the United States for establishing a defense on the grounds of insanity. As defined by the English judiciary in 1843, the rules require proof "that at the time of committing the act, the party accused was laboring under such a defect of reason from disease of the mind, as to not know the nature and quality of the act he was doing, or if he did know it, that he did not know he was doing what was wrong" (Brooks, 1974, p. 149). As understanding of mental processes has increased, the terms "insanity" and "psychosis" have become less meaningful as either legal or medical terms.

Insanity is a legal description of behavior that reflects some form of mental illness and a resulting incapacity. The model of the insanity defense developed by the American Law Institute (ALI) states that "the actor is excused because of mental illness if he did not have a capacity to either appreciate what he is doing or to control his actions." Thus, the McNaghten test basically provides one excuse, that is, "I didn't know what I was doing" or "I didn't know what I did was wrong." The second type of excuse is found more clearly in the ALI formulation, "I couldn't help it" (Brooks, 1974, p. 112). At the present time, the McNaghten test is used as the sole test in fewer than half the states but is one of the standards in most jurisdictions. As of 1971, the ALI test has been adopted by statute in seven states and by decisions in three more. On the federal level, six courts of appeal have adopted the test as is and two others have made minor modifications.

The insanity defense touches upon citizens' ultimate social values and beliefs and seeks to draw a line between those who are to be held morally responsible, blameworthy, free-willed, punishable, and capable of being deterred and those who are not. The key to the defense of not guilty by reason of insanity is how people are dealt with after acquittal by reason of insanity. Traditionally, there have been strong legal disincentives to the insanity defense, such as indefinite confinement on a locked ward for the criminally insane in a state mental institution (Wexler, 1977). With increasing realization that the insanity defense simply establishes a reasonable doubt about sanity at the time of the crime, courts have begun to find unconstitutional those statutes that authorize automatic commitment to institutions of those persons found not guilty by reason of insanity. Thus, with the emergence of statutory and constitutional limits on lengths of commitment, defendants raising an insanity defense are becoming less concerned with the possibility of an indefinite hospital confinement based on the legal protection of due process and equal protection.

The court, in responding to the mentally ill offender, not only needs to address issues relating to pressing charges, sentencing, and setting parole in a way that is just, but must grapple with some unique issues relating to the individual moral responsibility. Correctional facilities also are faced with some unique problems in dealing with the mentally ill offender.

Corrections

Jack, a twenty-one-year-old, is booked into the jail on charges of assault. He has some surface cuts on his wrist and has uncontrollable fits of crying. Because of paperwork, it will be six days before he can go to the state hospital for a pretrial competency hearing.

Ann, a middle-aged woman living in skid row district, while actively psychotic assaults a passerby with her purse, claiming the man has been following her and threatening her life. In jail, she refuses antipsychotic medications and rapidly deteriorates.

These two individuals, although they have not been sentenced, are being detained in jail, which is part of the correctional system. "Corrections" refers to all agencies of social control that attempt to rehabilitate and neutralize deviant behavior of adult criminals and juvenile delinquents for the protection of society. Institutions such as prisons, reformatories, and jails are included in this area, which is a series of programs and community facilities combining social control and rehabilitation objectives (for example, pretrial diversion, diversionary programs from jail and bail, halfway houses, work release, study release, referral to residential mental health treatment programs, and alcohol and drug programs.)

Jail, as part of this mélange, is somewhat unique in a number of respects. It includes three groups of individuals: those awaiting trial, those convicted and awaiting sentence, and those serving sentences. Thus, it is the only part of the criminal justice system where people may be detained even if they have not been convicted, as is true for Jack and Ann. The jail is also unique as a correctional setting in that most jails are managed by the local sheriff's department, with a primary allegiance to the law enforcement component of the criminal justice system. When law enforcement personnel, who are responsible for detecting crime and apprehending offenders, are also responsible for jails to which individuals can be sentenced, it is not surprising that jails have suffered from a poorly defined role in the criminal justice system (Nielsen, 1979).

In addition to receiving only limited attention in criminal justice research and practice, the jail has been neglected in viewing the interface between corrections and community mental health. The jail has particular significance for community mental health, because, unlike the prison, it is located in a community and must look to its environs for service supports, such as the staff of halfway houses and residential treatment centers. Because many of the mentally ill arrestees (one third to one half) are misdemeanants, the jail represents a focal point for the mentally ill. The jail, according to Joseph Rowan of the American Medical Association, is turning into a second-rate mental hospital (Wilson, 1980). Parole and probation services also represent important components of the correctional system's relationship to community mental health because individuals on probation or parole are expected to utilize community resources to aid in functioning.

Returning to the two vignettes, one can see some of the problems involved with the mentally ill in the criminal justice system. In Jack's case, because he has been charged with a felony, there is no way he can be considered for involuntary commitment. Thus, he can get out of jail only by way of a pretrial competency hearing. His situation points up the differential treatment between persons charged with felonies and misdemeanors. In the case of a misdemeanor, the person may be dropped off at a hospital and ordered to return to court or jail after receiving treatment. Felons, however, must always be escorted by a correctional guard. This security requirement influences the kind of treatment they receive.

Ann's situation poses a different set of problems. The police are able to arrest her, but once in jail, she cannot be treated against her will. The only three situations where medical and mental health care personnel can override the person's will is the case of attempted homicide, suicidal behavior, or extremely psychotic behavior. Mental health professionals dislike the bind created by such limiting constraints on service delivery. An individual like Ann may not be disabled to the point that she can be involuntarily committed, so the staff simply must wait until she deteriorates to the point at which she can be.

Interrelationships Among System Components

The range of decision making available to criminal justice personnel becomes increasingly narrow as the mentally ill person moves through the system. The law enforcement officer has perhaps the broadest scope of discretion in deciding whether or not to arrest; the correctional officer has only limited discretion in classifying and/or counseling inmates in a penal institution.

Community resources and diversion programs are important factors that influence how far an individual penetrates the criminal justice system. Diversion, particularly as it relates to the mentally ill, illustrates the "sieve" effect of the process. More persons are investigated than are arrested, more arrested than charged, more charged than tried, and more tried than convicted. Like a sieve, the process is designed to provide a number of screens, each eliminating cases that are inappropriate for the final imposition of criminal sanctions. In the case of the mentally ill arrestee, we might expect even fewer cases to lead to trial and conviction. A large percentage of the mentally ill offenders is diverted to community facilities for treatment. As a result, the community mental health worker is faced with a set of issues and concerns that may not be present in the typical mental health client population.

Issues in Treating the Mandated Client

The general lack of involvement by the community mental health centers with the mentally ill offender is widely known. Although numerous explanations abound, the overriding issue seems to be the difficulty of treating the client in terms of the chronic nature of the disorder and the involuntary nature of the treatment process. In a review of twenty-six community mental health centers and their relationship to the criminal justice system, Modlin, Porter, and Benson (1976, p. 716) noted: "Many mental health personnel are skeptical of the legal offender's treatability. They point out that he is often without personal motivation toward treatment and is coercively referred by a judge or probation officer. Because of the nonvoluntary nature of the service, often times workers feel that it is not possible to do therapy with a client who is not interested."

Criminal justice professionals suggest that all individuals are ambivalent concerning their behavior. Thus, although one may not voluntarily seek mental health services, one can still benefit from them when under court order. Some mental health professionals may feel that some court-mandated clients can benefit from therapy, such as those convicted on shoplifting or drunk driving. Because these individuals are more typically in the mainstream of society and their act was atypical enough to warrant court-ordered treatment, they may benefit from services even though on an involuntary basis. However, the larger number of clinicians seem to feel they have nothing to offer individuals labeled "sociopath." This raises another issue as to the treatability of different kinds of people in the criminal justice system. As one psychiatrist was quoted: "They are all alcoholics, drug users, or psychopaths, three of the categories we have the least success in helping" (Modlin, Porter, and Benson, 1976, p. 716). The issue of treatability really cannot be sorted out until we look at the different kinds of mentally ill people in the criminal justice system. Issues of treatability speak not only to the client's particular needs and problems, but also to the practitioner's skills and interests.

In looking at individuals with mental health problems in the community, we must include both individuals on parole or probation and individuals detained in jail. At the present time, there is little empirical data suggesting the kinds of mental health problems that individuals on probation or parole as a whole tend to exhibit. Discussion with individuals involved in administering such programs indicates that the vast majority of individuals on parole or probation, roughly 80 percent, are required by the court to receive treatment for alcohol, drug, or mental health problems. The population on which more is presently known is individuals in jail who are referred to social service projects in the jail. Petrich's (1976) study looked at clients served in a psychiatric clinic in the jail, which provided short-term, crisis-oriented psychiatric treatment and referral services (see Table 1, which indicates the psychiatric diagnosis for the inmates treated in the clinic).

Psychotropic medication, together with supports through day treatment, social living skills, housing programs, and active outreach, allows the majority of the chronically mentally ill to live in the community. Those diagnosed as manic-depressive can also function with medication in a socially acceptable manner in the community. Additionally, antidepressants and psychotherapy have been found to provide efficacious treatment for the suicidal and depressed. Drug dependency and alcoholism are likely to be addressed by specialized treatment agencies that can also reach out to the jail population, similar to mental health center outreach. Thus, even interpreting the statistics conservatively, we find the majority of individuals in jail can respond to medication, therapy, and community support systems provided by mental health workers. The combination of these services can help those in and out of jail manage their daily activities.

Table 1. Psychiatric Diagnoses for 524 Consecutive Psychiatric Patients, King County and Seattle City Jails, Seattle, Washington.

	Male		Female	
	Number	*Percentage*	*Number*	*Percentage*
Total	422	100[a]	102	100[a]
Schizophrenia	168	40	40	39
Antisocial personality	130	31	17	17
Drug dependency	114	27	11	11
Alcoholism	93	22	13	13
Mania	42	10	8	8
Depression	35	8	17	17
Miscellaneous	117	28	28	27

[a]Total percentage may exceed 100 because of multiple diagnoses for each patient.
Source: Petrich, 1976, p. 40.

Antisocial personalities include those who are referred to as psychopaths and are now considered sociopaths (that is, those who act with no concern for their action's consequence to others and are seen as severely lacking in ethical or moral development). Clinicians often use these labels to refer to anyone in jail or prison with a mental health problem. However, many psychiatrists and others insist this diagnosis is nothing more than a "wastebasket" category where cases that do not seem to fit elsewhere are put (Brooks, 1974). Halleck (1967) has noted that even within psychiatry there is a widespread disagreement as to whether psychopathy is a form of mental illness, a form of ego, or a form of fiction. Despite these diagnostic labels, there is a growing literature that suggests those who have been labeled with masochistic character disorders or personality disorders are actually borderline personalities and are in fact treatable in an intensive, highly structured residential setting (Shapiro, 1976; Vaillant, 1975).

The large number of chronically mentally disabled who end up in jails requires expanded job functions for the mental health worker. In addition to doing therapy, the worker may need to assist the person to gain financial assistance, to acquire housing, to seek vocational rehabilitation services, and to advocate for a host of other services.

Another issue raised in work with the court-mandated client is one of confidentiality. There is no doubt that the court and probation or parole officer need to know if a person is attending therapy sessions and making progress toward treatment goals. Under state law, if a probation officer asks a mental health worker how things are going in therapy, the mental health worker cannot tell that person without a release-of-information form. In order for this process to work smoothly, the probation officer must be clear about the kinds of information needed and aware of the time a mental health worker needs to comply with such requests. The court, as well as probation or parole officers, actually needs only a minimal amount of information about therapy, which need not raise serious questions around confidentiality. However, in order to make the criminal justice inquiries as unobtrusive as possible, the information needed should be gathered on the basis of legitimate and specific requests.

Part of a mental health practitioner's reluctance to work with criminal justice personnel is due to inappropriate referrals, which often may arise from ploys on the part of an attorney to have more time before the trial or represent an easy disposition by a prosecutor with an overcrowded docket. Mental health workers will need to educate the criminal justice system personnel on how to identify an appropriate referral and how to use the mental health system in a way that is useful for the client and productive for both systems. Because the referral to a mental health practitioner is for therapeutic as opposed to social control purposes, it is important for those in the criminal justice system to recognize that involvement with a mandated client also requires extra time and effort, including the visitation time and interviewing space. Although the jail is a smelly, noisy, crowded place lacking in privacy, evidence indicates that reaching people while in jail before seeing them on the outside results in a much greater likelihood of sustaining the treatment process and making significant progress (Nielsen, 1979).

The Needs of the Mentally Ill Offender

The mentally ill offender has some unique needs, often based on personal deficits and presumed criminal offenses. The mentally ill offender may return to the community from a state hospital ward for the criminally insane or be released from prison, but this discussion will focus on the mentally ill offender in jail and only secondarily consider the offender who is on probation or parole. As a group, mentally ill offenders frequently display the handicapping conditions of mental illness, substance abuse, and developmental disabilities, which contribute to their difficulties in surviving in the community and navigating through the mental health and criminal justice systems. Although individual needs vary according to circumstances, socioeconomic status, illness, and so forth, it is important to understand the common range of basic needs that must be met to enable these offenders to live in the community.

The mentally ill offender on probation or parole already is involved with an individual in the criminal justice system whose job it is to aid in linking him or her to services and providing a brokerage function. This function is usually provided by a probation or parole officer and in some cases by a community service worker, who mobilizes and manages community resources in such areas as employment, legal aid, financial counseling, health services, and counseling. Thus, the mentally ill offender on probation or parole has someone who will help secure needed services. At the present time, there is little research to indicate the different levels and kinds of services needed by the mentally ill on probation and parole. Although there is more knowledge of the general needs of individuals in jail, there is no clear picture of how these needs vary according to particular circumstances.

A study of nine King County hospitals, including the state hospital and the jail, was conducted in order to determine the number and types of mentally ill persons needing placement in long-term residential care each month (Stevenson, 1980). The mentally ill were defined as those persons suffering from schizophrenia, organic brain syndrome, major affective disorders, and depression and not those with character or personality disorders only. The overall finding was that in any given month, 61 percent of the mentally ill persons leaving hospital or jail needing residential care did not receive it. Of the existing facilities, congregate care is the most sought after and least available. In a given month, 72 percent of those needing congregate care were unable to obtain it. Persons from jail were recognized as making up a disproportionate number of people needing, but not receiving, residential care. Survey results estimated that persons from the jail constitute 17.8 percent of the need. A subset of those leaving jail whose access to housing is most limited is persons with assaultive and destructive behavior. Analysis of facility admissions criteria indicate that at best only six of the forty-seven facilities (10 percent of the beds) would accept a client with assaultive/disruptive behavior. Thus, housing is a high priority need of a large percentage of mentally ill offenders.

Additional research has been done in King County (King County Jail Services Project, 1978) to identify the range of needs displayed by dysfunctional offenders and assess the impact on case management and follow-up services. With the use of a drug case manager, three developmental disabilities case managers, and a mental health case manager in each of the mental health centers, formal agreements or service plans between the client and the case manager were developed as a means of clarifying and individualizing service goals for each client during a specific time period.

The study covered a four-month period during which time approximately 600 individuals were referred to the project. Of those referred, 290 were admitted into the program for case management services. The only offenders allowed into the project were those with disability levels that fell below 50 on the Global Assessment Scale (GAS). On the GAS, a measure assessing a person's overall psychological and social functioning, a score of 50 or below indicates major impairment. Although client referrals came from several sources, the largest single source of referrals was the criminal justice system. Of the 290 admitted clients, 178 were identified and referred by the jail social services staff. The state and county probation and parole officers accounted for 27 referrals; attorneys referred 32 clients; and 29 clients were referred by community mental health centers throughout King County. Community service agencies, family, and self-referrals accounted for the remaining 24 clients. Clients were assigned to centers according to the mental health catchment areas in which they resided. They were referred to the appropriate case manager by primary diagnosis of mental illness, developmental disabilities, and drug abuse. Of the 290 clients admitted to the project, 59 percent had a primary diagnosis of mental health, 23 percent had a primary diagnosis of developmental disabilities, and 18 percent had drug abuse as the primary diagnosis. Of the total 290 clients served, 83 percent had a primary or secondary diagnosis of mental illness; 27 percent were to some degree developmental disabled; and 30 percent were involved in drug abuse either as a primary or secondary problem.

Figure 1 indicates the percentage of client-identified social service needs. Study results indicate that the case-management model was successful in helping dysfunctional offenders gain access to community services. Greatest success was in meeting clients' legal needs, with less ability in securing the needed housing and vocational resources. In addition to assessing the services needed by mentally ill offenders in the jail, this study pointed out the need for case management services that bridge the gaps between the criminal justice and mental health systems. Thus, case managers' advocacy, coordination, and follow-up activities helped to reduce the stigma of the offender label and greatly facilitated the use of other services in the community. As a group, in addition to operating under the dictates of the court, case managers were able to work through the hostile and frequently tedious process of securing needed services from a host of autonomous service agencies often inconveniently located throughout the community.

Community Mental Health Center Roles

The mental health professional possesses valuable expertise related not only to treatment of clients, but also to educating criminal justice personnel, especially law enforcement officers. Although about half the requests for police assistance in urban areas involve domestic and family problems, the amount of knowledge and training related to mental health and human behavior is minimal. Mental health professionals can aid in educating law enforcement officers in

.Figure 1. Client-Identified Social Service Needs.

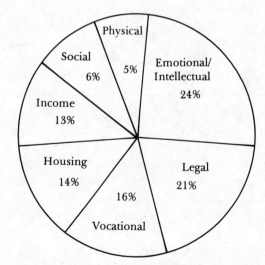

Source: King County Dysfunctional Offender Project, 1978.

assessing suicidal or homicidal potential, deciding whether a person should be detained for those reasons, and knowing how to handle such a person (Cumming and Edell, 1965).

The mentally ill offender may be among the most difficult people that law enforcement officers face. Thus, a mental health consultant can help by establishing procedures to arrange psychiatric examinations as part of an emergency commitment procedure or provide direct assistance in managing a difficult emotionally disturbed person (Mann, 1976). Often there is limited awareness of the community mental health resources available for assisting the person with behavioral and social problems. Given the amount of police officers' discretion, it is important that as many different options as possible are recognized. When it is not clear that there are alternative ways of handling a situation, the likelihood of arresting a person increases. Mental health consultation with police can include in-service training, family crisis management, community relations workshops, and case and/or program consultation.

Another group in need of mental health consultation and education services is jail staff. Jail staff members are often inadequately trained in human behavior and are frequently new to their jobs. They are usually ill prepared to recognize and manage psychotic and potentially suicidal inmates. With the use of mental health concepts and consultation from mental health professionals, jail personnel are better able to identify and refer difficult cases to mental health staff (Nielsen, 1979). The establishment of such consultative and educational services also provides a vehicle through which system changes can be made. Because jail facilities are usually crowded, they can aggravate psychological conditions and contribute to the appearance of psychiatric symptoms. Mental health consultants can advocate for modification of jail environments and procedures.

Another group that could benefit from educational and consultation services is legal professionals. The President's Commission on Mental Health (1978, p. 8), in looking at the justice system in community support systems, suggested: "Judicial personnel (judges, prosecutors, defense counsel, auxiliary staff) need to better understand the dynamics of human behavior, including mental illness and mental retardation, and reflect such insights not only in personal functioning but in operating procedures of the judicial agency (pretrial proceedings, adjudication, sentencing, civil litigation, diversion, and release on recognizance programs, and so forth)." Thus, the mental health professional can aid court officials to respond to the mentally ill offender in a manner consistent with modern mental health concepts and practices.

Direct Services

Just as it is possible to offer consultative and educational services to personnel involved in the three major areas of the criminal justice system, there are also numerous opportunities in all areas for direct service intervention. Treatment evaluation, assessment, and diversion require early intervention in order to help individuals in the criminal justice system. Evaluation of an actively psychotic person by a crisis intervention team before a preliminary hearing is crucial if the person is to have the problem identified. In addition to getting background information and assessing the current level of functioning and need, it is particularly important to identify whether there is a need for emergency treatment at a hospital or detoxification center, or if jail intervention or coordination is sufficient. Although mental health professionals might serve on the sheriff's staff in order to assess and screen individuals, in most communities, the police officer will make the assessment.

Mental health professionals can also be involved in the treatment process while the individual is in jail. For example, a Salt Lake City, Utah, community mental health center provided such services as chemotherapy, hospitalization, crisis intervention, long-term individual psychotherapy, and family and group psychotherapy (Nielsen, 1979). Offering services within the jail had a number of benefits. Individuals in jail are in a transitional state; the process of arrest and confinement frequently produces anxiety and personal discomfort otherwise lacking in the more chronic offender types. Thus, intervention by mental health professionals during this time may result in improvements in the offender's mental health that might not occur otherwise.

In addition to being a therapist, the case manager assumes the functions of brokering and advocating as clients attempt to get the necessary social services required for them to stay in a community. The President's Commission on Mental Health (1978) documents a vagrant population in south Berkeley, California, predominantly male with a median age of twenty-three, whose members have histories of hospitalization for mental illness and who are likely to be arrested and have contact with the criminal justice system. Given these difficulties, case managers needed aid to secure public assistance and provide an address for clients' checks, and to correspond with a "straight community" that provided free local telephone service to help people find lodging, food, and jobs, as well as phone contact for out-of-area relatives. These kinds of modifications and additions to mental health workers' roles and functions need to be made as we attempt to meet the needs of a population that in earlier days would not have sought help in the community.

Although this discussion focuses on mentally ill offenders in jails, inmates of prisons also have great and glaring needs. Because the family has proven to be an important variable in inmates' recidivism rates, it would seem appropriate for mental health workers to do preventive work with inmates' families when an inmate leaves the jail and also if and when the person returns. A method that has been useful with delinquents and that may also have a potential for the adult offender is the use of short-term behavioral family intervention, which is aimed at assessing the family actions that maintain the offender's behavior, modifying family communication patterns, and instituting a pattern of contingency contracting to modify a nonadaptive pattern (Alexander and Parsons, 1973). This kind of intervention may be particularly appropriate for the mentally ill offender who increases the stresses on the family and on his or her social network.

Administrative Decision Making

Given limited resources and energy, mental health administrators need to decide on the most effective way to interface with the criminal justice system. One would expect that such decisions would be based in part on workers' interests, monies available for different kinds of activities, staff expertise, and the locations of facilities. Concurrently with assessing internal resources, the administrator needs to consider the needs of the criminal justice system. Are mental health assessments currently conducted in the jail? What group is in the greatest need? What appears to be the most efficient approach to offering the most effective services for the minimum amount of dollars (for example, serving inmates' families or offering active outreach services for the more chronically mentally ill offender)?

Beyond the specifics of deploying staff and developing programs, administrators need to consider the role they can play in financing new and appropriate facilities. Congregate care facilities are needed if diversionary programs are to be available to the mentally ill offender. Thus, the administrator can go a long way in aiding the system by being involved in planning and program development and using political clout to garner funds for facilities and demonstration projects. So, too, is it important to recognize the jail as a community agency. Just as nursing home patients are patients of community mental health centers and are not denied health service delivered by another agency, the residents of local jails are entitled to outreach services from mental health centers. Both involve community residents who are entitled to community-based mental health services (Nielsen, 1979).

Conclusion

The mentally ill offender is increasingly recognized as an individual who too often falls between the cracks, failing to get the necessary treatment in either the criminal justice or mental health system. The mentally ill offender raises some unique and difficult issues. Community members fear the bizarre and unpredictable behavior of some mentally ill individuals, which can lead to the involvement of the criminal justice system. A related issue is that of defining insanity and the conditions under which a person is not morally responsible for his or her actions. The mentally ill offender's right to refuse treatment results in correctional professionals being unable to administer services. Tighter involuntary treatment laws, together with the lack of community residential facilities, result in jails becoming second-rate mental hospitals.

Just as the mentally ill offender poses unique issues for the criminal justice system, so, too, community mental health centers face some special issues. In the past, most individuals considered mentally ill and involved in the criminal justice system were seen as psychopathic personalities and very difficult to treat successfully. However, the deinstitutionalization of state hospitals has increased the variety of mental health disorders found in local communities, some of which have proven to be alleviated with medication, counseling, and training programs.

In order for the mentally ill offender to stay in the community, clinical and administrative professionals in mental health centers need to become more involved in the criminal justice system. Brokering functions in the areas of employment, legal aid, health services, and counseling are vital. Housing is a major gap in allowing individuals to remain in the community. Clinical staff offering training for criminal justice staff on the etiology, treatment, and handling of bizarre or violent behavior would be a strong contribution. From an administrator's perspective, the most effective way to interact with the criminal justice system will depend on staff interest, expertise, and resources. Regardless of the specific form of involvement, the administrator is in a position to support the coordination of efforts among the correctional, social service, and mental health systems.

As the deinstitutionalization movement continues, more and more people are being treated in the community. A growing proportion find their way into the criminal justice system. Only through their active involvement with the mentally ill offender can mental health professionals help prevent prisons and jails from becoming the new mental hospitals.

References

Alexander, J. F., and Parsons, B. D. "Short-Term Behavioral Intervention with Delinquents' Families: Impact on Family Process in Recidivism." *Journal of Abnormal Psychology*, 1973, *81*, 219–225.

Borgman, R. D. "Diversion of Law Violators to Mental Health Facilities." *Social Casework*, 1975, *56*, 418–428.

Brooks, A. D. *Law, Psychiatry and the Mental Health System*. Boston: Little, Brown, 1974.

Cohn, A. W. "The Criminal Justice Nonsystem." In J. A. Inciardi and K. C. Haas (Eds.), *Crime and the Criminal Justice Process*. Dubuque, Iowa: Hunt, 1978.

Cumming, E. E., and Edell, L. "Policeman as Philosopher, Guide, and Friend." *Social Problems*, 1965, *12*, 276–286.

Halleck, S. L. *Psychiatry and the Dilemmas of Crime: A Study of Causes, Punishment, and Treatment*. New York: Harper & Row, 1967.

Jacoby, J. E. "Dangerousness of the Mentally Ill—A Methodological Reconsideration." In C. J. Fredrick (Ed.), *Dangerous Behavior: A Problem in Law and Mental Health*. Rockville, Md.: National Institute of Mental Health, 1978.

Keilitz, I. *Screening and Evaluation of Client-Offenders: An Operational Definition*. (Report No. 1, Working Draft.) Williamsburg, Va.: National Center for State Courts, 1980.

Kerper, H. B. *Introduction to the Criminal Justice System*. St. Paul, Minn.: West, 1979.

King County Dysfunctional Offender Project. *Final Report*. Seattle, Wash., September 1978.

King County Jail Services Project. *Final Report.* Seattle, Wash., October 1978.

Mann, P. A. "Establishing a Mental Health Consultation Program with the Police Department." In J. Monahan (Ed.), *Community Mental Health and the Criminal Justice System.* New York: Pergamon Press, 1976.

Modlin, H. C., Porter, L., and Benson, R. E. "Mental Health Centers in the Criminal Justice System." *Hospital and Community Psychiatry,* 1976, *27* (10), 716-719.

Monahan, J. (Ed.). *Community Mental Health and the Criminal Justice System.* New York: Pergamon Press, 1976.

Montilla, M. R. "Environment for Community Corrections." In E. E. Miller and M. R. Montilla (Eds.), *Corrections in the Community.* Reston, Va.: Reston, 1977.

Nielsen, E. D. "Community Mental Health Services in the Community Jail." *Community Mental Health Journal,* 1979, *15,* 27-32.

Petrich, J. "Introduction of a Psychiatric Acute Care Clinic into a Metropolitan Jail." *Bulletin of the American Academy of Psychiatry and the Law,* 1976, *4,* 37-43.

President's Commission on Law Enforcement. *The Challenge of Crime in a Free Society.* Washington, D.C.: U.S. Government Printing Office, 1967.

President's Commission on Mental Health. *Report to the President.* Washington, D.C.: U.S. Government Printing Office, 1978.

Shah, S. A. "Dangerousness: A Paradigm for Exploring Some Issues in Law and Psychology." *American Psychologist,* 1978, *33,* 224-238.

Shapiro, E. R. "The Psychodynamics and Developmental Psychology of Borderline Patients: A Review of the Literature." *American Journal of Psychiatry,* 1976, *133,* 1305-1315.

Sosowsky, L. "Crime and Violence Among Mental Patients Reconsidered in View of the New Legal Relationship Between the State and the Mentally Ill." *American Journal of Psychiatry,* 1978, *135,* 33-42.

Stevenson, D. G. *Assessment of the Housing and Residential Care Needs of the Mentally Ill in King County and Recommendations for Action.* Seattle, Wash.: 1980.

Vaillant, G. E. "Sociopathy as a Human Process." *Archives of General Psychiatry,* 1975, *32,* 178-183.

Wexler, D. B. *Criminal Commitmemts of Dangerous Mental Patients: Legal Issues of Confinement, Treatment, and Release.* Rockville, Md.: National Institute of Mental Health, 1977.

Whitmer, G. E. "From Hospitals to Jails: The Fate of California's Deinstitutionalized Mentally Ill." *American Journal of Orthopsychiatry,* 1980, *50* (1), 65-74.

Wilson, R. "Who Will Care for the Mad and Bad?" *Corrections,* February 1980, pp. 5-17.

❧ 24 ❧

Working with
Abusers of Alcohol
and Other Drugs

Roger A. Roffman

The misuse of mood-changing drugs in mental health settings presents a challenge to the mental health manager. This chapter presents an overview of current knowledge about mood-changing drugs and their effects and describes drug-related issues that may emerge in mental health agencies. Terms are defined and various drug classifications are described. The chapter focuses on implications of drug-related problems for staff management and policy development in the drug treatment area of program operations and the interrelationship of drug and alcohol treatment. There are implications for management that affect supervision of staff as well as relationships with other community agencies.

The misuse of psychoactive substances by mental health agency clients and/or their relatives presents a challenge not only to the clinician but also to the administrator. In such settings, many persons are likely to be abusing alcohol, legal psychoactive drugs, illicit substances, or several of these in combination. Other clients are the spouses, children, or parents of substance-abusing individuals. Not infrequently, they are adversely affected through the relationship. Consequently, the proper assessment of client drug-related problems is a critically important service capability for effective case management. Considering the frequency with which alcohol or other drug abuse problems are hidden, at times as a function of client denial or the apparent predominance of other symptoms such as depression, accurate assessment becomes a highly pertinent issue. The attitudes, knowledge, and skills required for effective performance of this facet of client assessment are not generally acquired by the majority of mental health practitioners. Assuring that the agency is prepared to assess drug-related problems accurately, therefore, has administrative implications in reference to staff selection and role assignment, supervision and consultation, in-service training and continuing education, and interorganizational linkage.

Beyond assessment, the clinical challenge in treating the abuser of alcohol or other drugs is formidable. Both in their acute (for example, overdose, panic reaction, or toxic psychosis) and chronic (for example, physical debilitation, family problems, or legal difficulties) manifestations, abusers of psychoactive drugs are difficult persons with whom to work.

The drugs used in the treatment of emotional disorders are valuable components of service delivery in the mental health agency, although they are not always used in the best manner to maximize their potential while minimizing associated risk. Periodic reviews of drug utilization, including patterns of concurrent and/or consecutive nonchemical interventions in community mental health centers, are likely to be mandated under federal law in the future (Towery and Brands, 1979). Today's mental health executive is faced with policy decisions concerning the adequacy of the staff's drug-prescribing practices. The administrator may wish to consider the use of continuing education programs for professional staff in elevating the competence and knowledge of drug prescribers and other service providers whose responsibilities are likely to include monitoring client behavior for adverse drug reactions and/or improper prescribing or regimen noncompliance. To begin, some definitions of relevant terms may be useful.

1. *Psychoactive drug*—any chemical substance that alters mood, brain functioning, or perception; includes alcohol, legal and illegal drugs, solvents, and many compounds used in the treatment of emotional illness or disorder.
2. *Substance abuse*—the use of any psychoactive drug in a manner that adversely affects an individual's health, economic, social, or legal functioning (for example, arrests); includes illicit drug abuse, alcohol abuse and alcoholism, and the improper use of legal, therapeutic, psychoactive drugs.
3. *Dependence*—a psychological and/or physical "need" for the drug; other terms sometimes used include habituation, compulsive use, and addiction.

    *   *Psychological dependence*—an attitude or state of feeling in which the individual "needs" and uses the substance(s) to maximize well-being or functioning.
    *   *Physical dependence*—a physiological adaptation to the repeated administration of a substance, manifested by tolerance and a withdrawal syndrome.
4. *Tolerance*—a need for increasing dosages of a substance in order to achieve the desired effect.
5. *Withdrawal syndrome*—a set of symptoms, generally different for various classes of drugs, present when the body reacts to the abrupt cessation of regular drug use.
6. *Therapeutic psychoactive drugs*—agents used in the treatment of affective disorders, psychosis, and symptoms of emotional crisis or distress.

Classifying Psychoactive Drugs

Drugs can be classified in a variety of ways. The classification scheme used here groups them on the basis of their principal actions in affecting behavior.

Central Nervous System Depressants

Central nervous system (CNS) depressants include alcohol (to be discussed separately) and compounds used to treat anxiety, sleeping disorders, and convulsive disorders and to produce anesthesia. Although they differ in several respects, these drugs depress activity, ranging on a continuum from producing a state of slight lethargy or sleepiness through a rapid onset of sleep, inducing anesthesia, and, in the extreme, causing death from suppression of breathing and heart activity. These substances also share an alcohol-like behavioral action that contributes to their potential for nonmedical use as "recreational" agents.

Tolerance develops following repeated use of depressants, with cross tolerance to all other depressants (except the antihistamines-diphenylamines) automatically occurring as the body adapts to the chronic presence of any one drug in this class. The substances in this category also produce a characteristic set of withdrawal symptoms in individuals who abruptly cease taking the drug(s) after a fairly lengthy period of regular use. In certain instances, withdrawal from the CNS depressants can be life threatening. Therefore, medical supervision is mandatory, and patients withdrawing from these drugs may need inpatient care. In Tables 1 and 2, some of the more commonly prescribed and sometimes misused CNS depressants are listed.

Demand for CNS depressants from patients in both general medical and mental health settings can be quite persistent, with "shopping around" among physicians a common practice. Many individuals are apparently successful in acquiring repeated prescriptions for agents in this class. As a consequence, dependence on these drugs has been increasing, as has the rate of acute reactions seen in emergency rooms and crisis clinics.

Emergency problems associated with CNS depressants include overdose (deliberate or accidental), withdrawal symptoms, and temporary psychosis. The dangers associated with overdose can be severe, and therefore a suspected overdose calls for prompt medical supervision. Because the suicidal person contacting a therapist or crisis line may have ingested drugs in this category, it is necessary immediately to identify the nature of the individual's recent drug and alcohol intake and acquire medical evaluation of the data. One important implication for the mental health administrator is the need to assure that the staff knows how and when to acquire the needed data, to whom they should be presented in determining the existing degree of danger, and which resources to utilize for additional intervention.

Alcohol

Although alcohol is a CNS depressant, I discuss it separately because it deserves considerable attention in its own right. It is often said that one in ten

Table 1. Anti-anxiety Agents.

Drug Class	Generic Name	Trade Name
Benzodiazepines	Chlordiazepoxide	Librium
	Chlorazepate	Tranxene
	Oxazepam	Serax
	Diazepam	Valium
	Prazepam	Verstran
	Flurazepam	Dalmane
Diphenylamines	Hydroxyzine	Atarax
		Vistaril
Propanediols	Meprobamate	Equanil
		Kesso-bamate
		Miltown
	Tybamate	Tybatran

Table 2. Sedatives and Hypnotics.

Generic Name	Trade Name
Barbiturate Sedatives	
Amobarbital	Amytal
Butabarbital	Butisol
Heptabarbital	Medomin
Mephobarbital	Mebaral
Metharbital	Gemonil
Pentobarbital	Nembutal
Phenobarbital	Eskabarb
	Luminal
	Stental
Secobarbital	Seconal
Barbiturate Hypnotic	
Talbutal	Lotusate
Nonbarbiturate Sedatives	
Acetylcarbromal	Sedamyl
Chloral betaine	Beta-Chlor
Chloral hydrate	Felsules
	Kessodrate
	Noctec
	Somnos
Paraldehyde	Paral
Nonbarbiturate Hypnotic	
Ethchlorvynol	Placidyl
Ethinamate	Valmid
Glutethimide	Doriden
Methaqualone	Parest
	Quaalude
	Somnafac
	Sopor
Methylpentynol	Dormison
Methyprylon	Noludar

American drinkers becomes alcoholic, but the "fallout" resulting from alcohol abuse also includes occasional abusers of alcohol who are not alcoholic and the many other victims aside from the one doing the drinking (such as spouses, children, and employers).

Alcohol has a wide range of physical and emotional effects. Its physiological influence extends to the digestive system, where alcohol abuse is associated with high rates of cancer. The abuse of alcohol can have adverse effects on the neurological system, with deterioration in peripheral nerves and temporary or permanent organic brain syndromes. The cardiovascular system can be adversely affected, and it is estimated that perhaps 25 percent of alcoholics develop diseases of the heart. Alcohol also decreases the production of all types of blood cells, with associated adverse consequences. Body muscle is affected by alcohol, with a possibility that binge drinking can result in muscle inflammation or wasting.

Alcohol abuse can produce a wide range of emotional consequences. Disinhibition and increased feelings of self-confidence are common with moderate use, although many people who abuse alcohol experience elevated interpersonal problems as a result of poor judgment, greater expression of anger, more experience of sadness, and so forth.

Much of what has been said about tolerance and physical dependence with reference to the central nervous system depressants also holds with regard to alcohol. The symptoms of withdrawal are similar. Toxic reactions to alcohol may be due either to alcohol by itself or to its having been taken in conjunction with some other CNS depressant. Individuals overdosing from alcohol may actually be in danger of death due to respiratory and circulatory failure. This danger is heightened when several CNS depressants have been taken in combination.

As with the other CNS depressants, alcohol abuse can result in a temporary psychosis. The individual may present with symptoms of suspiciousness, actually to the point of paranoid delusions. Alcohol can precipitate persistent hallucinations, sometimes with voices that accuse the individual of some negative trait or activity. Most such individuals will improve considerably within a number of days, although medical evaluation for possible hospitalization is important.

The organic brain syndrome accompanying alcohol abuse can be a direct effect of the drug itself and/or associated, alcohol-related vitamin deficiencies. At relatively low levels of use, judgment and performance are impaired as a consequence of alcohol. At high levels of use, most individuals will show considerable confusion and disorientation. Elderly individuals and those with preexisting brain disorders will be less tolerant of alcohol and will therefore present with organic brain syndrome manifestations at lower dose levels. A number of organic pictures are associated with chronic heavy doses of alcohol. A fairly substantial percentage of nursing home patients with chronic organic brain syndrome have histories of alcoholism. Nerve cell damage and vitamin deficiencies as well as trauma may have contributed to this syndrome.

Because alcohol can impair the body's ability to absorb thiamine, individuals may suffer certain neurological problems. Also, decreased recent memory, confusion, and confabulation (Korsakoff's syndrome) may occur. Some individuals will rapidly improve when given an adequate replacement dosage of thiamine. Others may have permanent impairment.

The diagnosis of alcoholism requires a focus on life problems and an analysis of the possible manner in which one's drinking style has affected one's social, health, economic, legal, and family functioning. The diagnostician takes a very careful history, looking for evidence that excessive or inappropriate drinking has been associated with an abnormal marital or family history, moving violations in an automobile, frequent school- or job-related problems, and possible harm to health (for example, cirrhosis or heart disorder).

Far more alcoholics probably go undetected in mental health and general medical settings than are identified through an appropriate history-taking and assessment process. Gradually, as physicians and those in the allied health fields become more knowledgeable about and sensitive to alcohol and drug problems in their patients, the overlooking of alcoholics will decrease. At this point, however, it appears that the detection of and appropriate intervention in such problems is at a very low level.

In the backgrounds of many mental health clients who are not themselves alcohol abusers can be found very significant difficulties with their spouses, parents, or children who *are* alcohol abusers. The impact on the children of an alcoholic can be particularly severe. Not infrequently, such children will fear disclosing to the therapist an aberrant drinking pattern in the parent, possibly due to lack of understanding or fear or guilt. These persons commonly suffer as victims, having been caught in an unhealthy relationship. Moreover, as the alcoholic improves, his or her family members are likely to need assistance in adjusting to a new life-style. Survival for such family members has often meant the learning of skills and behaviors, which they must "unlearn" as the alcoholic person improves.

In summary, adequate diagnostic assessment in mental health settings must include preparation of the clinician to reach beyond the obvious and actively search for indicators that alcohol or other forms of drug abuse may be extant in the client or in somebody close to the client. The administrator must be sure that clinicians are sensitive to the need for such thoroughness in assessment, skillful in being able to carry out this function, and given the time to implement it. In-service training is important, as is the identification of alcoholism professionals in the community who can serve as referral resources or as consultants.

One of the major "themes" that create friction between mental health specialists and professionals in the field of alcoholism is the degree of emphasis given to the issue of drinking among clients with multiple problems. Some ex-alcoholic alcoholism professionals have lamented that when they were still actively drinking alcoholically, they were seen as clients by many mental health professionals who either chose not to probe into their drinking history or assumed that whatever problems in drinking existed would disappear once the emotional disorder at its roots was resolved. Alcoholism professionals will argue that the drinking must be dealt with *first*. Avoiding that as the primary objective may lead the alcoholic client to build an additional reserve of justification to continue drinking, partly on the basis that a professional mental health clinician has not seen fit to encourage the patient to do any differently.

This critical "theme" between the fields also has another important aspect. A fairly substantial number of alcoholics appear to have begun their alcoholic drinking secondary to some other disorder that in fact is the primary cause. When alcoholism exists as a result of some other primary cause, it is referred to as "secondary alcoholism." Alcoholism in the absence of preexisting major psychiatric problems can be diagnosed as being primary. Secondary alcoholism is most likely to be seen with either antisocial personality or affective disorder as the primary disorder (Schuckit, 1979).

Both in relation to primary antisocial personality and primary affective disorder with secondary alcoholism, it is imperative that mental health clinicians not miss the associated drinking pattern. Moreover, the necessity for referral of such individuals to appropriate facilities for treatment of alcoholism must be clearly understood by the clinical staff. In-service training should include exposure to each of the treatment modalities employed in alcoholism rehabilitation as well as Alcoholics Anonymous. Again, the importance of adequate staff training and available consultation and referral resources must be emphasized.

Client motivation for treatment is often low. The effective therapist should be able to convey to the tentative client an accepting attitude, an understanding of the client's emotions, and a clear intention not to be misled from identifying the role played by alcohol in relation to the problem. A trained clinician should also be skillful in helping those in the client's environment, such as family members, employer, or the clergy, in influencing the individual to undertake treatment. This is a critically important "gatekeeper" role for the mental health practitioner. Training of selected staff personnel in the specific skills of working with the alcoholic's network needs to be a high priority precisely because of the numbers of clients likely to need this service.

Opiates and Opiatelike Analgesics

Pain-killing narcotic drugs (analgesics) and those used in the treatment of diarrhea and cough are included in this classification. A list of representative drugs is presented in Table 3. Among the opiates are naturally occurring substances (opium, morphine, and codeine), semi-synthetic substances (heroin), and completely synthetic substances (Darvon and Demerol).

Predominant effects of these drugs are reduction or elimination of pain, production of a state of drowsiness, alteration of mood, and, at higher doses, clouding of mental functioning. These drugs produce rapid tolerance with repeated use, and cross tolerance to drugs in this class is also found. Individuals who regularly take these drugs can quickly become physically dependent.

"Street" use of drugs in this class has at various points in the last century become severely problematic. Addiction subcultures in the United States have periodically expanded considerably to produce "waves of addiction" that grew and then receded. The very substantial profits made by dealers in opiate drugs

Table 3. Opiates and Opiate-like Analgesics.

Generic Name	Trade Name
Opium	
Heroin	
Morphine	
Codeine	
Hydromorphone	Dilaudid
Oxycodone	Percodan
Methadone	Dolophine
Propoxyphene	Daricin
Meperidine	Demerol
Diphenoxylate	Lomotil
Pentazocine	Talwin
	Fortral

have created incentives for market expansion and the corruption of public officials. Crime associated with opiate dependence has also represented a major social problem, with the costs of illicit opiates being so high that dependent individuals are likely to engage in a criminal life-style in order to support their dependence.

A fairly substantial proportion of street opiate users in the United States are young, male, and members of minority groups. Nonmedical use of opiate drugs is not limited, however, to those who fit the street user profile. Illicit use by physicians, nurses, and other health professionals who have routine access to these drugs has been a problem. Recent research has described a subpopulation of users who are middle or upper class and occasionally use opiates illicitly over an extended period of time without becoming physically dependent. Not a great deal is known about these individuals who "chip" with heroin and other opiates, although it is likely that their patterns of life stability are stronger than those of the more typical street user.

Dependence on opiate drugs has commonly been perceived as an irreversible pattern associated with chronic relapse. The Vietnam experience has forced some revision in that perspective, however. Because many American soldiers became physically dependent on opiates while in Vietnam but few continued using them after they returned to the United States, the irreversible nature of opiate dependence has been questioned. A subculture of deviance probably never developed in Vietnam. Individuals who used the drugs there probably defined their use as temporary and justifiable, given the context.

Treatment prognosis for those opiate abusers who are caught up in a subculture of deviance is quite poor. Most individuals treated for opiate dependence relapse within two years following discharge from treatment. However, following repeated treatment exposures, the rate of abstinence increases over time. The mortality rate is also quite high, with causes of death including suicide, homicide, accidents, diseases, and infections. Emergencies associated with drugs in this class are usually due to overdose and/or allergic reactions. Both are potentially life threatening and require immediate medical attention. Fortunately, narcotic antagonists exist that can quickly reverse an opiate overdose.

As is the case with withdrawal from the barbiturates, individuals who have become dependent on the opiates and are withdrawing are likely to be in considerable psychological distress. A marked drive for the drug will exist, with the individual feeling an intense need for a new dose within a few hours of the last injection. Physical symptoms of withdrawal tend not to be life threatening; they begin within eight to twelve hours of the last dose and peak within two to three days. An individual in withdrawal is likely to manifest restless sleep, dilated pupils, loss of appetite, goose flesh, back pain, tremor, incessant yawning, weakness, gastrointestinal upset, chills, muscle spasm, and abdominal pain. During these several days of withdrawal, the individual will be very irritable. Although these symptoms are very prominent during two or three days following cessation of use, withdrawal from opiates actually goes on for many months. Discomfort during this more protracted period may help to explain the very high rate of relapse among formerly dependent individuals.

Opiate abusers are very likely to have a number of medical problems associated with their drug taking. Problems such as skin infections, hepatitis and other liver abnormalities, gastric ulcers, and anemias are commonly found. The need for concomitant medical attention for opiate abusers during mental health intervention is therefore important.

Opiate abusers are likely to be younger than alcoholics, are more likely to be referred by the criminal justice system, and will have a greater history of antisocial problems. The challenge to the clinician in making an accurate assessment while effectively educating the individual about his or her drug problem and encouraging rehabilitation will be considerable.

Since the early 1960s, methadone detoxification and maintenance have been fairly widespread. Methadone is a synthetic substance that itself is addicting but that has several advantages over heroin. It can be taken orally and lasts much longer than heroin. Individuals placed on methadone maintenance are given some respite from the life-style of the hustling junkie, with the objective of using this time to build improved social, vocational, and family functioning.

In many parts of the United States, therapeutic "communities" offer programs that emphasize a self-help approach, employing an intensive, highly structured, live-in environment that seeks to rebuild an individual's character by a process of peer confrontation and support. As is the case with methadone, therapeutic communities are helpful for many individuals, but retain fewer than half of those beginning treatment.

Central Nervous System Stimulants

Commonly abused stimulant drugs are listed in Table 4. The drugs in this class include the amphetamines, cocaine, and a number of other substances that share the property of stimulating the central nervous system. Relatively few medical conditions are treated with drugs in this category. Cocaine has utility as a local anesthetic. Other drugs in this class are used in the treatment of narcolepsy and hyperkinesis. Their use in weight control has largely been discontinued because

Table 4. Central Nervous System Stimulants.

Generic Name	Trade Name
Amphetamine	Benzedrine
Benzphetamine	Didrex
Caffeine	
Chlorphentermine	Pre-Sate
Cocaine	
Dextroamphetamine	Dexedrine
Diethylpropion	Tenuate, Tepanil
Fenfluramine	Pondimin
Methamphetamine	Desoxyn, Fetamin
Methylphenidate	Ritalin
Phenmetrazine	Preludin
Phentermine	Ionamin, Wilpo

people rapidly develop tolerance to them, they are ineffective over the long run, and their potential for abuse is significant.

CNS stimulants cause euphoria and a reduction in fatigue and the need for sleep. Appetite reduction, increased energy, possible interference with normal sleep patterns, and a reduction in distractibility in children with hyperkinetic syndrome are commonly found effects. An increased ability to focus or concentrate is often cited as a reason for using these drugs.

Tolerance develops quite rapidly, with the possibility that individuals who are regularly using stimulants will quickly seek elevated dosages. Although withdrawal has not classically been defined as presenting major physical threat, there is little question but that individuals who have been chronically abusing stimulants will experience a set of adjustment difficulties upon cessation, including apathy, irritability, depression, and possible suicidal ideation.

Profiles of stimulant abusers include both those individuals who begin their use within a medical context, such as weight control, and those who acquire stimulants such as amphetamines or cocaine through illicit channels for recreational purposes. In either case, emergency problems associated with these drugs include panic reactions, temporary psychosis, and a number of possible medical difficulties. Physical effects associated with abuse include a rapid heart rate, palpitations, anxiety, nervousness, and hyperventilation. As a consequence, individuals who are taking large amounts of stimulants can experience temporary panic associated with the belief that they are experiencing a heart attack, losing control, or becoming psychotic.

Overdosing with stimulants can result in convulsions, markedly elevated blood pressure, a very high body temperature, and possibly cardiovascular shock. Psychological dimensions of excessive doses can include a high rate of suspiciousness, repetitive stereotyped behaviors, picking at various objects and parts of the body, and grinding of the teeth (bruxism).

Temporary psychotic conditions are associated with stimulant abuse. A high level of paranoid delusions and suspiciousness may be manifested, and hallucinations involving auditory, visual, or tactile experiences (feeling things crawling on one's skin) can occur. Individuals experiencing paranoid delusions associated with stimulants can become quite violent, resulting in unprovoked outbursts of aggression. Following cessation of stimulant abuse, individuals are at considerable risk for depression that may involve suicidal ideation and/or attempts. As a consequence, very careful mental health assessment and appropriate intervention is important in the first month of abstinence following a long period of stimulant abuse.

Cannabis

Marijuana, one of several products derived from the Cannabis plant, generally refers to its flowering tops and leaves. The plant material is quite complex, containing at least 419 individual chemicals. Among these are the cannabinoids, 61 currently identified chemicals unique to Cannabis. Delta-9-tetrahydrocannabinol (THC, for short) is believed to be the principal psychoactive cannabinoid in the plant.

Pharmacologists generally classify marijuana by itself because it is not a stimulant or a depressant or a narcotic, although it can produce behavioral symptoms similar to those produced by the other kinds of drugs. The psychoactive effects of marijuana vary, depending on how much is taken, its potency, the setting, and the individual's mood and expectations. The most commonly experienced reaction to small doses is a state of mild intoxication. When a normal dose has been taken, the individual generally has a pleasurable feeling of well-being. (Because potency of marijuana on the illicit market varies, it is difficult to be precise about what constitutes a "normal" dose. For my purposes, a normal dose is approximately three to five inhalations from a cigarette made from marijuana that costs $60 or less an ounce. For the more expensive, and thus generally more potent, marijuana, a normal dose might be one or two inhalations.) Often the person feels more talkative, humorous, and perhaps contemplative. It is common for the person to experience an increased enjoyment from music, food, and perhaps color and touch. Distortion of these senses, however, rarely occurs.

Another common experience is momentary forgetfulness. For example, a person might find that he or she suddenly cannot remember what has just been said in a conversation and needs to work a bit harder on concentration. These are not permanent effects, but last only for the short period of time the person is using marijuana. People using marijuana tend to experience time as passing somewhat slower than normal; that is, if they are asked to estimate how much time has passed in a certain interval, they may overestimate the amount.

A less common but occasional effect of marijuana is the temporary experience of anxiety or fearfulness. Most often when this occurs, it is in the person who has never before used this drug and is consequently a bit apprehensive about the new feelings she or he is experiencing. It may also occur in the experienced user who has taken high-potency marijuana.

Very few physical effects are experienced while using marijuana. An increase in pulse rate occurs, but not to the extent that it presents a problem, with one important exception. There is evidence that in persons with impaired heart function (angina pectoris), engaging in physical effort while using marijuana may result in chest pain. Among the other physical effects associated with the use of marijuana are a reddening of the eyes, a decrease in the secretion of tears, a reduction in intraocular pressure, dryness of the mouth and throat, and an increase in the diameter of air passages of the lungs. In some individuals, a lowering of blood pressure is found. Several of these physical effects have relevance for possible therapeutic uses of marijuana.

Scientists have learned that tolerance to marijuana develops with prolonged use. This means that the heavy user will be likely to increase the amount taken over time due to the body adjusting to the frequent presence of the drug. A larger dose becomes necessary in order to achieve the effect earlier produced by a smaller amount.

Under conditions of typical street use of marijuana, physical dependence does not occur. However, stopping after prolonged heavy use may result in a period of readjustment with symptoms such as irritability, restlessness, appetite disturbance, and difficulty sleeping.

The notions of several decades ago that marijuana caused criminality, aggressive behavior, and harder drug use have been dismissed. The progression theory that marijuana leads to use of "harder" drugs has not been documented, although there is a statistical correlation between the use of marijuana and the use of other drugs. Marijuana intoxication has been found to result in a decrease rather than an increase in expressed and experienced hostility. It is in relation to driving performance that the marijuana-intoxicated state is of greatest concern. Impairment in driving ability often occurs even with low dose levels.

There is no evidence that marijuana causes mental illness. However, it is unwise for those with diagnosed schizophrenia to use marijuana because of the risk of precipitating an acute psychotic episode.

The effects of marijuana in relation to memory, sense of time, tasks involving reaction time, conceptual formulation, learning, perceptual motor coordination, and attention have been examined in laboratory conditions. It appears that marijuana affects each of these only during the hours in which the individual is using the drug. However, in the context of frequent marijuana use by students, these effects can have serious implications for learning ability. Although some individuals report a subjective feeling of greater learning while "high" in the classroom, the evidence from research contradicts that perception. Because there are data from national surveys that as many as 10 percent of high school seniors are daily marijuana users, the disruption of knowledge acquisition and classroom functioning accompanying this pattern of marijuana use must be considered a social problem of considerable magnitude.

Several long-term effects have been actively studied in recent years. Among them are the following:

1. *Pulmonary effects.* One long-term effect for which there is considerable evidence is the impairment of lung functioning resulting from regular use. There is no direct evidence at this time that smoking marijuana causes lung cancer. However, there is reason to expect that extended use may ultimately be discovered to result in the occurrence of this disease. Marijuana smoke has been found to contain larger amounts of cancer-producing hydrocarbons than does tobacco smoke. Another possible pulmonary effect pertains to the impairment of antibacterial defense systems in the lungs following exposure to marijuana smoke.

2. *Reproductive effects.* Impairment may result in diminished sperm count and motility in males as well as possible interference with fertility in females. These effects may be of particular significance for the marginally fertile. Experimental studies also raise the possibility that regular marijuana use in the female may result in an increased risk of reproductive loss, for example, fetal resorptions or abortions.

3. *Effects on the immune response.* Whether prolonged use of marijuana results in a reduction of the body's natural defenses against illness has been the subject of several studies. The results are as yet inconclusive, with different researchers reporting contradictory evidence.

4. *Effects on chromosomes.* Chromosomal alterations, either through increases in the number of abnormal chromosomes or a reduction in the number of chromosomes in some body cells, have been a matter of concern because of the potentially serious implications related to genetic transmission. At this time, there is no convincing evidence that marijuana use causes clinically significant chromosome damage.

5. *Alterations in cell metabolism.* Possible alterations in cellular metabolism, particularly in the production of DNA and RNA, which are involved in cell reproduction, have also been studied. Among the difficulties that could potentially exist in this regard are an increased susceptibility to cancer and erratic cell growth in marijuana users. Another possibility is that marijuana might have value in inhibiting human cancer growth or in preventing organ rejection in human organ transplant surgery. The current status of research in this area does not warrant definitive conclusions.

6. *Brain damage.* A 1971 British study raised the possibility that brain atrophy (shrinkage) might be a consequence of chronic marijuana use. Subsequent studies, using more advanced research procedures, have failed to verify this hypothesis.

7. *Intellectual functioning.* Indications that chronic marijuana use may impair intellectual functioning have come from overseas studies, which have major limitations due to their quality. Research on American users has not led to the finding of intellectual impairment, although most of these studies have been done with highly motivated college students using relatively small amounts of marijuana for short periods of time. The frequently mentioned concern that prolonged use leads to an "amotivational syndrome," or loss of ambition and goal directedness, has not been demonstrated in research studies.

Several potential therapeutic uses of marijuana and/or related compounds are currently under investigation. The most promising of these is nausea and vomiting control in relation to chemotherapy treatment for cancer. Other potential therapeutic uses being studied include the treatment of glaucoma, convulsive activity in epileptics, anxiety, pain, depression, asthma, anorexia (an eating disorder), and muscular spasticity in paraplegics and patients with multiple sclerosis. In each of these areas, additional research will be necessary before conclusions can be drawn.

Hallucinogens

Hallucinogens alter consciousness with the production of abnormal sensory inputs of a predominantly visual nature. Table 5 lists representative hallucinogenic drugs. This category includes naturally occurring (psilocybin and peyote) and synthetic (LSD) hallucinogenic agents. There is a history of hallucinogenic drug use in many cultures dating back for thousands of years.

The predominant effects of hallucinogenic drugs include an increased awareness of sensory input and a subjective feeling of enhanced mental activity. Environmental stimuli appear to be experienced in a somewhat distorted manner; bodily images appear to be altered; introspection is perceived as considerably enhanced; and, not uncommonly, individuals claim to experience previously unacknowledged connections between themselves and their surroundings.

Physical effects include dilated pupils, elevated blood sugar, a fine tremor, facial flushing, and increased blood pressure and body temperature. Rapid tolerance, which rapidly reverses, is manifested to hallucinogenic agents. Physical dependence does not appear to occur.

Commonly, drugs sold as hallucinogenic agents in the street culture are misrepresented. Individuals believing they have purchased LSD are often getting what they paid for, but much of the material represented as being mescaline or peyote is either an inert substance or some other hallucinogenic agent. Adulterants are commonly found mixed with hallucinogenic chemicals. As a consequence, it is not safe to assume that any particular sample will have a predictable outcome; the variability is too large for the buyer to be assured of content and quality.

LSD is a very potent drug producing hallucinations that last from four to twelve hours. The actual experience of being "high" depends upon the dose, the individual's emotional and mental preparation, prior experience, and the environmental context.

The peyote cactus yields mescaline, which is also a commonly used hallucinogen. The effects of mescaline are similar to those of LSD, although there is a slower onset and a frequent occurrence of unpleasant side effects such as nausea and vomiting.

Psilocybin is a hallucinogenic chemical found in certain mushrooms, many of which grow in abundance in the Pacific Northwest. The onset of effects is rapid, generally within fifteen minutes. The overall psilocybin "high" lasts for perhaps five to six hours. DOM or STP is a synthetic hallucinogen and resembles

Table 5. Hallucinogenic Drugs.

Generic Types	Examples
Indolealkylamines	LDS
	Psilocybin
	Psilocyn
	Dimethyltryptamine (DMT)
	Diethyltryptamine (DET)
Phenylethylamines	Mescaline (peyote)

Phenylisopropylamines	2,5-dimethoxy-4-methyl-
	      amphetamine (DOM or
	      STP)

Related drugs	Phencyclidine (PCP)
	Nutmeg
	Morning glory seeds
	Catnip
	Nitrous oxide
	Amyl or butyl nitrite

LSD in its effects. The drug is less potent than LSD, however. Effects begin usually within one hour of ingestion and disappear within seven to eight hours.

Emergency problems associated with hallucinogenic agents include panic reactions, flashbacks, and toxic reactions. The panic attack or anxiety reaction is manifested by an individual who is acutely frightened, often hallucinating, and worried about losing control and sanity. Generally, such reactions occur in individuals who are novice users or those who have unexpectedly received a very potent dose. Treatment generally does not include using medication but rather reassuring the individual over a period of hours while the drug reaction is wearing off. Placing the individual in a comfortable and warm physical environment is also important. There is considerable risk in using antipsychotic medications for hallucinogenic panic reactions. In the event that the hallucinogenic agent is STP, the antipsychotic medication may actually enhance the psychoticlike symptoms, rather than reduce them.

Flashbacks, or the experience of drug effects days or weeks following drug ingestion, are generally reported in association with hallucinogenic agents. Victims of flashbacks often fear that they have experienced permanent brain damage and understandably are likely to be quite anxious and perhaps paranoid. The possible mechanism causing flashback activity is the retention in the body of drug metabolites, which become reactivated, perhaps as a result of a new drug-taking experience or an emotional crisis. Individuals may experience hallucinations while having a flashback and may also have feelings of depersonalization or severe emotional reactions. Treatment generally includes reassurance that this set of symptoms will gradually reduce and education about the probable mechanisms underlying the flashback. The individual will also need instruction to avoid medications that are likely to have a mood-changing effect.

Toxic reactions to hallucinogenic agents include a loss of contact with reality and such physical symptoms as palpitations, increase in blood pressure and temperature, perspiration, and blurred vision. Convulsive activity is also a potential effect. The individual may manifest many of the same symptoms of a panic reaction when experiencing an overdose. Medical supervision is important and careful monitoring for at least twenty-four hours is necessary. For STP or PCP, the period of monitoring may need to be for as long as two weeks in the event of a toxic reaction. Psychotic reactions associated with hallucinogens generally clear rapidly. Again, STP and PCP may be exceptions, with longer periods of psychoticlike symptoms being manifested.

Phencyclidine (PCP), also called angel dust, needs some discussion in its own right. Originally introduced as a general anesthetic agent, it is currently used as a veterinary anesthetic but is no longer used in medical care of humans. Its common use as a street drug has resulted in a number of behavioral problems. This drug can be taken through smoking, oral ingestion, or injection. It is easily produced by amateur chemists. Physical effects associated with PCP include increases in blood pressure, heart rate, respiratory rate, and muscle rigidity. Other physical effects include sweating, flushing, drooling, and pupillary constriction. An individual may experience dizziness, reduced coordination, and slurred speech.

Psychological effects at low doses include a feeling of euphoria. At higher doses the individual is likely to experience a drunken state, numbness of the extremities, and delusions. Violent behavior has been reported with PCP intoxication on numerous occasions. At very high doses, convulsive activity may lead to death. Toxic reactions to PCP have been fairly commonly reported and may represent a potentially fatal threat at higher dosage levels. The individual may be psychologically detached and unresponsive to external stimuli or may present in a highly excited and potentially violent and hostile manner. Paranoid and/or manic behavior may occur, with psychotic symptoms lasting from a day to perhaps as long as a month. Hospitalization on a closed psychiatric ward may be necessary if individuals are potentially harmful to themselves or to others.

Glues, Solvents, and Aerosols

Glues, solvents, aerosols, and similar substances that may be abused for mood-changing effect are listed in Table 6. All these drugs produce depression of the central nervous system. The fact that they are readily available, inexpensive, legal, and easy to conceal makes them attractive to some individuals, particularly adolescent delinquents. Generally, the mood-changing effect begins within minutes and lasts for an hour or less. Individuals feel giddy and light-headed. Amnesia may occasionally be experienced during the height of the inhalation episode.

Physical effects associated with acute intoxication may include irritation of the eyes, sensitivity to light, double vision, ringing in the ears, coughing, and irritation of the lining or mucous membranes of the nose and mouth. Individuals may feel faint, may experience nausea and vomiting, may suffer from diarrhea, and may show irregularities in heartbeat.

Table 6. Glues, Solvents, and Aerosols.

Generic Types	Examples
Glues	Toluene, naphtha, acetates, hexane, benzene, xylene, chloroform
Cleaning solutions	Trichloroethylene, petroleum products, carbon tetrachloride
Nail polish removers	Acetone
Lighter fluids	Naphtha, aliphatic hydrocarbons
Paints and paint thinners	Toluene, butylacetate, acetone, naphtha, methanol, ethanol
Aerosols	Fluorinated hydrocarbons, nitrous oxide
Other petroleum products	Gasoline, benzene, toluene, petroleum ether

Tolerance to these drugs develops and disappears quite rapidly. There do not appear to be withdrawal effects, and therefore these substances are not believed to be physically dependence producing. The kinds of emergencies seen with solvent abuse include toxic reactions, medical complications, and organic brain syndromes. Panic reactions, when they occur, tend to be very short-lived. The physical distress involving a toxic reaction is potentially life-threatening, including respiratory depression and cardiac irregularity. Rapid loss of consciousness and sudden death may occur. Individuals inhaling solvents deeply from a plastic bag may suffer the risk of death from suffocation.

Psychological consequences of toxic reactions include anxiety and some level of mental impairment. Violent outbursts during intoxication are possible, and the individual will need to be treated with supportive care, including controlling behavior for the short time intoxication lasts.

Treatment of the Multidrug Abusing Client

Individuals who are heavily abusing a combination of mood-altering substances occasionally find their way into treatment in a mental health agency. It is important in dealing with such individuals first to determine whether there is any primary physical dependence to one or more substances. Second, the possibility of a preexisting psychiatric disorder must be considered. Third, the culture that characterizes the individual needs to be determined in assessing whether a street-oriented treatment environment, as opposed to a more conventional context, would be appropriate. Casual users of marijuana, hallucinogens, cocaine, and other psychoactive substances may be coerced into seeking treatment, perhaps by concerned parents or by the criminal justice system. Careful assessment needs to be given to the presence or absence of major health or life problems accompanying the individual's drug-taking patterns. If the essential difficulty is law violation, the treatment offered ought not to be the same as rehabilitation geared toward the individual with a major dependence difficulty. Rather, the casual user in difficulty with the legal system may need to learn better decision-making skills. Of course, the fact of legal coercion does not rule out the possibility of an individual having a major drug dependence problem. In such instances, the legal system's oversight of the individual may be effectively used as leverage in promoting client involvement in treatment. Residential therapeutic communities often are appropriate treatment contexts for the heavily involved multidrug abuser whose socialization has been to a street culture.

Conclusion

A wealth of information has been compiled concerning the types, effects, and usages of various psychoactive drugs. Out of the facts and findings on which this chapter draws, four principal implications emerge for mental health administrators. The first is that mental health clinicians need to be adequately trained to conduct assessments of clients' drug and alcohol histories in order to identify and properly serve substance abusers and/or their families. Second, medical evaluation of individuals who are potentially in jeopardy from toxic reactions, withdrawal, or other medical emergencies is necessary. All clinical staff members must know what criteria require a referral to or consultation with a physician. Third, the prescribing of therapeutic psychoactive medications brings with it a host of potential difficulties. All clinical personnel in mental health centers should be trained to identify signs of adverse drug effects, with the goal of bringing such matters to the attention of the prescribing physician. In-service training in mental health centers is vitally important for this team function to operate properly. The fourth implication is that the potential misuse of therapeutic psychoactive drugs also warrants a systematic internal review process through which drug prescribing is periodically reviewed on a case-by-case basis as well as for purposes of establishing mental health agency policy.

References

Honigfeld, G., and Howard, A. *Psychiatric Drugs: A Desk Reference.* (2nd ed.) New York: Academic Press, 1978.

Roffman, R. A. "Addiction Concepts and the Vietnam Experience." *The Urban and Social Change Review,* 1976, *9* (2), 16–18.

Schuckit, M. A. *Drug and Alcohol Abuse: A Clinical Guide to Diagnosis and Treatment.* New York: Plenum, 1979.

Towery, O. B., and Brands, A. B. *Psychotropic Drugs: Approaches to Psychopharmacologic Drug Use.* Washington, D.C.: U.S. Government Printing Office, 1979.

ੴ 25 ੴ

Occupational
Therapy Services in
Mental Health Programs

Sylvia Harlock

Occupational therapy services related to aftercare and sheltered workshops provide a valuable dimension to mental health programs for marginally functioning chronic clients. When mental health administrators understand and utilize occupational treatment plan approaches, occupational therapy services can be implemented most advantageously. This chapter will familiarize managers with the most salient characteristics of occupational therapy philosophies, principles, and practices. Specific evaluation and treatment approaches are described and examples of occupational therapy services are given.

Occupational therapy involves the treatment of clients with cognitive, social emotional, and/or physical problems. In the early 1900s, a number of people recognized the therapeutic value of structured activity programs for the institutionalized mentally ill. Almost at the same time, a separate group recognized that participation in activities could hasten the recovery of the physically injured. Persons representing these two roots merged in 1917 to form the National Society for the Promotion of Occupational Therapy. The purpose of the association was "the advancement of occupation as a therapeutic measure, the study of the effects of occupation on the human being, and the dissemination of scientific knowledge of this subject" (Hopkins and Smith, 1978, p. 10). The profession has remained dedicated to this basic focus, as is reflected in the definition of occupational therapy adopted by the American Occupational Therapy Association in 1977: "Occupational therapy is the application of purposeful, goal-oriented activity in the evaluation, problem identification, and/or treatment of persons whose function is impaired by physical illness or injury, emotional disorder, congenital or developmental disability, or the aging process, in order to achieve optimum functioning, to prevent disability, and to maintain health" (Reed and Sanderson, 1980, p. 4).

Since the beginning of the profession in 1917, many advances have been made in understanding the function of goal-oriented activity in a person's life and in designing treatment methods to assist in the healthy development and rehabilitation of the ill and injured (Cynkin, 1979; Hopkins and Smith, 1978; Reed and Sanderson, 1980).

Occupational therapy traditionally has been offered in hospital inpatient psychiatric units, community mental health center day treatment programs, residential treatment facilities (including halfway houses), alcohol treatment programs, sheltered workshops, nursing home and conglomerate care facilities, home health agencies, and geriatric daycare programs. To a lesser degree, occupational therapy also has been available through outpatient psychiatric/mental health programs, drug treatment programs, special educational programs for the mentally disturbed in the school system, jails and prisons, community-based social service programs for special populations or groups (such as child abusers or juvenile delinquents), and through private practitioners. The types of medical and social diagnoses that occupational therapists have traditionally treated have corresponded to the types of clients encountered in these settings.

This division would appear to reflect a medical–social division rather than a division based on the client's need for a service such as occupational therapy. There are probably several factors that account for this. Occupational therapy has historically been closely aligned with medicine, but is more recently becoming prominent in educational and community-based social service treatment agencies/programs.

A second factor underlying these service utilization patterns is somewhat related to the first, in that occupational therapy has in the past been viewed as adjunctive to the medical profession. The occupational therapist provided the activities under the physician's prescription, and the physician provided the primary therapy. This has been changing over the past fifteen to twenty years; occupational therapists have become responsible in their own right for evaluating and treating the client in collaboration with the team.

A third factor lies in the demographic characteristics of the members of the profession. Until the past few years, over 90 percent of the field was composed of therapists who were female, in their middle twenties, with bachelor's degrees in the field. The majority left the field after a few years of employment to assume the role of homemaker-mother. The trend has changed. More men are entering the field; women are working in the field longer; and an increasing percentage of therapists are completing master's degrees in occupational therapy and related fields. The longer the work experience and the higher the educational attainment, the more likely it is that therapists will develop internal knowledge bases unique to the profession, enabling them to function independently and to design new service delivery programs.

A fourth factor is reimbursement patterns. Insurance coverage and program funding for mental health programs have been notoriously poor. Among the mental health professions, insurance coverage for occupational therapy has been slow in coming. But this situation is changing. Across the nation, hospital inpatient occupational therapy, and in many states outpatient services as well, are now usually reimbursable.

In the future, we are likely to see occupational therapists moving increasingly into the role of primary therapist, moving into outpatient and community-based social service programs, expanding their involvement from working primarily with clients with psychiatric diagnoses to including those with social diagnoses (for example, child abuse and juvenile delinquency), and providing more consultation to other disciplines, families, and paraprofessionals.

There are two levels of entry into the field of occupational therapy, one at the registered occupational therapy level and another at the certified occupational therapy assistant level. The two main routes that correspond to these levels are the bachelor's degree and the associate-level degree, respectively. Both involve educational and fieldwork training and passage of national certification examinations, but at different levels of depth and somewhat different levels of focus of content. Most client evaluation and program planning is done by the registered occupational therapist, with the certified occupational therapist functioning in an assistant role. Consultation is done by the registered occupational therapist. Thus, the registered occupational therapist is involved in management of a service and supervision of other personnel. The registered occupational therapist receives some coursework in management and supervision, but it is expected that a therapist have two to three years of clinical work experience before assuming the role of chief of a service. Many master's-level occupational therapy educational programs offer the opportunity to focus on advanced educational training in administration and management.

The field of occupational therapy is developing very rapidly. In 1978, there were thirty-six schools offering bachelor's-level degrees in occupational therapy, sixteen offering master's-level degrees, and one offering a doctoral program (American Occupational Therapy Association, 1978). The emphasis is currently on the development of more master's- and doctoral-level educational programs. There has also been a recognition of the need for more research in the field. A Research Division was created in the National Office of the American Occupational Therapy Association in 1979, and a program has been instituted to offer technical guidance and grant procurement assistance to therapists in the field. With an increasing percentage of therapists obtaining advanced degrees in occupational therapy and related fields, involvement in research will increase. The national organization, the American Occupational Therapy Association, is a strong organization in terms of facilitating the development of the field.

Clients' Problems of Concern to Occupational Therapy

Occupational therapy is concerned with individuals who have difficulty functioning in their daily lives. They have difficulty carrying out their physical or psychosocial/emotional daily living activities, work activities, and/or play/leisure activities.

Independent Living/Daily Living Skills

Independent living/daily living skills (including self-care) refer to the skill and performance of physical and psychological/emotional self-care, work, and play/leisure activities to a level of independence appropriate to age, disability, and lifespace (cultural background, value orientation, and physical and social environment).

Physical Daily Living Skills. Physical daily living skills refer to the skill and performance of daily personal care, with or without adaptive equipment. The category includes but is not limited to the following:

1. *Grooming and hygiene*—the skill and performance of personal health needs, such as bathing, toileting, hair care, shaving, applying makeup.
2. *Feeding/eating*—the skill and performance of sequentially feeding oneself, including sucking, chewing, swallowing, and using appropriate utensils.
3. *Dressing*—choosing appropriate clothing, dressing oneself in a sequential fashion, including fastening and adjusting clothing.
4. *Functional mobility*—moving oneself from one position or place to another, including skills necessary for activities such as bed mobility, wheelchair mobility, transfers (bed, car, tub, toilet, chair), functional ambulation, with or without adaptive aids, use of public and private travel systems, such as driving own automobile and using public transportation.
5. *Object manipulation*—handling large and small common objects, such as calculators, keys, money, light switches, doorknobs, and packages.

Psychological/Emotional Daily Living Skills. Psychological/emotional daily living skills refer to the skill and performance in developing one's self-concept/self-identity, coping with life situations, and participating in one's organization and community environment. It includes but is not limited to the following:

1. *Self-concept/self-identity*—the cognitive image of one's functional self, which includes but is not limited to
   - Clearly perceiving one's needs, feelings, conflicts, values, beliefs, expectations, sexuality, and power.
   - Realistically perceiving others' needs, feelings, conflicts, values, beliefs, expectations, sexuality, and power.
   - Knowing one's performance strengths and limitations.
   - Sensing one's competence, achievement, self-esteem, and self-respect.
   - Integrating new experiences with established self-concept/self-identity.
   - Having a sense of psychological safety and security.
   - Perceiving one's goals and directions.

2. *Situational coping*—handling stress and dealing with problems and changes in a manner that is functional for self and others, which includes but is not limited to
   - Setting goals, selecting, harmonizing, and managing activities of daily living to promote optimal performance.
   - Testing goals and perceptions against reality.
   - Perceiving changes and need for changes in self and environment.
   - Directing and redirecting energy to overcome problems.
   - Initiating, implementing, and following through on decisions.
   - Assuming responsibility for self and consequences of actions.
   - Interacting with others, dyadic and group.
3. *Community involvement*—interacting within one's social system, which includes but is not limited to
   - Understanding social norms and their impact on society.
   - Planning, organizing, and executing daily life activities in relationship to society, including such activities as budgeting, time management, social role management, arranging for housing, nutritional planning, assessing and using community resources.
   - Recognizing and responding to needs of families, groups, and complex social units.
   - Understanding and responding to organizational/community role expectations as both recipient and contributor.

Work. Work refers to skill and performance in participating in socially purposeful and productive activities. These activities may take place in the home, employment setting, school, or community. They include but are not limited to the following:

1. *Homemaking*—meal planning, meal preparation and cleanup, laundry, cleaning, minor household repairs, shopping, and use of household safety principles.
2. *Child care/parenting*—includes but is not limited to physical care of children and use of age-appropriate activities, communication, and behavior to facilitate child development.
3. *Employment preparation*—precursory job activities (including prevocational activities), which include but are not limited to
   - Job-acquisition skills and performance.
   - Organizational and team participatory skills and performance.
   - Work-process skills and performance.
   - Work-product quality.

Play/Leisure. Play/leisure refers to skill and performance in choosing, performing, and engaging in activities for amusement, relaxation, spontaneous enjoyment, and/or self-expression. This includes but is not limited to the following:

1. Recognizing one's specific needs, interests, and adaptations necessary for performance.
2. Identifying characteristics of activities and social situations that make them play for the individual.
3. Identifying activities that contain those characteristics.
4. Choosing play activities for participation, such as sports, games, hobbies, music, or drama.
5. Testing out and adapting activities to enable participation.
6. Identifying and using community resources.

Sensorimotor Components

Sensorimotor components refer to the skill and performance of patterns of sensory and motor behavior that are prerequisites to self-care, work, and play/leisure performance. The components in this section include neuromuscular and sensory integrative skills, including perceptual motor skills.

Neuromuscular. Neuromuscular refers to the skill and performance of motor aspects of behavior. This includes but is not limited to the following:

1. *Reflex integration*—enhancing and supporting functional neuromuscular development through eliciting and/or inhibiting stereotyped, patterned, and/or involuntary responses coordinated at subcortical and cortical levels.
2. *Range of motion*—using maximum span of joint movement in activities, with and without assistance, to enhance functional performance.
3. *Gross and fine motor coordination*—muscle control, coordination, and dexterity while participating in activities.
4. *Strength and endurance*—using muscular force within time periods necessary for purposeful task performance, which involves but is not limited to progressively building strength and cardiac and pulmonary reserve, increasing the length of work period, and decreasing fatigue and strain.

Sensory Integration. Sensory integration refers to skill and performance in development and coordination of sensory input, motor output, and sensory feedback. This includes but is not limited to the following:

1. *Sensory awareness*—perceiving and differentiating external and internal stimuli.
2. *Visual-spatial awareness*—perceiving distances between and relationships among objects, including self.
3. *Body integration*—perceiving and regulating the position of various muscles and body parts in relationship to each other during static and movement states.

Cognitive Components

Cognitive components refer to skill and performance of the mental processes necessary to know or apprehend by understanding. This includes but is not limited to the following:

1. *Orientation*—comprehending, defining, and adjusting oneself in an environment with regard to time, place, and person.
2. *Conceptualization/comprehension*—conceiving and understanding concepts or tasks such as color identification, word recognition, sign concepts, sequencing, matching, association, classification, and abstracting.
3. *Cognitive integration*—applying diverse knowledge to environmental situations.

Psychosocial Components

Psychosocial components refer to skill and performance in self-management and dyadic and group interaction.

1. *Self-management*—expressing and controlling oneself in functional and creative activities.
   * *Self-expression*—expressing one's feelings and interpreting and using a variety of communication signs and symbols.
   * *Self-control*—modulating and modifying present behaviors and initiating new behaviors in accordance with situational demands.
2. *Dyadic interaction*—relating to another person.
3. *Group interaction*—relating to groups of three to six persons or more.

Therapeutic Adaptations

Therapeutic adaptations refer to the design and/or restructuring of the physical environment to assist self-care, work, and play/leisure performance. This includes selecting, obtaining, fitting, and fabricating equipment and instructing the client, family, and/or staff in proper use and care of equipment. It also includes minor repair and modification for correct fit, position, or use.

Prevention

Prevention refers to skill and performance in minimizing debilitation. It may include programs for persons where predisposition to disability exists, as well as for those who have already incurred a disability.

Underlying Skills

The performance of any one of these activities requires the development of a large number of specific skills. Thus, when encountering clients with problems in these areas, the therapist looks for problems in the underlying skills. These underlying skills may be grouped into the following categories: psychosocial skills, cognitive processing skills, and perceptual-motor and sensory integration skills.

The psychosocial skills category covers the skills involved in developing and using a self-concept that is constructive for self and others, expressing and controlling oneself in functional and creative activities, coping with problems, and interacting with others in dyadic and group situations. This category reflects a wide variety of social-psychological, psychoanalytic, and humanistic perspectives on how human beings function (Hall and Lindzey, 1970; Hollander and Hunt, 1971; Lieberman, 1977; Reilly, 1974). Problems in knowing one's own strengths and limitations, realistically perceiving one's own and others' needs, setting goals and directions for one's own life, having command of a range of ways of expressing oneself, being able to conceptualize problems in terms of needed behavioral change and action, being able to set limits on self and others, and knowing and performing a variety of tasks and social/emotional role behaviors in a group are examples of the types of problems that become the focus of evaluation and treatment in occupational therapy. All mentally ill and mentally retarded clients have some problems in these areas (Freedman and Kaplan, 1967; Hopkins and Smith, 1978; Rowe, 1970).

Cognitive processing covers the mental skills involved in orientation, conceptualization, comprehension, and integration. This category reflects psychological perspectives on how human beings function (Ginsburg and Opper, 1969; Hall and Lindzey, 1970; Posner, 1973). Problems in concentration, attention span, memory, and ability to generalize and utilize problem-solving strategies are examples of the types of problems that become the focus of evaluation and treatment. A wide variety of mentally ill and mentally retarded clients exhibit cognitive processing difficulties (Freedman and Kaplan, 1967; Hopkins and Smith, 1978; Rowe, 1970).

The perceptual-motor and sensory integration skills reflect a neurophysiological perspective on how the human being functions (Guyton, 1971; Luria, 1973). An individual has a number of sensory mechanisms for receiving sensory input, a complicated neurophysiological system for processing that input, and motor mechanisms for expressing the output. The neurophysiological processing mechanisms enable the individual to attend to or disregard stimuli, interrelate simultaneously received stimuli, and utilize those stimuli to direct and coordinate movement. Some of the processing mechanisms involve cortical (higher brain) levels, some subcortical. Most of this sensorimotor processing takes place without one's conscious awareness at the subcortical level. Problems of hypersensitivity to stimuli such as touch or sounds, abnormal balance or equilibrium responses, hyperactive motor behavior, uncoordinated motor behavior, and poor perception of body schema are examples of the types of problems that signal general sensory integration difficulties. Only recently has this approach been applied to evaluation and treatment of the mentally ill, particularly with the person with a diagnosis of chronic schizophrenia. It is an approach that has been used recently also with children with learning disorders and with autistic children (Ayers, 1973; de Quiros and Schrager, 1978; King, 1974).

Occupational Therapy Evaluation and Treatment Approaches

Occupational therapy evaluation involves an analysis of the client's performance goals, strengths, deficits, and environment. Information is gathered through interviews with the client and significant others and observation of the client's performance in activities or tasks selected to elicit specific information (Azima and Azima, 1959; Hopkins and Smith, 1978; Kohlman-McGourty, 1979; Mosey, 1973; Reed and Sanderson, 1980; Takata, 1969). This information is interpreted and decisions are made regarding treatment based on the treatment philosophy and theory of human behavior espoused by the therapist and agency. Occupational therapy shares basic treatment philosophies with other mental health professions. Although occupational therapy treatment usually reflects the ideas of more than one treatment philosophy and theory of human behavior, I shall discuss the following theories separately for the sake of clarity: social-educational learning theory, cognitive theory, developmental theory, psychoanalytic theory, behavior modification theory, and sensory integration theory.

Social-educational learning theory is really a conglomeration of theories sharing the assumption that the client has skill deficits and/or dysfunctional learned performance patterns and needs to be helped to acquire skills and/or more functional performance patterns. One learns by being able to observe good models, by being instructed and directed in the performance of an activity/task, and by receiving corrective feedback from self and others. Actual practice is an important part of learning (Bandura, 1977; Binder, Binder, and Rimland, 1976; Hollander and Hunt, 1971; Langsley and Kaplan, 1968). In this approach, the occupational therapist models the kinds of performance desired, provides structured activity-learning experiences for the client, and gives the client corrective feedback on his or her actual performance (Auerbach, 1974; Broekema, Danz, and Schloemer, 1975; Heine, 1975; Hopkins and Smith, 1978; Llorens and Rubin, 1967).

Cognitive theory is based on the assumption that human beings are rational creatures whose ideas about the world and analysis of a given situation serve to elicit emotions and direct behavior. The way to change feelings and behavior is to change the person's analysis of the situation and general views of the world (Binder, Binder, and Rimland, 1976; Haley, 1976; Kendall and Hollon, 1979). In using this approach in occupational therapy, attention is paid to the fact that ideas are abstract statements of how one views things. Observation and discussion of a specific activity/task experience provide the opportunity to analyze the execution of those ideas. Observation of the implementation of one's ideas is an essential step in evaluating, expanding, and changing one's ideas (Fidler, 1969; Hopkins and Smith, 1978; West, 1959).

Developmental theory is based on the assumption that a human being evolves through sequential stages of development and that if a stage is skipped or inadequately mastered, performance in later stages will be hampered (Ginsburg and Opper, 1969). Occupational therapy treatment involves analyzing the client's level of mastery in the various performance areas essential to daily functioning and providing the opportunity to master performance tasks sequentially from an already acquired level of mastery (Hopkins and Smith, 1978; Mosey, 1973; Reilly, 1974). A similar theme is expressed in the humanistic psychology literature without the strict adherence to the sequential ordering of performance tasks. The general idea of the humanist is that the human being will naturally develop and evolve, given the opportunity, a secure environment, and continuously successful achievement (Binder, Binder, and Rimland, 1976; Hall and Lindzey, 1970; Rogers, 1965).

Psychoanalytic theory is based on the assumption that the human being has innate drives that must be expressed in socially acceptable ways and that the mechanisms by which these innate drives are controlled and channeled are, to a large extent, unconscious (Bellak, Hurvich, and Gediman, 1973; Freedman and Kaplan, 1967; Searles, 1960). Occupational therapy treatment focuses on an analysis of socially acceptable expression of inner needs, use of ego defenses in a manner that is helpful for the individual, and development of ego skills. Treatment provides the client with activities and interpretations that channel expression, strengthen desirable defense mechanisms, interfere with undesirable defense mechanisms, and facilitate development of ego skills (Becker and Page, 1973; Fidler and Fidler, 1963; Hopkins and Smith, 1978; Llorens and Rubin, 1967).

Behavior modification theory is based on the assumption that classical and instrumental conditioning can change behavior (Binder, Binder, and Rimland, 1976; Patterson, 1971). Activities provided in occupational therapy and/or the client-therapist relationship may serve as the medium for behavioral expression and change or may serve as stimuli and reinforcers for behavioral change (Cermak, Stein, and Abelson, 1973; Hopkins and Smith, 1978).

Sensory integration theory is based on the premise that manipulation of the sensory input can have a corrective effect on the functioning of sensory integrative mechanisms, a necessary component to successful cognitive and motor performance and the performance of daily life activities (de Quiros and Schrager, 1978). Occupational therapy provides direct sensory stimulation and/or activities that contain the appropriate sensory stimuli and sensory integrative tasks (Ayers, 1973; King, 1974; Watzlawick, 1978).

Each of these approaches may be used as the primary evaluation and treatment approach or in combination with others. In all of the perspectives, the provision of and direction in activities and tasks are combined with interpretive discussion by the occupational therapist with the client. A wide range of activities may be used as a focus for discussion and participation, depending upon the client's treatment needs and goals and the resources of the facility and therapist.

Strengths Inherent in the Emphasis on Activity Performance

Although the occupational therapy approach overlaps that of the other mental health professions, there are some unique strengths and contributions inherent in occupational therapy. Occupational therapy involves the analysis of activities and tasks in terms of the cognitive, sensorimotor, emotional, and social components in order to select and adapt activities to meet the therapeutic needs of clients with various disabilities. There is considerable emphasis on the therapeutic use of activities and tasks, which derives from an understanding and treatment of both the physically disabled and the mentally ill. Most of the other mental health professions emphasize the understanding and treatment of the mentally ill, with little emphasis on the physically disabled.

Psychotherapy is essentially a verbal mode of treatment. The occupational therapy emphasis on activity and task performance adds the nonverbal, performance dimension. A verbal description of an action is a representation of the action; it is not equivalent to the action. Distortions occur due both to the act of observing and to the inadequacies of the verbal tool used to describe the action. In the action mode, things that are not apparent in the verbal mode often become obvious. For example, in an evaluation of the interaction of a mother-father-adolescent son family, the family was asked to do a collage together. It quickly became obvious to the family and therapist how interaction actually transpired. Without even discussing it, the family divided up the paper (the territory) into three parts. Mother and son hesitated until father glued pictures on the paper, identifying his territory. Next the son staked out his, and mother quietly took what was left. All expressed verbally and in the pictures chosen for the collage great feelings of loneliness, of being misunderstood, of not knowing what was expected by the others, and, in the case of the son, of aggressiveness within his territorial bounds (weapons aimed at father's portion of the collage). The family visually recognized how they had approached the task and were able to discuss their typical approach to interaction with each other.

An activity not only provides the opportunity for a range of modes of expression, but it provides the opportunity in a group for multiple simultaneous expression. In a psychotherapy group session, one person speaks at a time while others are expected to listen and sequentially build on the theme or topic. In an activity treatment session, everyone may be simultaneously carrying out a piece of what becomes a product of the whole group. Within one activity, the variety of tasks and skills required is great. The visibility of one's contribution is great. The symbol of integration of the group is also visibly apparent. For many client groups, the wide range of opportunity for expression, contribution, and concrete-to-abstract symbolism of experience is needed.

A third value in the analysis and use of activities and tasks in therapy is the opportunity it provides for implementing ideas. What do two different people mean by "being self-reliant"? Illustration with a number of concrete situational events is frequently necessary to ensure that two people mean the same things by the same abstract terms. Many of the problems mentally ill clients face are encapsuled in abstract terms: The client needs to be more "assertive," to be more "open" about his or her feelings, to be more "direct" in his or her feedback, to deal with "shorter-term" goals, to be more "organized," and so on. Implementation of these directives can be modeled in concrete activity sessions. The client's attempts to perform in accordance with the directive can be observed by both the client and therapist, and the consequences can be immediately observed and discussed by client, therapist, and others participating.

For clients who have severe difficulties generalizing from one situation to another, it may be important for the therapist to provide a structured daily living program for the client in the actual environment in which the client is to perform the activities and tasks involved. These clients may do very poorly in applying information gained in verbal psychotherapy to their daily lives.

Developing skill in motor performance takes practice. Activity sessions and activity or task assignments give clients opportunities to practice behaviors they want to acquire. The fact that both the therapist and client can observe the performance in activity treatment sessions provides the additional benefit of the opportunity for immediate corrective feedback.

Illustrative Program Descriptions

I describe two occupational therapy programs, one located in a community-based rehabilitation setting (day treatment and sheltered workshop) and one in a crisis-oriented, short-stay, acute care inpatient facility (hospital), to illustrate the organization and staffing of occupational therapy treatment programs.

Community-Based Facility. The community-based facility (Hepler, 1980) offers transitional rehabilitation services for psychiatrically disabled adults having severe to moderate handicaps. The services are designed to assist clients in gradually moving from a dysfunctional, dependent condition to a state of independent living and employment in business and industry. Based on their level of functioning, clients are assigned to one or two primary programs: the social adjustment or vocational adjustment programs.

The social adjustment program serves the more dysfunctional clients with mental health counseling, psychotropic medication adjustment, practical living skills training, housing relocation assistance, and prevocational services. The vocational adjustment program focuses upon higher functioning clients and provides vocational adjustment counseling, work adjustment training, job sampling, job placement, and supportive follow-up. As they become more functional, clients transfer from the social adjustment program to the vocational adjustment program and eventually into independent living and nonsubsidized jobs in industry and business. Clients may also enter the vocational adjustment program directly. Real-life industrial experiences are offered as part of the vocational adjustment program (sheltered workshop). Work, for wages, in such industrial operations as small-parts assembly, packaging, light manufacturing, sewing and serging, collating, paper recycling, document destruction, and excelsior production provides opportunities for work evaluation and training on the premises. Job placement and supportive follow-up services take place throughout the larger metropolitan community.

Over 200 clients are served in the facility annually. About 10 percent of these each year move into independent living and working situations. Some clients stay over a period of two to three years; some move on to other programs. A slow rate of progress is expected and achieved by most of the clients. A wide range of diagnoses is seen, with schizophrenia being by far the most common. Frequently, over half the clients have histories of psychiatric problems that extend over five or ten years, including occasional hospitalization. Work histories are usually minimal or nonexistent. Most of the clients are single, Caucasian, and live in group homes or independent living situations. The median age is about twenty-eight, with a range of eighteen to fifty-five years.

The clinical treatment staff consists of three social workers, three occupational therapists, a vocational counselor, a psychologist, a nurse, and six social science bachelor-level persons. Many of the staff work in both the social adjustment and vocational adjustment programs.

The occupational therapy section is in charge of the practical living skill training services and is heavily involved in the housing relocation assistance, prevocational evaluation, and work adjustment and job sampling services. Two registered occupational therapists and a certified occupational therapy assistant are employed full-time. In addition, two full-time occupational therapy fieldwork students (assistant and bachelor level) rotate through the facility, one of each every three months. The students come from schools throughout the nation and have completed their academic training, but have not taken their certification examinations.

One registered occupational therapist works primarily in the social adjustment program. Approximately two hours each day is spent evaluating clients in independent living and prevocational skills. A full evaluation takes approximately two to three hours. Another two hours is spent supervising or coleading, with the certified occupational therapy assistant or the occupational therapy fieldwork students, practical living skills training groups. The groups last anywhere from one-half to one and one-half hours, are given one to three times a week, and focus on such areas as personal hygiene, food and nutrition, cooking, money management, home management, transportation, communications, use of leisure time, sensory integration treatment, and time management. One to two hours each day is spent in the vocational adjustment program evaluating clients for placement in the sheltered workshop program of the facility, adapting work tasks to meet clients' physical, emotional, and social needs, supervising the occupational therapy students and other employees in their work with the clients, and assisting with the design and management of this part of the program. The occupational therapist assists the vocational adjustment program director with analysis of job samples in relation to clients' training needs, development and redesign of client work evaluation forms, and so on. The remaining two to three hours is spent in agency meetings, program planning, reporting, and occupational therapy management tasks.

The other registered occupational therapist works primarily with individual clients whose needs for individual therapy are greater than what can effectively be accommodated in the regular group sessions, whose needs must be met on-site in a community setting, or whose needs occur out of phase with the regularly scheduled program (for example, client needs money-management or apartment-location assistance, and those groups are not scheduled to be offered for a month). The focus of treatment is still practical living skill, prevocational and job placement evaluation, training, and support, however.

Acute Care Facility. The acute care facility (Kohlman-McGourty, 1980) is a twenty-one bed, crisis-oriented, short-stay facility, operating at a 93 percent average occupancy rate and serving patients with a wide range of psychiatric diagnoses on a voluntary admission basis. The unit is part of a large teaching hospital located in a metropolitan area. The program is oriented toward crisis intervention, adjustment in medication, and referral and discharge planning.

Approximately sixty to eighty patients are served each month. Of these, about 20 percent stay two to three days, 10 percent three to four weeks, and the vast majority about a week. Most patients have low to middle socioeconomic backgrounds. They are referred to the unit through the emergency service of the hospital; by private therapists and mental health professionals; and by friends, family, or self. Some, when they leave the hospital unit, are referred to other services, such as community mental health centers, some are referred to private therapists, and some are simply discharged.

The clinical treatment staff consists of the usual spectrum of professionals found in the psychiatric unit of a teaching hospital: a psychiatrist, a psychologist, two social workers, two occupational therapists, and a nursing staff of twenty-four (including sixteen registered nurses). Patients are referred to occupational therapy for evaluation and treatment in the areas of functional living skill and performance, cognitive skills and performance, psychological functioning skill and performance, social skill and performance, and sensory integration performance. Patients with problems in any of these areas (over 90 percent of the patients) are assigned to regularly scheduled occupational therapy treatment groups for further problem identification and problem solving, and/or receive discharge planning/home treatment counseling from the occupational therapist to assist them in dealing with their problems. Treatment groups vary in their focus, but the following groups are typical of what is usually offered: assertiveness, time management, exercise, goals, life changes, and task. The treatment groups meet for one to two hours and are scheduled two to three times per week. Because of the evaluative nature of the group focus, high turnover in patients, and size of most of the groups (six to ten patients), groups are cooled by the two occupational therapists or by the occupational therapist and a nurse. The combined sixty hours of clinic-related time per week is thus spent in the following manner: 25 percent on patient evaluations, 35 percent on patient treatment and discharge planning, 25 percent on team communication and planning, and 15 percent on occupational therapy planning and patient home visits.

Case Illustrations

Two cases will be presented to illustrate the implementation of occupational therapy services. The first involves evaluation, treatment, and discharge planning for a young woman admitted to a short-term hospital inpatient psychiatric treatment facility (Sheffer, 1980). In this illustration, focus is placed primarily on occupational therapy treatment. The second case involves a boy in a day-treatment program for severely emotionally disturbed children (Hense, 1980). The discussion of the boy's treatment includes information on how occupational therapy is integrated into the agency's total day treatment program.

Case 1: Sarah, Acute Care Hospital Setting

Sarah was a twenty-three-year-old, single, white female admitted with a diagnosis of depression and severe separation anxiety involving her mother. The patient was living at home just prior to admission to the hospital. She was interviewed and asked to complete the following three items of evaluation: a schedule listing the activities in which she had engaged on a day typical of the week immediately preceding admission, with notation of whether she wanted or had to do each of the activities, whether she saw each as a self-care, work, or play activity, and whether she felt she had done each well or poorly; a drawing of a subject of her choice; and a drawing of herself and her family doing something together.

Results of the interview and evaluation showed that Sarah had average or better intelligence; could apply information gathered in a discussion situation to a performance situation fairly well, although activity treatment sessions were helpful for illustrative purposes; had fairly strong motivation to work on and solve her problems; and had good insight into her moderately severe problems but poor insight into problems related to handling anger and handling her family's possessiveness of her. As a result of identification of specific problems, the following treatment plan was designed with Sarah:

A. Develop skills necessary to live independent of family
  1. Self-care
    a. Mental health. The main focus is to develop awareness of her own needs for independence, self-expression and recognition from others, and to overcome skill deficits in being able to meet her own needs in this area. Examples of behaviors to work on are
      • Identifying the need for assertive expression.
      • Acquiring constructive methods of saying "no," setting limits on others, and expressing anger.
      • Learning how to ask for and deal positively with feedback from others.
      • Learning to recognize when she is beginning to feel anxious, sad, and depressed and learning constructive ways to keep from becoming more depressed and isolated, such as involving herself in activities and social situations in which she feels confident.
      • Identifying the characteristics of activity and social situations in which she feels confident versus anxious.
    b. Social skills. The main focus is to acquire awareness of her strengths and deficits in social skills and improving skills, particularly in relation to the types of people she would need to relate to if living independently (peers, employers, teachers, and fellow students). Examples of behaviors to work on include
      • Learning how to initiate casual conversation, how to quickly find out a stranger's interests, and how to let others know her own interests.

- Learning to feel comfortable sharing her opinions even though other persons might disagree or just not respond, learning that social participation, not necessarily agreement, is often the goal of social interaction.
- Learning to handle social situations with male peers, appropriate but safe ways to initiate contact and set limits, what are neutral topics and activities one can use to keep the situation from becoming too close without having to end the interaction.
  c. Practical living skills. The main focus is on the acquisition of factual information needed for independent living, such as
  - How to find an apartment.
  - Renter's rights and resources in case of difficulties with a landlord.
  - Money management and simple budgeting methods.
2. Work. The main focus is upon vocational exploration, including
   - Identifying past work experiences that were/were not enjoyable and successful.
   - Identifying types of work that might be potentially enjoyable, where training necessary to do them would be available, and possible obstacles to acquiring the training.
3. Play/leisure. The main focus is on developing the awareness of play activities and situations she did/did not enjoy and on identifying opportunities in her own local community for pursuing these interests and/or acquiring new ones on discharge.
B. Discharge planning. The main focus of hospitalization is on identification of Sarah's own goals, strengths and deficits, support and stress elements in her environment, and evaluation of the type of postdischarge treatment needed.

The main approach to treatment was one of self-discovery and self-planning, with high expectation for independent work and follow-through by the patient. Sarah was guided by the therapist in discussions and in experiential learning situations to areas of difficulty. She was asked to assess her own strengths and deficits, to identify and practice in the hospital ways of overcoming these deficits, and to seek opinions, suggestions, and help from other patients in this process. Sarah participated in assertiveness training, communication, money management, and nutrition planning task groups in her hospital occupational therapy treatment program. In a discharge-planning treatment group, Sarah developed her own home program, which consisted of a weekly time schedule and identification of sequential tasks necessary for moving from her home situation to living in an apartment, working part-time in a florist shop, and attending college part-time. The home program was designed to enable her both to transfer her learning from the hospital to her community setting and to provide guidelines for further development of self-awareness and independent living skill acquisition. Sarah was discharged after fourteen days of hospitalization, with weekly follow-up outpatient sessions with the occupational therapist and psychiatrist.

Case 2: Joey, Child Day-Treatment Program

Joey, a nine-year-old white male quite small for his age, was accepted for treatment in a day-treatment program because of highly ritualized, compulsive behavior, low social skills, extreme withdrawal, and noncompliance. He lived with both parents and one older sibling and participated in day treatment five days a week, six hours a day. The program in which he was involved was offered jointly through a community child mental health setting and a public school district to meet the unique therapeutic and educational needs of severely emotionally/behaviorally disturbed children in a long-term setting. Joey was part of a self-contained classroom of ten children with a special education teacher and assistant in which focus was on developing academic skills and acceptable classroom behaviors. He received individual and small-group therapy with a social worker who worked on psychodynamic issues and social skills training. The social workers also saw Joey's parents to deal with family dynamics and parenting skills. Occupational therapy services were available to Joey on a regular basis. The various disciplines involved worked together as a team to coordinate treatment for Joey.

As with the majority of the population served in Joey's program, he had sensorimotor and daily living skill deficits, which the occupational therapist addressed. Development delays and sensorimotor deficits greatly compound the problems of emotionally disturbed children. They may have such poor coordination they can have no success playing with peers; they may have great difficulty screening out irrelevant visual or auditory stimuli; they may be unable to perceive consistencies in their environment due to poor visual processing; and they may jump or get angry when touched. All of these serve to lower frustration tolerance and increase the number of failures for highly impulsive children. This, in turn, results in low self-esteem.

The occupational therapist evaluated Joey with standardized tests for visual-motor integration and for motor coordination. Clinical observations were made of sensory integration deficits, and information on daily living skills was gleaned from a screening tool, the parents, and the interdisciplinary team. Results were as follows:

- *Motor skills*—weak trunk and leg muscles; could hop only two to three times per foot; five to six years below age level on balance, total body coordination, and use of hands on fine motor tasks.
- *Daily living skills*—could not tie shoes; bathed about one quarter of self; unable to write address correctly; poor at calendar and time skills.
- *Sensory integration skills*—poor processing of vestibular system stimuli; hyperreactive to touch; great difficulty moving arms across vertical midline of body; poor at stabilizing joints; great trouble smoothly carrying out nonhabitual movement.
- *Other observations*—knew right and left at age-appropriate level; group skills nonexistent; initially refused even to stand in same room as rest of group; stiff trunk, almost no spontaneous neck or trunk rotation.

Gross motor skill delays, sensory integration deficits, and limited self-help skills (to be addressed later in treatment) were selected for occupational therapy treatment.

Joey was seen two to three times a week in occupational therapy, first individually, then in small groups. Motor activities and games were used within a behavior modification superstructure consistent with interactional and behavioral demands in other parts of his program. The games and exercises used were adapted to help enhance his central nervous system processing at an appropriate developmental level. As he gained in skill level, his self-esteem improved. This enabled him to be seen in small groups to aid in his social development and provide more models for learning motor skills. Once Joey was comfortable working in small groups and began seeking acceptance from peers, daily living skill needs were addressed in a small-group format, with actual practice of activities, playing of games that built on skills being taught, and some peer-group pressure and support. One of three rewards was used to encourage Joey's participation: three to five minutes of free choice activities at the end of the treatment session; points earned during treatment, which were traded for a small prize or sticker at the end of group; or points earned during treatment that carried over to the classroom for a reward at the end of the day.

At the time of his termination from the program three years later, Joey (age twelve) had made significant gains:

- *Motor skills*—improved from four-year-old level to nine-year-old level.
- *Daily living skills*—with strong enough contingency, would bathe and change clothes daily, shampoo own hair; could write address, use calendar, count varying coins up to fifty cents, tell time up to five-minute intervals.
- *Sensory integration skills*—still showed signs of poor vestibular system processing, but could tolerate stimuli longer; able to tolerate touch for longer periods; still resistant to moving arms across midline of body; much improvement in moving smoothly through space.
- *Other observations*—able to participate for long periods of time in group sessions with three to six peers in parallel play; able to play interactively with others for five minutes at a time.

The strong progress Joey made in not only his motor skills and daily living skills but also his social skills speaks to the success of a highly structured, action-focused program. At the end of three years, a change in his home placement was made and referral to another treatment facility was necessary. Further treatment for developmental delays, socialization, and self-care training was recommended. A thorough outline of the progress he had made, the reinforcers and programs that resulted in optimal cooperation, and suggestions for appropriate treatment tasks and activities were forwarded to his next placement.

Role of Occupational Therapy in Agency Management

The primary focus of this chapter is what occupational therapy has to offer the clients in the agency. However, a very brief overview of the role of occupational therapy in agency management is also important. An agency manager or administrator is concerned about the degree of overlap and uniqueness of the different mental health professions, the reimbursement potential of the different services, and the assurance of uniformity and quality of performance of persons within a profession.

The degree of overlap and uniqueness among the different mental health professions is difficult to assess. In the 1960s, the trend was to blur roles as much as possible. The trend today has swung back toward capitalizing on the uniqueness of each of the professions. From the previous illustrations, it is apparent that there is some overlap between occupational therapy and service provided primarily through verbal psychotherapy. Overlap also occurs between occupational therapy and the other activity therapies, such as recreation therapy, music therapy, and art therapy. Two characteristics separate occupational therapy from the other therapies. First, the medical and human development theory base in the training of the occupational therapist is much more extensive than in the other therapies. Second, occupational therapy focuses on the use of a broad spectrum of activities and tasks, but the other therapies have been built on the specific activity modalities corresponding to the name of the therapy. This makes occupational therapy a more versatile service than the others.

The area of reimbursement potential has been a primary concern of state and national occupational therapy associations in the past few years, and significant strides have been made in improving the coverage of occupational therapy services by third-party payers. Efforts will continue in this direction to ensure that occupational therapy services are included in state and national program regulations.

A professional organization, through educational program accreditation and individual therapist certification, and a state, through licensure, can regulate minimum qualifications of persons entering and practicing in a field. This is one way that a profession and government can help an agency administrator provide uniformity and quality of performance of treatment personnel in the agency. All occupational therapy educational programs are acredited by the American Occupational Therapy Association. In addition, the entry-level national certification examinations are updated regularly. This ensures a minimal level of knowledge and skill at the entry level. The profession is currently considering the development of a continuing certification examination as well. Approximately 20 percent of the states have state licensure laws covering occupational therapists. The licensure laws usually incorporate the requirement that occupational therapists pass the appropriate national certification examination, rather than a separate state examination. Once therapists have been employed in a particular agency, their performance may be monitored through quality assurance programs within the agency. Many occupational therapists do participate in Professional Standards Review Organization quality assurance, utilization review, and other programs.

Future Directions of the Field

The delivery of occupational therapy services is expanding into a wider range of social and educational service agencies and programs. The development of aftercare living and sheltered workshop programs in the community for the marginally functioning or chronic clients is likely to receive increasing attention in the near future. With its focus on the design of structured living and work environments, occupational therapy should gain in importance in this area.

References

American Occupational Therapy Association. *Member Handbook.* Rockville, Md.: American Occupational Therapy Association, 1978.

American Occupational Therapy Association. *Uniform Terminology System for Reporting Occupational Therapy Services.* Rockville, Md.: American Occupational Therapy Association, 1979.

Auerbach, E. "Community Involvement." *American Journal of Occupational Therapy,* 1974, *28,* 22.

Ayers, E. *Sensory Integration and Learning Disorders.* Los Angeles: Western Psychological Services, 1973.

Azima, H., and Azima, F. J. "Outline of a Dynamic Theory of Occupational Therapy." *American Journal of Occupational Therapy,* 1959, *13,* 215–221.

Bandura, A. *Social Learning Theory.* Englewood Cliffs, N.J.: Prentice-Hall, 1977.

Becker, R. E., and Page, M. S. "Psychotherapeutically Oriented Rehabilitation in Chronic Mental Illness." *American Journal of Occupational Therapy,* 1973, *27,* 34–38.

Bellak, L., Hurvich, M., and Gediman, H. K. *Ego Functions in Schizophrenics Neurotics, and Normals.* New York: Wiley, 1973.

Binder, V., Binder, A., and Rimland, B. (Eds.). *Modern Therapies.* Englewood Cliffs, N.J.: Prentice-Hall, 1976.

Broekema, M. C., Danz, K. H., and Schloemer, C. U. "Occupational Therapy in a Community Aftercare Program." *American Journal of Occupational Therapy,* 1975, *29,* 22–27.

Cermak, S. A., Stein, F., and Abelson, C. "Hyperactive Children and an Activity Group Therapy Model." *American Journal of Occupational Therapy,* 1973, *26,* 311–315.

Cynkin, S. *Occupational Therapy.* Boston: Little, Brown, 1979.

de Quiros, J. B., and Schrager, O. *Neuropsychological Fundamentals in Learning Disorders.* San Rafael, Calif.: Academic Therapy Publications, 1978.

Fidler, G. S. "The Task-Oriented Group as a Context for Treatment." *American Journal of Occupational Therapy,* 1969, *23,* 43–48.

Fidler, M. A., and Fidler, J. W. *Occupational Therapy.* New York: Macmillan, 1963.

Freedman, A., and Kaplan, H. (Eds.). *Comprehensive Textbook of Psychiatry.* Baltimore: Williams & Wilkins, 1967.

Ginsburg, H., and Opper, S. *Piaget's Theory of Intellectual Development.* Englewood Cliffs, N.J.: Prentice-Hall, 1969.

Guyton, A. C. *Basic Human Physiology.* Philadelphia: Saunders, 1971.

Haley, J. *Problem-Solving Therapy: New Strategies for Effective Family Therapy.* San Francisco: Jossey-Bass, 1976.

Hall, C., and Lindzey, G. *Theories of Personality.* New York: Wiley, 1970.

Heine, D. E. "Daily Living Group." *American Journal of Occupational Therapy,* 1975, *29,* 628–630.

Hense, B. Personal communication. Seattle, Wash., 1980.

Hepler, N. Personal communication. Seattle, Wash., July 18, 1980.

Hollander, E. P., and Hunt, R. G. *Current Perspectives in Social Psychology.* New York: Oxford University Press, 1971.

Hopkins, H. L., and Smith, H. D. (Eds.). *Willard and Spackman's Occupational Therapy.* (5th ed.) Philadelphia: Lippincott, 1978.

Kendall, P. D., and Hollon, S. C. (Eds.). *Cognitive-Behavioral Interventions.* New York: Academic Press, 1979.

King, L. J. "A Sensory Integrative Approach to Schizophrenia." *American Journal of Occupational Therapy,* 1974, *28,* 529–536.

Kohlman-McGourty, L. "Kohlman Evaluation of Living Skills." Presentation at the Mental Health Assessment Institute, American Occupational Therapy Conference, Detroit, Mich., April 1979.

Kohlman-McGourty, L. Personal communication. Seattle, Wash., July 25, 1980.

Langsley, D. G., and Kaplan, D. M. *The Treatment of Families in Crisis.* New York: Grune & Stratton, 1968.

Lieberman, J. N. *Playfulness: Its Relationship to Imagination and Creativity.* New York: Academic Press, 1977.

Llorens, L. A., and Rubin, E. *Developing Ego Functions in Disturbed Children.* Detroit: Wayne State University Press, 1967.

Luria, A. R. *The Working Brain.* New York: Basic Books, 1973.

Mosey, A. C. *Activities Therapy.* New York: Raven Press, 1973.

Patterson, G. R. *Families,* Champaign, Ill.: Research Press, 1971.

Posner, M. I. *Cognition.* Glenview, Ill.: Scott, Foresman, 1973.

Reed, K., and Sanderson, S. *Concepts of Occupatinal Therapy.* Baltimore: Williams & Wilkins, 1980.

Reilly, M. (Ed.). *Play as Exploratory Learning.* Beverly Hills, Calif.: Sage, 1974.

Rogers, C. *Client Centered Therapy.* Boston: Houghton Mifflin, 1965.

Rowe, C. J. *An Outline of Psychiatry.* (5th ed.). Dubuque, Iowa: Brown, 1970.

Searles, H. F. *The Nonhuman Environment.* New York: International Universities Press, 1960.

Sheffer, M. Personal communication. Seattle, Wash., 1980.

Takata, N. "The Play History." *American Journal of Occupational Therapy,* 1969, *23,* 314–318.

Watzlawick, P. *The Language of Change.* New York: Basic Books, 1978.

West, W. (Ed.). *Psychiatric Occupational Therapy.* Dubuque, Iowa: Brown, 1959.

⚜ 26 ⚜

Serving the
Developmentally Disabled

Robert T. Fraser

Although in some states mental health and developmentally disabled services have been integrated, historically program administrators in mental health agencies have not been concerned with serving the developmentally disabled and have not been knowledgeable about their needs or the services available to them. This chapter describes the major legislatively defined disabilities, the pychosocial needs of the developmentally disabled, current service provisions and gaps, and future directions for providing mental health services for the developmentally disabled. Managers need to maintain ongoing communication with agencies that specifically serve the developmentally disabled in order to coordinate mental health programs and create new outreach programs for these clients.

The developmental disabilities (DD) terminology is of relatively recent origin, born with the Developmental Disabilities Services and Facilities Construction Act of 1970, PL 91-517. This act basically defines developmental disability as one that is attributable to mental retardation, epilepsy, cerebral palsy, or some other condition related either to mental retardation or another neurological condition requiring similar treatment. The emphasis was on a continuing disability originating before the age of eighteen that presented a substantial handicap to life functioning. Breen and Richman (1979, pp. 3–4) emphasize the importance of understanding the development of this definition and provide the following data:

1. In 1970 Social Security figures showed mental retardation, cerebral palsy, and epilepsy to be the leading causes of disability in adults whose handicap originated in childhood. These three disorders accounted for 80 percent of all adults disabled in childhood receiving Social Security benefits. . . .
2. There is ample evidence of multiple handicaps and of the overlapping of the three conditions clinically. Of the 750,000 individuals with cerebral palsy, two-thirds are mentally retarded. An estimated 20 percent to 30 percent of

epileptic individuals are mentally retarded (Conley, 1973). Of institutional-ized mentally retarded persons, one-half have seizure disorders.

Capute (1974) states that one third of those with developmental disabilities have one handicap, an additional third have two handicaps, and the remainder have three or more disabilities. Although recent legislation emphasizes long-term functional and noncategorical disabilities originating before the age of eighteen, there is continuing categorization. The 1975 act added the categories of autism and the reading disability known as dyslexia, if associated with other developmen-tal disabilities.

The 1975 Developmental Disabilities Bill of Rights Act (PL 94-103) seeks to guarantee the rights of developmentally disabled populations in the area of educa-tion and treatment (Martin, 1978). These rights relate to access to services, fairness in diagnosis, equal protection of the law in preventing inappropriate labeling or classification in the educational process, and the development of individual writ-ten educational plans. Other rights include the right to notice in regard to the criteria for entrance into a program before the person is processed and data collec-tion begun (relates to individual or guardian as appropriate). After notice, consent must be given by the individual concerned or competent other in a voluntary fashion, following review of all pertinent information about program risks and benefits. If consent is not given, the developmentally disabled person or the guard-ian involved has the right to an agency hearing accompanied by a lawyer. At any time in this process, the client and/or concerned guardian have a right to see the client's records.

Additional rights that have been provided through legislation include free-dom from abuse, which includes the right to refuse particular therapies and drug regimens, equitable pay for institutional work, and protection from physical abuse and "abusive contingencies" in behavioral management programs. The categories of personal rights and community rights involve, respectively, basic rights to marry and/or to live in a residential community. These legal rights of the developmentally disabled provide chiefly a structure for accountability—unless funding levels are more closely tied to the performance of the various institutions and community agencies, there will still be problems with compliance (Martin, 1978).

The Developmentally Disabled Assistance and Bill of Rights Act (PL 95-602) of 1978 represents the most comprehensive effort to reduce the categorical aspects of previous legislation by defining a developmental disability as (1) a severe, chronic disability attributable to a mental or physical impairment; (2) manifested before the individual reaches age twenty-two; (3) likely to continue indefinitely; (4) resulting in substantial limitation in *three* or *more* of the follow-ing areas to include self-care, receptive and expressive language, learning, mobil-ity, self-direction, capacity for independent living, and economic self-sufficiency; and (5) reflecting the person's need for a combination and sequence of special interdisciplinary or generic care, treatment, or other services of lifelong or ex-tended duration and individually planned and coordinated. This definition includes mental retardation, epilepsy, cerebral palsy, autism, severe learning disabilities, spina bifida (cleft spine), the severely hearing disabled, and the blind. This act also makes the local developmental disabilities service agency responsible for an individually written "habilitation plan" detailing the manner in which services are to be provided, with intermediate and long-term service objectives and the criteria for evaluating success toward reaching these objectives.

The Principle of Normalization

Much of the recent legislative modifications are a result of the impact of "normalization" philosophy and strategies that have become prevalent in our country over the last decade. This principle was originally explicated by Nirje (1969) in relation to normalizing the life experiences and daily activity patterns of the mentally retarded, based upon a Scandinavian model. Wolfensberger (1972) extended the normalization principle to a more specific examination and restructuring of human service delivery systems that need to establish and maintain behavior, interactions, and physical appearances for potentially deviant populations that are as *culturally normative* as possible. Wolfensberger describes the accountability tool called the Program Analysis of Services Systems (PASS), which involves forty-one ratings with which to evaluate a program and its physical facility. It is based on the premise that in order to normalize the lives of the mentally retarded and other potentially deviant populations, one must begin by normalizing the systems that serve them.

The profound effect of the normalization principle has been felt in the areas of housing and education as related to the goals of a "least restrictive living environment" and access to mainstream education. As more developmentally disabled individuals move from institutions to more "independence-oriented" community residences and enter the "normal" educational facility or classroom, it can be anticipated that the demands on the mental health system for consultation and individualized services will increase. This growing demand is the interactional effect of both the needs of these individuals and the inadequate facilities/resources in the community needed to ease their adjustment.

Overview of Specific Developmental Disabilities

Mental Retardation

> Sandi is a thirty-five-year-old mildly mentally retarded (IQ 57) female who lives in the community with her elderly parents. She attends a day activity center, but otherwise has no social interaction because her parents restrict her to the home—largely to assist with household tasks. She loves her parents and experiences guilt in wanting to leave home, but feels it is important for her own socialization and independence. The young woman verbalizes these difficulties with staff and peers at the day activity center. Role playing in one-to-one counseling and group sessions assisted Sandi to verbalize

these concerns to her parents. Social work staff of the center also worked with the parents in easing Sandi's transition to a group home in town (Walker, 1980, p. 293).

The American Association on Mental Deficiency (Grossman, 1977) defines Sandi's degree of mental retardation as significantly subaverage. This categorization includes individuals having an IQ score of 70 or below determined prior to the age of eighteen, existing simultaneously with deficits in adaptive life behaviors. The American Association on Mental Deficiency (AAMD) classifies the retarded into the four categories of mild, moderate, severe, and profound retardation. Halpern (1980) indicates that the Stanford-Binet and Wechsler scales are the most widely accepted and utilized instruments for assessing the relationships between intelligence quotient and level of impairment, as in Table 1.

Although there are different ways to characterize retarded behavior, across such life functions as independent functioning, physical development, communication, social development, economic development, occupation, and self-direction, Table 2 illustrates only three of these areas for those fifteen years of age or older in the mildly and profoundly retarded groups.

A significant amount of mislabeling has occurred in the identification of those with mental retardation because of the inability of traditional IQ tests to account for ethnic and subcultural differences. Mercer (1973) has identified a method for assessing the intelligence and adaptive behavior of minority group members, including blacks and Chicanos. Additionally, institutionalized persons tend to produce test scores lower than normals because of a lack of life exposure. In a similar manner, conditions associated with poverty and poor educational systems would also increase the risk of mild mental retardation, and Halpern (1980) notes that twice the number of mentally retarded can be identified in the lower socioeconomic class as in the middle and upper classes combined.

There are a number of known causes of mental retardation, including prenatal injury, gross brain damage after birth, premature birth, infection (for example, rubella), intoxication, metabolic errors (phenylketonuria), nutritional deficits, and cultural deprivations. In some cases, a syndrome such as Down's, which results in an individual having slanted eyes, a tongue thrust, and coarse hair, can be related to a specific medical cause, such as a trisomy of chromosome 21 (three rather than the usual two chromosomes). Halpern (1980) indicates that less than 25 percent of those diagnosed as mentally retarded have a clearly attributable medical cause. Wortis (1970) indicates that of the diagnosable cases, Down's Syndrome is the most commonly diagnosed.

If we use a standard IQ test score below 70 as a discriminator, approximately 3 percent of the population would fall within the retarded range (Ca.pute, 1974, p. 558; Halpern, 1980, p. 2). Halpern (1980, p. 4) estimates that 85 percent of the mentally retarded population are mildly retarded (IQ 55-70), 12 percent are moderately retarded (IQ 40-55), and the remaining 3 percent are either severely or profoundly retarded (IQ below 40).

Unless a child has overt physical symptoms or apparent deficits in adaptive behavior, retardation is often not diagnosed until he or she reaches school. Ideally,

Table 1. Relationships Between IQ and Level of Impairment.

| Level | Obtained Intelligence Quotient | |
	Stanford-Binet	Wechsler
Mild	68–52	69–55
Moderate	51–36	54–40
Severe	35–20	39–25
Profound	19 and below	24 and below (extrapolated)

Table 2. Comparison of Adaptive Behavior of the Mildly and Profoundly Retarded.

Independent functioning	Physical	Communication
Mild		
Exercises care for personal grooming, feeding, bathing, toilet; may need health or personal care reminders; may need help in selection or purchase of clothing	Goes about local neighborhood in city or campus at institution with ease, but cannot go to other towns unattended; can use bicycle, skis, ice skates, trampoline, or other equipment requiring good coordination	Communicates complex verbal concepts and understands them; carries on everyday conversations, but cannot discuss abstract or philosophical concepts; uses telephones; writes simple letters
Profound		
Feeds self with spoon or fork, may spill some; puts on clothing but needs help with small buttons and jacket zippers; tries to bathe self but needs help; partially toilet-trained but may have accidents	May hop or skip; may climb steps with alternating feet; rides bicycle; plays dance games; may throw ball and hit target	May have speaking vocabulary of over 300 words and use grammatically correct sentence; if nonverbal, may use many gestures to communicate needs; understands simple verbal communications; speech sometimes indistinct

assessment is conducted by professionals in a state developmental disabilities agency, in a university-affiliated child development and mental retardation center, in other university departments (psychology or special education), or by privately licensed psychologists. It is important that a professional, experienced with the pertinent developmental disability, conduct the assessment, along with a team assessment involving medical, educational, social work, and psychology professionals. Assessment should have both a diagnostic and prescriptive emphasis.

Epilepsy

Ed, age forty-five, has generalized tonic-clonic (grand mal) seizures that are well controlled by Dilantin. Ed was sent to a residential institution for the retarded by his father, a medical doctor, at the age of nine. He was referred to the institution because of "hyper-activity" and occasional absence (petit mal) seizures. In his early teens, he was transferred to a state mental institution. It appears that Ed was well assimilated into the daily activities at the institution. Although his seizures (which developed into the grand mal form) were relatively well controlled and his "hyperactivity" ceased, he remained at the institution for twenty-two years. His testing upon release indicated above-average intellectual functioning and no psychopathology—the release coming as part of the state's deinstitu-tionalization push to the community. Presently, Ed refuses to work because of concerns about loss of his federal subsidy and his ability to maintain a job. He lives in a congregate facility, traveling the city by bus for diversion (adapted from case notes, Regional Epilepsy Center, Harborview Medical Center, Seattle, Washington).

This case is representative of some of the social isolation and referral prob-lems experienced by those with seizure conditions. The neurological disability of epilepsy can be described as a tendency for recurrent, excessive, and irregular discharges of neurons within the brain. The term "epilepsy" is derived from the Greek word for seizure. There are two major categories of seizures: generalized and partial. Generalized seizures primarily involve the tonic-clonic (grand mal) and absence (petit mal) seizures. The tonic-clonic seizures consist of two stages: a tonic stage in which the person becomes rigid and falls to the ground and a clonic stage in which the person undergoes a series of convulsions. The average tonic-clonic seizure lasts approximately two minutes, with the person being able to return to normal activities in a period of time varying from a few minutes to several hours. In contrast to the tonic-clonic seizure, the absence or petit mal seizure involves a short disruption of consciousness in which people cease whatever they are doing and stare straight ahead. Recovery is almost immediate for this type of seizure, which is often unrecognized by the person having the seizure or others in the area. Absence seizures generally occur in children, and about 40 percent develop gener-alized tonic-clonic (grand mal) seizures. Other types of generalized seizures exist, such as myoclonic jerks and akinetic or atonic seizures, which are less common.

Partial seizures usually have a focus in the brain's cortex. Seizure symptoms are related to the specific lesions and disturbed areas that are located in particular portions of the brain. The hands and fingers are commonly affected due to aber-rant discharging in the motor cortex. In general, a part of the brain is being affected in partial seizures; involvement of both hemispheres characterizes gener-alized seizures.

Partial complex or psychomotor seizures, which originate in the temporal lobe, are the most common of the partial seizures. This type of seizure can result in feelings of fear, emotional distress, anger, auditory and visual hallucinations, and/or automatic motor movements (fumbling with one's hands, lip smacking, clutching at clothing, or wandering behavior). These are partial seizures with complex symptomatology. Other seizures seem to begin as partial seizures, affect-ing a particular portion of the body, and then generalize. These are called partial seizures, secondarily generalized.

First-aid measures for those experiencing seizures are very basic. In the case of the generalized tonic-clonic (grand mal) seizure, it is helpful to guide the person to the ground and place a pillow or a piece of clothing under the person's head. With other seizures, most of the first aid involves monitoring a person during the seizure and reorienting him or her when the seizure is over.

The etiology of a person's epilepsy can be very difficult to determine. The causes vary widely and to some degree can be associated with specific types of epilepsy. For example, petit mal epilepsy has been proposed as an expression of an autosomal dominant gene with unusual characteristics that is nearly completely expressed during mid to late childhood. Partial complex seizures seem to be principally caused by scarring of the temporal lobe during the birth process. Other lesions in the brain that cause epilepsy can be a result of a stroke, head trauma, or a tumor. Additional causes include prenatal factors such as infectious diseases in the mother (for example, rubella) or other postnatal factors (such as the parasitic infections of encephalitis or meningitis).

The incidence given for epilepsy in the population has tended to vary between 1 and 2 percent. In the adult population with uncontrolled seizures, the generalized tonic-clonic (grand mal) seizures and partial complex (psychomotor) seizures appear to be the most common. Others (absence or partial seizures, secondarily generalized) are less common.

Medical evaluation of the person with epilepsy is best conducted by a neurologist. Evaluation includes the taking of the neurological history, physical examination, and a series of electroencephalograph (EEG) recordings (ideally a wake and a sleep EEG). A new advance in neuroradiology, the computerized axial-tomography (CAT) scan, has been of assistance in rapidly scanning for abnormal structures within the brain. It is also valuable to involve a neuropsychologist in order to gain more specific information of brain-related deficits caused by seizures over time. The neuropsychologist can also provide additional data relating to the seizure's focus based upon examination of the testing results.

Blood serum levels are routinely taken and monitored for those placed on a regimen of anticonvulsant medications. The common approach is to use one primary anticonvulsant drug appropriate to the seizure type, with others being used only if imperative. Despite advances in the development of new anticonvulsants, it is estimated that about half the population with epilepsy continues to experience seizures.

Cerebral Palsy

> Bill, age twenty-three, has an athetoid form of cerebral palsy and is diagnosed as having a paranoid thought disorder. Because of his inability to maintain a reality orientation in a work activity center, Bill was returned to his residential center. This was done with the approval of the local developmental disability agency, but no effort was made to replace the day work program with any type of program/service. Staff at the residential center, although not highly skilled in dealing with this type of resident, made attempts at devel-

oping a behaviorally oriented program for this individual. Although some adjustment gains have been made, Bill has remained without a day program for more than a year, with no mental health intervention services being provided by the DD agency (adapted from case notes, United Cerebral Palsy Regional Center, Seattle, Washington).

Bill's case is representative of the service gaps that often exist for those with cerebral palsy. Many agencies are unprepared or simply do not make an effort to provide services to members of a population that can have serious mobility and communication difficulties. Molnar and Taft (1973) note that the term cerebral palsy implies there is a motor disorder that is secondary to a static brain lesion that occurred prenatally, perinatally, or postnatally in early childhood.

Cerebral palsy symptoms include spasticity, athetosis, rigidity, ataxia, tremor, atonia, dystonia, and mixed types. Spasticity is the most common form of the disability. It occurs when the stretch reflex is inhibited and is manifested in three ways: an excessive response to rapid stretch of the involved muscles when the tendons are tapped by a reflex hammer during a clinical examination, one or more "bouncing" contractions (clonus) occurring spontaneously when the muscle is stretched and held by force, and stereotyped postures assumed as a result of persistent muscle contraction in certain muscles (Easton and Halpern, 1980). An example of typical postures would be a continual bending posture of the knees, wrist, and elbows reflecting constricted mobility.

The motor disorders in cerebral palsy can also be categorized according to the parts of the body affected: quadriplegia—four extremities; diplegia—lower extremities, mildly affected upper extremities; monoplegia—one extremity; hemiplegia—both limbs on one side; paraplegia—lower extremities alone; triplegia—three extremities. This topographical classification is most often applied to the spastic type of cerebral palsy. Among those with the spastic form of the disability, hemiplegia is most common, with monoplegia and triplegia being the most rare (Molnar and Taft, 1973).

Although the symptomatology of cerebral palsy will vary from patient to patient, it involves involuntary motor movements that become evident as an individual attempts a purposeful motor action (Easton and Halpern, 1980). It can initially involve one limb but then generalize to other limbs or the trunk of the body. It appears that athetoid movements tend to increase with anxiety and during the adolescent period (Molnar and Taft, 1973). Dystonia, a situation in which a person experiences increased muscle tone occurring concomitantly in both muscles and their antagonists, may be associated with athetosis and called tension athetosis. Dystonia, however, can also occur alone or as a component of spasticity (Easton and Halpern, 1980).

Other forms of cerebral palsy include *rigidity*, involving an inhibiting, excessive muscle tone; *atonia* (hypotonia), in which muscle tone can be almost absent; or *ataxia*, in which a person has real difficulty in accurately positioning a limb. These other forms of cerebral palsy are rare and occur among less than 10 percent of those with cerebral palsy.

Cerebral palsy can have a number of complications that raise numerous treatment concerns. These associated disabilities include respiratory infections, scoliosis (curvature of the spine), degenerative joint disease, contractions (limitations of joint range of motion), visual and auditory impairments, and deformities.

Causes for cerebral palsy can also be broken down into different categories: prenatal, natal, and perinatal. Prenatal causes include maternal infections, Rh incompatibility, anoxia, toxicity, and to a minor degree, genetic causes. Perinatal causes can include hemorrhage and anoxia related to difficulties in the birthing process, prematurely putting the infant at risk (Easton and Halpern, 1980; Molnar and Taft, 1973). Postnatal causes again include anoxia, vascular incidents, brain trauma, and infections such as meningitis.

Molnar and Taft (1973) estimate that the incidence of cerebral palsy ranges between 1.6 and 5 per 1,000 population under twenty-one years of age in the United States. Easton and Halpern (1980) estimate that the incidence of the disability is closer to 0.5 percent of the population. The majority of those with cerebral palsy have the spastic form of the disability; the second largest group has mixed forms of the disability; and the third largest group is those with the athetoid type of cerebral palsy.

The impairing effects of cerebral palsy on physical and mental capabilities require a comprehensive medical, functional, and psychosocial evaluation. Medical evaluation is best conducted by a neurologist and can also involve assessment of the patient's potential seizure activity. Other evaluations include nutritional, dental, hearing, visual, and respiratory concerns performed by the appropriate professional.

Functional evaluation can include assessments by physical therapists, psychiatrists, and/or occupational therapists regarding the breadth of motor movement and precision related to the patient's motor control. If the patient has skeletal problems or contractures, a referral may be made to an orthopedic specialist for further evaluation. The ability to communicate is assessed by a speech pathologist. Psychosocial evaluation is frequently conducted by a psychologist who is familiar with cerebral palsy. This professional can modify traditional testing as necessary in order not to penalize the patient with motor dysfunction or other disability-related deficits. In some cases, a test will be administered several times or a job-sample/work-tryout assessment is used to secure information for treatment planning. Treatment in cerebral palsy can require the coordination of a wide range of approaches, including medications for better muscle control, orthopedic surgery, various exercise regimens, and counseling.

Autism

Jack is a nine-year-old autistic boy who lives with his family. He has extreme communication problems, is hyperactive, and is given to temper tantrums and solitary, rocking behavior. The child also has experienced absence (petit mal) seizures, which appear to be fairly well controlled with medication. Jack has caused innumerable problems for his parents and placed a severe strain on their marriage. His father has been subject to bouts of alcoholism during recent years. Last summer while being cared for by an older brother, Jack started a fire in the kitchen while toying with the stove. He panicked and ran upstairs. A substantial portion of two downstairs rooms was burned before the older brother could quell the blaze. At last report, Jack was being seen by a behaviorally oriented psychologist at a children's hospital and making some behavioral gains (adapted from case notes, Regional Epilepsy Center, Harborview Medical Center, Seattle, Washington).

Identifying the causes of autism and prescribing treatment strategies is still rudimentary in contrast to some of the other disabilities. Wiegerink and Pelosi (1979) emphasize that autism is a neurointegrative disorder and not a function of parenting style. Coleman (1978) classifies autism's symptoms under three categories: (1) onset before thirty-six months of age, reflecting an inability to relate to others, abnormal perception of sensory stimuli, a propensity for "sameness" and compulsive behavior, severe language retardation, and motility disturbances and stereotypes (hand flapping, rocking, facial grimaces); (2) autistic behaviors coupled with childhood schizophrenia with onset at age three or later; and (3) neurological impairment such as hydrocephalus and autistic characteristics. Most autism research relates to the classic autistic characteristics without the complication of additional disabilities. Considerable attention is given to the lack of language among those with autism.

Although a number of causes have been postulated and research initiated in a number of areas, there is nothing conclusive regarding etiology at this time. The causes of autistic symptoms are generally considered to be multiple in origin and prenatal or perinatal, but they remain unclear. Autism has been associated with a number of central nervous system abnormalities, including infantile spasms, genetic neurochemical anomalies, rubella, phenylketonuria, and varicella encephalitis. There have been very few studies on the incidence of autism in the population. Coleman (1978, p. 117) says that the two studies that have been done suggest an incidence of about 0.05 percent.

Because of the lack of understanding of autism, a team evaluation is important. Professionals involved could include a psychiatrist, neurologist, neuropsychologist, social worker, speech educator, speech pathologist, and nutritionist.

Mental Health Needs of the Developmentally Disabled

There are a number of mental health and social adjustment needs that are specific to members of different developmentally disabled groups and their significant others. Initially, parents must learn to cope with the loss of an ideal child, develop realistic expectations, and seek a balance in their parent-child interactions to avoid isolating the child or showering the child with an abnormal amount of attention. Parents can harbor extreme guilt related to their bringing the child into the world and therefore often need professional assistance and/or community support during this period of adjustment.

Brain impairment is commonly accompanied by psychological and behavioral problems. Rutter, Tizard, and Whitmore (1970, p. 33) estimate that the prevalence of psychiatric disorder is more than twice as high among children with neurological abnormalities (24 percent) than among children with physical disabilities and no neurological disorder (9 percent) or within a normal sample of children (6 percent). Cognitive and neuromuscular deficits, in addition to impoverished environments, can result in significant communication difficulties. Those who are more severely impaired among the developmentally disabled can have numerous physical difficulties (for example, skeletal, respiratory, or dental) that cause recurring trauma not only to the individual, but to parents and significant others.

One of the most salient problems that seems to affect all developmentally disabled groups relates to establishing a "route to independence" for the young adult with this type of disability. Strax (1976) emphasizes that in some cases the young adult is simply sheltered and overly protected. Even for those individuals whose parents try to assist by normalizing interactions, there can still be difficulties, such as risk taking and minimal opportunities to learn coping behaviors.

Mental Retardation. When serving the mentally retarded, one must work with the parents and/or entire family. Some parents will need particular assistance during the child's first year of life to cope with feelings of anguish and confusion over the future. Parents are often not informed early enough or, when they are informed, are given incomplete information (Farber, 1959). Farber and Ryckman (1965) also indicate that grandparents can have difficulty in accepting the disabled child and be a source of stress to parents. Intervention can also assist in preventing neglect and/or increased responsibility being placed on older children in the family (Gayton, 1975).

Walker (1980) emphasizes three basic needs of the retarded client: the need for someone to listen, the desire to make independent decisions, and the need for an accepting support system. Whatever the level of impairment, certain needs for affection and the fear of failure often need to be addressed. The range of personality problems is as varied as that found among normal children. Many of the psychosocial problems of the retarded can, however, be remedied through their acquiring skills of social competence in a number of daily living areas, including self-care and vocational, interpersonal, and independent living.

Cerebral Palsy. Those with cerebral palsy and their significant others can experience a number of emotional problems, especially related to the individual's verbal limitations, visual-perceptual difficulties, joint and skeletal problems, auditory impairment, or other neurological deficits. Given the functional limitations of those with cerebral palsy, parents and others can have a propensity to be overly solicitous (for example, accompanying the child everywhere and reducing expectancies in relation to household chores) (Anderson, 1973). A study by Shere and Kastenbaum (1966) revealed that mothers were actually fostering passivity in their severely disabled children with cerebral palsy and perceiving passive behavior as characteristic of the "good" and "happy" child. Easton and Halpern (1980) indicate that the solicitousness of others in the environment can assist in shaping egocentric behaviors in the young adult with the disability. A pathological degree of family support around the child with cerebral palsy can be commonly observed.

The pattern of neurological assets and deficits can make therapeutic intervention particularly confounding in working with adults with cerebral palsy. For example, some aspects of verbal ability can appear normal while comprehension is impaired or visual-perceptual deficits present significant limitations (Bergsma and Pulver, 1976). Other neurological impairments and social deficits can result in excessive perseveration on tasks and rigidity in problem-solving approaches (Easton and Halpern, 1980).

There is no question that the daily experiences encountered by those with cerebral palsy can be extremely disconcerting (for example, segregated classes for those with severe physical disabilities, physical therapy sessions interrupting daily activities, ambulation difficulties, respiratory problems, and difficulties with self-care). Behavioral problems can result because of these experiences and the frustrations of not being able to communicate verbally or physically with others. Those with cerebral palsy have the same needs as other persons, and they can be addressed through relatively short-term psychosocial interventions.

The parents of those with cerebral palsy can have particular difficulty with the time-honored physician's advice to "treat your child like a normal child" (Freeman, 1970). According to Bergsma and Pulver (1976, p. 23), parents "must walk a tightrope between acceptance of the fact that he (the child) is different from other people and insistence that he should be like them." These parents can benefit from counseling that helps to develop guidelines for establishing expectations in the home, enriching the child's environment, integrating the child into the community, or improving motor and sensory skills.

Epilepsy. Rodin, Shapiro, and Lennox (1977, p. 36) found that of the 369 patients with epilepsy evaluated, less than 25 percent had epilepsy only. The remainder of this sample had additional psychological problems, neurological deficits, specific neurological handicaps, and other behavioral problems. Those with epilepsy only seem to adjust well in school and vocational settings, but those with associated disabilities, specifically brain impairment, seem to have encountered the most difficulties in general life adjustment.

Those with early onset of the disability will have greater psychosocial problems. Some studies (Bagley, 1972) indicate that the response from the environment is a greater factor in an individual's maladjustment than neurological deficits. If the individual with this disability does not have a chance to adjust to the disability, it becomes apparent that it is even more difficult for others to acclimate to seizure occurrences. People with epilepsy will often feel that their social life is curtailed, their ability to marry is restricted, their educational progress is impeded, and that job discrimination is a significant life impairment (Edwards, 1974). One of the most significant limitations epileptics encounter is the legal inability to drive, and some surveys have indicated that as much as 80 percent of this disability group can be subject to this limitation (Edwards, 1974, p. 241). This limitation reinforces isolation and results in the loss of numerous opportunities to develop social skills.

Anticonvulsant medications can have a number of unpleasant side effects that can also affect psychosocial functioning. An additional problem with the anticonvulsants is that although they are necessary for adequate seizure control, their continued usage can foster drug dependency and can be embarrassing to the individual. Although there do not appear to be specific personality or psychological disorders associated with epilepsy, Betts, Merskey, and Pond (1976) indicate that depression was the most common diagnosis for psychiatric admission. Epilepsy can present some diagnostic problems inasmuch as hysteric reactions and seizure disorders can often be confused, and some aggressive outbursts can actually be associated with the confusion resulting from subclinical seizures (Scott, 1978) or postseizure confusion.

Although still somewhat controversial, there is considerable support for a pattern of psychological problems associated with psychomotor seizures. Bear and Fedio (1973) used a behavioral rating profile and patient self-reports to establish that those with right temporal lobe seizures can have a tendency toward emotive or behavioral aberrancies (for example, flashes of anger, sadness, elation, or rigidity in thinking). Those with left temporal seizures can have a propensity toward intellectual ruminations, religiosity, and a sense of personal destiny. Other general characteristics observed among those with temporal lobe epilepsy include humorless sobriety and hypergraphia. An individual having temporal lobe involvement with associated psychological difficulties may not be a viable candidate for the traditional verbal therapies.

Those least affected by the disability and nearly normal were found to be the least open in discussing the disability and had the poorest self-image (Hodgman and others, 1979).

Autism. The etiology of autism is poorly understood and the diagnosis is surrounded with a considerable amount of confusion. The prognosis is generally poor. DeMeyer and others (1973, p. 223) indicate that 1 to 2 percent recover to normal, 5 to 15 percent were found to function at a borderline level, 16 to 25 percent were at a fair level, and 60 to 75 percent were at a poor level; 42 percent remained institutionalized. Margolies (1977) notes that these data were established before behavioral approaches to treatment were widely used, but they are basically discouraging data. It is not particularly surprising that a wide range of treatment approaches has been attempted with this population, including electroconvulsive shock, custodial isolation, psychoanalytic therapy, operant conditioning, and megadose vitamin therapies (Schlopler and Reichler, 1971).

The children who do make gains tend to be mildly autistic and have better language abilities and perceptual motor skills. It appears that this group can also profit from positive environmental changes (DeMeyer and others, 1973; O'Gorman, 1978). Behavior therapy approaches have met with some success, especially in the area of speech gains, although seldom is real conversational fluency achieved. O'Gorman (1978) indicates that the more sustained gains have been made when the mother was involved in maintenance of the therapy.

The Challenge for Community Mental Health Programs

Fischer (1980) has reviewed a number of the obstacles encountered in attempts by community mental health programs to reach out to the developmentally disabled. It can be particularly difficult to reach out to a group that already has one stigmatizing disability and is not necessarily receptive to addressing mental health problems. Parents and care givers can be similarly supportive of these individuals and contribute to the denial of mental health problems by maintaining territorial control over all forms of care. It can often be difficult for the mental health practitioner to assist a DD client and the primary care giver. In addition, mental health clinicians need to confront their own feelings about the inability of the developmentally disabled to use traditional talk therapies, as well as their perceptions of unappealing appearance because of the nature of the disability. The following community mental health services can be developed to meet the mental health needs of the developmentally disabled.

Comprehensive Treatment. Referral procedures need to be established with pertinent health care specialists who can meet the primary treatment needs of those with developmental disabilities (neurologists, speech pathologists, and so forth) by a mental health clinician who is responsible for *referral services,* not only to health care specialists, but to resources involved in residential, social, and other independent living services for DD populations.

Diagnostic Services. If not available from staff in a mental health program, such services will need to be purchased from an outside consultant. Diagnostic work can involve neuropsychology evaluation, assessing adaptive levels of behavior (Schwartz and Allen, 1974; Windmiller, 1977), and other modifications to traditional psychological testing (Ellis, 1978; Keats, 1965; Meyers, 1973). A clear understanding of all the medical aspects of the disability is presupposed prior to any intervention.

Short-Term Intervention Programs. A substantial proportion of those with developmental disabilities can have their mental health needs satisfied with relatively short-term interventions, involving eclectic approaches (role playing, psychoeducational approaches coupled with homework, and so forth). Walker (1980) recommends time-limited approaches involving six to ten sessions, although conceding that periodic subsequent follow-up sessions are imperative for members of this population.

Behavior Therapy Programs. The prevalence of brain impairment experienced by members of this population and other severe behavioral or learning deficits make the behavioral therapies a very useful form of treatment (Bernstein and Karan, 1979; Ross, 1972). Adaptive behavior has been taught to those with developmental disabilities in the areas of personal care, social skills, communicative skills, and job skills. This can involve a wide spectrum of behavioral tools such as modeling, positive reinforcement, prompting, shaping, and extinction procedures. Behavioral approaches have shown particular promise in working with the autistic child (Lovaas, Schreibman, and Koegel, 1974; Margolies, 1977; Marzuryk, Barker, and Harasym, 1978; Schlopler, Brehm, Kinsbourne, and Reichler, 1971).

Family Intervention Programs. Although not every family needs family counseling, the need is prevalent and often thinly disguised. These interventions can help parents deal with feelings of guilt, denial, or grief; clarify changes in the relationship and coping strategies; and deal with possible effects on siblings. Developing parent networks or groups can be especially helpful in working in these areas.

Parent/Paraprofessional Training Programs. The training of parents, significant others, or institutional paraprofessionals can be an invaluable adjunct to mental health therapy for the developmentally disabled. Parental and paraprofessional involvement can range from carrying out specific behavioral instructions to full participation as a cotherapist based on behavioral analysis training and involvement in the planning and conducting of treatment (Berkowitz and Graziano, 1972; Schlopler and Reichler, 1971; Tymchuk, 1975). A review of behavioral training programs for parents indicates that mothers are most frequently trained, operant treatment approaches are most commonly used, and aggressive or hyperactive behaviors very often are targeted for change (Berkowitz and Graziano, 1972).

Sex Education Programs. Although perhaps more appropriately categorized under social competence or adaptive behavior training the sexual education needs of the developmentally disabled should be emphasized. Sexual adjustment issues are crucial in view of the natural biological needs of these individuals, frequent physical limitations, isolation from social learning experiences, and cognitive deficits. At the Hvidovre Denmark Center for those with epilepsy, the sexual education program involved a small-group format with a staff leader/facilitator for each group (Kuhlman, 1979). Groups were separated into several levels based upon the participants' cognitive abilities and degree of life exposure.

These components provide an outline of mental health services and treatment strategies for the developmentally disabled. This is not to exclude provision of other important services, such as genetic counseling or school consultations, but to provide a good core service program. In some states, mental health agencies are mandated to provide a wider spectrum of services to developmentally disabled groups. In addition, a number of community facilities, including group homes and congregate care facilities, could benefit from mental health consultation in relation to normalizing the environment, developing group counseling programs, and establishing behavioral training programs.

Conclusion

There are many service-delivery problems for the developmentally disabled, including lack of transportation, changing service eligibility procedures, inadequately funded programs, and poor services accountability (Bernstein and Karan, 1979). Community facilities serving the developmentally disabled do not generally receive the mental health services that they need and do not have the money to purchase such services.

In attempting to serve the developmentally disabled better, mental health agencies can initiate several basic steps to increase access to mental health services: (1) outreach services to primary caregivers, general practitioners, pediatricians, and other medical personnel to make them aware of their patients' mental health needs and to make appropriate referrals to community resources and (2) ensuring coordinated services and communication between mental health agencies and agencies serving the developmentally disabled by delineating areas in the provision of mental health services and *scheduling cross training* among the various professionals involved in serving the developmentally disabled.

Other programs of value to the developmentally disabled can be identified through contact with the local developmental disability agency. An eligible person may not be aware of programs' existence or may repeatedly fall through the service cracks. State protection and advocacy officers for the developmentally disabled can be an excellent resource in ensuring that individuals receive needed services. Boggs (1978) has presented a complete taxonomy of the programs affecting the developmentally disabled.

It is important for community mental health agencies to meet the mental health needs of the developmentally disabled. The next decade should produce a number of innovative mental health services, coordinated efforts between agencies, and novel consultation arrangements in order to serve better the developmentally disabled citizens of our country.

References

Anderson, E. M. *The Disabled Schoolchild: A Study of Integration in Primary Schools.* New York: Barnes & Noble, 1973.

Bagley, C. "Social Adjustment and the Adjustment of People with Epilepsy." *Epilepsia,* 1972, *13,* 33–45.

Bear, D. M., and Fedio, P. "Quantitative Analysis of Interictal Behavior in Temporal Lobe Epilepsy." *Archives of Neurology,* 1973, *34,* 454–476.

Bergsma, D., and Pulver, A. E. (Eds.). *Developmental Disabilities: Psychological and Social Implications.* New York: Liss, 1976.

Berkowitz, B. P., and Graziano, A. M. "Training Parents as Behavior Therapists: A Review." *Behavior Research and Therapy,* 1972, *10,* 297–317.

Bernstein, G. S., and Karan, O. C. "Obstacles to Vocational Normalization for the Developmentally Disabled." *Rehabilitation Literature,* 1979, *40* (3), 66–71.

Betts, T. A., Merskey, H., and Pond, D. A. "Psychiatry." In J. Laidlaw and A. Richens (Eds.), *A Textbook of Epilepsy.* London: Churchill Livingstone, 1976.

Boggs, E. "A Taxonomy of Federal Programs Affecting Developmental Disabilities." In J. Wortis (Ed.), *Mental Retardation and Developmental Disabilities: An Annual Review.* Vol. 10. New York: Brunner/Mazel, 1978.

Breen, P., and Richman, G. "Evolution of the Developmental Disabilities Concept." In R. Wiegerink and J. W. Pelosi (Eds.), *Developmental Disabilities: The DD Movement.* Baltimore: Brookes, 1979.

Capute, A. J. "Developmental Disabilities: An Overview." *Dental Clinics of North America,* 1974, *18,* 557–577.

Coleman, M. "The Autistic Syndromes." In J. Wortis (Ed.), *Mental Retardation and Developmental Disabilities: An Annual Review.* Vol. 10. New York: Brunner/Mazel, 1978.

Conley, R. W. *The Economics of Mental Retardation.* Baltimore: Johns Hopkins University Press, 1973.

DeMeyer, M. K., and others. "Prognosis in Autism: A Follow-Up Study." *Journal of Autism and Childhood Schizophrenia,* 1973, *3,* 199–246.

Easton, J. K. M., and Halpern, D. "Cerebral Palsy." In W. Stolov and M. R. Clowers (Eds.), *The Handbook of Severe Disabilities.* Washington, D.C.: U.S. Government Printing Office, 1980.

Edwards, V. E. "Social Problems Confronting a Person with Epilepsy in Modern Society." *Proceedings of the Australian Association of Neurologists,* 1974, *11,* 239–243.

Ellis, D. "Methods of Assessment for Use with the Visually and Mentally Handicapped: A Selective Review." *Child: Care, Health, and Development,* 1978, *4,* 397–410.

Farber, B. *Effects of a Severely Retarded Child on Family Integration.* Monographs of the Society for Research in Child Development, No. 71. Chicago: Society for Research in Child Development, University of Chicago, 1959.

Farber, B., and Ryckman, D. B. "Effects of Severely Mentally Retarded Children on Family Relationships." *Mental Retardation Abstracts,* 1965, *11,* 1–17.

Fischer, M. *Procedural Manual for Mental Health Counselors and Consultants Working with the Disabled.* Olympia, Wash.: State of Washington Division of Developmental Disabilities, 1980.

Fraser, T., Erikson, K., and Thompson, J. "The Role of Specialized Vocational Services in Comprehensive Treatment of the Individual with Epilepsy." Paper presented at the Epilepsy International Symposium, Vancouver, B.C., Canada, September 1978. (ERIC Document Reproduction Service, ED 168 267)

Freeman, R. D. "Psychiatric Problems in Adolescents with Cerebral Palsy." *Developmental Medicine and Child Neurology,* 1970, *12,* 64–70.

Gayton, W. F. "Management Problems of Mentally Retarded Children and Their Families." *Pediatric Clinics of North America,* 1975, *22,* 561–570.

Grossman, H. J. (Ed.). *Manual on Terminology and Classification in Mental Retardation.* Washington, D.C.: American Association on Mental Deficiency, 1977.

Halpern, A. S. "Mental Retardation." In W. Stolov and M. R. Clowers (Eds.), *The Handbook of Severe Disabilities.* Washington, D.C.: U.S. Government Printing Office, 1980.

Hodgman, C. H., and others. "Emotional Complications of Adolescent Grand Mal Epilepsy." *Journal of Pediatrics,* 1979, *95,* 309–312.

Keats, S. K. *Cerebral Palsy.* Springfield, Ill.: Thomas, 1965.

Kuhlman, A. Personal Communication. Hvidovre, Denmark: May 14, 1979.

Lovaas, O. I., Schreibman, L., and Koegel, R. "A Behavior Modification Approach to the Treatment of Autistic Children." *Journal of Autism and Childhood Schizophrenia,* 1974, *4,* 111–129.

Margolies, P. J. "Behavioral Approaches to the Treatment of Early Infantile Autism: A Review." *Psychological Bulletin,* 1977, 249–264.

Martin, R. "Legal Regulations of Services to the Developmentally Disabled." In

M. S. Berker and others (Eds.), *Current Trends for the Developmentally Disabled.* Baltimore: University Park Press, 1978.

Marzuryk, G. F., Barker, P., and Harasym, L. "Behavior Therapy of Autistic Children: A Study of Acceptability and Outcome." *Child Psychiatry and Human Development,* 1978, *9* (2), 119-125.

Mercer, J. *Labeling the Mentally Retarded.* Berkeley: University of California Press, 1973.

Meyers, C. E. "Psychometrics." In J. Wortis (Ed.), *Mental Retardation and Developmental Disabilities: An Annual Review.* Vol. 5. New York: Brunner/Mazel, 1973.

Miller, E. A. "Cerebral Palsied Children and Their Parents: A Study in Child-Parent Relationships." *Exceptional Child,* 1958, *24,* 298-302.

Molnar, G. E., and Taft, L. T. "Cerebral Palsy." In J. Wortin (Ed.), *Mental Retardation and Developmental Disabilities: An Annual Review.* Vol. 5. New York: Brunner/Mazel, 1973.

Nirje, B. "The Normalization Principle and Its Human Management Implications." In R. Kugel and W. Wolfensberger (Eds.), *Changing Patterns in Residential Services for the Mentally Retarded.* Washington, D.C.: President's Committee on Mental Retardation, 1969.

O'Gorman, G. "Childhood Autism." *Practitioner,* 1978, *221,* 365-371.

Richman, G., and Breen, P. "The Developmental Disabilities Council and Its Membership." In R. Wiegerink and J. W. Pelosi (Eds.), *Developmental Disabilities: The DD Movement.* Baltimore: Brookes, 1979.

Rodin, E. A., Shapiro, H. L., and Lennox, K. "Epilepsy and Life Performance." *Rehabilitation Literature,* 1977, *38,* 34-39.

Ross, R. T. "Behavioral Correlates of Levels of Intelligence." *American Journal of Mental Deficiency,* 1972, *76,* 545-549.

Rutter, M., Tizard, J., and Whitmore, J. (Eds.). *Education, Health, and Behavior.* London: Longmans, 1970.

Schlopler, E., Brehm, S., Kinsbourne, M., and Reichler, R. J. "Effect of Treatment Structure on Development in Autistic Children." *Archives of General Psychiatry,* 1971, *24,* 415-421.

Schlopler, E., and Reichler, R. J. "Parents as Co-Therapists in the Treatment of Psychotic Children." *Journal of Autism and Childhood Schizophrenia,* 1971, *1* (1), 87-102.

Schwartz, B. J., and Allen, R. M. "Measuring Adaptive Behavior: The Dynamics of a Longitudinal Approach." *American Journal of Mental Deficiency,* 1974, *4,* 424-433.

Scott, D. F. "Psychiatric Aspects of Epilepsy." *British Journal of Psychiatry,* 1978, *32,* 417-480.

Sellin, D. F. *Mental Retardation: Nature, Needs, and Advocacy.* Boston: Allyn & Bacon, 1979.

Shere, E. S., and Kastenbaum, R. "Mother-Child Interaction in Cerebral Palsy: Environmental and Psychological Obstacles to Cognitive Development." *Genetic Psychology Monographs,* 1966, *73,* 255.

Smead, V. S., and Goetz, T. M. "Special Classroom Placements for E.M.R. Children: Guidelines for Community Mental Health Personnel." *Community Mental Health Journal,* 1979, *15* (1), 17–26.

Strax, T. "Adolescence: A Period of Stress and Search of Identity." In D. Bergsma and A. E. Pulver (Eds.), *Developmental Disabilities: Psychological and Social Implications.* New York: Liss, 1976.

Tymchuk, A. J. "Training Parent Therapists." *Mental Retardation,* 1975, *13* (5), 19–22.

Walker, P. W. "Recognizing the Mental Health Needs of Developmentally Disabled People." *Social Work,* 1980, *25,* 293–297.

Wiegerink, R., and Pelosi, J. W. *Developmental Disabilities: The DD Movement.* Baltimore: Brookes, 1979.

Windmiller, M. "An Effective Use of the Public School Version of the AAMD Adaptive Behavior Scale." *Mental Retardation,* 1977, *15* (3), 42–45.

Wolfensberger, W. *The Principle of Normalization.* Toronto, Ontario: Institute on Retardation, 1972.

Wortis, J. (Ed.). *Mental Retardation: An Annual Review.* Vol. 2. New York: Grune & Stratton, 1970.

⚥ 27 ⚥

Mental Health
Services for Women

Naomi Gottlieb

The mental health community has been slow in moving beyond traditional ideas about women in the family and in society and their related mental health problems. This chapter identifies new perspectives and information about women related to two conclusions: (1) that whatever the problem presented or the service offered to women, gender differences and women's special circumstances need to be considered and (2) that new research and practice experience have called into question some basic assumptions about women clients and their mental health needs and have developed new intervention modalities attuned to different assumptions. With this information, program managers should promote changes through more in-service training for staff based on new data about women's special needs, planning for the creation of new programs and promoting organizational changes to guarantee the nonsexist delivery of mental health services.

The long-range goals of this chapter are to encourage services to both men and women that are not bound by stereotyped thinking about either sex and that offer expanding alternatives that hold promise for enhanced mental health to both groups. The focused attention here on women is based only in part on the predominance of women among the clients of mental health agencies. Though issues that affect the majority of clients would be important per se, the emphasis here is the result of the current social phenomenon of a new perspective and burgeoning information about women. Questions have been raised generally about women's role in society by political activists and writers associated with the women's movement, and, more to the point here, the accumulating research of many scholars and the practice experience of mental health professionals suggest different explanations for and different resolutions of women's problems. My immediate purpose here is to present those perspectives and service approaches for women, but I hope the same process will evolve for men as well (that is, the questioning of long-held assumptions and the development of new interventions for men who seek mental health services). The long-range goal is nonstereotyped services for all clients. My emphasis on women is appropriate and needed in its own right and I view it as a step toward that goal.

There are reasonable questions being raised about the way women's mental health problems are addressed today. The kind of doubts surfacing about many current approaches need to be clear before I proceed to a statement of a revised perspective on women. As one example, a very frequent concern that women of all ages bring to mental health professionals is depression. This problem is usually approached primarily as an individual, intrapsychic phenomenon, etiologically based in the individual's circumstances and psychology. Although the incidence of depression among women is two or three times that among men (Seiden, 1976, p. 1117), most mental health interventions are not based on the common features of all women's experiences that could explain this greater incidence. One could view this greater frequency of depression as a coincidence unrelated to pervasive social phenomena affecting women as a group. It seems more reasonable, however, to question the continued and total explanation of the etiology in separate histories one by one. I shall present an alternate view.

As a second example, the recently termed "displaced homemakers" phenomenon describes the woman who, because of divorce, separation, or widowhood, needs to reenter the work world after a considerable period in the homemaker role. Lack of job skills and of basic social skills needed to handle a work situation, low self-esteem, and little sense of independence characterize the woman in such circumstances. The option frequently selected in services to such a woman emphasizes her as an individual and deals with the ways she can cope, feel more assured, and change her situation. As important as is the individual understanding, missing in such a view are questions about factors present in the childhood experiences of many girls that do not foster needed job and social skills, about factors in the marriages of many women that do not foster independence, and about factors that isolate women from one another. Alternative perspectives that build on commonalities suggest different mental health services.

Third, the usual therapeutic situation in a mental health setting, by its very nature, may be a deterrent to the woman client's greater sense of mental well-being. In that situation, based on the medical model, the mental health professional, with whatever degree of direction or indirection he or she assumes with the client, will most probably be viewed by the woman as an expert on whom she will be dependent while in treatment. This circumstance may repeat the lifelong pattern of dependence and powerlessness in the social realm that many women experience. The treatment situation thereby often does not counteract a major source of a woman's difficulties.

These illustrations introduce a fuller exposition of an alternative perspective and highlight two main issues: (1) Frequently occurring problems, such as depression and the displaced homemaker phenomenon, can be understood more completely in terms of a socialization process most women experience. That understanding suggests treatment approaches based on these commonalities. (2) The milieu in which service is offered can repeat past negative socializing influences.

The alternative view will develop these themes further and case illustrations will particularize their application. These alternate views will stress the importance of socialization processes and the experiences women share. This perspective in no way implies that the individual woman's particular needs, her idiosyncratic circumstances, behavior, and feelings, are to be ignored. My perspective assumes the compelling impact of women's common experiences and looks there first for explanations of difficulties and for implications for treatment. The stand recognizes different personal adaptations from individual to individual but advocates a first and continuing look at the effect of those factors that women share, that derive from societal expectations, and that often have deleterious effects on women's mental health.

Because much of the professional training of mental health practitioners has focused on the individual and his or her personal circumstances, a compelling argument needs to be made about the importance of a social view. The social perspective I shall discuss emphasizes commonalities in groups of people, based, to a great extent, on societal expectations. Although mental health professionals frequently reassure clients that their emotional problems are not unique to them, the client often does not hear that there are societal reasons for some of the problems most women share.

Socialization of Women

With many individual and ethnic variations, women as a group experience the world differently from men. The major expectation is that women will make their contribution to society through their nurturing, interpersonal skills and that women's achievements will be reflected from other people rather than based on their own accomplishments.

From the onset and continuing throughout childhood and adolescence, parents expect that girls will find their most important fulfillment in life from the roles of wife and mother. The attributes needed for those roles differ from those needed by the boy whose major life role will be the economic provider for the family. The necessary characteristics for the major feminine role—ability to nurture others, dependence on the male provider, sense of responsibility for the emotional well-being of the family, passivity, and unassertiveness—are encouraged from the beginning.

Persons important to the developing female child send this message in various ways. Though the actual differences between male and female at birth have been discovered so far to be quite limited (Maccoby and Jacklin, 1974), differences between the behavior of girls and boys as they mature are noteworthy. From their early months, female infants are encouraged, far more than boys, to have close bonds with adults and to gain satisfaction, far more than boys, from interpersonal ties (Goldberg and Lewis, 1972; Moss, 1972). Boys are expected to be more exploratory and autonomous, girls to stay close by, both sets of attributes in keeping with their adult roles. Observations of children's behavior in preschool and classroom situations (Baumrind and Black, 1967; Joffee, 1971) confirm that, from their early years, girls and boys manifest distinctively different attitudes and behavior related to their future roles. Parallel observations of the forces that encourage these distinctions can be found in textbooks (Wietzman, Hokada, and Ross, 1972; Women on Words and Images, 1972), behavior of classroom teachers (Chasen, 1974; Levy and Stacey, 1973), and in the media and advertising (Vincent, 1971). Such community efforts as citizens' groups to counteract sex-role stereotyping in schools attest to the pervasiveness of such practices.

By adolescence, girls expect that marriage and children will define their lives. Erikson's (1968) conceptualization of identity formation proposes that the adolescent girl will establish her identity through the man she later chooses. There may be differential acceptance of the formulation, but in any event, and in a practical sense, a woman's life is determined largely by her husband's economic situation, the geographical location of his work, his name, often his social group, and, by and large, the decisions he makes that affect the family. That personal experience is reinforced daily by the larger society, in which women see repeatedly that power and control in most areas are exerted exclusively by men. Young girls learn early that their entry into marriage and their later economic and social well-being will depend on continuing to please their husbands, and their own status will depend on how well they minister to the emotional and day-to-day needs of their families.

The family ties are primary for women and work is secondary. The work they are encouraged to do is very limited in its range and closely reflects home-related tasks (for example, nursing, teaching, and social work). Adams (1971) refers to this as the "compassion trap." Though most women work throughout much of their adulthood and an ever-increasing number of married women work, those jobs provide 56 percent of the salaries of men (Moser, 1974, p. 15). Women work for appreciable periods of time—on the average, two twenty-year-old mothers, one with one child and one with four children, can expect to work for twenty-five and seventeen years, respectively (Kreps, 1971, p. 4)—but that work is not considered a career. Women expect and accept lower pay than men and also must adapt to a series of discontinuities in their work life. Some of these discontinuities result from divorce or widowhood and a period of single parenthood, but even in a long-term two-parent family, the work discontinuities for women are marked. A man will be at work "for an unbroken block of some forty years between leaving school and retirement" (Kutza, 1975, p. 6), but women will be in and out of the labor force, depending on home circumstances. Though there is considerable evidence that women are not just brief visitors to the work world, their work discontinuities have received little attention (Kreps, 1971).

Women are viewed primarily as having private, not public, lives. Work outside the home is far less important than family roles. Psychological therapy offered to women frequently concentrates on how well women can be returned to normal functioning in that private world, with far less attention to the public arena.

Whole areas of women's lives have not been considered important because of the emphasis placed on their role in the nuclear family. For example, exceptions to the woman in the two-parent family, the single-parent mother and the lesbian, have not been accepted as valid social phenomena until very recently. Even for the woman who has been a homemaker in a two-parent family, the extended period of time when she is no longer in that role has been virtually ignored. The woman who marries at twenty and who has a life expectancy of eighty will live forty-five years past the time her youngest child is a full-time student and thirty-two years after the marriage of that youngest child (Kirsh, 1974). She can also expect to survive her husband by a number of years (Payne and Whittington, 1976). Thus, the primary role for which women have been prepared—that of wife and mother—is not called for during a major portion of their lives.

Ethnic differences need to be underscored in this discussion. In some cultures, the expectation of "feminine" qualities may be even more emphasized (for example, the passive woman in Asian culture) or the dominance of the male stressed (as in the "macho" aspect of Chicano culture). But in others there are contrary circumstances, such as in black society, where the expectation that women will work is strong (Solomon, 1980). Comparatively little is known about how the experiences of nonwhite women differ from their white counterparts. I assume that the world of ethnic minority women is different from ethnic minority men. What is known about these groups to date would confirm this, but the extent and subtleties of these differences have yet to be documented.

Perhaps the most important aspect of this brief review of the socialization of women is that, until recently, it was assumed that this set of societal expectations by and large did not constitute a problem for women. Women certainly experienced problems—their presence in great numbers in the offices of psychiatrists, psychologists, and social workers was testament to this—but their problems were considered individually determined. The difficulties were the woman's; there was not a problem with the consequences of the expected role.

Another way to look further at the implications of that role would be to enumerate those traits and abilities that are most likely to foster mental health. The mentally healthy person, one would conjecture, has basic material wellbeing; a good sense of self-esteem and self-value; a range of social skills and attitudes enabling her or him to show and accept affection, cope with problems, express feelings, and be appropriately assertive; a sense of mastery in a number of areas; work that is valued; and independence and autonomy (Broverman and others, 1970). This does not exhaust the list of preferred attributes to mental health, but it is a starting point to estimate how women fare, given their social role.

We know that women have a more limited set of social and work skills than men. They tend to be self-critical (Berlin, 1980) and nonassertive (Richey, 1980). They are rewarded for being feminine, though persons exhibiting both feminine and masculine traits (androgynous individuals) are far more able to adapt flexibly to a variety of situations (Bem, 1974). Women spend considerable portions of their lives in employment that has little status and is not valued monetarily. Although women's family role is ostensibly honored by the society, the persons hired to substitute for them (daycare workers and household employees) are paid very poorly for their work. Studies of married women by Bernard (1972) show them to be more depressed than married men, and she conjectures that marriage is a different phenomenon for women than for men, resulting in wives feeling submissive and helpless. Groups of women (single parents, lesbians) are made to feel that their status is not acceptable and needs to be corrected by a change in marital circumstances for the single parent and in sexual orientation for the lesbian. Older women are severely affected by retirement policies that leave them the poorest segment of society and by a lack of preparation for the activities of a good portion of their adult lives when they are left roleless.

Much of what is expected of women, it would seem, does not lend itself to their mental health. This is not to say that many of the qualities looked for in women are undesirable or unhealthy. The ability to nurture, to express feelings, and to show concern for others are wholesome traits, and, in fact, proponents of androgynous characteristics in all persons believe that the mental health of men would be enhanced if they were to adopt these feminine qualities. Men, of course, also have a list of traits that society has stereotyped for them—competitiveness, achievement, and aggressiveness. The problem for women is that the "feminine" traits have been emphasized to the exclusion of other qualities and skills more adaptable to a range of situations. The other problem for women is that, in comparison with "masculine" traits, women's sex-typed qualities are devalued in this society in arenas that count: important decision making, positions of power and influence, and work that is valued and paid well.

A better understanding of these gender-related issues has been achieved because previously closed questions are now being studied. Rossi (1964) has suggested that social scientists have been reluctant to study the issues society treats as closed, for example, how women feel about motherhood or how men feel about the necessity of work. New insights are developing now as some of these questions have been posed and the effects of stereotyping reviewed. Though innate sex differences appear to be minimal, we may not know the true differences between women and men until we raise boys and girls in an effectively nonsexist manner. For now, it seems safe to assume that the considerable differences seen between female and male adults are not attributable to inherent differences. As one practical indicator, increasing numbers of women enter fields nontraditional to them when affirmative action plans are implemented. This would confirm that the previous low representation of women was not innately but societally determined. Greater numbers of women have not suddenly or innately acquired the ability to be lawyers, engineers, or architects; social barriers have been lifted to permit women to develop and use a wider range of abilities.

Changes to rectify past effects can in themselves be problematic. The suggestions that women's work role becomes more important, that men develop more nurturing qualities, that women become more assertive and assume more decision-making power will not be implemented casually. Those persons, particularly couples, now trying to make those changes find it far from easy. However, considering the consequences of the status quo for women's health, the uncertainty of attempts to dilute stereotyping is a lesser hazard. More to the point here, women's mental health in the foreseeable future will be affected by society's current expectations. This chapter is thus concerned with how the interventions of mental health staff can be used to help women cope with these continuing effects.

Case Examples

With respect to the following case examples, several caveats are in order. First, socialization issues will appear repetitively since the focus of the chapter is the pervasive effects of social expectations. Such effects will be shown, however, to be manifested in different ways in individual situations. Second, the intention is not to stress any particular intervention; rather, the sample of approaches will be used illustratively. Other specific interventions for similar clients could easily be fashioned. Third, many of the suggested approaches will be seen as conscious attempts to counteract the effects of stereotyped socialization.

After presenting only a few essential elements in each client situation, the first intervention plan to be outlined will be that used by a mental health worker whose framework is an individually oriented model with comparatively little attention to women as a group or to effects of the socialization processes. Following this, I shall present an alternate approach based on the societal model I have discussed (see Radov, Masnick, and Hauser, 1980, for a similar format). The second presentation will be made in somewhat more detail to provide a fuller exposition of how treatment is shaped by this perspective. Discussions following the case examples will highlight several themes found in the cases.

Depressed Woman. The client is twenty-nine; recently divorced; has two children, ages seven and three; and is employed as a secretary. She reports periods of severe depression, particularly around her responsibilities for her children.

Current intervention: The therapist prescribes an antidepressant for the depressive symptoms and establishes a supportive relationship in which the client can achieve insight into her ambivalence about her children. The previous marital problem is discussed so that future relationships with men can be improved.

Alternative intervention: Viewing the depressive symptoms as an expression of a negative sense of self and "learned helplessness" (Seligman, 1974) and of reality pressures, the therapist focuses on cognitive restructuring to encourage less self-critical views and more positive self-statements. The therapist comments on the messages all women receive about their exclusive responsibility for the family's well-being and plans with the client for pleasant breaks for herself. The client is referred to a woman's support group for both psychological support and (if the group arranges trading childcare responsibilities) practical relief for the children's care.

The previous marital situation is discussed, as are new relationships with men, but emphasis is also placed on the importance of a better work situation, on the specific stresses of inadequate income, and on the values of relationships with woman friends.

Woman with Marital Problems. The client is thirty-eight; married to a construction foreman; has two sons, sixteen and fourteen; works part-time as a sales clerk. She reports marital difficulties, particularly in their sexual relationship. She appears anxious to understand her part in the marital problems, though her husband, whom she describes as very dominating, refuses to participate.

Current intervention: Encouraged by the client's interest in understanding herself, the therapist focuses on relevant aspects of the client's past—her relationships with her parents and their roles in the family. The therapist helps the client to see the connection between her present marital relationship and her role in relation to her parents, including the negative attitudes about sexuality they imparted to her.

Alternate intervention: Aware of the client's eagerness for help and self-understanding, the therapist is nonetheless concerned that the client could easily become a long-term "good client." The therapist is alert to the passive role that the woman plays vis-à-vis her dominant husband and builds into their work together a purposeful plan to encourage a sense of power and self-assertion in the client. The client's passive acceptance of her husband's statement that she has a sexual problem, as well as her inability to articulate her own sexual needs, are seen as important elements in the sexual difficulties. The therapist uses assertion training as part of the individual work and refers the client to a women's assertion-training class. There the client develops further skills but also understands, in the work with other women, the societal expectation that women will be unassertive. In individual counseling, the client considers the possible impact of her increased assertiveness on the marriage and the choices she will need to make related to that impact. The counselor also refers the client to books on female sexuality written from a woman's perspective so that she can understand that sexual desires and satisfactions of males and females are often different.

Abused Woman. The client is twenty-four, with two young children, married to a man who is physically abusive to her. He is extremely apologetic after each battering episode and has threatened suicide if she leaves him.

Current intervention: The therapist acknowledges that the husband has a serious problem but, because he refuses help, proposes that the woman work on her part of the problem. She is encouraged to look at what she might be doing that provokes his battering. The alternative of divorce is discussed, as is the client's guilt about the impact of this on her husband. The therapist urges the client to gain some understanding of her reasons for staying in the relationship so that she might alter the relationship with her husband and so that, if she decides to leave, she does not repeat this situation with another man in the future.

Alternate intervention: The therapist emphasizes the client's right to protect herself from physical harm and helps the woman to see how, like most women, she feels a need to take care of and protect family members over and beyond her own needs. The therapist also relates the woman's acceptance of abuse to her low sense of self-esteem and uncertainty of a life on her own. Discussions of how she can receive both practical sources of support and increased self-esteem from work outside the home are part of the therapy. In the therapist's group with other abused women, the client sees that she shares with others the experience of being controlled by an exceedingly jealous and abusive husband and alters her previous conception of herself as "crazy" because she put up with his extreme behavior. She realizes that other women also feel they are only half-persons without a relationship to a man, but from the direct experience with another woman in the group who has left an abusive situation, she begins to see that it is possible to develop an identity separate from her husband.

Displaced Homemaker. The client is fifty, her children are grown and living separately; and she has just gone through divorce, initiated by her husband. Because her husband did not want her to work during their marriage, she has only done volunteer work in the past. She has generally stayed close to home and is fearful of venturing far from her familiar surroundings. She has no regular source of income and needs to work.

Current intervention: The therapist focuses first on the immediate situation of employment and income, suggesting several community agencies for practical assistance. The client is given support for efforts to seek work. Therapy is also concerned with the difficulties that occurred in the marriage and the client's feelings about her husband's divorce action, and she is helped to see her role in the problem.

Alternate intervention: In focusing on the immediate situation, the therapist refers the client to a special job training program for displaced homemakers. As the client reports back positively on hearing other women in the program talk of their common experiences as women, the therapist emphasizes how her role in the marriage met what society expected but how she now needs to develop skills for which that role did not prepare her. The therapist makes clear to the client that their work together, to be helpful, should allow the client to begin to make her own decisions, to have a sense she can be an independent person.

Much of the therapy time is spent in role rehearsals for employment-related activities, about which the client has many fears. The client worries that the prospects for marriage seem dim, and the therapist stresses the potential in the client to have a satisfying life, with work and both female and male friendships, should she not remarry.

Lesbian Client. The client, age twenty-five, a computer programmer, identifies herself as a lesbian, and states that her problem is the difficulty of visits with her seven-year-old daughter, who lives with her former husband, to whom the client has relinquished physical custody. The daughter appears resentful and rebellious whenever they are together.

Current intervention: The therapist encourages the client to think through her feelings about the custody decision, though the client indicates that, by and large, she is satisfied this was the best decision for her. The therapist does not press her to reconsider, but suggests discussions about her ambivalence concerning her daughter. The therapist also encourages the client to consider her lesbianism as a factor in her relationship with both her daughter and her former husband.

Alternate intervention: The therapist focuses on the visiting situation as a parent-child problem and helps the client to develop strategies to deal with her daughter's behavior. The client's feelings about her daughter are part of this discussion. The therapist accepts the client's statement that the custody issue is resolved for her. The client is referred to a lesbian mother's group for the benefit of shared experiences with other lesbians in similar child custody circumstances.

Themes in Intervention

Widening the Arena of Women's Lives

Certain themes have recurred in the case situations. The first is that women feel, and many therapists reinforce the belief, that their life situation is essentially defined by the men to whom they are attached. In these examples, the therapist in the current intervention sections focuses on present or future relationships with men to the exclusion of other aspects of the woman's life. The woman thus receives one more message, and from a person in authority, that, in fact, the marriage or intimate relationship is *the* crucial aspect of her circumstances and that her continuing mental health derives exclusively from the success of that tie. In addition, there may be little said in these discussions about certain aspects in that relationship that call for her to assume behaviors, such as passivity and dependence, that do not promote mental health. Not only is the focus predominantly and sometimes exclusively on the tie to a man, the possibility is disregarded that what is traditionally expected of the woman in such a relationship can be a problem for her mental health. In addition, there is frequently very little said about the importance of work to women, and particularly the effects on her of work discontinuities.

Admittedly, the client herself may stress the relationship with husband or lover as the key one. In the alternate approach discussed here, it is suggested that the therapist attempt to widen the women's emotional resources and introduce broader social dimensions to the problem.

Alternate therapy tries to create a greater arena for a woman's life (work as well as family, other activities separate from both, friendships with other women) and recognizes that usual expectations and limited roles create problems. In each instance cited in the alternate approaches, the therapist consciously enlarges the discussions to counteract social limitations on women. Sometimes, when appropriate, the therapist will comment directly on societal pressures, as in the cases of the depressed woman and the displaced homemaker. In others, merely raising the issues separate from the family can indicate to the client that those areas are valid aspects of her life that can contribute to her mental well-being.

Another important socialization factor related to the immediate family is the often exaggerated sense of responsibility the woman assumes for the emotional needs of her family. Not only is that sense of responsibility exacerbated when family problems arise, as in the abused woman's situation, but it can be unwittingly exploited in therapy. The stress the therapist places on the woman's participation in problems of intimates can easily be interpreted by the woman as further evidence that, as she had assumed, she is clearly and almost solely responsible for the emotional upsets in her family. Alternate therapy would not absolve women from the effects of their contribution to interpersonal difficulties, but by deliberate and overt attention to the effects of socialization, can help the woman to see the realistic extent of her responsibility.

A subtheme related to the primacy given to the marital relationship is that deviations from the heterosexual nuclear family are devalued. Single-parent families, 90 percent of them headed by women, have only recently been given attention and study (Brandwein, 1974; Burden, 1980) and have traditionally been viewed as a temporary situation until women remarry. The single-parent family has been considered an aberration; the cure, another marriage. The support needed to maintain the mother and her children is not part of public policy; the salaries most women earn cannot decently provide for a family; and there is a tendency for the woman client and her therapist to see marriage as the only solution at hand. Not only in the single-parent example cited earlier, but in the case of the displaced homemaker and the woman with the marital problem, there is the issue of how women will manage without men to support them. The alternate therapist helps the woman to see an independent life as a real possibility, to seek supports to make it feasible, and to gain pleasure from her own abilities to be independent. These therapeutic activities need not come from a conviction that women are better off without men. To the contrary, the alternate therapist may be convinced that only when women can experience independence and autonomy will they be able to enter mutual and strengthening relationships with men, not based on dependent needs or on psychological, economic, or societal pressures.

Related to the usual emphasis on the nuclear family and women's relationships with men is the attitude toward the lesbian client. Although the major professional associations have made clear (though only very recently) that homosexuality is not considered a psychological disorder, it is easy to assume that when the lesbian client experiences a problem, her sexual orientation is somehow a factor. The previously cited case discusses that theme, as well as the related one of a mother's decision to relinquish the custody of her children, another example of an affront to traditional views about the family.

Connecting Women with Other Women

A second theme in the cases is the alternate therapist's conscious attempts to connect women with one another. Contrary to the stereotype of the "kaffee klatsch" or the gossipy women's circle, women have been isolated from each other relative to frank exposure of important areas of their lives, particularly an awareness of those areas affected by their common socialization. Facilitators of women's groups report on the eye-opening quality of women's realization that other women, and indeed most women, experience the same expectations, the same kinds of relationships with men, and the same attitudes about work (Wyckoff, 1977). In the same vein, in individual therapy, there is value when the woman therapist acknowledges that she too has been shaped by this society's expectations and that all women, including the woman therapist, are dealing in some way or another with those effects.

The displaced homemaker and the abused woman's cases are meant to reflect the phenomenon of shared group experiences about socialization. The importance of those shared experiences lies not only in the reassurance to the individual woman that she is not a lone sufferer but that her responses are valid. The group support and insights can constitute the permission women need to break out of old roles. The sharing of practical notions and psychological support can make the difference for women trying to be more autonomous either on their own or in ongoing relationships. Selected use of recent feminist literature can also help women understand commonalities among all women.

Women and Power

Third, several of the cases were used to illustrate the issue of power, defined here as control over important areas of one's life. As discussed, society delegates little public power to women and within the family situation assumes that men will have a major power position. Therapy can be seen by the woman as another instance in which a person in authority is in a position of power relative to her. Because therapists usually do not see this as an issue or, if they do, see professional control as appropriate, the factor is ignored and the assumption made that a period of dependency is necessary to the outcome of the treatment.

An alternate view of power is recommended if one accepts the position that women have been deprived of such power and that a sense of mastery and control over one's life circumstances is one of the essential prerequisites to mental health. This alternate view assumes that an unequal power balance is inherent in the therapy situation and that for the benefit of the woman client, the therapist, without relinquishing his or her position deriving from professional expertise, needs to exert a conscious effort to make the issue explicit and encourage autonomous activities within the therapy situation. In the marital problem discussed, because of the woman's passive role with a dominant husband, the alternate therapist surfaces this issue. In the case, example of depression, in which "learned helplessness" is seen as a causative factor, an effective antidepressant can come from acting on a new sense of mastery encouraged in therapy.

Women as "Good Clients"

As a fourth theme, there is a combination of characteristics seen frequently in women that result in their being considered "good clients." More than men, they are likely to acknowledge personal problems, seek help for them, talk more freely, and respond to a person in authority with compliance (Phillips and Segal, 1969). There is a natural tendency for therapists to view all these traits as positive and useful in the therapeutic encounter. The problematic aspect of these behaviors is that when women are seen as "good clients," as in the marital problem case, therapy can be inappropriately extended and, more important, the possibility for women to act more independently can be lost. When women's behaviors are seen as determined by the expectation that they will be compliant in such main areas as unequal power, limited roles, and devalued work, then therapy that does not counteract the compliant expectation becomes just one more instance of it. This poses a dilemma for many therapists because the verbal, amenable client makes therapy easier and often asks the therapist to exercise exactly that power. In the same vein, there is a tendency to see assertiveness as an attribute inappropriate to women, rather than as a strength needed to manage independently. A different view and a conscious effort to encourage other behaviors in women come with the understanding that a sense of control and legitimization of questioning and assertive behavior can promote health.

Special Nature of Special Problems

The final theme, touched on in the illustration of the depressed woman, concerns classes of problems in which labels for women have been used with little awareness or research into the special nature of these problems. The female alcoholic and the menopausal woman are two such examples. Recent study has identified that the alcohol- or drug-abusing woman has a different entry into and experience with chemical dependency than her male counterpart (Gottlieb, 1980). That understanding has come from the fairly new attention given to women as a separate group. Treatment programs devised especially for women with chemical dependencies have also brought to light, through services that counteract women's socialization, how traditional programs, either mixed-sex or for women alone, have served to reinforce stereotypes and have masked women's special needs. The menopausal woman has been seen as a problem because, by and large, individual physicians and research studies have reported on clinical populations, thereby excluding whole groups of women who do not experience difficulties during menopause. Even in clinical populations, menopausal problems have not been viewed as "real" problems (Page, 1977). Programs that assume a different view about women in the menopausal years have discovered latent strengths rather than problems (Page, 1977). Other studies indicate that many women's menopausal problems are quite different from their physicians' interpretations of them (Bart and Grossman, 1976).

Researchers have, in fact, brought into question a whole set of assumptions about the problematic nature of women's reproductive system (Lennane and Lennane, 1973). A more complete understanding of normal female sexuality, quite altered from the traditional view, has been gained in recent years (Koedt, 1970) and sex-related problems given a new perspective. In the process, it has become clearer how women and girls have been inappropriately implicated in phenomena related to sexuality. For example, rape was viewed traditionally as a sexual and not a violent act; incest was the result of the young girl's sexual provocations; the sexual behavior of adolescent girls was dealt with differently from that of boys by the justice system (Crow and McCarthy, 1979). As another example of a special problem, the aging process, with its attendant economic, social, and psychological stresses, has been found to be a different experience for women than for men (Lowenthal, Thurnher, and Chiriboga, 1975).

These themes culled from the examples and now taken together can be summarized in four main recommended attributes of alternate, nonstereotyped therapy for women: (1) Therapy needs to recognize those deleterious effects of the socialization process. (2) Therapy needs to encourage greater life options for women. (3) Therapy needs to empower women as much as possible. (4) In each class of problem treated, gender differences need to be assumed and investigated.

Agency Example

Specialized mental health services can be offered in such a way as to incorporate the attributes of nonstereotyped interventions. For example, in 1973, the Women's Institute in Seattle was established by a small group of social work educators and practitioners. Though the following description of services has been drawn from the experience of this one agency, the account could be considered typical of many alternative counseling programs developed in recent years (Gottlieb, 1980). The Women's Institute offers a combination of individual counseling, group counseling, and educational services. Women can begin at the institute in any of these areas and often will alternate between the three modes.

At the outset of a request for individual counseling, the woman client is encouraged to take an autonomous role. In the initial phone call or intake interview, she is informed of her right to gain information about both the agency and the counselor so that she can decide whether this is the appropriate person and organization. The initial interview is viewed as a mutual exploration process, and the client is advised of her right to evaluate the counselor, including asking specific questions about the counselor's professional background and practice orientation. Efforts are made to demystify the counseling process through the worker's clear and frequent discussion of her practice methods and of the choices the client can continually exercise. The worker tries to equalize the power differential between herself and the client by such procedures as the use of first names, self-disclosure about the commonalities women experience, and continual attention to the client's right to decide about important issues in the counseling process.

In assessing each situation, the worker assumes that societal expectations and discrimination will play an important role in any woman's problem. Aware of the narrow roles usually assigned to women, the worker will explore many options with the client (for example, the importance of work and the value of experiences and relationships outside the family, especially with other women). Because women's expected social roles limit their repertoires of skills, women will be referred to institute classes to learn needed skills, such as assertion training, time and financial management, risk taking, and self-criticism reduction. To counteract the isolation of women from one another, women clients will be referred to groups of other women (sometimes just to a group of two) if the worker believes that two clients with similar problems can learn from each other. Often the client will enter larger groups, such as those for battered women or for single parents, to receive both psychological and practical supports. The assumption of these group experiences is that women have much to learn from one another and that mutual learning can be more useful than the assistance of the expert to a sense of autonomy in women. In all services offered, value is placed on the woman's right to be strong and assertive and not submissive.

The agency's administrative arrangements help to create an atmosphere in which women's rights are respected. The professional staff operates on a consensus model and through several mechanisms increases both the credibility and other options of the office staff. For example, the office manager takes part in administrative decision making, engages in a mutual evaluation process between the board and staff, and is encouraged to assume paraprofessional responsibilities with client groups. This atmosphere of respect for women's capabilities is reflected in the office staff's interaction with women clients.

Administrative Changes

A mental health facility administrator can take several steps to introduce alternative, nonstereotyped services for women. The first is the need for in-service training for staff. Many staff members were trained prior to the time of these recent insights and new empirical data about women's special needs. Administration, board, and staff members need to be convinced that this new information affects the lives of the majority of their clients and that alternate therapies can be useful. The resources for improved knowledge about women can come from the literature (see the References) and from the experience of innovators of new programs. In most cities, the staff of such alternate agencies as feminist therapy services, shelters for abused women, rape relief centers, lesbian resource agencies, centers for menopausal women, and female sexuality institutes can provide the required expertise. In-service training can consist of workshops, courses, and individual consultations conducted by such knowledgeable persons.

The important new perspectives on rape, abuse, incest, and other problem areas central to women's lives have been pioneered by paraprofessionals even more than professionals. The in-depth work with rape victims, for example, provides awareness of certain aspects of the rape-trauma syndrome that most professionals have not addressed.

Stress also needs to be placed on how to minimize the therapist's authority position in the usual medical model of therapy because this may not encourage the woman client's autonomous stance. Emphasis needs to be placed on a thorough understanding of social inequities and attention paid to reality situations. For example, the young single parent's depression may be largely based on her dilemma on how to maintain her family on her low salary or how to get some practical relief from the constant care of her children. Without attending to these factors, the therapist may be ignoring major etiological factors in the woman's depression (Radloff, 1975).

Second, the administrator must plan to create new programs especially for women. A primary example is the women's support group for consciousness raising, for assertion training, for specific supports, such as for the single parent, the displaced homemaker, and the abused woman. The experience of alternate treatment centers in the drug treatment field suggests that any kind of inpatient or day-treatment programs with mixed groups must avoid pigeonholing women into stereotyped roles (Gottlieb, 1980). From studies of women and men in groups, it is known that women act less assertively (Richey, 1980). In many mixed-sex treatment programs, women will be expected to assume traditional roles (for example, household maintenance as an exclusive task for women in residential treatment centers). Program planners must make conscious efforts to counteract these expectations.

Third, and perhaps most difficult to achieve, the service organization should itself be nonsexist in its orientation and operation if staff members are to be expected to offer nonstereotyped services. A mental health agency in which there is inequity between men and women as far as positions held, salaries received, and decision making will be a difficult place to implement nonsexist service for clients. Women staff who accept or must work in a setting in which they are paid less than men for their work or in which they are subject to sex-stereotyped behaviors and attitudes will find it very difficult to encourage their women clients to be assertive and take more control over their lives. Men staff members and administrators who have not become aware of the effects of sex inequities in their own workplace will have little consciousness that inequities are an issue for their women clients. Clients who see that only men are in positions of power in an agency or note, for example, that in a cotherapy situation the male therapist takes the lead over the female therapist will have no role model to fashion their own more assertive behavior.

These aspects of organizational life are not easy to alter. A necessary first step is the awareness that women experience the world differently from men and that important aspects of that experience may not be good for their mental health. Staff members need to be convinced that there is an issue here. This is not only a professional matter because the awareness of gender differences affects everyone personally. Changing organizational life and altering therapeutic interventions to correct inequities based on sex is no mean task.

The particular ways administrators may choose to begin (or, in some instances, continue) the process will vary. Staff discussions, consciousness-raising sessions, use of outside consultants and trainers, and adding to library resources can be used with different timing and for different purposes from agency to agency. Depending on the agency clientele, varying attention will be given to the much-needed understanding of the differences that exist for ethnic minority women around all the issues discussed in this chapter. Agencies will also need to consider how new insights about women will affect their theoretical orientations and practice interventions. There has been no attempt in these discussions to suggest that one particular methodology is necessitated by the new knowledge about women's needs. However, it would be naive to propose that customary interventions will be unaffected by increased convictions about women's distinctive needs. The individual therapist will need to make his or her own judgment about the necessary changes.

Conclusion

It would be handy to be able to conclude this chapter with a summary of a series of studies that prove that the alternate interventions suggested here are, in fact, more effective than usual therapies for the treatment of women's mental health problems. Those data are not available, though we have several indications along the way.

First, we know of the increasing awareness of a whole range of problems not in the public consciousness a few years ago: sex inequities and sex harassment in the workplace, family violence and sexual assault, the condition of the single parent, lack of public power for women. Communities and organizations that have made services accessible to respond to these problems have been flooded with instances of inequities.

There are important society-wide changes that will affect all families and women in particular—the noteworthy increase in labor force participation of women, the delay in age at marriage, the lowered birth rate. Therapists who continue to base their understanding of women on a perspective that predates these changes do so at the risk of ignoring reality.

Second, we have a body of knowledge accumulating about gender differences that raises many questions about long-held assumptions and suggests alternate approaches for individual problems. A number of disciplines contribute to that literature—psychology, sociology, social work, health services—through the work of increasing numbers of women scholars in those fields. Some of that literature has been cited in the discussions and appears in the References.

Third, there are a limited number of empirical studies that have tested out some of the propositions advanced in the new literature and some of the treatment methods proposed. For example, it has been shown that women who work outside the home recover from depression more readily than those who do not (Weissman and others, 1971), suggesting that activity in multiple roles is health promoting. A treatment program for women who were drug abusers that included care for their children was found to be more effective than a program that did not address the need for child care (Schwingl, Martin-Shelton, and Sperazi, 1980). These kinds of investigations need to be replicated and expanded so that there is an increased empirical base for the perspective advanced in this chapter.

Enough is known at this point to bring into question the bases of services to women. This chapter has documented the need for the challenge and provided the rationale for and some specifics of alternate approaches.

References

Adams, M. "The Compassion Trap." In V. Gornick and B. Moran (Eds.), *Women in Sexist Society*. New York: Basic Books, 1971.

Bart, P., and Grossman, M. "Menopause." *Women and Health*, 1976, *1*, 3–11.

Baumrind, D., and Black, A. "Socialization Practices Associated with Dimensions of Competence in Preschool Boys and Girls." *Child Development*, 1967, *38*, 291–327.

Bem, S. "The Measurement of Psychological Androgyny." *Journal of Consulting and Clinical Psychology,* 1974, *42,* 155–162.

Berlin, S. "Cognitive-Behavioral Interventions for Problems of Self-Criticism Among Women." *Social Work Research and Abstracts,* 1980, *16,* 19–28.

Bernard, J. *The Future of Marriage.* New York: World, 1972.

Brandwein, R. "Women and Children Last: The Social Situation of Divorced Mothers and Their Families." *Journal of Marriage and the Family,* 1974, *36,* 498–509.

Broverman, I. K., and others. "Sex-Role Stereotypes and Clinical Judgments of Mental Health." *Journal of Consulting Psychology,* 1970, *34,* 1–7.

Burden, D. "Women as Single Parents: Alternate Services for a Neglected Population." In N. Gottlieb (Ed.), *Alternative Social Services for Women.* New York: Columbia University Press, 1980.

Chasen, B. "Sex-Role Stereotyping and Prekindergarten Teachers." *Elementary School Journal,* 1974, *74,* 220–235.

Crow, R., and McCarthy, G. *Teenage Women in the Juvenile Justice System: Changing Values.* Tucson, Ariz.: New Directions for Young Women, 1979.

Erikson, E. *Identity: Youth and Crisis.* New York: Norton, 1968.

Goldberg, S., and Lewis, M. "Play Behavior in the Year-Old Infant: Early Sex Differences." In J. Bardwick (Ed.), *Readings on the Psychology of Women.* New York: Harper & Row, 1972.

Gottlieb, N. "Women and Chemical Dependency." In N. Gottlieb (Ed.), *Alternative Social Services for Women.* New York: Columbia University Press, 1980.

Joffee, C. "Sex Role Socialization and the Nursery School: As the Twig is Bent." *Journal of Marriage and the Family,* 1971, *33,* 467–475.

Kirsh, B. "Consciousness-Raising Groups as Therapy for Women." In V. Franks and V. Bartle (Eds.), *Women in Therapy: New Psychotherapies for a Changing Society.* New York: Brunner/Mazel, 1974.

Koedt, A. "The Myth of the Vaginal Orgasm." In S. Firestone and A. Koedt (Eds.), *Notes from the Second Year: Women's Liberation.* New York: Radical Feminism, 1970.

Kreps, J. *Sex in the Marketplace: American Women at Work.* Baltimore: Johns Hopkins University Press, 1971.

Kutza, E. *Policy Lag: Its Impact on Income Security for Older Women.* Occasional Paper 6. Chicago: School of Social Service Administration, University of Chicago, 1975.

Lennane, K. J., and Lennane, J. "Alleged Psychogenic Disorders in Women—A Possible Manifestation of Sexual Prejudice." *New England Journal of Medicine,* 1973, *288,* 288–292.

Levy, B., and Stacey, J. "Sexism in the Elementary Schools: A Backward and Forward Look." *Phi Delta Kappan,* 1973, *55,* 105–109.

Lowenthal, M., Thurnher, M., and Chiriboga, D. *Four Stages of Life: A Comparative Study of Women and Men Facing Transitions.* San Francisco: Jossey-Bass, 1975.

Maccoby, E., and Jacklin, C. *The Psychology of Sex Differences.* Stanford, Calif.: Stanford University Press, 1974.

Moser, C. "Mature Women: The New Labor Force." *Industrial Gerontologist,* 1974, *1,* 14–25.

Moss, H. "Sex, Age, and State as Determinants of Mother-Infant Interaction." In J. Bardwick (Ed.), *Readings on the Psychology of Women.* New York: Harper & Row, 1972.

Page, J. *The Other Awkward Age: Menopause.* Berkeley, Calif.: Ten Speed Press, 1977.

Payne, B., and Whittington, F. "Older Women: An Examination of Popular Stereotypes and Research Evidence." *Social Problems,* 1976, *23,* 488–504.

Phillips, D., and Segal, B. "Sexual Status and Psychiatric Symptoms." *American Sociological Review,* 1969, *34,* 58–72.

Radloff, L. "Sex Differences in Depression—The Effects of Occupation and Marital Status." *Sex Roles,* 1975, *1,* 249–265.

Radov, C., Masnick, B., and Hauser, B. "Issues in Feminist Therapy: The Work of a Women's Study Group." In N. Gottlieb (Ed.), *Alternative Services for Women.* New York: Columbia University Press, 1980.

Richey, C. "Assertion Training for Women." In S. Schinke (Ed.), *Community Application of Behavioral Methods: A Sourcebook for Social Workers.* Chicago: Aldine, 1980.

Rossi, A. "The Equality of Women: An Immodest Proposal." *Daedalus,* 1964, *93,* 607–652.

Schwingl, P., Martin-Shelton, D., and Sperazi, L. "The First Two Years: A Profile of Women Entering Women, Inc." In N. Gottlieb (Ed.), *Alternative Social Services for Women.* New York: Columbia University Press, 1980.

Seiden, A. "Overview: Research on the Psychology of Women. II. Women in Families, Work, and Psychotherapy." *American Journal of Psychiatry,* 1976, *133,* 1111–1123.

Seligman, M. "Depression and Learned Helplessness." In R. J. Friedman and M. M. Katz (Eds.), *The Psychology of Depression: Contemporary Theory and Research.* Washington, D.C.: Winston, 1974.

Solomon, B. "Alternative Social Services and the Black Woman." In N. Gottlieb (Ed.), *Alternative Social Services for Women.* New York: Columbia University Press, 1980.

Vincent, G. "Sex Roles in Television Programs." Unpublished manuscript, School of Social Welfare, University of California, Berkeley, 1971.

Weissman, M., and others. "The Social Role Performance of Depressed Women: Comparison with a Normal Group." *American Journal of Orthopsychiatry,* 1971, *41,* 390–405.

Wietzman, L., Hokada, E., and Ross, C. "Sex Role Socialization in Picture Books for Pre-School Children." *American Journal of Sociology,* 1972, *77,* 1125–1150.

Women on Words and Images. *Dick and Jane as Victims: Sex Stereotyping in Children's Readers.* Princeton, N.J.: Women on Words and Images, 1972.

Wyckoff, H. *Solving Women's Problems.* New York: Grove Press, 1977.

꙳ 28 ꙳

Programs
for the Elderly

Nancy R. Hooyman
Stephanie J. FallCreek

Even though the particular mental health needs of the elderly have received attention recently, older persons continue to comprise a small percentage of those actually served by mental health agencies. This chapter outlines basic needs of older persons for mental health services, issues of clinical interventions, service and community network considerations, and implications for training and service delivery. The challenge to mental health managers is to develop community-based programs utilizing, wherever possible, the natural helping networks. Creating a place for geriatric mental health services within the mental health agency is seen as a first step toward developing a range of community mental health services linked to the network of aging services.

The mental health needs of the elderly have long been neglected, as partially evidenced by the fact that less than 4 percent of the clients of community mental health centers are over sixty-five (Weinberg, 1976, p. 18). Despite the passage of the 1975 amendment to the Community Mental Health Center Act requiring centers to develop programs for the elderly, most community mental health centers have been slow to respond to the mental health needs of this rapidly increasing segment of our population. In fact, mental health professionals have been accused of being ageist, less willing to invest resources in the elderly than in children and young adults. Other barriers to the service utilization by the elderly are their lack of awareness of services and their own negative attitudes toward mental health programs; most centers do not have outreach efforts geared toward the elderly and many older people face transportation difficulties. A further problem is the failure of Medicare and Medicaid to reimburse for long-term outpatient mental health services for the elderly (Patterson, 1976).

In addition to these obstacles, resources for mental health in general are being sharply curtailed at the same time that the elderly's mental health needs are likely to increase. For example, older people who have been able to function in their homes primarily because of chore and home health services may find their level of functioning impaired by cuts in services. For the frail or vulnerable elderly who are particularly prone to being hurt by budget cuts, institutionalization may be their only resort. Birren predicted at the 1975 National Conference on the Mental Health of the Elderly that, "Even if mental health professionals were to devote their full time to the older population, it is doubtful whether they could meet today's needs as defined by some reasonable standard of professional care" (National Institute of Mental Health, 1976). The prospect of adequately meeting these needs in the 1980s seems even more remote. Despite this gloomy resource picture, mental health professionals must be knowledgeable about the elderly's mental health needs and develop cost-effective programs and services to meet them.

The delivery of geriatric mental health services should include a recognition of the following continuum of care sites: home health care day programs, public housing, halfway houses, board and care facilities, nursing homes, general hospitals, and private mental health facilities. Each of these sites may range along a continuum from no specialized geriatric programs or personnel, to some specialized geriatric services, to a team of geriatric specialists acting as consultants, to regionalized geriatric services. Several basic programmatic and service-related issues need to be addressed regarding the balance between direct and indirect services, mental illness and mental health orientations, facility-based and outreach-focused services, services related to acute or chronic care, services offered through formal or informal support systems, and age-integrated versus age-segregated services (National Institute of Mental Health, 1976). These issues will be addressed throughout this chapter.

Demographic and Social Trends

The single most important demographic fact impacting on mental health services for the elderly is that the U.S. population as a whole is aging. Because of medical advances, primarily in the earlier years, more people are living to face the challenges of old age. Nearly 25 million Americans (13.9 million women, 9.6 million men) or 11.2 percent of the population are over sixty-five, an increase from 20 million or 9.8 percent a decade ago. A man reaching sixty-five today has an average life expectancy of 13.9 years, a woman, of 18.3 years. The proportion of the population sixty-five and over varies by race and ethnic origins: 11 percent for whites, 8 percent for blacks, and 4 percent for persons of Spanish origin (Lowy, 1979, p. 27). By the year 2020, in large part because of the effect of the baby boom, individuals over sixty-five years of age will constitute approximately 32 million or over 15 percent of the population.

A major consequence of an aging population is an increased demand for health care and social services. The population over sixty-five accounted for 25 percent of the federal budget (including Social Security) or $112 billion in fiscal 1978. Moreover, the population of the very old, who generally need the most services, will be increasing more rapidly in the years ahead. In 1970, less than one in five Americans was eighty or older; in twenty years, it will be one in four. This growth in the vulnerable or frail elderly, who generally have at least one chronic condition and require multiple health and social supports, is particularly significant for the field of geriatric mental health. As Butler has noted, "We haven't, in some cases, been adding a lot of life to people's years," ("As Lives . . . ," 1979). Our culture, which emphasizes youth and productivity, tends to view the rapid increase in the elderly population and older people themselves as a problem. The problem, however, can be traced to many of the conditions facing older people, such as poverty, chronic disease, mental illness, substandard housing, and social isolation. Thus, a major challenge for geriatric mental health program managers is to develop a multiproblem and multidisciplinary approach to improving the quality of the elderly's lives in terms of their health, psychosocial, and economic needs.

Numerous myths and stereotypes surround the aging process. The older person is often portrayed as passive, asexual, sick, and ineffective. The biological model of aging has tended to equate aging with disease. Most research has been conducted on the sick elderly, with decline viewed as the key concept of later life. Contrary to these myths, the majority of older people are mobile; are in contact with family, friends, or neighbors; and live in the community. Although 85 percent of the elderly have one or more chronic conditions, 81 percent are physically capable of getting around on their own without assistance. Only 5 percent of the elderly are in institutions; for those who are attempting to remain in their own homes, their families provide 80 percent of their home health care. Less than 10 percent suffer some degree of dementia. Needless to say, there is tremendous diversity within the population over sixty-five. There is a need to recognize the different rates of the aging processes, as well as differences by gender, socioeconomic status, age (for example, the young-old of fifty-five to sixty-five or the old-old of over eighty years), race, and geographic location.

Mental Health Needs of the Elderly

The aging process inevitably brings some normal and intrinsic losses and stresses, such as sensory losses. Other losses are superimposed by society, such as loss of status, work, and income. Most older people adjust to these losses, even though they may experience grief, guilt, loneliness, or anxiety in response to them. For many elderly, however, mental illness may be the outcome of these stresses. Five percent of the elderly in the community have been estimated to be severely disturbed, 15 percent neurotic, and 10–15 percent to experience mild to moderate degrees of impairment (Weinberg, 1976, p. 18).

The major mental health problems of the aged are senility and depression. These are very different types of diseases, but they have symptoms that sometimes make them hard to distinguish diagnostically. Half or more of the institutionalized elderly suffer from some form of senility (Rosenfeld, 1978, p. 127). The incidence of depression runs as high as 50 percent for older people with physical illnesses (Glassman, 1980, p. 292). The symptoms of depression among the elderly are similar to those among younger people; yet often the psychological symptoms defined as serious in young adults are considered nontreatable symptoms of "normal aging" in the elderly. The processes leading to depression among the elderly, however, appear to differ from that of younger adults. For older people, depression seems to result from loss of self-esteem as the environment changes or as their reduced body efficiency prevents them from adapting to meet their needs. The incidence of depression is highest among elderly unable to work, impaired by physical disabilities, under a doctor's care, and suffering financial hardships.

Diagnostic problems with the elderly are frequent because concurrent mental, physical, and social problems abound and can give rise to similar clinical symptoms. In evaluating an older person, practitioners need to be especially alert to the possibility of depression because the confused and disoriented behavior of depression is similar to chronic brain syndrome and because depression is the most treatable of all mental disorders. Unfortunately, many depressed older people may be misdiagnosed as senile and institutionalized rather than given appropriate treatment for depression. The diagnosis of "chronic organic brain syndrome" may be used erroneously to describe depression.

This large number of older persons needing help for depression is confronted with a relatively short supply of providers and an insurance system antithetical to long-term psychotherapeutic approaches. Given these constraints, what therapeutic approaches with the elderly hold promise? Blum compared the effects of theme-oriented psychotherapy, psychoanalytically oriented psychotherapy, and counseling with one another and with psychopharmacological treatment of depression and found that all of the approaches have merit (Rosenfeld, 1978).

Other types of functional disorders are less common than depression. Schizophrenia rarely develops for the first time in late life, but represents a lifelong pattern. Affective psychoses, such as involutional melancholia, manic-depressive psychoses, and paranoid states, tend to occur most in the age range fifty-five to sixty-five. Neuroses include anxiety neuroses, hysterical neuroses, obsessive compulsive and phobic neuroses, and hypochondrial neuroses, but their incidence among the elderly is not disproportionately high.

Other treatable mental health problems of the elderly include suicide, alcoholism, and drug abuse. The elderly account for approximately 25 percent of reported suicides, with rates highest for white males in their eighties and for white women in middle age. Practitioners must respond to an older person's threats of suicide because older people are less likely to fail in their suicide attempts than younger people are (Butler and Lewis, 1977).

Alcohol and drug abuse among the elderly has tended to be ignored by both gerontologists and mental health professionals. Multiple medications, overmedication, or medication as the only form of treatment are the most common types of drug abuse. The elderly consume more than 25 percent of all prescribed drugs and an even larger percentage of over-the-counter drugs. A 1977 study by the National Institute of Alcoholism and Drug Abuse found that the elderly often take psychotropic drugs in combination with other prescription drugs or with alcohol. Of those surveyed, 33 percent used between two and four prescription drugs and 50 percent used alcohol in combination with drugs. With the physical changes brought on by the aging process and the increased number of drugs used, the possibility of drug interactions and negative side effects is great. Doctors often do not explore alternatives to drug therapy, but instead provide a prescription as "the answer," which results in "pacification through drugs" (Butler, 1975).

Prevention, detection, and intervention efforts regarding alcoholism among the elderly have also been limited. The National Institute on Alcohol and Alcohol Abuse estimates that 10 percent of men and 2 percent of women over sixty-five are alcoholics. In some nursing homes, the rate of alcoholism may be as high as 20 percent (National Institute on Alcohol and Alcohol Abuse, 1979, p. 4). Although these estimates may appear low compared to the general population, the impact of alcoholism on the elderly is probably greater than on younger people because the elderly are more likely to react adversely to alcohol (Schuckit, 1980). The general effect of excessive alcohol consumption on an older person is to hasten the aging process; alcoholism increases susceptibility to various illnesses and tends to reduce the life span. Rates of alcoholism among the elderly are higher for widowed persons and for individuals with other health problems. As many as 20 percent of elderly medical inpatients and 10–15 percent of elderly outpatients have serious life problems related to alcohol (Schuckit, 1977, p. 369).

Problems of early detection and diagnosis are the greatest barrier to the treatment of elderly alcoholics. What is perceived as frailty, senility, or confusion may, in fact, be alcoholism. The most common crises associated with the onset of problem drinking in older persons are bereavement, retirement, social isolation, and boredom. In older alcoholics, the commonly associated mental health problems are depression, low self-esteem, anxiety, and hostility (Rathbone-McCuan and Roberds, 1980).

The psychosocial elements of alcoholism in older populations are important factors to be considered in diagnosing an older person. The symptoms of older alcoholics may not necessarily be the "classic" alcoholic symptoms of shakes, blackouts, seizures or hallucinations, dangerous or aggressive public behavior, or the sheer amount of alcohol consumed. The early symptoms may be depression, self-neglect, social withdrawal, or difficulties in relationships. Assessment criteria regarding older alcoholics should consider risk factors such as middle age, developmental tasks, divorce, bereavement, retirement, social isolation, and health problems. A "high index of suspicion" is needed to diagnose older alcoholics, especially women, because they are likely to complain of physical, emotional, and life difficulties rather than allude to any drinking problem (Schuckit and Morrissey, 1979).

Chronic brain syndrome is the mental health problem most commonly associated with older people and, as mentioned earlier, the most often misdiagnosed. According to Busse (1976, p. 5), 4–6 percent of people over sixty-five demonstrate signs of chronic brain disease; the incidence is higher among women.

Chronic brain syndrome covers two specific psychiatric disorders: senile dementia and psychoses associated with cerebral arteriosclerosis. Cerebral arteriosclerosis, or hardening of the arteries, may assume psychotic proportions where the patient's behavior includes screaming, pacing, and roaming.

The cause of senile dementia is not yet known, except that brain cells die and the brain shrinks, causing a breakdown in intellectual capacities, such as loss of short-term memory and abstract thinking capacities. The onset is gradual, but the deterioration is rapid. Alzheimer's disease or severe memory loss was formerly thought to be separate from senile dementia, but now is believed to be similar, to begin among younger age groups, and to account for 50–75 percent of the dementia cases.

The approach to chronic brain syndrome is one of management and of making the patient as comfortable as possible. A simplified, orderly environment with moderate stimuli, recreational and occupational therapy, and techniques to preserve orientation is recommended. Many victims of organic brain syndrome also suffer from depression and additional psychological and physical problems. If these "excess disabilities" are minimized through proper treatment, many older people can show gains in daily behavior, even if their underlying physiological condition is not improved. Group psychotherapy has been found to be beneficial for both patients and family members (Weinberg, 1976).

In contrast to chronic brain syndrome, acute brain syndrome may occur at any age, brought on by an external event, illness/infections, systemic poisoning such as drug reactions, or malnutrition. Careful assessment is essential because the confusion, disorientation, and memory lapses are comparable to those with chronic brain syndrome, but acute brain syndrome is treatable.

An estimated 15 percent of patients with organic brain syndrome are considered to have the acute form and therefore to have readily reversible conditions (Rosenfeld, 1978, p. 137). Both reversible and irreversible brain disorders may occur in the same person, making the problem of treatment and diagnosis even more difficult. If a reversible brain syndrome is assumed by the practitioner to be a chronic brain disorder, the elderly patient is apt to be institutionalized without active treatment and without hope of discharge.

Mental Health Needs of Women, Minorities, and the Frail Elderly

The incidence and consequences of mental health problems tend to vary by sex, ethnicity, and age. Currently, there are approximately 146 older women for every 100 older men, with women over age sixty-five the fastest growing segment of the U.S. population. Older women are more likely than older men to be poor, to live alone, to be socially isolated, and to have chronic health problems. They are likely to be culturally denigrated and to incorporate the negative cultural view of themselves. Depression, alcoholism, and drug misuse are more common among older women than among older men. Therapeutic modalities used with younger women, such as psychotherapy and certain behavior modification approaches, often have not been adequately tested for their effectiveness with older women

(Rathbone-McCuan and Hart, 1979). In general, comparatively little research has been conducted on older women's mental health needs because gerontological research often does not separate out gender and gerontologists have only recently addressed the needs of older women.

Even less is known about the mental health needs of minority elderly, whose position is one of triple jeopardy—old, poor, and minority. It is known that minority elderly are more likely to live in poverty and to have more chronic health problems than white elderly; the resultant role losses suggest that minority elderly would be extremely vulnerable to functional disorders. In addition, minority elderly undoubtedly face greater barriers to obtaining services. Butler and Lewis (1977) describe how racial prejudice and discrimination affect both the quality and the amount of mental health care available to minority elderly. Often such discrimination is not deliberate, but results from the fact that the majority of mental health program staff have only a limited understanding of and experience with the culture, life experiences, and needs of elderly minorities. Others have noted that for minority elderly, the problem is not overinstitutionalization, but underinstitutionalization or inappropriate institutionalization (Gelfand, 1979–1980; Schafft, 1979).

The likelihood of minority elderly being adequately served by both community-based services and institutions apparently depends on the presence of minority staff, the physical accessibility of the services to minority communities, and the attitudes and cultural sensitivity of staff toward minorities. In outreach efforts to minority aged, assessments of mental health status that are responsive to variations in ethnic culture need to be developed, staff must be trained to be culturally sensitive, and members of minority communities should be involved in the formulation and delivery of new mental health services.

The population over age seventy-five, or the frail elderly, presents a major challenge to the mental health system to develop appropriate support systems. Although more likely to be institutionalized, a large percentage of frail elderly attempt to remain in the community, often cared for by children or other relatives who are in their sixties and among the young-old. Their needs are complex and long-term, often requiring multiple health and social services. The emotional aspects of their chronic illnesses may be as debilitating as their actual physical impairments. The incidence of chronic brain syndrome and depression is likely to be higher among the frail elderly than among the young-old.

A mental health problem until recently identified among the frail elderly is that of familial abuse and neglect. Women over age seventy-five who are dependent upon family care givers are especially vulnerable to neglect or abuse. Abuse includes the deliberate infliction of physical harm as well as physically endangering neglect. Abusers tend to be husbands and adult children, more often daughters.

Three major hypotheses have been advanced to explain the occurrence of abuse: that abuse is the historical and normative behavior for family members; that the care giver is suffering from mental illness, alcoholism, substance misuse, or mental retardation and therefore lacks the appropriate judgment to provide care; or that abuse is one outcome of various stresses, especially the burden of providing twenty-four-hour care to a dependent older person. Clearly, these explanations have quite different implications for interventions for the victim and family care givers. If stress on the care giver appears to be the cause, then an appropriate intervention would be to mobilize community support systems in order to reduce the care-giving burden. In cases where abuse is the norm or the result of the care giver's pathological behavior, the focus would be on removing either the abuser or victim and finding alternative living arrangements. Both interventions require that providers be aware of the possibility of abuse, develop appropriate case detection techniques and protocols, and be knowledgeable about community support resources.

Mental Health Needs by Location

In 1977, Eisdorfer examined the delivery of mental health services in the United States, with special reference to the aged. He concluded that the "drop in psychiatric inpatient care episodes in state and county hospitals was associated with a substantial increase in the total number of other types of patient care episodes" (p. 316). Further, he concluded that a clear age patterning existed. Persons under thirty-five years of age were likely to receive outpatient services; those over thirty-five were more likely to be treated in a mental hospital.

Elderly patients in state mental hospitals represent two types, which have different implications for diagnosis and prognosis and therefore for treatment. Long-term residents were admitted to a mental hospital early in life and grow old there. The recently admitted generally have developed mental illness for the first time in late life. Unfortunately, both groups have often been treated the same, even for those with reversible brain syndrome. The treatment of the aged patient in large public state hospitals raises questions about the effectiveness of regulations to ensure their right to receive active therapeutic treatment. All too often the "active therapeutic treatment" is only a variation of medication regimes or a new treatment that is standard for all age groups who are assigned to chronic care wards.

While the geriatric population in state mental hospitals has dropped by half from 1960 to 1973, in part because of the enactment of Medicaid in 1965, the chronically ill elderly population has increased substantially in nursing homes (LaVor, 1977). Because nursing home requirements under Medicaid were more flexible than provisions for patients in state mental hospitals, the growing proprietary nursing home industry could absorb many "deinstitutionalized" patients and be reimbursed by Medicaid. The states, in turn, could receive matching funds, thus easing fiscal problems. Many older people with mental disorders are admitted to nursing homes without any contact with the mental health system and without adequate assessment of their mental health needs. In addition, the majority of nursing homes are ill equipped to care for or treat the elderly mentally ill patient. It has been estimated that up to 30 percent of those occupying nursing home beds are psychiatric patients; in addition, such care is expensive (Eisdorfer, 1977, p. 316). As Weinberg (1976, p. 17) notes, "To transfer a person from a state hospital to a nursing home is not to deinstitutionalize him, but merely to transfer him from one kind of institution to another." In fact, the custodial atmosphere of some nursing homes may be more restrictive of personal freedoms than some state hospitals. In addition, people with severe organic mental impairments are likely to experience decline or death after being moved to a nursing home (Rathbone-McCuan and Hart, 1979).

Despite the passage of Public Law 94–63, mandating the provision of services to the elderly, community mental health centers have not adequately addressed the service gaps created by deinstitutionalization. In part, this results from the tendency of mental health centers to focus on persons who actually seek help from the center, rather than to reach others in the community through consultation, education, or primary prevention services. Another barrier is the elderly's sense of self-reliance and their reluctance to perceive themselves as having "psychological problems" that require help (Patterson, 1976).

A number of other barriers prevent the elderly from effectively utilizing community mental health centers. One has been the professional staff's attitude toward older people and their limited knowledge of the aging process. Many mental health practitioners have viewed older people as depressing and unsatisfying to work with, as unworthy of the investment of their effort, and as unlikely to change. The impact of Freudian treatment orientations upon attitudes toward working with the elderly has been extensive (Butler and Lewis, 1977). Little effort has been made to adapt therapies used with younger adults to be appropriate for older populations. For example, Rathbone-McCuan and Hart (1979) documented the use of socialization group programming and chemical therapy for older women, rather than task-centered and behavioral therapies, which tended to be used with younger women. Therapists may also experience countertransference with an elderly patient, evoking their own unresolved conflicts with their parents or their own fear of death (Butler and Lewis, 1977). In a 1975 survey of psychiatrists, only 2 percent of their patients were sixty to sixty-four years of age and 2 percent were over sixty-five years (Weinberg, 1976, p. 18). As Butler remarked, "Psychiatrists have tended to avoid the elderly like a plague" (Butler, 1975, p. 234).

Theories of Aging

In addition to these institutional, fiscal, and attitudinal barriers to the development of comprehensive mental health programs for older persons, various theories of aging have influenced the design of social and health services and the formulation of specific clinical interventions. These theories are disengagement, activity, subcultural, developmental, and exchange.

The geriatric mental health practitioner needs to assess the extent to which different theories influence his or her interventions. Whether one believes that aging is a withdrawal from active participation (disengagement theory), that activity is essential to successful aging (activity theory), that how one ages depends upon lifetime habits of coping (developmental theory), or that environmental supports are necessary to compensate for diminished exchange resources (exchange theory) clearly affects the ways in which mental health professionals relate to an older person and the kinds of interventions they are likely to use.

Disengagement theory, the most controversial, has perhaps had the most negative effects in terms of segregating service systems for the elderly (Cumming and Henry, 1961). Reflecting the commonsense observation that older people are more subject to ill health and the probability of death than their younger counterparts, Cumming and Henry asserted that a process of mutual withdrawal normally occurs in order to ensure both an optimum level of personal gratification and an uninterrupted continuation of the social system. For example, older people move out of social roles in order to make room for younger persons, to maintain a balance between their own reduced energies and demands, and to conserve their emotional resources in order to prepare for death. The assumption that disengagement is universal, inevitable, and functional for both the older person and society has been widely criticized.

In contrast, activity theory presumes that activities must take place to offset the losses of old age, preserve morale, and sustain self-concepts. People are assumed to remain socially and psychologically fit by keeping active (Havighurst and Albrecht, 1953). Accordingly, services should be developed specifically for old people, such as golden age club activities and other age-segregated leisure pursuits. A limitation of activity theory is that little attention has been directed to the differences between types of activities on an individual's ability to exert any significant control over either the roles themselves or the performance of those roles. Accordingly, activity theory has received only limited empirical support and has been criticized as an oversimplification.

In contrast to the assumption of activity theory that people continue to adhere to middle-aged standards as they age, the subcultural perspective asserts the development of a distinctive aged subculture (Rose, 1965). Individual involvement in an aged subculture depends on the solidarity of the age group itself, plus the nature and extent of contacts retained with the total society through families, the media, employment, or the older person's own resistance to aging. Disagreement surrounds the question whether an aged subculture will evolve to the point where older people become a voting bloc; it is agreed, however, that a strong relationship exists between peer group participation rates and the adjustment process of the elderly (Hochschild, 1973; Rosow, 1967).

The developmental perspective of aging conceives of personality as continually evolving, with adjustments at each successive stage reflecting earlier coping strategies as well as the matrix of current environmental factors. To meet the tasks of living, people develop distinctive behavioral and psychological responses, which those with whom they interact come to identify as their personality (Havighurst, 1968). Most developmental psychologists also see a gradual turning inward over the life course, with older people being less attentive to external events and more attuned to their own inner states.

Exchange theory, applied to aging, provides an especially useful perspective (Dowd, 1980; Martin, 1971). Exchange theory, similar to activity or disengagement theory, predicts decreasing participation with age in major social institutions. The basis of this prediction, however, is qualitatively distinct from these other theoretical approaches. According to exchange theory, differential possession of and access to the resources necessary for equitable social exchange strongly influence the elderly's participation in all social institutions. The elderly are systematically deprived of valued resources and of access to acquiring new resources needed for favorable social exchanges because of societal conditions, not through any responsibility of their own. For example, a mandatory retirement policy deprives older workers of material resources, relational and personal characteristic resources (for example, the opportunity to develop friendships among co-workers), and resources based on authority. Compliance is often the only commodity older people have to bargain with in the marketplace in order to win acceptance and support from others (Blau, 1973).

We find an exchange theory perspective to be useful. Currently, a large segment of the public perceives the costs of maintaining older people as independently as possible as outweighing the benefits or contributions. If mental health programs were developed to strengthen the older person's resources for self-maintenance and to enable continuing community contributions, this perception would perhaps be changed to reflect the value of roles by older people in our society. Mental health program managers need to examine the extent to which their agency's programs and policies may unwittingly aid in diminishing the older person's resources for social exchange. The focus thus becomes one of empowering older people and developing their resources to create opportunities for balanced exchange relationships.

Types of Geriatric Mental Health Programs

The mental health program managers and staff have numerous factors to consider in planning to implement or expand a program for older persons. The range of mental health problems among older persons suggests the need for a multifaceted, multidisciplinary program strategy. At least three basic approaches are called for in a comprehensive community mental health program for older persons:

1. *Direct therapeutic services* to provide counseling and therapy for individuals and groups with mental health problems.
2. *Education and prevention activities* among older persons and service providers, for example, classes, seminars, media presentations, and so forth, about existing and potential mental health problems and methods for preventing, recognizing, and treating them.
3. *Consultation and training* with both service providers and natural helpers to recognize and deal with mental health problems among clients.

Direct Therapeutic Services

Provision of direct therapeutic services is the most frequent approach to older people's mental health needs. A comprehensive assessment is critical and should include an evaluation of the emotional, cultural, and socioeconomic factors affecting older people, their nutritional habits, their use of medications and alcohol, and circumstances surrounding the onset of their symptoms, their patterns of medical care, and their social networks.

Most models for direct service delivery have been group treatment approaches within institutional settings (Feil, 1967; Finkel and Fillmore, 1971; Saul and Saul, 1974; Steury and Blank, 1978). Such groups generally serve as a socializing agent, as a medium of staff contact, as a means of reality orientation, as a stimulus to motivation, as a provider of roles, and as a diagnostic agent. Groups within institutional settings can be classified as orientation groups, task groups, and therapy groups. At admission to an institution, groups are especially useful as a means to orient older persons and their families in adjusting to role changes. Maintaining or healing family relationships is essential at this point.

A wide range of task groups exists within most institutions. One function of task groups is to increase the residents' opportunities for self-governance. Decision-making and leadership skills cannot be fostered through purely recreational groups. Instead, decision-making structures that can influence the administration, such as resident councils, need to be developed. Opportunities for older adults to be centrally involved in planning and carrying out their own recreational activities should exist, rather than only having programs "presented" to them.

Remotivation therapy, an effective therapy technique within hospital and nursing home settings, was developed in the 1950s for nursing personnel in state mental hospitals. A series of fifty-minute sessions provide for group interactions in five steps: a climate of acceptance, a bridge to reality (for example, reading poetry or introducing current events), sharing the world we live in through reinforcement of appropriate responses to the topic discussed, appreciation of the work of the world through linking the topic discussed to past interests outside the institution, and a climate of appreciation in which patients are reinforced (Toepfer, Bicknell, and Shaw, 1974). Schoolchildren can be effective remotivation therapists (Butler and Lewis, 1977). Goals for such therapy might be motivation to live; improvement of communication skills, of self-awareness, of social skills and social identity, and of self-control; and development of a sense of camaraderie and identity within the setting.

Reality orientation is effective in preventing, halting, or reversing disorientation and memory loss in confused patients. Reminiscence, or life review, can help the elderly revitalize a past sense of self-esteem, reinforce a sense of identity, and allay anxieties associated with signs of decline. The life review can reintegrate the personality, give new meaning to one's life, and help mitigate one's fears of death. But constructive outcomes of the life review are not inevitable. The reviewer may experience depression, panic, guilt, and constant obsessional rumination (Butler and Lewis, 1977). The treatment goal should be to help the older patient make appropriate use of reminiscence. Both the amount and content of reminiscing provide important diagnostic clues about the client's self-image, the amount of stress experienced, and the types of relationships desired.

Education and Prevention

Although many of these treatment techniques are effective, the mental health professional's task has broadened beyond the provision of therapy to include the mobilization of community resources for the benefit of its members (President's Commission on Mental Health, 1978). Such efforts recognize that linkages between informal community resources and the formal mental health service system can therapeutically benefit clients.

Accordingly, a promising area for education and for prevention of mental health problems among the elderly is the mobilization of social networks or the informal social supports of family, friends, neighbors, peers, and local community organizations. A variety of economic, social, or emotional services and information may be exchanged along the linkages of informal personal networks. In contrast to traditional social service delivery systems, exchanges among informal social networks are not formalized, but utilize people's caring about each other and their natural helping tendencies to respond to daily needs, ranging from household chores to crises such as sickness or hospitalization.

The value of network building to promote mental and physical well-being has been demonstrated for other age groupings. For example, the outcome of an individual's response during difficult times is influenced not only by the degree of stress and the individual's ego strength, but also by the quality of emotional support provided by the natural network (Caplan and Killilea, 1976). The absence of social supports can increase one's susceptibility to disease (Cassell, 1976). Gerontologists have long emphasized the importance of emotional support for relatives, friends, and neighbors for older people's well-being. Indeed, current budget reductions point to the necessity of better utilizing informal community resources for the elderly.

Several programs around the country have begun to strengthen and/or build social networks as an intervention to promote the elderly's physical and mental well-being. These interventions can be categorized as personal network building, volunteer linking, mutual aid network, neighborhood helpers, and community empowerment (Froland, Pancoast, Chapman, and Dimboku, 1979); all of them involve a collaborative effort between formal agencies and informal supports.

Personal network building seeks to strengthen the existing ties among the network of an individual in need, often by utilizing natural helpers (for example, friends, neighbors, relatives, peers with similar problems, postal workers, grocery clerks, public utilities workers, apartment house managers, and local merchants). These helpers can provide the following kinds of social support: emotionally sustaining help, such as contact with a trusted party during stressful periods; problem-solving behavior, such as providing new information or direct assistance; indirect forms of assistance, such as simple availability and listening; and advocacy. Older people may be more likely to turn to these natural networks for information and skills because they are more accessible and more likely to be trusted than the formal service delivery system.

A community mental health approach based on identifying and strengthening natural networks would involve expanding or mobilizing the skills and resources of the social network, which the older person does not yet view as supportive. Helping networks need to be created where they do not exist. For example, in an effort to reach isolated elderly, the community mental health center staff in Spokane, Washington, trains fuel oil dealers, meter readers, fire department staff, taxi drivers, and postal carriers to watch for situations and symptoms that indicate the frail elderly's needs for mental health services (*Information and Assistance . . .* , 1980).

Another approach recognizes the importance of healthy family ties, particularly because families provide 80 percent of the in-home care, often without support or respite for their care-giving efforts. The Natural Support Program, sponsored by the Community Service Society in New York City (Mellor and Getzel, 1980), the Family/Friends Support Project of the Ebenezer Society in Minneapolis (Gray and others, 1980), and the multigenerational family project, As Parents Grow Older, developed through Child and Family Services in Ann Arbor, Michigan (Silverman, Brache, and Zelinski, 1981), provide counseling, information, skills training, and mutual aid both to the older person and to family members. When family members are better prepared to provide care and therefore experience less stress, the improved care-giving relationship is assumed to benefit the mental and physical well-being of the older family member.

Volunteer linking seeks to develop a new or enhanced support system for the individual. For example, through Oregon's Northeast Salem Community Association (NESCA), volunteers from local churches develop familylike networks for chronically mentally ill persons (*Networks for Helping . . .* , 1978). Peer counseling and support systems, such as through the Turner Geriatric Clinic in Ann Arbor, Michigan, have involved older volunteers in the provision of mental health services, including health education about topics such as memory problems, stress, and nutrition. Peers provide individual counseling, the organization of small support groups, and referral and information services in a rural area (Select Committee on Aging, 1979). At the Nebraska Center for Aging, trained peer counselors facilitate assertiveness and problem solving in their clients. A variety of outreach programs have utilized elderly neighbors to go into homes to assess problems visually (Toseland, Decker, and Bliesner, 1979). For example, in Iowa's Project Be-My-Guest, women from local churches reach out to friends, neighbors, and relatives and accompany them to agencies to explain available services (Select Committee on Aging, 1979). A review of peer counselor and outreach programs concluded that such efforts provide group support and expanded opportunities for leadership roles (Campbell and Chenoweth, 1980).

When peer counselors are utilized, direct staff involvement in service delivery is often decreased, and the role of staff members as educators, consultants, and trainers to the peer counselors is emphasized. Because such a redefinition of professional roles and responsibility may be difficult for some staff members, time needs to be allocated to developing an effective working partnership between professional staff and older volunteers.

A third approach aims to create or promote supportive capacities within *mutual help groups*. Such groups engage in joint problem solving and emphasize reciprocity in their exchange of resources. Examples include Widows to Widows Information and Support services, which are in many cities, and the Benton Mutual Help Model, which was implemented in a rural area. Data gathered on the Benton model indicate that participants experienced increased friendship and helping relationships and reinforcement of social roles with a community orientation. Participants stated that the mutual help groups' major benefits were reduction of loneliness and increase in psychological supports (Ehrlich, 1979).

The focus on *neighborhood helpers* attempts to strengthen existing self-help in a given neighborhood locality. The Senior Block Information Service in San Francisco uses social networks to develop low-income elderly's leadership and self-help capacities. Elderly volunteers, delivering a monthly newsletter, are regularly in contact with other elderly residents, linking them to resources and strengthening their problem-solving skills (Ruffini and Todd, 1979).

A neighborhood care program has been proposed to strengthen natural helping through respite care, neighborhood aides, neighborhood elder-sitting pools, and a neighborhood block home as a place where elderly neighbors could turn for assistance. Neighborhood aides could routinely canvass the neighborhood, report problems, visit homebound elderly, and provide a link to community services (O'Brien and Whitelaw, 1978).

Under a *community empowerment* approach, the formal agency helps to build the community's capacity for problem solving and for action. A mental health outreach program that empowered an inner-city community is the Neighborhood Family in Miami, Florida. This model assumes that older people in the community can work together as a family to alter stressful personal and environmental conditions and can benefit emotionally from the familylike interactions. The Neighborhood Family was initiated by a staff gerontologist at the Jackson Memorial Hospital, Community Mental Health Services. Rather than establish a clinical outpatient program, the one staff person started with older people in a target area, who defined the problems and services and requested psychiatric assistance for approximately 15 percent of the membership. The staff person chose to work alone in order to reinforce the necessity for every elderly member's participation in decision-making roles. When staff were later added to the consumer-based and community-administered body, they functioned as members of the "family," not apart from it as "staff" (Ross, 1980).

Such education and prevention approaches require staff with both teaching and community organization skills. A mental health agency itself cannot possibly provide individual or even small-group attention to the majority of older persons in the community. Agency staff must generate enthusiasm for the concepts, information, and skills they wish to share, must mobilize already existing community resources to provide a vehicle for education and prevention activities, and must communicate effectively with persons who lack knowledge of the mental health system and experience with treatment of mental illness.

Consultation and Training

A consultation and training approach utilizes many of the skills identified in the description of education and training. The goals, however, may differ. As a consultant, the staff person's role is to share expertise and knowledge in a way that enhances the consultee's ability to solve problems and deliver services to older persons. This may, for example, utilize teaching and training in clinical skills, community organization, needs assessment, and resource mobilization. For example, service providers and caretakers for older persons need to be familiarized with mental health concerns, to develop skills in recognizing and managing mental health problems in their client population, and to utilize available community resources. Outreach for consultation can be directed toward a variety of settings, including residential care facilities, social services, and recreational facilities such as senior centers and nutrition sites, and toward providers of specific services such as home chore agencies and legal aid organizations.

Because accurate information about the prevention, incidence, and treatment of mental health problems of older persons is lacking among service providers, the mental health agency offering consultation and training has numerous choices about where to focus its efforts. One community agency, the Southeast/ Mission Geriatric Service, has included residential long-term care facilities, congregate meal sites, senior centers, public health departments, home health agencies, and acute and convalescent care hospitals in its ongoing educational assistance consultation program (Ruffini and Urquhart, 1979–1980).

Depending upon the mental health agency's resources, the consultation and training program might focus sequentially on various components of the service provider community. For example, beginning with those already engaged in delivery of services to older persons in residential care settings, the mental health agency could provide intensive training to professional staff in the identification and appropriate management of common mental health problems. Subsequently, the mental health agency staff, acting in a consultative role, could support the residential facility professional staff to deliver in-service training to paraprofessional staff involved in client care on a day-to-day basis. After appropriate staff members have been familiarized with basic information, the mental health agency staff person could participate directly as a consultant in monthly case conferences with service providers or could provide ongoing consultation as needed to the staff person chairing these sessions. This model is developmental in nature, requiring the allocation of more resources in the initial stages, with an emphasis on the mental health agency staff as trainers, and evolving toward mental health agency staff as consultants.

Another model focuses on consulting with the providers within the natural helping network. These providers are not likely to be "professionally trained" in helping; yet they face many of the same challenges professionals encounter, and perhaps an even broader range of problems because they are in the neighborhood. The consultant thus works to assist the natural helper to deal effectively with a range of problems with minimum professional assistance (Collins and Pancoast, 1976).

All the approaches and strategies discussed rely to some extent on the use of a network of services for the aged. The Older Americans Act of 1965, as amended (OAA), initially created this network, which largely consists of organizations funded and managed, at least in part, through local Area Agencies on Aging (AAA). The AAA is responsible for planning, pooling, and coordinating local resources to create a comprehensive service system for the elderly. The AAA always administers funds for programs supported by the Older Americans Act and often has responsibility for allocating funds from other public and private sources, such as United Way or federal revenue sharing.

The aging network includes many direct service programs, such as nutrition, transportation, social services, and recreation. Agencies receiving these funds range from public senior centers sponsored by municipal recreation departments, to private, for-profit home health care agencies, to demonstration projects operated by hospitals and universities. Also included in this part of the aging network are agencies and groups that do not receive direct support for OAA funds, but nonetheless do provide direct services to older persons, such as private charitable organizations, city-funded programs, and advocacy groups. For example, groups such as the Silver-Haired Legislature of Georgia and the Senior Lobby in Washington have joined the network to influence legislation relevant to older persons.

Ways to utilize effectively the members of the aging network in developing a mix of direct services, consultation, and education/prevention can be illustrated by the case of a community mental health center that lacks a formalized geriatric program. In many centers where existing resources appear fully utilized for other population groupings, it is commonplace that one staff person sees most of the small number of elderly clients. Although generally lacking geriatric specialization, such staff members would often be interested in undertaking additional responsibilities in geriatric mental health. In such cases, the mental health agency's options for program development are numerous. Setting priorities among program delivery possibilities and sequencing their development present a major challenge. Some major issues in making these decisions include:

1. The overall mental health agency program plan and how any geriatric component fits into that plan.
2. The mental health agency's immediate and future goals for a geriatric program.
3. Staff readiness (expertise) and receptivity to the geriatric program.
4. Resources available, including informal social supports.
5. Whether to serve primarily the visible frail elderly or the more isolated frail elderly, who are the most difficult to reach and potentially require the most intensive treatment.
6. The mixture of direct and indirect mental health services to be delivered (for example, consultation with other service providers and institutions, interinstitutional case consultation involving staff from various sites).

In order to plan for maximum effectiveness, several kinds of information are essential. First, the manager must be aware of the composition of the older population in the catchment area—their numbers, their general economic situation, their general health status, the nature of special population clusters (such as the presence of non-English-speaking elderly). The area agency's information and assistance specialist can help in providing this information. Second, knowing the nature of existing programs and resources allows for developing services without duplication, identifies potential providers of in-service training, and allows coordination of mental health services with related systems. Such information, which is essential in determining the mix of direct and indirect services, is also generally available from the local area agency. Third, understanding the range of treatment modalities and service delivery strategies effective with this group will reduce the risk of poor service utilization and reduced treatment outcomes.

Outreach activities could be the place for the community mental health center to begin a program for expanding its services to older persons. Outreach activities, of course, are diverse, and include home visits to individual clients who are experiencing a mental illness and need inpatient treatment, identification of high-risk individuals and groups who could utilize educational, prevention-oriented seminars provided in natural gathering places, and relationship-building efforts with service providers who will be a source of referral.

Choosing to emphasize outreach immediately takes the community mental health center away from its institutional home, moving activities into the community, increasing the center's visibility, and establishing an expectation that services will be delivered to some extent in the community. If staff resources are scarce, and if professional staff members are committed to one-to-one and small-group therapy as the primary treatment modality, then the disadvantages of a strong geriatric outreach program may outweigh the advantages.

Under ideal conditions, as more older people are identified and receive services, a base would be built for advocating for additional resources for mental health. If this ideal does not materialize, however, program managers would nonetheless have the experiential data base to make informed judgments about the viability of geriatric mental health programs in their particular catchment areas.

Table 1 suggests how the experience and expertise of the aging network members might be used to provide needed resources for different aspects of a community mental health center program. Where sufficient resources are not available from members of the aging network, the program manager may explore the following: reimbursement from agencies served by consultants, sliding scale fees for service to older people and their families, and providing services through the corporate sector. When resources are diverted from other established activities, the rationale for any policy and program changes must be clearly communicated to staff, consumers, and the general public.

Conclusion

The challenge to mental health agencies to develop, deliver, and maintain services to older persons is clear. A significant problem exists, in terms of both the

Table 1. Problems Addressed by Aging Network Resources.

Presenting or Potential Problem	Intervention Method	Linkage Organization	Aging Network Resource
Lack of contact with reality (client) Patient management (provider)	Remotivation therapy (client) Staff training (provider)	AAA	Access to facilities with receptive clients and staff
Depression	Individual group counseling	AAA-funded home repair program Meals on wheels	Referrals Referrals
Chronic brain syndrome/acute brain syndrome	Management and/or detection and/or treatment	Congregate-living setting; over 60 community health clinics	Staff to be trained; referrals
Outreach to isolated	Training peer counselors, outreach workers	Retired Senior Volunteer Program Senior Center	Ongoing program support Volunteers facilities
Inadequate preparation for transitions (for example, wife to widow)	Educational group (prebereavement; widow's group)	Nutrition site Senior Center Legal Services	Population facility Cofacilitator from staff Referrals
Lack of community mental health center familiarity with local resources for older persons	Community mental health center staff in-service training	AAA/State Unit on Aging	Trainer

numbers of older persons affected or likely to be affected by mental health problems and the severity of the problems experienced, ranging from the highest suicide rate of any age group to severe depression accompanied by or manifested by decreasing physical and mental competence. As the numbers of the old-old in the population grow absolutely and proportionally, this challenge will increase as well. How can the mental health agency assist the community to meet the older person's mental health needs without reinforcing the stereotyping of this same population as sick, servile, and feeble? The manager and agency staff need to plan and develop programs based in the community, utilizing wherever possible the natural resources available, such as older persons as peer counselors, neighborhood self-help and mutual aid groups, and families as sources of support. The manager must encourage recognition of the mental health needs of older persons and a respect for mental health services—therapeutic, preventive, and consultative—in both the professional community and the general public. The mental health agency can build, step by step, activity by activity, a geriatric mental health program that is responsive to community needs, cognizant of using available resources maximally, and long lasting with the support of the community it serves.

The program manager has a vital, though not always visible, role in providing mental health services to older persons. The manager must create and maintain an appropriate place for a geriatric component within the larger organization. This requires knowledge of the mental health needs of older persons and possibilities for addressing them, as well as awareness of and sensitivity to the agency staff's prior and continuing commitments to other population groups. With limited resources, the manager must help to shape a program that serves those whose needs may not be most visible, for which there may be little popular support, and for which financial support may be difficult to obtain. The manager is thus challenged to be creative, aware of the options, flexible in responding to both staff and community interests and skills, and realistic in building a program and delivering services that maximize the ability of the commmunity for its members to enhance mental health, prevent mental illness, and meet the needs of those in crisis.

References

"As Lives Are Extended, Some People Wonder If It's Really a Blessing." *Wall Street Journal*, October 25, 1979.

Birren, J. E. *The Psychology of Aging*. Englewood Cliffs, N.J.: Prentice-Hall, 1964.

Blau, Z. S. *Old Age in a Changing Society*. New York: New Viewpoints, 1973.

Busse, E. "The Clinical Challenge of the Elderly: Some Areas of Concern and Special Interest." *Issues in Mental Health Services*. Rockville, Md.: National Institute of Mental Health, 1976.

Butler, R. N. *Why Survive: Being Old in America*. New York: Harper & Row, 1975.

Butler, R. M., and Lewis, M. *Aging and Mental Health*. (2nd ed.) St. Louis, Mo.: Mosby, 1977.

Campbell, R., and Chenoweth, B. "Peer Support System." Paper presented at the 33rd Annual Meeting of the Gerontological Society, San Diego, Calif., November 1980.

Caplan, G., and Killilea, M. *Support Systems and Mutual Help*. New York: Grune & Stratton, 1976.

Cassell, J. "The Contribution of the Social Environment to Host Resistance." *American Journal of Epidemiology*, 1976, *104* (21), 107–123.

Collins, A. H., and Pancoast, D. C. *Natural Helping Networks: A Strategy for Prevention*. New York: National Association of Social Workers, 1976.

Cumming, E., and Henry, W. E. *Growing Old: The Process of Disengagement*. New York: Basic Books, 1961.

Dowd, J. "Aging as Exchange: A Preface to Theory." *Journal of Gerontology*, 1975, *30*, 584–599.

Dowd, J. *Stratification Among the Aged*. Monterey, Calif.: Brooks/Cole, 1980.

Ehrlich, P. *Mutual Help for Community Elderly: Mutual Help Model*. Carbondale: Southern Illinois University Press, 1979.

Eisdorfer, C. "Evaluation of the Quality of Psychiatric Care for the Aged." *American Journal of Psychiatry*, 1977, *134*, 315–317.

Feil, N. "Group Therapy in a Home for the Aged." *Gerontologist*, 1967, *7*, 192–195.

Finkel, S., and Fillmore, W. "Experience with an Older Adult Group at a Private Psychiatric Hospital." *Journal of Geriatric Psychiatry*, 1971, *4* (2), 188–199.

Froland, C., Pancoast, D., Chapman, N., and Dimboku, P. "Professional Partnerships with Informal Helpers: Emerging Forms." Paper presented at the Annual Convention of the American Psychological Association, New York City, September 1979.

Gelfand, D. "Ethnicity, Aging, and Mental Health." *International Journal of Aging and Human Development*, 1979–1980, *10* (3), 289–298.

Glassman, M. "Misdiagnosis of Senile Dementia: Denial of Care to the Elderly." *Social Work*, 1980, *25* (4), 288–292.

Gray, K., and others. "Reimbursing Family/Friends for Home Care: A Demonstration Project." Paper presented at the 33rd Annual Meeting of the Gerontological Society, San Diego, Calif., November 1980.

Havighurst, R. J. "A Social-Psychological Perspective on Aging." *Gerontologist*, 1968, *8* (2), 67–71.

Havighurst, R. J., and Albrecht, R. *Older People*. New York: Longman, 1953.

Hochschild, A. R. *The Unexpected Community*. Englewood Cliffs, N.J.: Prentice-Hall, 1973.

Information and Assistance Program, Elderly Services. Spokane, Wash.: Spokane Community Mental Health Center, December 1980.

LaVor, J. *Long-Term Care: A Challenge to Service Systems*. Washington, D.C.: U.S. Department of Health, Education, and Welfare, 1977.

Lowy, L. *Social Work with the Aging*. New York: Harper & Row, 1979.

Martin, G. "Power, Dependence and the Complaints of the Elderly: A Social Exchange Perspective." *Aging and Human Development*, 1971, *2* (2), 108–112.

Mellor, J., and Getzel, G. "Stress and Service Needs of Those Who Care for the Aged." Paper presented at the 33rd Annual Meeting of the Gerontological Society, San Diego, Calif., November 1980.

National Institute of Mental Health. *Issues in Mental Health and Aging*. Vols. 1–3. Rockville, Md.: National Institute of Mental Health, 1976.

National Institute on Alcohol and Alcohol Abuse. *The Elderly: A Study of Legal Drug Use by Older Americans*. Services Research Monograph Series. Washington, D.C.: U.S. Department of Health, Education, and Welfare, 1979.

Networks for Helping: Illustrations from Research and Practice. Proceedings of the Conference on Networks, Portland State University, Portland, Ore., November 1978.

O'Brien, J., and Whitelaw, N. *Planning Options for the Elderly*. Portland, Ore.: Institute on Aging, Portland State University, 1978.

Patterson, R. "Community Mental Health Centers: A Survey of Services for the Elderly." In National Institute of Mental Health, *Issues in Mental Health and Aging*. Vol. 3: *Services*. Bethesda, Md.: National Institute of Mental Health, 1976.

President's Commission on Mental Health. *Report to the President from the President's Commission on Mental Health.* Washington, D.C.: U.S. Government Printing Office, 1978.

Rathbone-McCuan, E., and Hart, V. "Therapeutic Neglect of Older Women in Mental Health Services." Paper presented at the 33rd Annual Meeting of the Gerontological Association, Washington, D.C., November 1979.

Rathbone-McCuan, E., and Roberds, L. "Treatment of the Older Female Alcoholic." Paper presented at the 26th Annual Meeting of the Western Gerontological Society, Anaheim, Calif., 1980.

Rose, A. M. "The Subculture of the Aging: A Framework in Social Gerontology." In A. M. Rose and W. A. Peterson (Eds.), *Older People: Their Social World.* Philadelphia: Davis, 1965.

Rosenfeld, A. *New Views on Older Lives: A Sampler of NIMH-Sponsored Research and Service Programs.* Bethesda, Md.: National Institute of Mental Health, 1978.

Rosow, I. *Social Integration of the Aged.* New York: Free Press, 1967.

Ross, H. *How to Develop a Neighborhood Family: An Action Manual.* Miami, Fla.: University of Miami, 1980.

Ruffini, J., and Todd, H. F., Jr. "A Network Model for Leadership Development Among the Elderly," *Gerontologist,* 1979, *2* (19), 158-162.

Ruffini, J., and Urquhart, P. "A Comprehensive Geriatric Mental Health Service in San Francisco." *International Journal of Mental Health,* 1979-1980, *8* (3-4), 101-116.

Saul, S., and Saul, S. "Group Psychotherapy in a Proprietary Nursing Home." *Gerontologist,* 1974, *14* (5), 446-450.

Schafft, G. "Nursing Homes and the Black Elderly." Paper presented at the Annual Meeting of the Gerontological Society, Washington, D.C., November 1979.

Schuckit, M. "Geriatric Alcoholism and Drug Abuse." *Gerontologist,* 1977, *17* (2), 168-174.

Schuckit, M. "Alcoholism and the Elderly." *Advances in Alcoholism,* 1980, *16,* 1-3.

Schuckit, M., and Morrissey, E. "Drug Abuse Among Alcoholic Older Women." *American Journal of Psychiatry,* 1979, *136* (4B), 607-610.

Select Committee on Aging. *Innovative Developments in Aging: Area Agencies on Aging.* Washington, D.C.: U.S. House of Representatives, 1979.

Silverman, A., Brache, C., and Zelinski, C. *As Parents Grow Older: A Manual for Program Replication.* Ann Arbor: Institute of Gerontology, University of Michigan, 1981.

Steury, S., and Blank, M. *Readings in Psychotherapy with Older People.* Rockville, Md.: National Institute of Mental Health, 1978.

Toepfer, C., Bicknell, A., and Shaw, D. "Remotivation as Behavior Therapy." *Gerontologist,* 1974, *14* (5), 451-453.

Toseland, R., Decker, J., and Bliesner, J. "A Community Outreach Program for

Socially Isolated Older Persons." *Journal of Gerontological Social Work*, 1979, *1* (3), 211–225.

Weinberg, J. "Community Programs for the Elderly: Alternatives to Institutionalization." In National Institute of Mental Health, *Issues in Mental Health and Aging.* Vol. 3: *Services.* Rockville, Md.: National Institute of Mental Health, 1976.

☙ 29 ❧

Child and Adolescent
Mental Health Services

Peter J. Pecora
Maureen A. Conroyd

*Planning and managing children's mental health services requires an under-
standing of diagnostic assessment and treatment planning, along with skills
in program coordination and communication involving parents, the
schools, and collateral contacts. These issues and skills can be understood in
terms of a continuum of services that includes prevention, outpatient services, day treatment, crisis or runaway shelters, group homes, and inpatient
psychiatric services. This chapter highlights the critical administrative
issues managers face in delivering mental health services to children in a
variety of settings and in responding to the problems of financial constraints, staff training, program coordination, and service accountability.*

- There are approximately 72.4 million children, age eighteen and under, in the
  United States (U.S. Bureau of the Census, U.S. Department of Commerce,
  1981).
- From 5 to 15 percent of children from the ages of three to fifteen experience
  persistent and socially handicapping mental health problems (President's
  Commission on Mental Health, 1978; Robins, 1978).
- Based on a 5 percent prevalence estimate, nearly 3.6 million children in the
  United States experience significant mental health problems.
- In 1975, only 655,000 children under the age of eighteen were admitted to
  mental health facilities (Calhoun, Grotberg, and Rackley, 1980).

Note: We wish to acknowledge the assistance of Marion Cassafer and our colleagues who provide children's mental health services in King County, Seattle, Washington. Special appreciation is
extended to Young Soon Lukoff, M.D., child psychiatrist; Patrick Burke, M.D., medical director of
inpatient psychiatry unit, Children's Orthopedic Hospital; Linda Rappond, M.S.W., director of the
shelter; and Debra Tombari, M.S.W., coordinator of involuntary treatment at Fairfax Hospital.

- Of the 2,300 mental health clinics in the United States, an estimated 200 are child guidance clinics where only 40 percent of the children admitted receive any treatment, and the remaining 60 percent receive no more than a diagnosis (Goldsmith, 1977).

Clearly, the statistics indicate a need for more mental health services for children and adolescents. At the same time, there is a critical need for an increased number of mental health personnel who are specifically trained to work with children and adolescents. The gap between service need and available personnel is especially acute because of the dramatic increase in the misuse of psychoactive drugs, including alcohol, among youth and a nearly threefold increase in the suicide rate of adolescents (President's Commission on Mental Health, 1978). Despite the trend toward deinstitutionalization and community support services, there still remains a scarcity of high-quality residential and group care facilities for the treatment of autistic, psychotic, retarded, multihandicapped, violent, or suicidal children and adolescents. With the continuing shortage of funding and the increasing complexity of child and adolescent problems, the integration of existing child mental health and child welfare services is necessary in order to promote family-oriented day-treatment and home-based services (Bryce and Lloyd, 1981; Maybanks and Bryce, 1979).

Mental Health Needs and Disorders

Distinguishing the basic mental health needs of children from those needs that are culturally specific is difficult. The needs of children and adolescents are closely related to the norms and expectations of the community and environment that affect the child, the adolescent, or the young adult (Kagan, 1976). Despite this difficulty, at least four basic mental health needs of children can be identified.

Needs. Early cognitive stimulation and learning experiences using the five senses in daily living comprise one mental health need. Motor activity and stimulation are important for language development, for general cognitive skills, and for coordinating sensorimotor activities (Salasin and others, 1977). Having a stable, loving, and trusting relationship with an adult comprises a second basic need of children and adolescents. This need relates to the concept of psychological parenthood, or the continuous, stable emotional support over time of at least one parent or parent surrogate (Bowlby, 1969, 1973; Goldstein, Freud, and Solnit, 1973; Yarrow, 1964). Children need the security that comes from being reasonably safe from severe bodily or emotional harm and having a trusting relationship with an adult. Children are amazingly resilient and vary greatly in their ability to withstand hardship, but their emotional or intellectual development may be retarded or damaged if they are deprived of a stable, loving, or trusting relationship with an adult (Rutter, 1979a). As Salasin and others (1977) have noted, infants who are taught by the words, feeling states, or the behavior of caretakers that they are unwanted or a burden may develop failure-to-thrive syndrome, which can include anorexia, weight loss, and listless, withdrawn behavior.

A third mental health need involves a child's opportunities to gain a sense of competence and self-esteem. Children may lack a sense of competence and self-esteem because of inappropriate labeling, a lack of attention, or erroneous stereotyping of potential abilities because they are female, minority, or from a low-income family (Salasin and others, 1977). Opportunities to gain self-esteem help prevent the emergence of a failure syndrome that can appear in connection with rebellious or antisocial behavior designed to gain attention, power, revenge, or merely to cope with the situation.

Because of the interaction between physical well-being and mental health, the failure to meet a child's basic health care needs can be viewed as the fourth mental health need (Berlin, 1975). These basic needs include adequate health care for the mother during pregnancy, a balanced diet, adequate medical and dental care, adequate housing and clothing, and protection from physical and other hazards. Although good physical health does not guarantee adequate mental and emotional health, physical problems can lead to mental or emotional problems.

The four mental health needs of cognitive and experiential stimulation, parental emotional support and protection, opportunities to gain a sense of competence and self-esteem, and the role of physical health are all related to Bronfenbrenner's (1979, p. 60) observation that child learning and development are "facilitated by the participation of the developing person in progressively more complex patterns of reciprocal activity with someone with whom that person has developed a strong and enduring emotional attachment, and when the balance of power gradually shifts in favor of the developing person." Mental health services for children and adolescents should be designed with a conscious recognition of both mental health needs and problems, so that services can help to promote the child's total health while addressing specific intellectual, emotional, behavioral, or physical disorders.

Disorders. The term "mental disorder" related to child or adolescent dysfunctioning is taken from the *Diagnostic and Statistical Manual of Mental Disorders* (DSM III) (American Psychiatric Association, 1980, p. 6) and defined as "a clinically significant behavioral or psychological syndrome or pattern that occurs in an individual, and that is typically associated with either a painful symptom (distress) or impairment in one or more important areas of functioning (disability). In addition, there is an inference that there is a behavioral, psychological, or biological dysfunction, and that the disturbance is not only in the relationship between the individual and society." Disorders vary according to age, sex, and social circumstances. Mental health problems are more common in boys. Admission rates for boys were 65 percent higher than those for girls in outpatient services, but only 9 percent higher in inpatient services (Calhoun, Grotberg, and Rackley, 1980, p. 65). In addition, mental health problems are more frequently identified for both sexes during adolescence than during early childhood. Children living in poverty are at particularly high risk for mental health problems. Children from female-headed families are admitted to outpatient mental health facilities at four times the rate of children from two-parent families. Mental health experts believe that the difference in admission rates is because of the higher stresses associated with single parenthood. One major cause of stress is that female-headed families have median incomes less than half those of husband-wife families (Calhoun, Grotberg, and Rackley, 1980). In some cases, poverty may interact with other factors in the promotion of mental disorders. Children living in inner-city areas have higher rates than children living in small towns or rural areas (President's Commission on Mental Health, 1978).

The most common problems leading to mental disorders in children are emotional problems, behavioral problems, and impairments or delays in the development of normal functions. Generally, emotional disorders such as fears, anxiety, depression, obsessions, and hypochondriasis occur with the same frequency in boys and girls, but conduct disorders related to poor peer relationships, aggressiveness, theft, and destructiveness are significantly more prevalent among boys (President's Commission on Mental Health, 1978). Developmental mental health problems include special learning difficulties, such as reading and arithmetic disorders, and are found much more commonly in boys. These disorders, along with selected ones of the more prevalent physical disorders, are described in the next sections. Descriptions are based on definitions given in DSM III.

Behavioral Disorders

1. *Attention deficit disorder.* This disorder is characterized by signs of inappropriate inattention and impressivity, sometimes identified as Hyperkinetic Syndrome, Hyperactive Child Syndrome, Minimal Brain Damage or Dysfunction, and Minimal or Minor Cerebral Dysfunction. Excess motor activity frequently diminishes in adolescence. Attention deficit disorders are common, occurring in as many as three percent of American children twelve and under. Boys are ten times more likely to have this disorder than girls.

2. *Conduct disorders.* The essential feature of conduct disorders is a repetitive and persistent pattern of conduct in which either the basic rights of others or major age-appropriate societal norms or rules are violated. Conduct Disorders are more serious than ordinary mischief and pranks of children and adolescents. Four DSM-III subtypes are: Undersocialized and Aggressive; Undersocialized and Nonaggressive; Socialized and Aggressive; and Socialized Nonaggressive. The most common disorders are the Socialized and Nonaggressive, and the Undersocialized and Aggressive. Both subtypes are far more common among boys than girls.

Emotional Disorders

1. *Anxiety disorders.* This subclass includes three disorders in which anxiety is the predominant clinical feature. Separation Anxiety Disorder is evidenced by excessive child anxiety on separation from major attachment figures or from home or other familiar surroundings. Onset may be as early as preschool age but the most extreme form, involving school refusal, seems to begin about ages 11 and 12 with males and females equally likely to exhibit these symptoms.

Avoidant Disorder of childhood or adolescence is characterized by a persistent and excessive shrinking from contact with strangers of sufficient severity so as to interfere with social functioning in peer relationships. Yet the child has a clear desire for affection and acceptance, and has relationships with family members and other familiar figures that are warm and satisfying. This disorder may develop as early as two and one-half years. In contrast to Avoidant Disorder, Overanxious Disorder is evidenced by excessive worrying and fearful behavior that is not focused on a specific situation or object, and that is not due to a recent stressful experience. Typical age at onset is not known but this disorder is more common in boys than in girls.

2. *Other emotional disorders.* Another significant emotional disorder is Reactive Attachment Disorder of Infancy, which reflects poor emotional development (for example, lack of age-appropriate signs of social responsiveness, apathetic mood) or physical development, such as failure to thrive. Onset occurs before eight months of age and is usually due to inadequate caretaking.

Other emotional disorders include Schizoid Disorder (defect in the capacity to form social relationships), Elective Mutism (continuous refusal to speak in all social situations), Oppositional Disorder (pattern of disobedient, negativistic and provocative opposition to authority figures), and Identity Disorder (severe subjective distress regarding inability to reconcile aspects of self into a relatively coherent and acceptable sense of self).

Physical Disorders

1. *Eating disorders.* This subclass of disorders is characterized by gross disturbances in eating behavior, including Anorexia Nervosa, Bulimia, Pica, Rumination Disorder of Infancy, and Atypical Eating Disorder. The essential features of Anorexia Nervosa are intense fear of becoming obese, disturbance of body image, significant weight loss, refusal to maintain a minimal normal body weight, and amenorrhea (absence or suppression of menstrual discharge). The disturbance cannot be accounted for by a known physical disorder or illness such as an intestinal virus or blockage. Anorexia Nervosa occurs predominantly in females (95 percent); and as many as one out of two hundred fifty females between twelve and eighteen years may develop this disorder.

In contrast, Rumination Disorder in Infancy usually starts between three and twelve months of age and involves the repeated regurgitation of food, with weight loss or failure to gain expected weight. This disorder generally develops after a period of normal functioning, is potentially fatal, and is equally common in male and female infants and children.

2. *Stereotyped movement disorders.* This disorder involves abnormality of gross motor movement, such as tics or involuntary rapid movements of a functionally related group of skeletal muscles or the involuntary production of noises and words. Transient tics are recurrent involuntary, repetitive, rapid movements which can be voluntarily suppressed for minutes or hours. Boys are three times as likely to have this disorder and 12 to 24 percent of school-aged

children have had a history of some kind of a tic. Other stereotyped movement disorders include Chronic Motor Tic Disorder (duration of at least one year), Atypical Tic Disorder (for tics unclassifiable by other categories) and Atypical Stereotyped Movement Disorder such as head banging, rocking, or repetitive hand movements that are distinguished from tics because they are voluntary and are not spasmodic.

3. *Other disorders with physical manifestations.* Other disorders with physical manifestations include: Stuttering (speech), Functional Enuresis (urination), Functional Encopresis (defecation), Sleepwalking Disorder, and Sleep Terror Disorder.

Developmental Disorders

1. *Pervasive developmental disorders.* Developmental disorders are characterized by distortions in the development of psychological functions related to social skills and language such as maintaining attention, perception, reality testing, and motor movement. More than one basic area of psychological development is affected at the same time and to a severe degree. Infantile Autism is one type of Pervasive Developmental Disorder and reflects a lack of responsiveness to other people (autism), gross impairment in communicative skills, and bizarre responses to various aspects of the environment. Frequently emerging within the first thirty months of age, this rare disorder (two to four cases per ten thousand) is three times more common in boys than in girls.

2. *Specific developmental disorders.* Specific Developmental Disorders affect a single specific function and children behave as if they are passing through an earlier normal developmental stage, because the disturbance is a delay in development, not a distortion. Specific Developmental Disorder is a controversial classification since many of the children with these disorders have no other signs of psychopathology. Impaired functions include reading (Developmental Reading Disorder), arithmetic (Developmental Arithmetic Disorder), language (Developmental Language Disorder), speech (Developmental Articulation Disorder), and combinations of the above (Mixed Specific Developmental Disorder).

Other Child and Adolescent Disorders

Related child and adolescent disorders include Substance Use Disorders, which are dependence on drugs, including alcohol and nicotine as well as illicit drugs. While most children dependent on drugs do not have conduct disorders, children with conduct disorders have especially high rates of drug involvement. Other less prevalent child and adolescent disorders include Organic Mental Disorder, Personality Disorder, Schizophrenia, and Somatoform Disorders (see DSM-III for definitions and diagnostic information).

Service Delivery Issues

Planning and managing children's mental health services requires an understanding of issues related to diagnostic assessment and treatment planning, program coordination and communication, parent involvement, school involvement, and collateral contact. These issues are described in the context of the range of services that comprise a mental health service delivery system.

Assessment and Treatment Planning. The task of assessing the psychosocial and physiological functioning of the individual child and formulating impressions from which to proceed remains the most significant step in any successful mental health delivery system. This task is twofold (Dangerfield, 1980, p. 9):

> 1. To make an estimate as accurate as possible of the degree of dysfunction experienced by the child; to assess how far this behavior deviates from what would be considered as typical or normal behavior for the age; and to decide whether the child is handicapped by his or her family, personal, or interpersonal circumstances.
> 2. To make an estimate as accurate as possible of the probability for change within the individual child or family. To what extent can the child participate and make changes that will make his or her life better? If the probability is low, what are the factors that contribute to the poor prognosis, and what treatment can increase the probability of change?

The assessment of the child and family members receiving counseling includes a clinical diagnosis to determine the level of functioning and emotional disturbance of each person. Some useful assessment tools include the Global Assessment Scale (GAS), *Diagnostic and Statistical Manual of Mental Disorders* (DSM III), and Diagnostic Profile (GAP). Children are affected by a variety of elements, including level of family functioning, educational handicaps, developmental delays, emotional deprivation, and racial discrimination. Thus, it is important for the mental health professional to evaluate the child and family in the totality of their experience.

The mental health service delivery system should avoid treating children like miniature adults. For example, the amount of time the agency allows for an intake evaluation should not be based on the adult treatment model, which is inadequate and inappropriate for children. A child's assessment must include a detailed family social history, a psychosocial developmental history of the child, a mental health status exam, separate interviews with the parent(s) and child(ren), and significant collateral contacts, such as public schools, child protective services, and juvenile court services. Children usually present a pattern of behavior that is symptomatic of their underlying emotional difficulties. A therapist needs to ascertain carefully the nature of these emotional problems. Specific issues, like depression or suicidal ideation, may be fairly obvious in adults, but are expressed more subtly in children. A thorough diagnostic evaluation is necessary to formulate treatment goals and objectives for the child and family. Treatment interventions must relate to significant aspects of the problem, and inaccurate assessments can lead to poor treatment. Poor treatment is not only a waste of time and money, but can further demoralize an already discouraged client.

Children's mental health services provide an opportunity to prevent future adult problems, as well as to break the chain of events that may lead to family breakdown or the requirement to place a child in an institution. It is particularly important for parents, childcare staff, or physicians working with the child on a daily basis to use diagnostic information carefully and to work together using a common goal or plan.

Funding and Reimbursement Policy. Funding is another major issue in mental health service delivery. The amount of funding usually influences the types of services provided and the types of client populations served. For example, some federal and state funds are provided only for treatment of seriously disturbed children, based on stringent eligibility criteria for financial reimbursement. Because the cost of service to children usually exceeds the amount of financial reimbursement, service priorities that offer treatment to clients who are able to pay a significant portion of their fee or who are able to receive financial support through public auspices, such as Medicaid, may be established. However, the children of the "working poor," who neither qualify for Medicaid nor can afford full fee, are often unable to receive necessary services. To avoid excluding these families, carefully designed sliding fee scales should be used whenever possible.

Another critical issue concerns reimbursement policies. In clinical practice, 50 percent more staff time is required to treat a single child than to treat a single adult. Most policies stipulate payment for a "face-to-face" contact with the child; however, reimbursement for significant collateral contact is inadequate or nonexistent. Cooperative relationships must be maintained with the child's schoolteacher, caseworker, or court-appointed guardian ad litem to ensure quality of care for the child, but the current fee-for-service reimbursement rates in many states discourage mental health staff from providing adequate diagnostic, case management, or outreach services.

Communication and Coordination. Channels of communication between the various social agencies serving children must be developed and maintained. The mental health needs of children would be better served through improved coordination of children's programs such as child welfare, juvenile justice, family court, the schools, vocational training, and medical assistance. In many states, there is no foundation in organizational structure or policy for establishing a unified statewide approach for meeting the mental health needs of children and families. Such agencies as the Division of Mental Health, Bureau of Children's Services, Division of Juvenile Rehabilitation, Division of Developmental Disabilities, and Office of Public Instruction often do not work together with a common goal or direction. Instead, there seems to be an ongoing struggle for survival within each separate service as they compete for funds. This contributes to the lack of a unified, goal-oriented planning and integration of services at the clinician level.

Community-Based Care. Hospital beds for children should be located in the child's own community. Because of a lack of community residential services for the involuntarily committed child, children can be held in hospitals long after the acute phase of their illness. Community services such as the home-based care offered by homemakers or home health agencies would allow the child to be maintained at home with professional supervision.

Parent Services. Many current mental health systems need to emphasize parenting skills as a way of treating children. Parents need special skills to care adequately for emotionally disturbed children in the home. Parenting classes, in-home training, and thorough follow-up or aftercare services are useful for maintaining children in their own homes. Furthermore, adoption subsidy programs in many states provide state money and medical support to families who wish to adopt children with mental or physical health problems. To assist these parents with effective child rearing, many states pay for diagnosis and treatment planning in order to care for these children. However, it is ironic that while innovative adoption subsidy programs exist, there is a shortage of services for children living in their own homes who have emotional problems. The lack of such supportive assistance encourages families to relinquish mentally ill and emotionally or behaviorally disturbed children to the state.

Mental Health Services in Schools. Children's mental health services in the public schools frequently address problems of adolescent pregnancy, truancy, alcoholism, drug abuse, sexual abuse, child abuse, and suicide. Although school systems usually refer children with serious problems to community mental health agencies, a child is frequently too tired after a full day of school to participate in a mental health program. Half-day school programs combined with day treatment may be necessary for these children (Larsen, Van Hook, and Anderson, 1980). Unfortunately, some school districts are wary of identifying a child's mental health need if they bear the legal responsibility to provide for that need (as they do under Education for the Handicapped Child, Public Law 94–142). Furthermore, teachers do not receive the training and sometimes lack the confidence necessary to refer disturbed children for screening and evaluation.

Elementary school counseling programs seek to work with children at an early age regarding self-concept, understanding of others, and communication. Some community mental health agencies provide consultation and training to teachers, counselors, and school administrators (Morse, 1975). The need for a relationship between community mental health agencies and schools is becoming even greater as schools lose counselors because of funding problems.

Child Mental Health Services

The severity of the child's problem, availability of resources, motivation of family, and public laws influence the type of service a child and his or her family utilizes. Thus, a comprehensive mental health delivery system needs to incorporate a wide range of services and treatment strategies. "Care needs to be exercised so that the delivery system is not shaped around the worker's bias of what is the best form of treatment. Rather, the delivery system must have a number of options so that needs of the child and his or her family can be assessed, and they can then be referred to the treatment strategy that meets the need. For example, within the mental health delivery system there should be opportunities for a strong family therapy focus needed by some children and families, and play therapy or individual treatment needed by others. Hence, there needs to be ease of access for the child and his family into the specific treatment strategy that is deemed best" (Dangerfield, 1980, pp. 8–9).

Mental health services therefore should be organized in such a way that a child can utilize any service or combination of services as his or her treatment needs change (see Figure 1). This continuum of mental health services is also related to such essential child and family social services as protective services and foster care.

Figure 1. A Continuum of Mental Health Services for Children and Adolescents.

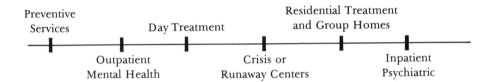

Preventive Services

One cannot discuss mental health services without emphasizing the importance and cost-effectiveness of preventive services. For example, if all pregnant women were guaranteed access to good prenatal and perinatal care, many instances of mental retardation and other childhood disorders such as fetal alcohol syndrome could be prevented. In addition, family-centered childbirth practices hold promise for reducing child abuse and neglect through strengthened parent-child bonding (Garbarino, 1980). Similarly, if future parents were routinely exposed to parent education and childcare activities in school, some of the unrealistic expectations that can lead to poor parenting and child abuse could be prevented.

In fact, much of the stress and disruption that causes family breakdown could be prevented if mothers and fathers had access to part-paid maternity leaves, quality, low-cost daycare, and homemaker services in times of stress (President's Commission on Mental Health, 1978). In-home care serves the function of ameliorating family distress by providing practical help to the family. A homemaker can provide emotional support while helping parents to improve their childcare techniques and home management skills. A lay volunteer can befriend a lonely, isolated parent and provide him or her with warmth, nurturing, and instructive role modeling. Partial care out of the home can be an essential auxiliary service to maintain healthy family functioning. Childcare centers that provide emotionally supportive education, as well as custodial care for preschool children and school-age children and supportive services to parents, are important for promoting the mental health of children and families.

Educational classes or support groups sponsored by mental health agencies, schools, churches, and community groups also represent preventive services. These classes or groups can focus on concerns within the family, such as divorce or remarriage, communication, substance abuse, and sexuality. Other preventive measures include periodic developmental assessments, employee-assistance programs, and programs for preparing workers for economic instability (Price and others, 1980).

Yet no matter how many preventive measures our society adopts, there will always be children who require special help. A network of psychiatric, pediatric, counseling, special education, and occupational training services is needed. These services must reflect the ways in which children's needs differ from those of adults and should promote a continuing relationship between the child and his or her family.

Outpatient Services

Mental health services provided to children and families on an outpatient basis are usually offered once a week for fifty minutes. Because the child is a minor, the provision of counseling requires that the parent or guardian give written consent to treatment, pay the client fee, provide the transportation, assure the child's regular attendance, and actively participate in the treatment plan. The parents' motivational level is instrumental in treating the child.

It is difficult to state unequivocally which children need outpatient services. However, some of the stressful factors affecting children are lack of nurturing; inadequate interpersonal relationships; frequent family moves; parent(s) working outside the home; loneliness; loss of a significant person or pet because of death, separation, or emotional detachment; illness, injury, or disability of a significant person in their life; and special learning needs based on neurological or emotional impairment. None of these situations, in and of itself, is harmful to the character development of the child. What is important is how the child perceives the situation and how well the child is able to cope with diverse life changes. Many of the emotional or behavioral problems resulting from these stressful factors can be addressed through outpatient counseling services.

Some of the critical issues in the planning and administration of outpatient programs include the uniqueness of children's mental health services, work load expectations, and funding resources. The uniqueness of children's services is reflected at the time of a request for service, when it must be determined which adult has legal custody, which adult needs to be included in treatment planning, and which adult will be responsible for transportation, fee payment, and attendance. Successful treatment may require individual play therapy or a socialization group for the child and parent participation in such services as marital counseling, parent education counseling, or individual or group therapy. Because this approach usually requires two sessions per week, which many parents are unable to afford, treatment sessions are usually "shared" between parent and child.

Although the child is the "identified problem," other family members are often involved, and their commitment to change may also be necessary. Often these children are the "symptom bearers" of the stress and tension in the home. In addition, the child might live with only one parent, neither parent, or both parents in separate households. Other significant adults, such as foster parents or relatives, may also need to be involved in treatment sessions.

Another management issue to be considered is the determination of work load standards for child and family mental health services. Basing work expectations on an adult outpatient model ignores the complexity of providing children's services. Costing out a unit of service and predicting with accuracy how many units of service (client hours) can be billed and what kind of revenue will be generated are all critical administrative tasks. For example, the provision of children's services usually requires extensive collateral contacts, in addition to the involvement of the family with such referral sources as the schoolteacher, probation officer, pediatrician, or child protective service (CPS) social worker. Written and verbal follow-up reports on the treatment progress may also need to be written or gathered by staff. Diagnostic evaluations may also be requested by family or juvenile court. Clinical records and therapists may be subpoenaed by the court to provide information about the child's welfare. Case consultation is also necessary when there are several professionals providing treatment to different family members, as in cases of incest. These support services are essential components of a children's service program.

Staff resources are the greatest investment in the delivery of children's mental health services. Specialized professional child therapy training is inadequate to meet the needs of child mental health staff. Thus, good clinical supervision and consultation is essential to augment professional training and experience. Many programs employ a child psychiatrist to provide psychiatric evaluations and psychologists to conduct psychological testing. Due to the complexity and severity of children's cases and the pressure of the work environment, care must be taken to create a positive, stable work environment. Because finances are limited, intangible benefits need to be created (for example, flexible hours, in-service training, and involvement in a community project). Staff members need time to "debrief" difficult situations by consulting with a colleague and adequate facilities and space, such as a childsafe play therapy room with simple toys and games.

Funding is also a critical issue in the management of a children's program. Because of limited funding, agency administrators need to be careful when setting funding priorities with the staff and board to specify what portion of the children's population will be served. The severity of the problem, age of the child, nature of service delivery, and community needs must be taken into account.

Day Treatment

Further along the continuum of children's mental health services designed to provide "the least restrictive treatment environment" are day-treatment services for children and adolescents. Such programs offer a range of services to clients who need less than twenty-four-hour-per-day care but require more than outpatient treatment. In most states, day treatment is offered on the basis of at least three hours per day and at least three days per week. Day-treatment services include individual, family, and group therapy; socialization and recreational activities; academic tutoring; parent counseling; and medication management.

The children and adolescents referred to day-treatment programs are usually severely or acutely disturbed or behaviorally disabled with personality or conduct disorders. They can also be developmentally delayed because of physical or neurological impairment and environmental deprivation. Day-treatment services are viewed as an alternative to hospitalization, and the treatment modality varies according to the age of the child and the nature of the disorder. For example, an adolescent program for youth aged thirteen to seventeen years may focus on such treatment issues as autonomy, separation, and psychosocial maturation. A program for children from five to twelve years of age may emphasize interpersonal relations in their immediate environment, such as family, school, and peers. A preschool program for children two and a half to five years may focus on parent-child interaction as the primary treatment intervention.

The goal of the day-treatment program is to increase the child's capacity to adapt to his or her environment, to improve his or her functioning level, and to aid the child in becoming a more integrated person. It is essential that parents be involved in their child's treatment program.

Critical management issues for a children's day-treatment program relate to personnel selection, community relations, and ancillary resources. Staffing patterns of child and adolescent programs vary considerably. Some models use only master's degree professional staff; others use only paraprofessionals. Most programs use a combination of well-trained professionals, paraprofessionals, and student interns. Good clinical training and supervision is necessary to guide the team in a unified treatment approach. It is also beneficial to incorporate different disciplines on a team. For example, occupational therapists have unique skills and knowledge regarding sensory integration, visual and auditory perception, and motor skills. A child psychiatrist can provide psychiatric evaluation and consultation.

Staff members need time on a daily basis to review the child's progress, to discuss any relevant changes in the family, to adjust individualized treatment plans, and to coordinate with relevant community professionals. The stress and constant demands of working with this client population need to be offset by flexible hours, periodic closing of the program, and varied staffing patterns.

Community relations are an important consideration in planning a day-treatment program. It is advantageous to develop a supportive working relationship with the school district. Some programs have a combined educational/therapeutic milieu; others are physically separated. Schools can facilitate special education programs by providing special resources for children, releasing time to attend the program, and mainstreaming children back into regular classes. Some schools can offer in-kind contributions, such as classroom space, gym, playground, supplies, special consultants, and psychological testing. Issues such as eligibility criteria, program guidelines, confidentiality, parent involvement, staff supervision, and fee collection need to be addressed.

Because these children and youth are often at risk and need ancillary services, it is important to maintain ongoing relationships with hospital staff, child protective services, court personnel, and crisis outreach teams. Contacts with state and local funding agencies are also important to arrange for reimbursing the cost of services. Transportation and parental involvement are also key issues in ensuring the child's full participation. Some agencies secure donated vans; some school districts allow the use of their buses; and some mental health programs purchase a van and begin the therapeutic involvement at the time the child is picked up at home.

Crisis and Runaway Centers

The Juvenile Justice and Delinquency Prevention Act passed by Congress in 1974 contained the Runaway Youth Act (Title III). This act established a national model for providing services to runaway youth. The philosophy reflected in this model drew from the experiences of the youth drop-in centers and crisis hotlines of the previous decade. The model focuses on youth participation in decisions that will affect their lives.

A crisis center offers temporary shelter to a young runaway, involving short-term respite care to meet physical needs (housing, food, safety) and emotional needs (supportive counseling). Youth who need a crisis home frequently come from severely dysfunctional families in which many have been physically and/or sexually abused. Many of these youth come from homes that reflect a lack of caring and stability. Youth "run" to seek adventure, refuge, or a better life, and most are disappointed. Although the age range varies in different states, runaway youth eligible for care are usually between the ages of thirteen and seventeen. By law, runaway youth are usually allowed to remain in a shelter for a brief period of time, such as twenty-four hours, while parental or guardian consent is obtained. With parental consent, the youth may remain in the crisis shelter for up to seven days while a more permanent plan is worked out. Such plans include returning home, short-term or long-term licensed foster care, group homes, residential treatment, or independent living. During the stay in the center, emphasis is placed on the runaway taking responsibility for his or her own actions. Activities that require participation include household chores, academic work, group sessions, and intensive therapeutic sessions with the youth's family and appropriate community professionals.

A major management issue is the lack of resources for long-term care. Although many of these youth are unable to return home, they could improve their functioning level if offered a stable, secure living arrangement. In fact, even the clinical description of them is changing from borderline emotionally disturbed to life-style disturbed. This reflects a less pathological view of their social functioning. However, because of some of the learned behaviors of these young people, it is difficult for some of them to remain in the same program designed to help them (for example, frequent curfew violators or runaways are kicked out of the shelter). Thus, many of these young people, especially those who are already wards of the state, become revolving-door clients—moving from runaway street life, to temporary shelter, to foster care, to runaway street life. Although most of these children are between thirteen and fifteen years of age, some are as young as ten years old.

In addition to operating with limited resources, crisis center staff usually espouse participatory management principles for communication, decision making, and planning. But these staff members also need thorough training and supervision. Most are young adults who work twenty-four-hour shifts, four days a week, in order to maintain the essential ingredients of crisis response and outreach found in most crisis centers. Administrators need to be cognizant of the stress inherent in providing these services. One way staff can gain recognition and support is through agency affiliation with state and regional coalitions or the national Network of Runaways and Youth Services.

Residential Treatment and Group Home Services

Residential treatment centers and group homes provide treatment in a group care therapeutic environment that "integrates daily group living, remedial education, and treatment services on the basis of an individualized plan for each child, exclusively for children with severe emotional disturbances, whose parents cannot cope with them and who cannot be effectively treated in their own homes, in another family, or in other less intensive treatment-oriented child care facilities" (Child Welfare League of America, 1975, p. xvii).

In the past, a distinction has been made between group homes and residential treatment centers. Group homes are more of a community-based service and treat children in a more open setting; residential treatment centers serve children who are more disturbed. However, many of the more professional group home programs are successfully treating severely disturbed children. According to Whittaker (1977), most of the children in residential treatment and group care represent a multiplicity of interpersonal, emotional, learning, familial, and physiological problems. Common diagnostic labels include infantile autism, attention deficit disorders, childhood schizophrenia, conduct disorders, personality disorders, and developmental disorders.

When looking at children in both group care and residential treatment, a functional classification of the commonly observed problems can be developed to include intrapersonal, interpersonal, and external categories (Whittaker, 1979). The first problem category relates to intrapersonal problems such as poorly developed impulse control (for example, low frustration tolerance, limited ability to postpone gratification), poorly developed modulation of emotion (inability to handle the normal range of human emotions), and low self-image. Interpersonal problems comprise the second major category. These include relationship deficits (inability to form meaningful relationships with peers and helping adults) and family pain and strain (dysfunctional family behavior or relationships). The third major problem category concerns children's external problems. Special learning disabilities (for example, minimal brain damage, dyslexia) and limited play skills are two major external problem areas. Although the diagnostic labels and problem categories differ, these children have in common failure to develop emotional, social, and/or physical competence (White, 1959, 1979) and therefore need a therapeutic milieu found in a residential treatment center or group home. Residential treatment and group home programs should focus on growth and development in the child's total life sphere, rather than the remediation of psychiatrically defined syndromes or the extinction of certain problematic behaviors (Whittaker, 1979).

Administrators and planners of residential treatment and group home programs should be concerned with such major issues as continuity of care, definition of purpose, visibility, interventions linked to the purpose of a program, and public accountability (Whittaker, 1979). "Continuity of care" refers to the recent efforts to promote deinstitutionalization and home-based services and the need to create effective linkages between residential and community-based programs related to family, peer group, school, and church. In specifying their purpose and goals, residential treatment and group homes need to function as family support systems, rather than treating the child in isolation from his or her family and community. To facilitate a child's adjustment back into the community, parents should be involved in the child's treatment. Child and family support systems involving the program and community institutions, such as schools, recreational organizations, employment agencies, and churches, should be established.

Related to continuity of care and definition of purpose is the issue of visibility. Because residential treatment programs should be highly interconnected with the community, large and remote institutions are undesirable for the following reasons: (1) They tend to be built in outlying areas, and their remoteness can lead to a separation of children from their families and community. (2) They tend to create a need for regimen and routine that far exceeds that necessary in a family living environment. (3) They have a greater likelihood and danger of developing deviant subcultures. (4) They often stigmatize the staff and children as they perpetuate the myth that the children they serve are inherently different from the rest of us. "Just as we would not build a skyscraper in a residential neighborhood, we should not build residential facilities which are grossly out of harmony with their surrounding communities" (Whittaker, 1978, p. 33).

In addition to the use of small facilities, parents and childcare workers should be involved as central actors in the helping process because these persons know the most about the children in their care. Programs should be designed to maximize the collaboration between childcare staff and parents. Residential treatment and group care programs should be teaching skills for living, as well as using assessment and treatment procedures that are behaviorally specific and directly applicable to the real-life environments that children encounter in their homes.

The fourth area of concern involves linking treatment methods with program objectives. Too often, residential treatment and group home programs are preconceived because of theoretical biases. Consequently, programs often change their treatment focus and methods with changes in treatment directors or personnel. Presently, no single theory or set of practice methods can address the needs of a program that focuses on the total range of child development and the ecology of a child's world (Whittaker, 1979). Therefore, program managers and staff need to evaluate continuously the appropriateness of cognitive, behavioral, and psychoanalytic intervention methods for use within their treatment environment.

The fifth area of concern relates to public accountability. Residential treatment and group home programs should be able to demonstrate what it is they do in simple, clear, and jargon-free terms the general public can understand. All program staff, from the maintenance personnel to the director, should be able to explain the program purpose and methods. In addition, sound evaluative procedures should be built into all programs so that we can learn which service strategies are most effective with particular types of children and settings (Phillips and others, 1978; Velasquez and McCubbin, 1980). Furthermore, the criteria for defining successful treatment should reflect multiple measures instead of a single criterion, such as recidivism, school grades, or life satisfaction. Mental health program managers need to view residential treatment centers and group homes as important components in a network of services for meeting children's mental health needs.

Inpatient Hospitalization

There were an estimated 25,252 patients under eighteen years of age admitted to the inpatient services of state and county mental hospitals in 1975 (Meyer, 1977, p. 9). Approximately 55 percent were diagnosed as having transient situational disturbances and behavior disorders; 18 percent were diagnosed as schizophrenic; and 10 percent were diagnosed as personality disorders (p. 1). Children and adolescents can be admitted voluntarily to inpatient hospitalization programs, and in some states adolescents can be involuntarily committed.

Voluntary inpatient hospitalization provides twenty-four-hour care for children with severe emotional problems, which may be accompanied by serious medical problems such as diabetes, asthma, or epilepsy. Usually these children are in a crisis situation or represent complex treatment problems that are not amenable to more traditional resources. Some of these children are psychotic, and some of them have been diagnosed as having conduct disorders. Many of them have a history of being physically and/or sexually abused and have been removed from their homes. They also can be referred to the hospital from foster homes and residential treatment facilities when their behavior becomes unmanageable or when they are a danger to themselves or others.

During hospitalization, the following comprehensive medical and clinical services can be provided: diagnostic assessment; physical, neurological, and psychiatric examination; medication evaluation; psychological testing; and specialized services such as occupational therapy, recreational therapy, or socialization skill groups. Along with individual and family treatment, efforts are made to develop an individualized academic program and to provide clinical consultation to schools. Children usually receive inpatient care for six to twelve weeks and then are discharged to their natural homes, foster homes, or residential treatment facilities.

In contrast to voluntary hospitalization, involuntary hospitalization of adolescents requires a legal commitment and a legal proceeding offering evidence that the young person is a danger to himself, herself, or others or in some cases gravely disabled. In most states, a commitment request can be made for seventy-two hours (excluding weekends), fourteen days, or ninety days. At the end of each time period, evidence validating the request must be presented to a judge. An average length of stay for involuntary commitment is ten to twelve days. These adolescents are often referred because of their high-risk suicidal state; many are psychotic.

A critical administrative issue for inpatient care is the lack of appropriate resources to help children and their care givers after they are discharged from the hospital. These children have developed severe behavioral problems. Most have poor academic performance, poor ability to relate socially, and poor impulse control and judgment. Many children vent their frustration and anger through aggressive behavior. They present difficult behavioral management problems for parents, foster parents, or group home care givers. If placement in a residential facility is a viable choice, the child must meet specific eligibility criteria and wait until there is an opening. If foster care is a viable placement, then special services need to be given to the family to help members cope with an extremely difficult child. Individualized parent management training and support services can help maintain an emotionally disturbed child in foster care. Without adequate supervision, multiple foster care placements may occur, which further impede the child's social, emotional, and academic growth.

In addition to the appropriate use of resources, channels of interdisciplinary team authority and communication need to be structured and explicitly stated for an effective inpatient service. The medical prescription, clinical treatment, academic program, and behavioral management plan must be incorporated into an integrated approach. Strategic interventions with families and the use of medication require staff cooperation and acceptance. Additional clinical training may be given through supervision, consultation, and specialized in-service training programs.

Another management issue for an inpatient program is the staffing pattern. The unit operates on a seven-day, twenty-four-hour cycle. Generally, the greatest activity is during the day, and very few children are admitted to the program in the evening. Thus, most staff schedules are focused on the 7 A.M. to 11 P.M. time period. If the two shifts overlap, there is more shared responsibility during busy times and more opportunity created for effective communication with unit members. Some programs have experimented with flexible hours, such as ten-hour shifts four days per week.

A critical element in the management of the involuntary hospitalization program is staff selection. Highly qualified, experienced people who can effectively intervene in a crisis situation and mobilize family resources are needed. A physician to prescribe medication and complete psychiatric evaluations is needed. A forensic psychologist will complete a legal determination, and it is recommended that family therapists be used to stabilize the family system and to help family members cope constructively with this stressful situation.

After the initial admission, a therapist will meet with the patient and his or her family for both individual and family treatment sessions. A diagnostic evaluation will be prepared for the court; a management plan will be developed for the nursing staff; and appropriate referrals will be made for specialized examinations (for example, neurological) as necessary. After the initial seventy-two hours, several treatment dispositions can be considered: The patient can choose to remain in the hospital as a voluntary patient; the patient can be referred to a mental health agency or a private therapist for continued counseling; the patient can be discharged; or a request for fourteen-day hospitalization can be submitted if the designated criteria are met. If involuntary hospitalization is continued, the frequency and duration of the treatment with the individual and family are intensified. In addition, various other support services may be offered, such as socialization groups, skill-building classes, education, or occupational or physical therapy. Most adolescents are discharged home, although a few who are categorized as "gravely disabled" might be detained for ninety days because of a severely disordered thought process or an inability to handle basic self-care. An appropriate discharge plan might include a residential treatment facility.

Future Directions

In the last decade, much progress has been made concerning services for children with mental disorders. The DSM III classification scheme is an important contribution to the assessment of mental health functioning because of its many different diagnostic perspectives. Practical prevention programs are being developed in a variety of program areas (Price and others, 1980). Furthermore, researchers are identifying factors related to how some children do not seem to be damaged by stress or abuse (Rutter, 1979a, 1979b). This information can then be used to design targeted interventions for strengthening a child's psychosocial functioning.

Progress is slowly being made toward developing better assessment tools for children of various ages and backgrounds. Still needed, however, are simple and reliable assessment tools that can be used by nonspecialist workers in a wide range of services. Techniques for evaluating family functioning and a child's psychosocial environment in different sociocultural settings are also in short supply (President's Commission on Mental Health, 1978).

Techniques are also needed for integrating services. Effective treatment programs require a close working relationship among the treatment center, other social service agencies, parents, and various community supports. Strategies are needed for overcoming the organizational and funding barriers to improved linkages between mental health and other service sectors at a time when the need for these linkages is increasing with funding cutbacks.

Changing demographic trends in America also have implications for child mental health. Knowledge and skills necessary to serve ethnic minorities effectively have always been in short supply. With increases in the number of Hispanic and Asian families, the demand for more culturally relevant mental health services has also risen. In addition, seasonal and migrant farmworkers and their children, many of whom belong to racial minorities, represent a population anywhere from 250,000 to 6 million that has been almost completely excluded from mental health care (Larson, 1979). The constant mobility from place to place in search of work prevents them from obtaining any care, let alone continuity of care. Similarly, the dramatic increase in the number of divorces and single-parent families has not gone unnoticed by child mental health personnel. Treatment strategies for working with troubled children of divorced parents will remain an important priority.

As with adult mental health services, developing comprehensive service systems that are responsive to children in local areas is difficult. There are children who have severe mental disabilities that will persist throughout their lives. Some of these children will require a sheltered environment; some need a variety of services; and others need only periodic assistance. There are chronically disabled children capable of achieving a high level of independent functioning if a full range of community services, from group homes to income assistance, is made available. Without such a network of services, children will continue to suffer in their own homes or in institutions. Thus, more carefully planned and adequately supported efforts are necessary to keep children in their families and communities.

The personal and social supports that currently exist in our neighborhoods and communities are one of the great resources for maintaining mental health and for preventing the development of serious mental disabilities. For example, many young people with mental and emotional problems who come to the attention of the juvenile courts benefit from supportive neighborhood activities such as recreation and arts programs, educational supplements, and the community-based residential programs that serve as alternatives to incarceration in correctional institutions (President's Commission on Mental Health, 1978). Furthermore, most people initially turn to families, friends, neighbors, schools, religious institutions, self-help groups, and voluntary associations when they have problems. An effective long-range approach to promoting child and family mental health would be to enhance the ability of these supports without impairing their autonomy and natural strengths.

References

American Psychiatric Association. *DSM III—Diagnostic and Statistical Manual of Mental Disorders.* (3rd ed.) Washington, D.C.: American Psychiatric Association, 1980.

Berlin, I. (Ed.). *Advocacy for Child Mental Health*. New York: Brunner/Mazel, 1975.

Bowlby, J. *Attachment and Loss*. Vol. 1: *Attachment*. London: Hogarth Press, 1969.

Bowlby, J. *Attachment and Loss*. Vol. 2: *Separation Anxiety and Anger*. London: Hogarth Press, 1973.

Bronfenbrenner, U. *Ecology of Human Development*. Cambridge, Mass.: Harvard University Press, 1979.

Bryce, M., and Lloyd, J. C. (Eds.). *Treating Families in the Home: An Alternative to Placement*. Springfield, Ill.: Thomas, 1981.

Calhoun, J. A., Grotberg, E. H., and Rackley, W. R. *The Status of Children, Youth, and Families 1979*. Washington, D.C.: U.S. Department of Health and Human Services, 1980.

Child Welfare League of America. *1975 Directory of Member Agencies*. New York: Child Welfare League of America, 1975.

Dangerfield, D. E. *A Final Report to the Children's Services Coordinators—King County Mental Health Centers*. Bellevue, Wash.: Eastside Community Mental Health Center, 1980.

Garbarino, J. "Changing Hospital Childbirth Practices: A Developmental Perspective on Prevention of Child Maltreatment." *American Journal of Orthopsychiatry*, 1980, *50* (4), 588–597.

Goldsmith, J. M. "Mental Health Services for Children." In *Encyclopedia of Social Work*. Vol. 2. Washington, D.C.: National Association of Social Workers, 1977.

Goldstein, J., Freud, A., and Solnit, A. J. *Beyond the Best Interests of the Child*. New York: Free Press, 1973.

Kagan, J. "The Psychological Requirements for Human Development." In N. B. Talbot (Ed.), *Raising Children in Modern America: Problems and Prospective Solutions*. Boston: Little, Brown, 1976.

Larsen, E., Van Hook, R., and Anderson, J. "Community Mental Health Services to Children." In *Mental Health Subcommittee Report*. Presented to the Washington State Senate Committee on Social and Health Services. Olympia: Washington State Legislature, July 1980.

Larson, A. *Migrant and Seasonal Farmworkers: Summary of Problems. A Report Prepared for the Federal Regional Council, Region X*. Seattle: U.S. Department of Labor, Employee Standards Administration, Region X, May 1979.

Maybanks, S., and Bryce, M. (Eds.). *Home-Based Services for Children and Families: Policy, Practice and Research*. Springfield, Ill.: Thomas, 1979.

Meyer, N. G. "Diagnostic Distribution of Admissions to Inpatient Services of State and County Mental Health Hospitals, United States, 1975." *Mental Health Statistical Note No. 138*. Washington, D.C.: National Institute of Mental Health, 1977.

Morse, W. C. "The Schools and the Mental Health of Children and Adolescents." In I. Berlin (Ed.), *Advocacy for Child Mental Health*. New York: Brunner/Mazel, 1975.

Phillips, E. L., and others. *Program Development, Staff Training, and Practical Evaluations at Boys Town, 1975–1977*. Boys Town, Nebr.: Father Flanagan's Boys Home, 1978.

President's Commission on Mental Health. *Report to the President*. Vols. 1–3. Washington, D.C.: U.S. Government Printing Office, 1978.

Price, R. H., and others (Eds.). *Prevention in Mental Health—Research, Policy and Practice*. Beverly Hills, Calif.: Sage, 1980.

Robins, L. N. "Mental Disorders in Childhood." Working paper cited in President's Commission on Mental Health, *Report to the President*. Vol. 2. Washington, D.C.: U.S. Government Printing Office, 1978.

Rutter, M. "Maternal Deprivation, 1972–1978: New Findings, New Concepts, New Approaches." *Child Development*, 1979a, *50*, 283–305.

Rutter, M. "Protective Factors in Children's Responses to Stress and Disadvantage." In M. Kent and J. E. Rolf (Eds.), *Primary Prevention of Psychopathology*. Vol. 3: *Social Competence in Children*. Hanover, N.H.: University Press of New England, 1979b.

Salasin, J., and others. *Challenges for Children's Mental Health Services*. McLean, Va.: Mitre Corporation, 1977.

U.S. Bureau of the Census, U.S. Department of Commerce. *1980 Census of the Population*. Washington, D.C.: U.S. Government Printing Office, 1981.

Velasquez, J. S., and McCubbin, H. I. "Towards Establishing the Effectiveness of Community-Based Residential Treatment: Program Evaluation by Experimental Research." *Administration in Social Work*, 1980, *3*, 337–359.

Weintrob, A. "Changing Population in Adolescent Residential Treatment: New Problems for Program and Staff." *American Journal of Orthopsychiatry*, 1974, *44*, 604–610.

White, R. W. "Motivation Reconsidered: The Concept of Competence." *Psychological Review*, 1959, *66*, 297–333.

White, R. W. "Competence as an Aspect of Personal Growth." In M. Kent and J. E. Rolf (Eds.), *Primary Prevention of Psychopathology*. Vol. 3: *Social Competence in Children*. Hanover, N.H.: University Press of New England, 1979.

Whittaker, J. K. "Child Welfare: Residential Treatment." In *Encyclopedia of Social Work*. Vol. 1. Washington, D.C.: National Association of Social Workers, 1977.

Whittaker, J. K. "The Changing Character of Residential Child Care: An Ecological Perspective." *Social Service Review*, 1978, *52* (1), 21–36.

Whittaker, J. K. *Caring for Troubled Children: Residential Treatment in a Community Context*. San Francisco: Jossey-Bass, 1979.

Yarrow, L. J. "Separation from Parents During Early Childhood." In M. L. Hoffman and L. W. Hoffman (Eds.), *Review of Child Development Research*. Vol. 1. New York: Russell Sage Foundation, 1964.

❧ 30 ❧

Mental Health Promotion and Primary Prevention

Barbara J. Friesen

This chapter suggests that the development of prevention and promotion in mental health services begins with the positive attitudes of administrators and staff. Once an openness is present, the possibilities are available to undertake programming that seeks changes in individuals as well as promoting environmental changes. This continuum is described in terms of target populations, treatment methods, and worker roles. In addition, the tasks and processes for implementing mental health promotional programs are described. Managers need to be open to the ideas of promoting mental health and establishing prevention programs.

Prevention was first included as a national goal in the National Mental Health Act of 1946 (PL 79–487). This legislation provided for developing and assisting states in the use of the most effective methods of prevention, diagnosis, and treatment of psychotic disorders (Bloom, 1977). Mental health education had been a prevention strategy supported by the National Association of Mental Health since its inception in 1909. The purposes of mass public education were to increase public tolerance of the mentally ill and to provide information about positive mental health practices. Consultation had also been conceived as a prevention strategy since the 1920s, when psychiatric consultation to the public schools was promoted by the child guidance movement as a way of preventing juvenile delinquency.

The first federal financial support for preventive efforts was contained in the Community Mental Health Centers Act of 1963 (PL 88–164), which established federally funded community mental health centers and specified that consultation and education (C and E) be included as one of five mandated services. Although the range of prevention/promotion efforts has expanded considerably since 1963, consultation and education units in community mental health centers often serve as the prevention arm of these programs.

The provisions of the 1980 Mental Health Systems Act further advance the federal commitment to the "promotion of mental health." The legislation provides for the establishment of a mental health prevention unit within the National Institute of Mental Health in order to provide leadership in the following areas: establish national goals and priorities for the prevention of mental illness and the promotion of mental health; encourage and assist state and local agencies in achieving these goals; and develop and coordinate federal prevention policies and programs and assure increased focus on prevention and promotion activities with special grants. These federal initiatives are designed to support mental health centers in their efforts to strengthen and expand prevention programming.

Primary prevention/promotion activities have received relatively low priority in relation to clinical activities in community mental health programs. Although the reasons for the slow development of prevention services within the mental health field are complex and not fully understood, often cited barriers to prevention include lack of an adequate knowledge base (Kessler and Albee, 1975), inadequate resources and lack of constituency (Broskowski and Baker, 1974), competition with direct services for funding, and confusion about the targets and boundaries of prevention services (Snow and Newton, 1976).

Another impediment to the development of prevention programming appears to be a lack of administrative leadership and direction in this area. In a survey of staff in forty-three community mental health centers, Perlmutter and Vayda (1978) found that only 47 percent of respondents thought primary prevention was feasible. Of the total respondents, only 16.3 percent said that prevention was both feasible and operational in their center. Barriers to prevention programs cited included lack of expertise, lack of staff interest, limited resources, and inadequate definition of prevention services.

I view mental health prevention and promotion activities as critical components of the mission of community mental health agencies. In the short history of community mental health, there has been considerable ambivalence between the goals of prevention/promotion and the provision of services to people with identified problems. I clarify and critique this ambivalence in this module by using the concept of a continuum of service. Every clinical service carries within it the opportunity for mental health promotion, the chance to gather information about clients' common problems, and the seeds for developing innovative approaches to these common problems. Many potential "prevention" services exist within clinical situations; however, a prevention "ethos" is missing. Such an ethos would be demonstrated by mental health program staff activities that reflect "prevention thinking and actions" in all aspects of service delivery. The mental health administrator is pivotal in supporting the development of a prevention ethos among staff.

Perspectives on Prevention

Approaches to prevention in the mental health field have been pursued within three general perspectives. The first approach, modeled after classic prevention strategies in physical medicine, involves a search for specific causes of specific disorders. This line of inquiry is embodied in the public health model of prevention. A more recent emphasis, also patterned after the public health approach, moves away from the search for specific causes, and focuses more on multicausal factors, or stressors that may produce a variety of undesirable reactions, depending on individual circumstances. An emphasis on the promotion of health rather than the prevention of illness is the third perspective. This approach appears to hold promise for providing some guidance to community mental health programs in deciding which program development and service delivery strategies are feasible to undertake.

Public Health Model

Within the perspective of the public health model, health is defined as the absence of disease, and the health status of a given population can be estimated by examining the incidence and prevalence of specific disorders within that population. A primary focus is placed on identifying and isolating agents that cause or contribute to disorder in order to develop strategies for prevention and treatment. Target populations for prevention efforts are defined as those persons currently free from the disorder that the prevention program seeks to reduce or eliminate.

Specific Cause–Specific Disorder Approach. The specific cause–specific disorder model is patterned after the classic medical paradigm that has been used successfully in the prevention of many infectious and nutritional diseases in physical medicine (Bloom, 1979). It involves identifying a disease that is widespread and serious enough to justify the development of a prevention program, undertaking a series of studies to identify a theory of the path of disease development, and developing and evaluating a research-based experimental prevention program. Bloom (1979) points out that in order for this approach to be used effectively, there must be reliable methods for diagnosis so that it is possible to say whether a person does or does not have the disease. In addition, the diseases for which this approach has been effective have an identified necessary precondition or "cause," which can be removed or protected against.

The physical disorders for which this approach has resulted in effective prevention strategies include infectious diseases such as measles or mumps, for which vaccines can be developed; deficiency diseases, for which dietary or other supplements can be supplied; and conditions that result from exposure to toxic substances. Advances in knowledge about the prevention of physical diseases have contributed to the prevention of certain classes of associated mental disorder as well. Mental conditions related to exposure to specific substances such as poisons, chemicals, or certain drugs have been identified and can be prevented through avoiding exposure to these substances. Some conditions that may have mental or emotional consequences, such as neurological damage associated with measles, can be prevented through the control of the physical disease itself.

For many disorders currently classified as "mental or emotional," however, the necessary conditions for effective use of the classic prevention approach are not present. In many cases, reliable methods of diagnosis do not exist and/or no known single causal or contributing precondition can be identified. One reason for the difficulty in the development of reliable diagnostic methods is that mental or emotional disorders are most often socially defined. Unlike physical conditions, which can be objectively identified through measurement of temperature, changes in blood chemistry, or the identification of disease-producing organisms, the definition of mental disorder is intimately tied to the norms and expectations of a society. Thus, definitions of mental disorder may vary from culture to culture and may change over time within a given society. The elimination of homosexuality as a "psychiatric disease" category is an example of such a shift in social definition.

Multicausal Models/Life Stress Approaches. Although the classic prevention paradigm has led to advances in the development of prevention strategies for some physical and mental disorders, it has been less successfully applied to a number of other problems. For example, no single cause or precondition has been identified for disorders such as hypertension and coronary artery disease. These conditions are now thought to develop in relation to a combination of factors such as genetic predisposition, life-style and personal habits, and wider environmental forces. Similarly, a number of mental disorders may emerge through complex individual-environmental interactions.

Recent advances in knowledge have contributed to the recognition of the multicausal nature of many physical and mental disorders. The work of Selye (1956) on physiological adaptations of the body to external stressors, studies of Holmes and colleagues (for example, Rahe and Holmes, 1966), and the work of Dohrenwend and Dohrenwend (1974a, 1974b) on life stresses and on social and cultural influences on mental disorder are notable.

One major shift in thinking about prevention is a renewed interest in the relationship between physical and mental health. A related trend is the emphasis on the contribution of life stresses to the development of a variety of undesirable consequences (physical and/or mental). These advances are described by Bloom (1979) as a new prevention paradigm. Within this paradigm, it is assumed that all persons are vulnerable to life stressors and that almost any disorder or dysfunction may be associated with stressful life events. As Bloom (1979, p. 183) suggests, "Four vulnerable persons can face a stressful life event—perhaps the collapse of their marriage, or the loss of their job. One person may become severely depressed; the second may be involved in an automobile accident; the third may head down the road to alcoholism; and the fourth may develop a psychotic thought disorder, or coronary artery disease."

Within this view of prevention, the emphasis is shifted from identifying specific causal agents to identifying sources of stress that appear to have a strong relationship to the development of a number of undesirable consequences. This way of thinking about prevention is an important conceptual development for the mental health field. Elimination of the necessity for predicting which specific disorder will be prevented by a particular intervention removes many of the logical obstacles encountered within the classic prevention paradigm. In addition, there is a body of knowledge and skills that can be applied to this general prevention approach within the mental health field. A considerable amount of research literature examines the effects of specific life events, such as retirement or bereavement, seeks to identify vulnerable or at-risk populations, and discusses the outcomes of various prevention strategies.

Although the prevention of disorder has considerable appeal as an abstract social goal, prevention as a concept also has several features that may make it difficult to translate into mental health practice. When health is defined as the absence of disease, the overall goal of prevention activities is zero, a somewhat negative and discouraging goal for which it may be difficult to gain public support, particularly in the absence of methods that have been proven effective. In much of current prevention practice, it is also assumed that populations to which prevention strategies are targeted are those "without disorder"; so potential beneficiaries or prevention approaches are persons other than past or current clients of the mental health system. Other major difficulties in applying the concept of prevention of disorder to practice are problems related to the evaluation of prevention efforts, the logically difficult problems of measuring events that did not happen, and establishing that they would have happened if prevention intervention had not been provided. Such evaluation generally involves carefully controlled, long-term experimental studies that are beyond the technical and financial capacity of local mental health programs.

Although prevention as a concept is an important broad, long-range goal, because of the difficulties described, "health promotion" will often be a more useful framework for planning and developing a service delivery strategy at the local program level.

Health Promotion

The health promotion approach in the mental health field is rooted in a view of mental health as a continuum of degrees of wellness, rather than as the absence of defined disorder. The health promotion model begins with the point of view that all persons possess strengths and have the capacity to grow and learn, whatever their current degree of wellness. Thus, the goal of health promotion is positive and is aimed at increasing individual and community strengths and capacities. According to Ketterer, Bader, and Levy (1980, p. 264), "Promoting mental health means enhancing the competencies and well-being of individuals, groups, and communities through the application of multiple person-centered and system change efforts." These authors identify two general mental health promotion strategies: improving the well-being and strengths of normal and at-risk populations through competence-training strategies and modifying social policies, social systems, and environmental factors that impede the mental health and well-being of groups in the community.

Competence building is a key concept within the mental health promotion framework. Research in this area provides some persuasive evidence that helping people to build resources and adaptive strengths provides a defense against the development of a variety of problems. One interesting finding, for example, is that teaching cognitive and problem-solving skills to children not only increases their educational performance, but improves their social skills and behavioral adjustment as well (see, for example, Cowen, 1977; Shure and Spivack, 1972). Seligman's (1975) work on "learned helplessness" emphasizes the importance of mastery and the development of individual competence to cope with unpredictable and uncontrollable events.

In addition to a focus on increasing individual strengths, efforts have been made to describe and test the concept of "community competence." Iscoe (1974) identifies the characteristics of a competent community, which include such processes as the development of a wide range of choices, knowledge about how resources are acquired, and an increased capacity to solve its own problems. Although the person-centered and community-centered competence-promoting programs vary widely in approaches and techniques, they reflect a consistent theme, which can be summarized as "from helplessness to health."

Focusing on the promotion of mental health rather than on the prevention of illness is as much a difference in perspective as it is a departure from much of current prevention practice. In many instances, the interventions used may be very similar. For example, a program that helps people who are about to retire to anticipate and plan for the financial, social, and psychological changes they may face might be conceived as the prevention of a variety of possible disorders, such as depression, physical illness, or marital disruption. Or the emphasis might be on competence building, on increasing persons' capacity to anticipate and deal with a series of life changes that accompany retirement and the phenomenon of growing older in our society. Many of the actual techniques, such as life planning, analysis of leisure-time activities, and financial management, may be similar. The difference in perspective, however, is very important and more than merely a semantic shuffle. Particularly with regard to program evaluation, the burden is shifted from proving that something bad did not happen to demonstration of increased competence and well-being.

The promotion of health perspective provides a way to address directly some of the other barriers to prevention that have plagued the field. For example, lack of public support is frequently cited as a major problem (Broskowski and Baker, 1974). The development of a constituency for the prevention of mental illness is difficult because mental illness is not something that most people can identify with or imagine happening to them. The mentally ill are the "others," and it is unlikely that the public will have much investment in this goal, which is often seen as the domain of specialized experts. The promotion of individual and community competence and health, however, should have a wide appeal.

The evidence for public interest in health promotion and ways to improve the quality of life can be seen in the burgeoning health food and vitamin industry. The popular press is filled with advice about nutrition and how to cope with stress and other problems in living. Increased participation in exercise programs, weight-loss programs, self-help groups, consciousness raising, and personal-growth programs suggests that there is no lack of public interest in health promotion. A challenge for mental health programs, as well as organizations offering remedial services to those on the low-wellness end of the health continuum, appears to be how to increase the extent to which they are seen as centers for mental health.

Mental Health Services Continuum

Increased federal support for primary prevention and mental health promotion activities is a necessary but not sufficient condition for building health promotion and prevention into the fabric of community mental health programs. Fundamental questions about how best to fit prevention and promotion programming into the other tasks and functions of the mental health organization still remain.

The mental health services continuum I propose represents a departure from much of existing thought about prevention practice and program organization. Proponents of a prevention unit that is functionally (and sometimes physically) separate from the clinical or direct service components of the program argue that unless prevention is assigned to a specific staff, clinical demands will crowd out less urgent health promotion and prevention activities. To the extent that special skills are required, training can be more efficiently focused on workers with specialized and full-time prevention assignments. Paralleling this point of view is the argument that specialization results in higher quality of service and that mixing staff functions is confusing and inefficient.

All these concerns may have some basis in fact. The idea of a services continuum does not exclude the possibility of a separate prevention unit and specialized personnel. However, the inclusion of all mental health staff in the goal of increasing the health promotion and prevention focus of the center is necessary. If prevention and promotion are seen as auxiliary functions of the mental health program, we will continue to miss the rich opportunities for health promotion that are encountered daily by those engaged primarily in clinical service. As long as prevention/promotion practice is a vague activity carried out somewhere in the community (outside the community mental health center) by other people on unknown and unseen populations, it will remain a peripheral goal for a majority of mental health staff.

Mental health services can be conceived as a continuum along which specific services or programs can be arranged (see Figure 1). On the far left end of the continuum are direct services provided to individuals, families, and groups. The purpose of these interventions is to change or strengthen the functioning of individuals or family systems. At the far right end of the continuum are services aimed at modifying the physical and social environment of target populations or of the entire community. For the purposes of discussion, this continuum has been divided into four overlapping areas. Two of these areas (A and B) are aimed at individual, group, or family change; and the other two areas (C and D) focus on organizations, neighborhoods, and communities as change targets. The dimensions that may differentiate one area from another include the purpose of the

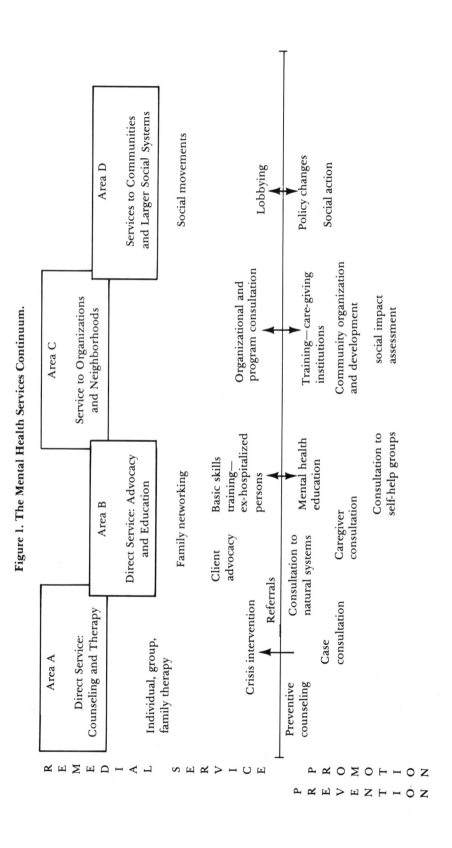

Figure 1. The Mental Health Services Continuum.

service, the size of the target or scope of the service, service methods, and worker roles. Movement from the left extreme of the continuum toward the right end is also generally accompanied by a higher degree of integration of mental health services into ongoing community processes and institutions.

Table 1 illustrates the distinguishing features of each of the four areas along the services continuum. It describes these services in terms of their major purpose or goal; the target population that constitutes the intended beneficiaries of service, both with regard to the number of people affected and the particular target problem involved; the methods or intervention used; the worker skills and roles involved in each type of service; service and program examples; and references to examples in the literature.

The areas overlap somewhat and are not meant to be arbitrary, but rather to illustrate a progression of services that range from those in Area A, which employ individual methods of bringing about changes in individuals, often within the walls of the mental health program, to activities in Area D, which are aimed at changing environmental conditions or reducing stressors that affect large numbers of people.

An advantage of looking at mental health services as a continuum lies in the ability to identify the purposes, methods, worker roles, and skills needed to provide services at each stage. The mental health manager can analyze the current services provided by the organization by locating them along the services continuum and can also project what changes in methods and roles would be necessary to provide service at some different point on the continuum.

Area A Services

The purpose of activities in Area A is to bring about change in individuals, either to solve specific problems or to strengthen individuals' ability to cope with current or future crises. The methods used include a variety of individual or group counseling or educational techniques. Because the services are usually provided by mental health staff specialists located within the mental health facility, they are largely separate from the ongoing life of the community, and the results of the services may be apparent to only a few people.

Examples of mental health services in this category include individual, group, and family therapy and many of the outpatient and inpatient services offered by mental health centers. Case consultation, which focuses on improving the treatment outcome for a specific client, also falls into this general category.

In addition to the many services generally known as treatment services that fall within Area A, a number of other services with a prevention or health promotion purpose, which share these characteristics, have also been developed. These services include such approaches as preventive counseling, crisis intervention, and referrals to other agencies.

Preventive counseling services help clients anticipate and plan for future situations that are known to be difficult for many people. A term frequently used in the prevention literature is "anticipatory guidance." These services are

Table 1. Distinguishing Features of Four Areas Along Continuum.

	Area A	Area B	Area C	Area D
Purpose	Bring about change in, strengthen individuals	Bring about change in, strengthen individuals	Modify environment, reduce stressors	Modify environment, reduce stressors
Target population	Individuals, families	Individuals, populations at risk	All members of a geographic area, organization	All members of a community, region
Methods	Individual, family, and group therapy Individual stress reduction, anticipatory guidance, and so forth	Educational approaches, networking, self-help, workshops, classes	Program consultation, organizational development, community organization	Policy analysis, lobbying, community development, social action
Worker roles	Counselor, broker, consultant	Educator, counselor, broker, mobilizer, consultant, program developer	Mobilizer, advocate, organizer, planner, administrator, consultant	Policy analyst, planner, advocate, researcher, community organizer
Services and program examples	1. *Preventive counseling:* first births, retirement, abortion 2. *Crisis intervention:* trauma, loss, separation, rape 3. *Referral to other agencies:* community support	1. *Consultation with natural support systems:* consult and support through family and friends 2. *Caregiver consultation:* to increase the skills of other providers: police, clergy, teachers 3. *Mental health education:* parent education, life planning 4. *Self-help groups:* kidney dialysis patients, overeaters, alcoholics	1. *Training emergency room personnel:* bereavement—loss for families 2. *Stress training:* teach employees to improve human service delivery 3. *Employee assistance programs:* focused on work stressors 4. Consult on unemployment and economic problem impact	1. Consultation on developing new juvenile code or model health legislation 2. Legislative lobbying for bills improving services or providing additional services
References	Appolone (1978)—Epilepsy Broussard (1976)—High-risk mothers Polak and others (1975)—Families and death	Collins and Pancoast (1976)—Natural helping networks Silverman (1976)—"Widow to widow" programs Vaughan and others (1975)—Family mental health maintenance	Boys (1977)—City employee training Tyler and Dryer (1975)—Social impact assessment	Schanie and Sundel (1978)—Media public education

provided when future events can be predicted, for example, the birth of a child, retirement, terminal illness, last child leaving home (the "empty nest syndrome"), or abortion.

Crisis intervention services are provided to individuals and families who have suffered a traumatic event, such as loss or separation. The purpose of these services is to promote the rapid resolution of the crisis situation, to assist individuals in coping with feelings, decisions, and problems of adjustment related to the event (Polak and others, 1975). Examples of situations in which crisis intervention may be appropriate include the death of a family member or close friend; loss of home, property, or financial security; rape; loss of limb or other serious physical disability; or divorce.

Referral of clients to other social agencies for service may also be a preventive strategy when that referral results in the provision of needed physical and/or psychosocial support that the community mental health program is unable to provide.

Area B Services

Services in Area B have the purpose of bringing about improved functioning of individuals or groups through providing skill building or other educational experiences. What differentiates these services from those in Area A is the greater scope (number of people affected) and an emphasis on reducing the extent to which ongoing leadership from mental health professionals is required. Community integration is enhanced by providing services outside the mental health facility or in collaboration with other community groups or institutions. Area B services often call for additional skills and roles beyond those needed for Area A.

Ketterer, Bader, and Levy (1980) describe three mental health promotion strategies that are primarily Area B activities: consultation to natural support systems, care giver consultation, and mental health education. Work with self-help groups is another important strategy in this area.

Area C Services

The mental health services provided in Area C are primarily aimed at organizational, neighborhood, and community change to create environments that promote growth and reduce stressors on individuals, families, and groups. Program consultation and training programs are frequently used to accomplish these purposes. In addition, advocacy, organizational development, social planning, community development, and community organization may be appropriate strategies.

The staff skills necessary to undertake Area C activities include program consultation skills, knowledge and skills in community organization and community planning, the ability to work with a variety of organizations to respond to community needs that no single organization can meet, and research skills associated with needs assessment, social impact assessment, and other information-organizing strategies.

Area D Services

Area D includes services and intervention that can affect whole communities or regions. Although this area overlaps somewhat with Area C, emphasis is given here to effecting policy changes or intervening in the economic and political sectors of the environment. Also included are community-wide public education efforts involving the media, such as those described by Schanie and Sundel (1978).

Implementing Mental Health Promotion Programs

This discussion of ways to expand mental health promotion services is built around several assumptions about the goals of community mental health programs and about the context within which these programs will be undertaken. I assume that mental health managers will see increased integration of mental health services into community processes and expansion of the scope and impact of services as a desirable outcome. Increasing the number of community members who benefit from mental health services is one way of stretching scarce resources, as well as a way of expanding the "community" emphasis in community mental health. Because there is unlikely to be a substantial increase in funding for mental health services, I also assume that health promotion activities will be carried out largely within current budgets and by existing staff. This formulation also places a large measure of responsibility for providing leadership in shaping the nature of community mental health programs with the mental health manager.

Managerial tasks and activities related to implementing mental health promotion programs include program assessment and planning, building staff, board, and community support, developing funding strategies, and developing an evaluation process.

Assessment and Program Planning

Before program planning is undertaken, a series of preliminary diagnostic tasks should be performed. These include manager's self-assessment of his or her commitment to mental health promotion, analysis of current service patterns, and examination of staff skills and interests in relation to proposed health promotion services. Major program planning tasks include identifying and selecting target populations and developing mental health promotion projects.

Two major purposes are served by an analysis of current service delivery patterns. First, it is necessary to understand "what is" in order to make informed choices about program changes. Program analysis is also one way of identifying areas where current services can be streamlined or consolidated in order to create some "resource slack" that can be used for program change. In particular, some program elements currently provided on an individual basis might be appropriately provided in groups. Services provided to individuals are often the most labor-intensive and the most expensive service mode. Careful analysis of services provided to individuals may suggest places where saving can be realized without sacrificing program quality. Examples of such areas might include components of the intake process that involve gathering or giving routine information, services such as relaxation training, which can be provided to groups of clients, or clients with common problems for whom group services are appropriate. Health promotion opportunities within current programs may also surface during a services assessment.

An assessment of staff interests and skills also serves a dual function. An inventory of staff capabilities and interests provides information for decisions about feasible prevention/promotion projects and training and staff development needs. Participation in the process of developing such an inventory may also increase staff interest and involvement in health promotion planning and program development.

One of the practical questions confronting mental health staff who have generated some ideas about expanding their prevention-promotion practice is how to link those ideas with the people or populations for whom the interventions are developed. Some suggestions for identifying and locating potential recipients of services include using

1. A social-problems approach in which a particular social problem is identified and interventions are designed to reduce the incidence of that problem.
2. A developmental-stage approach involving the identification of persons who are about to enter a life stage or status known to be stressful or problematic.
3. A crisis traumatic-event approach with emphasis on the provision of prompt crisis intervention to persons experiencing traumatic events.
4. An organizational geographic-boundary approach that defines the target population as all persons living or working within a given organization or geographic area.
5. A social-characteristics approach that identifies target populations for prevention and health promotion efforts on the basis of social indicators such as income, race, sex, or age, which have been shown to be correlated with a higher incidence of social problems.

These approaches are elaborated in Table 2.

Project Approach

The process of assessing staff interests and abilities, analyzing current service patterns, and identifying potential target populations may suggest a number of areas where change in emphasis and modes of service delivery are possible. Although major organizational restructuring is one approach to making these changes, it is likely to be too disruptive, to create a considerable amount of staff resistance, and is generally very difficult to manage. For these reasons, a project approach to increasing the prevention/promotion focus of the mental health organization can be a useful strategy. The project approach involves two major components: restructuring of job descriptions and expectations for individual

Table 2. Approaches to Identifying Target Populations.

Approach	Method	Examples	Advantages	Limitations
Social Problems	Persons are identified as being "at risk" of developing a particular disorder or social problem	Substance abuse Delinquency Child abuse Depression	Appeal to cause-effect logic Congruence with categorical funding practices Provides focus for developing special-interest group support	Difficulty of predicting problems in advance Dangers of inappropriate labeling Inadequate knowledge about causation Lack of tested interventions Evaluation barriers May be inefficient—persons who do not need them may receive services
Developmental Stage	Persons are identified as about to enter a life stage, or status, known to be stressful or problematic for many	Entry into school or work force Parenthood Last child leaving home Retirement	Labeling is minimized; emphasis on universal life transitions Emphasis on increasing competence; deemphasis on problem development Identification of potential service recipients relatively straightforward Growing research and intervention literature	Lacks appeal of problem prevention May not fit funding categories Eligibility/service recipient criteria decisions may be difficult May be inefficient—services may be provided to people who do not need them
Crisis/Traumatic Event	Individuals experiencing traumatic events are identified as target population	Sudden bereavement Rape Physical disability Separation or loss	Crisis intervention methods are well developed Special-interest group support often available Identification of potential service recipients relatively straightforward	Lack of trained personnel Complexity increased by need to collaborate with "front line" agencies (for example, police, hospitals)
Organizational/Geographic Boundary	All persons within an organization or geographic boundary constitute target population	Organizational change: schools, daycare centers, hospital emergency rooms Social impact assessment Community intervention: Unemployment Plant closing High crime or illness rates	Broad impact intervention with social system may benefit many members Labeling of individuals is avoided Circumscribed geographic area promotes focus, identification of members, residents	Specific goals/results may be difficult to define, identify; possible resistance from those with investment in status quo Effective interventions not well developed Evaluation difficulties related to unclear goals
Social Characteristics	Target populations identified on basis of social indicators (for example, sex, age, race, income) known to be correlated with high incidence of social problems, disorders	Special programs for women, AFDC recipients, elderly, children, minority group members	High visibility of target groups Often congruent with categorical funding Special-interest group support can be developed	Inappropriate labeling; goals/service recipients/impact may be difficult to identify May be inefficient Effective interventions not well developed Evaluation barriers

workers and planning and implementing a series of small, short-term projects within service units or at the agency level.

The importance of restructuring individual work assignments, job descriptions, and performance evaluation mechanisms cannot be overemphasized. Including the expectation that staff will devote time and energy to prevention/promotion activities is a sign that the agency administration is serious about such a change. It is also supportive of staff efforts because it legitimizes and makes central many activities that may have been seen previously as extra or peripheral, "not really a part of my job."

The expectations should be specific, perhaps in terms of number of hours per week, or they may be identified as specific activities where it is possible to identify assignments in advance. In order to maximize the extent to which staff will be investing in increased prevention/promotion activities, administrative expectations should be made clear. The expectation that staff will increase the level of prevention activity in their work load is taken as a given and is therefore largely nondiscretionary. Decisions about what activities to undertake, and the planning and implementation of these projects, however, should involve the full participation of staff, who can structure their activities around problem areas in which they have an interest and investment. This approach provides staff with an opportunity for professional development congruent with their own goals and needs.

At the unit or agency level, realistic short-term projects allow workers a chance to try out approaches they can undertake without a major long-term commitment of agency resources. Projects should be designed so that they can be feasibly managed within current staff abilities so they are not initially overwhelming. Short-term projects also have the advantage of providing relatively immediate feedback and a sense of accomplishment.

The nature of projects selected will vary with organizational circumstances and with staff interests and resources. One approach is to have individual staff members identify activities each will emphasize. For example, a staff member with an interest in promoting self-help or mutual aid groups for widows might contract to spend time visiting existing programs, gathering information about community resources, and planning for an individual project he or she could develop. Analysis of the issues faced by current and past clients may reveal common interests and needs that could be served by developing mutual aid groups initiated by mental health staff, but designed to become self-sustaining, with a small amount of consultation and support from staff.

It is likely that most of the projects developed by clinical staff will include activities involving services delivered to individuals, groups, and families, that is, those in Areas A and B of the services continuum. Expansion of activities from those in Area A involving current staff skills, and services provided within the center, to clinical, preventive, or health promotion activities provided in community settings will be no small step for many staff members. Persons who undertake projects that call for establishing collaborative relationships with other agencies and learning new skills and service methods will require considerable administrative encouragement, guidance, and support. This support may take a variety of forms, such as paving the way with other agency administrators, protection of time necessary to undertake projects, direct supervision or consultation, and provision of staff training opportunities.

Building Board and Community Support for Mental Health Promotion

The mental health manager's commitment to primary prevention and health promotion as an important and legitimate activity is the first necessary ingredient in obtaining support from the agency advisory or governing body. The manager must be able to provide concrete examples and plans and to project what these changes would mean for clients, for staff, and for relevant segments of the community. Maintaining an emphasis on health promotion and on increasing the visibility and relevance of the community at large is an important strategy.

Funding Strategies

The basic thrust of earlier suggestions for increasing the mental health program's activities in the prevention/promotion area has been reallocative, a realignment of service categories, and program emphases within the existing agency budget. The suggestions offered do not wholly involve "robbing Peter to pay Paul." Rather, an emphasis on group services rather than individual services where possible and maximizing professional impact by the development of service strategies that build in continuing nonagency support are advocated. Rueveni's (1979) family networking approach is an example of such a strategy.

In addition to realigning existing service delivery patterns, other resource-generating approaches include increasing reimbursement for prevention/promotion activities, locating alternative funding sources, increasing in-kind contributions, and developing joint programs with other community groups and organizations.

Evaluation of Prevention/Promotion Services

The need for evaluation of mental health programs in general and prevention/promotion programs in particular is a political (program survival) issue and is required in order to advance the effectiveness of mental health practice. Heller, Price, and Sher (1980) point out that some advocates of prevention may feel that a double standard is applied; the difficulties of evaluating prevention programs are highlighted while the questionable efficacy of much of clinical practice is ignored. Different standards *are* applied to prevention programs because they are relatively new, they are not rooted in the tradition of specific clinical disciplines, and they may be more difficult to justify to funding sources and the public because they are not aimed at immediate, visible problems.

The difficulty of engaging in long-term research, however, does not preclude mental health programs from conducting program evaluation studies that can contribute to the accumulating pool of knowledge about the process and outcomes of prevention practice. Heller, Price, and Sher (1980, p. 303) suggest that three major prevention components must be specified: the prevention target, consisting of the populations at risk and/or the risk situations that are expected to lead to vulnerability; the program or intervention, consisting of person- and/or environmental-oriented procedures to reduce vulnerability; and the expected outcomes.

The intended recipients of prevention/promotion interventions must be clearly identified. Prevention programs may be aimed at specific vulnerable populations or be focused on changing specific target situations. In each case, individuals constitute the ultimate target population, but, in the first instance, persons are identified as high risk because of specific population characteristics such as sex, age, race, family history, or economic status. In the second case, target situations known to be associated with higher risk are emphasized. For example, Heller, Price, and Sher (1980) note that well-controlled studies indicate that death, divorce, or separation from spouse places individuals at risk for both physical and psychological disability.

The evaluation process should be able to answer the following questions:

1. What specific end state is to be prevented or promoted?
2. What interventions could be expected to contribute to the reduced incidence of problems or improved positive outcomes?
3. Was the intervention successfully implemented?
4. What changes occurred as a result of the intervention? Were expected changes achieved? What other unanticipated changes were noted?
5. Were there any changes in nearby systems?
6. What were the financial, social, and political costs associated with the intervention?

The careful evaluation of prevention/promotion programs serves three major purposes: to contribute to program survival by increasing accountability for resources expended in this area, to improve program quality through the identification of useful and effective programs and interventions that should be retained and by pinpointing less useful or cost-effective program components that need modification, to add to the general knowledge base of prevention practice. In this regard, it is necessary to describe what was done, to whom, with what effect *and* to make that information available for other researchers and practitioners working in the prevention/promotion area through program reports or published program descriptions. Information about unsuccessful programs and description of the difficulties encountered in implementing prevention interventions is valuable and too often is not added to the existing knowledge pool.

Conclusion

This discussion of primary prevention in community mental health programs has included a brief history and examination of major conceptual approaches to mental health prevention programming. It is suggested that health promotion is a useful concept around which to organize local program development and mental health practice. Suggestions for implementing health promotion services in community mental health programs include attention to planning tasks, methods for building board and community support, and evaluation issues.

This treatment of primary-prevention practice is based on the belief that health promotion activities in mental health programs should and can be expanded and that mental health managers must provide the necessary leadership and impetus toward that end. Increasing the extent to which community mental health programs are centers for mental health rather than centers for mental illness requires a change in perspective and the involvement of all mental health staff in the development of an organizational prevention "ethos," or habit of thinking and working. Suggestions for achieving the goal of integrating health promotion practice into the fabric of mental health services include the use of a mental health services continuum as a tool for the assessment and planning of services. Because increased individual and community competence cannot be achieved through the efforts of the mental health system alone, collaborative efforts with other organizations and community interest groups are also emphasized.

References

Appolone, C. "Preventive Social Work Intervention with Families of Children with Epilepsy." *Social Work in Health Care,* 1978, *4* (2), 139–148.

Bloom, B. L. *Community Mental Health: A General Introduction.* Monterey, Calif.: Brooks/Cole, 1977.

Bloom, B. L. "Prevention of Mental Disorders: Recent Advances in Theory and Practice." *Community Mental Health Journal,* 1979, *15* (3), 179–191.

Boys, G. A. "A Systems Approach to Primary Prevention." Unpublished paper, Portland, Ore., 1977.

Broskowski, A., and Baker, F. "Professional, Organizational, and Social Barriers to Primary Prevention." *American Journal of Orthopsychiatry,* 1974, *44* (5), 707–719.

Broussard, E. R. "Primary Prevention Program for Newborn Infants at High Risk for Emotional Disorder." In D. C. Klein and S. E. Goldston (Eds.), *Primary Prevention: An Idea Whose Time Has Come.* Washington, D.C.: U.S. Department of Health, Education, and Welfare, 1976.

Collins, A., and Pancoast, D. *Natural Helping Networks: A Strategy for Prevention.* New York: National Association of Social Workers, 1976.

Cowen, E. "Baby Steps Toward Primary Prevention." *American Journal of Community Psychology,* 1977, *5* (1), 1–22.

Dohrenwend, B. P., and Dohrenwend, B. S. "Social and Cultural Influences on Psychopathology." *Annual Review of Psychology,* 1974a, *25,* 417–452.

Dohrenwend, B. P., and Dohrenwend, B. S. (Eds.). *Stressful Life Events: Their Nature and Effects.* New York: Wiley, 1974b.

Heller, K., Price, R. H., and Sher, K. J. "Research and Evaluation in Primary Prevention." In R. H. Price and others (Eds.), *Prevention in Mental Health.* Beverly Hills, Calif.: Sage, 1980.

Iscoe, I. "Community Psychology and the Competent Community." *American Psychologist,* 1974, *29,* 607-613.

Kessler, M., and Albee, G. "Primary Prevention." *Annual Review of Psychology,* 1975, *26,* 557-591.

Ketterer, R. F., Bader, B. C., and Levy, M. R. "Strategies and Skills for Promoting Mental Health." In R. H. Price and others (Eds.), *Prevention in Mental Health.* Beverly Hills, Calif.: Sage, 1980.

Perlmutter, F. D., and Vayda, A. M. "Barriers to Prevention Programs in Community Mental Health Centers." *Administration in Mental Health,* 1978, *5* (2), 140-153.

Polak, P., and others. "Prevention in Mental Health: A Controlled Study." *American Journal of Psychiatry,* 1975, *132* (2), 146-149.

Rahe, R. H., and Holmes, T. H. "Life Crisis and Major Health Change." *Psychosomatic Medicine,* 1966, *28,* 774.

Rueveni, U. *Networking Families in Crisis.* New York: Human Sciences Press, 1979.

Schanie, C., and Sundel, M. "A Community Mental Health Innovation in Mass Media Preventive Education: The Alternatives Project." *American Journal of Community Psychology,* 1978, *6* (6), 573-581.

Seligman, M. E. P. *Helplessness.* San Francisco: W. H. Freeman, 1975.

Selye, H. *The Stress of Life.* New York: McGraw-Hill, 1956.

Shure, M. B., and Spivack, G. "Means-Ends Thinking, Adjustment and Social Class Among Elementary School-Aged Children." *Journal of Consulting and Clinical Psychology,* 1972, *38,* 348-353.

Silverman, P. R. "Mutual Help Groups for the Widowed." In D. C. Klein and S. E. Goldston (Eds.), *Primary Prevention: An Idea Whose Time Has Come.* Washington, D.C.: U.S. Department of Health, Education, and Welfare, 1976.

Snow, D. L., and Newton, P. M. "Task, Social Structure, and Social Progress in the Community Mental Health Center Movement." *American Psychologist,* 1976, *31* (8), 582-594.

Tyler, J., and Dryer, S. "Planning Primary Prevention Strategy: A Survey of the Effects of Business Location on Indian Reservation Life." *American Journal of Community Psychology,* 1975, *3* (1), 69-76.

Vaughan, W., and others. "Family Mental Health Maintenance: A New Approach to Primary Prevention." *Hospital and Community Psychiatry,* 1975, *26* (8), 503-508.

❦ 31 ❧

Rural
Mental Health
Services

Ellen Russell Dunbar

Managers need to understand the relationship between the special qualities of rural life and the administration of mental health programs (for example, hiring persons who genuinely like rural people, giving staff adequate travel budgets, providing opportunities for professional growth, building budgets on the basis of local fiscal and human resources, and utilizing outside technical assistance and consultation from local and state officials). Because each rural setting is unique, program managers need to assess the special characteristics of their rural community and to be certain that their administrative styles fit rural mental health program needs.

Most rural settings are small places in big spaces, small systems covering large areas. Both the smallness and the largeness of rural places create special challenges for the mental health administrator, different from those faced by urban colleagues. Challenges are also created by the visibility of life in rural places and by cultures of rural areas. The high degree of visibility in which the rural mental health administrator must work creates unique service and organizational issues. There is not any one rural culture, but rural cultures are different from urban cultures. Both have great variation from one neighborhood, community, or region to another; yet each seems to merge into something that is either urban or rural.

Rural is not synonymous with disadvantaged, although recent efforts to bring attention to the problems of rural areas have emphasized disadvantaged rural populations (Flax and others, 1979; Schott, 1980; Weber, 1976). Rural people are very proud of their life-styles, and few would willingly trade for urban living. Likewise, rural mental health services are not poor sisters of urban mental health services, needing to be enriched with urban perspectives. It is, however, a relatively new institution still in the developmental stages. Mental health professionals are now learning about and adapting to the rural environment as they build programs to meet the specific and unique needs of the rural setting.

It is difficult to agree on a definition of rural. The U.S. Census Bureau defines any place with a population of 2,500 or less as rural and divides that between farm and nonfarm. A Standard Metropolitan Statistical Area (SMSA) is a county or group of contiguous counties that contain at least one, or part of a, city with a population of 50,000 or more. All other areas would, by elimination, be nonmetropolitan. These definitions overlap in that a town of 1,000 could be within a county designated as SMSA. Definitions of rural also vary in terms of the great diversity from one region to another and from one town to another (Flax and others, 1979). For this discussion, rural is defined as any area under 50,000 (nonmetropolitan) with sufficient distance from a metropolitan area to have separate traditions and human service systems.

This chapter describes three characteristics of rural areas that have relevance to mental health administration: size, visibility, and culture. Each of these will be related to the administrative functions of mental health, including service delivery, organizational maintenance, and professional advancement.

Characteristics of Rural Areas

Size

The low population density of nonmetropolitan areas generally results in small agencies, small budgets, small numbers of clients, and small staffs. Each staff person needs to be able to carry out a variety of different functions. Small agencies with small budgets do not have the flexibility to meet unexpected expenses. Small agencies divert people rather than money; if staff members are already overloaded with essential assignments, the administrator fills in with direct services tasks.

When the population is small, there are only a few individuals with any particular mental health problem in spite of the fact that the occurrence of mental illness appears to be greater in rural than in urban areas (Husaini and Neff, 1977; Mazer, 1976; Schwab, Warheit, and Holzer, 1972; Srole, 1972). Mental health staff persons are required to be generalists, prepared to handle "one of each" of a wide variety of presenting case situations, diagnoses, or involuntary commitments to the state hospitals. They need to be prepared to approach openly any situation, be it psychosis, incest, or adolescent rebellion, to begin the helping process. It is often difficult to find and recruit people with adequate experience and training to handle generalist practice.

Small organizations are less formal than large ones. There is less need to put things in writing because there is more opportunity for interpersonal communication. It can be seen as an insult to "put in writing" something that could be informally communicated to a staff person in the next office. It does not seem important to engage in case recording for clients who have been neighbors for several years. The informality of small organizations can conflict with the need for state and national organizations to maintain accountability for services and finances.

Although agencies and towns are small, the geographic area between towns may be quite large. Large rural catchment areas can reflect distances of 100 or 200 miles between the agency and the clients. It is difficult to respond to an emergency call when it comes from 150 miles away. Even routine services may require the client or mental health professional to travel some distance at a considerable cost in time and automobile expense.

The smallness of rural communities and the vastness of rural areas require different models of mental health service delivery and agency operation than those used in the metropolitan areas. State and federal mental health agencies often view rural areas with an attitude of superiority and demand conformity to urban service delivery approaches. The rural administrator must continuously negotiate between the expectations of the urban-oriented funding agencies and the organizational and service realities of small communities.

Visibility

Mental health agencies and professionals are highly visible in a small town. That visibility affects both personal life and professional practice. Professionals whose life-style is not compatible with the culture of the community may have a difficult time adjusting to life in the community or being accepted by the community. They may find they need to leave town periodically in order to enjoy a different life-style, or they may choose to do as they please, regardless of public attitudes, and thereby risk community rejection.

Likewise, professional practice is very visible. Word travels quickly about one's professional competence, incompetence, arrogance, or stupidity. Professional and personal life cannot be separated, as it can in an urban area. Even if immediate neighbors and friends are not clients, the professional will see clients in the market, at PTA meetings, in church, or in the next booth at the county fair. Visibility also creates difficulties for clients. Potential clients may stay away from mental health centers out of fear of being "discovered."

Culture

Although there are living experiences common to small towns, referred to as "rural culture," the differences within and among rural communities and population groups are greater than the commonalities. Any study of rural culture is limited to one or a few rural places or regions. For example, Hassinger and Whiting (1976) concluded that rural culture is related to agriculture, a finding that has little relevance to the towns that have depended upon mining for their economic base for several generations.

Research suggests that rural values emphasize subjugation to nature, fatalism, an orientation to concrete places and things, a view of human nature as basically evil, and an emphasis on primary relationships and family ties (Burdge and Rogers, 1972). Rural areas have also been described as having rigid, closed societies that are politically conservative and generally not open to new people or new ideas (Hassinger and Whiting, 1976; Reynolds, Banks, and Murphee, 1976). Any of these observations may or may not be true in a given locality. Therefore, it is important that all mental health managers undertake their own studies of the communities in which they live and work. Community values and culture provide guidelines for behavior and ways of seeing solutions for problems posed by the environment and the requirements of the social system (Flax and others, 1979). Values directly influence the community's response to mental health professionals and agencies.

Rural people relate to others on a personal, informal level rather than on a formal organizational level. The mental health professional gains acceptance and legitimacy as a person, rather than acquiring it when hired into an agency role. Some of that legitimacy may carry over to the agency, but not to other staff members. Each person must earn legitimacy through personal and professional behavior, on a person-to-person basis (Washington Human Resource Development Task Force, 1981). Research does not provide sufficient information regarding the criteria used by a rural community for making a judgment of an individual. Persons who have grown up in a rural community are socialized to know how those judgments are made. The newcomer needs to ask, observe, and listen rather than make assumptions based upon generalizations about rural attitudes. Again, community culture provides the guidelines for implementing effective mental health programs.

For example, rural communities informally regulate life's pace. Practitioners in rural areas often speak of "timing." Although urban life maintains a more or less regular rate of speed, rural communities are more likely to respond to the seasons or to the pace of nature (Luther, 1981). Sometimes, but not always, the pace of life is related to practical needs, such as harvesting or planting, or the ability to get over the mountain passes in winter. Other times it is style or manner. For example, some urban trained professionals need to learn how to talk more slowly if they do not want to "turn off" rural people.

Racism related to rural minority groups has not received sufficient research attention. There are myths that rural people are more racist than urban people. If racism were to be viewed in the context of living standards and conditions of poverty, rural minorities frequently suffer more than urban minorities due to unavailable and inaccessible services and the extent of rural poverty. In addition, geography plays an important role in the frequency of contacts between minorities and nonminorities. It is easier to avoid direct personal contact with racist whites in an urban area large enough for blacks, Indians, Chicanos, or Asians to develop separate institutions and social networks. Minorities in small communities may be more socially isolated and can experience profound rejection from individuals, social clubs, youth groups, churches, and other local organizations. Even within one community, different minorities may experience different treatment. The diversity of experience includes isolated migrant camps, midwestern farm towns that have no minorities, southwestern communities where Chicanos are in the majority, and northwestern counties comprised of Indian reservations and "white territory."

Whatever the culture of the particular rural community or how much it may differ from an urban area, it is likely to be transmitted directly rather than through formalized institutions. Mental health services are viewed and assessed in terms of the staff who provide the services rather than the reputation of the agency. The smallness, the visibility, and the personal nature of the relationships within rural communities influence the administration of mental health programs.

Service Delivery Issues In
Small Communities and Agencies

The small number of clients, small budgets, and limited resources call for adaptations and creative new approaches to providing mental health care and treatment (Huessy, 1972). Small communities cannot afford specialists to meet every need, and there is not sufficient demand. So rural practitioners need to be generalists. Mental health administrators must recruit and assign staff within small budgets in order to serve a small number of clients who reflect a wide variety of problems and live in far distant places.

It is difficult to recruit professional staff who are truly prepared to function as generalists. With few exceptions, graduate programs in the core mental health disciplines tend to promote specialist training. The rural administrator must often resort to hiring people without graduate training and preparing them with on-the-job training. Frequently, specialists are hired and either learn to adapt to the demands for generalist practice or return to the urban environment.

"Generalist," like "rural," is difficult to define. It is unlikely that one can find persons who can do everything extremely well or who know all one needs to know about a range of mental health problems. However, generalists are able to provide service in a wide variety of situations based on their skills in assessment, relationship building, and treatment planning. The client may be an individual, family, group, or community (Dunbar, in press). The generalist must reflect a flexible and open approach to a wide range of problems and situations. In addition, mental health staff need experience with different age groups and a variety of problems. Professionals who have specialized in one area, such as child psychology, gerontology, or drug abuse, may need considerable retraining and may find the adaptation difficult. The generalist practitioner needs to upgrade knowledge and skills continuously. For example, the mental health professional is frequently the only person in a rural community with any knowledge of psychotropic drugs, and therefore periodic training sessions are needed to update drug and diagnostic information. Local physicians and nurses should be included to enhance the overall capacity of the community.

Mental health professionals also need skills in assessing community life in order to utilize local resources effectively. For example, the practitioner needs to know the economics, politics, traditions, organizations, and informal networks in order to work effectively in the rural areas. These skills may be developed by the staff through periodic community needs assessments (Lamb, 1977; Warren, 1978).

To provide adequate service to far-flung rural people requires that staff move out of the offices to the places where people live. Many centers or agencies have set up satellite offices in the various small towns in their region (U.S. Department of Health, Education, and Welfare, 1978). Those satellite offices may be staffed by one person full time or by several staff for a day or a half day each week. The mode of staffing may depend upon staff members' interests and skills and the needs and size of the town. Some areas use circuit-riding specialists, such as a child psychologist visiting each town one day a week and the geriatric specialist on another day per week. A community needs assessment in each town would help determine what staffing arrangement is most desirable.

Because time and money are required for staff to travel, it is essential that mental health administrators budget for both. If travel time is not recognized as a legitimate and rewardable effort, staff members will become discouraged and burn out. The administrator needs to negotiate and advocate for recognition of travel needs, as well as the problems that occur when clients do not show up for appointments because of transportation difficulties. Staff travel efficiency has been increased by workers who carry tape recorders for dictating client records or for listening to training tapes while they are driving. Frequent regular intrastaff communication regarding travel plans can facilitate exchanges that may reduce the numbers of trips per person (Cedar and Salasin, 1979). Travel that is encouraged and supported can be exhilarating and morale building for staff members who are out interacting with people and involved in the total environment of the clients and their support system.

Visibility

Urban-oriented practice assumes an ability to maintain anonymity from clients when away from work, but the rural practitioner is visible to clients and nonclients at any time. Clients, too, are visible, and this visibility may affect the handling of staff assignments, confidentiality, and the care with which treatment decisions are made. Clients may worry about being seen entering a mental health center. There are times when practitioners meet clients in a neutral place, such as a local coffee shop, where they could be having a visit rather than "therapy." Many small town mental health agencies do not include the term "mental health" in their title, but use less specific names such as Community Service Center.

The administrator needs to maintain an atmosphere of flexibility and openness to various alternatives of case assignment. It is customary to refer clients to staff members where no prior relationship or knowledge existed. However, this is not always possible in small agencies. Advocating for the complete separation of personal life and professional therapeutic relationships is not realistic in rural practice. Where there is only one therapist, that person will help anyone who needs help. When there is more than one, they can agree on a referral policy that is feasible and relevant to the work situation.

Awareness of visibility also needs to be reflected in a rigid adherence to the principle of client confidentiality, especially in small towns, where community opinion is felt very directly. "Leaked" information can have a profound impact on a person's or family's life and can be very damaging. Once the confidentiality is broken, information travels quickly in the community and trust can be lost. The urban professional can probably get away with discussing confidential information with friends and family by disguising the name because the social and geographic distance is sufficiently great to protect the client from being known. This is not true in the small town, where even family members need to learn how to maintain confidentiality by not asking questions and by resisting the temptation to pass along information picked up on the "grapevine."

Administrators sensitive to the significance of maintaining confidentiality, especially written material, need to remind staff periodically to be alert to any slips in conversation and to orient clerical maintenance and volunteer staff to the importance of confidentiality. For example, in one town, people did not want to come to the agency because the secretary was "known to talk."

As a result, administrators need to be alert to the local reputations of potential employees.

Treatment success and failure are both visible. Visibility can work to the advantage and disadvantage of a program. Staff members new to a rural area need to proceed with caution by seeking advice from local residents, controlling enthusiasm for new ideas, and not being in a hurry to demonstrate competence. The rewards of client satisfaction and appreciation come in due time. When staff persons try to push new ideas without waiting to develop relationships or build some credibility and sense of timing, they get discouraged by what they perceive as resistance to change. What they are really facing is the fact that their actions are so visible that misstatements or insensitivities demonstrating a lack of knowledge of the community cannot be hidden. Every statement or behavior is out in the open to be judged by all, and therefore a little caution in the beginning is wise.

Mental health program managers need to orient new staff members to the wisdom of moving slowly at first. Experienced persons can be very helpful in this orientation process by demonstrating appropriate behavior as part of a nonthreatening staff team effort. In some agencies, new staff members work directly with an experienced worker for a period of time until they gain familiarity with the community and the agency. Unfortunately, many agency administrators feel that they cannot afford the staff time involved in two people working together; so they place new staff persons in the community to sink or swim. This unwise and inefficient deployment process can result in early staff burnout, as well as damaged agency public relations.

Rural Cultures

If an agency is to provide a service that will be acceptable and useful to people in rural areas, it will need to be creative in developing new approaches to service delivery. Community mental health staff are still struggling to move beyond the use of traditional "fifty-minute hours" requiring the client to come to an office. Although this approach works in some areas, it is not necessarily the preferred method of service delivery in rural areas. The personal, direct nature of relationships in rural communities requires that services be offered informally. As noted earlier, legitimacy is given to the professional rather than to the agency. Work relationships are also more informal, especially in relationship to opportunities to relate to colleagues outside the workplace (Eisenhart and Ruff, 1980). Staff members need a thorough knowledge of community customs and sense of timing, as well as an acquaintance with key citizens. Similarly, services to minorities need to be relevant to group customs and community expectations.

The professional person is legitimated after demonstrating competence and a willingness to be a full member of the community. The warm, friendly acceptance of people and their life-style is frequently gained by participating in community events, such as making floats for the community's favorite parade. Acceptance also comes from living a life-style that fits within the range of acceptable behavior in that community.

Mental health administrators establish their own legitimacy and provide the structure that will enable staff members to do the same. The structure would include staff assignments that give them opportunities to be in the community, such as participating in the Lions Club or giving a workshop on child abuse for elementary schoolteachers and medical professionals (Conklin, 1980). The need for staff members to meet community members is consistent with the agency goals of good public relations and the promotion of preventive, consultative, and educational services. Administrators need to match staff competencies and preferences with the interests and needs of community groups and organizations. For example, a county mental health agency had experienced a complete staff turnover, including the director. Three years later a city council member noted, with considerable doubt, that the mental health professionals did not seem competent, despite the observation that the likable director appeared to be doing the best he could. Although on further inspection it appeared that the staff members were competent, they had not been out into the community, but had been sitting in their offices doing therapy. The director apparently thought it would be sufficient for him to establish a public image and had not developed opportunities for staff to do the same.

Community activities need to be recognized and supported by administrators as well as delegated to staff. Brief reports will help the administrator keep up on community matters and will let the staff persons know that their efforts are recognized. Statistical reports need to include time spent at community events or talking with community people. A periodic report to the agency's board of directors from each staff person will give added significance to staff effort and will keep the board informed. While establishing and maintaining legitimacy, the staff is building knowledge and identity with the community culture. With this knowledge, they can better develop creative programs to meet local mental health needs.

Outreach to Minorities

Rural mental health agencies often find it difficult to reach out to the minority people in their service area. It is difficult to face the realities of racism and the fact that traditional approaches to therapy may not be relevant for rural minorities. The administrative task is to find ways to stimulate sensitive, relevant agency outreach. The direct expressions of racism can be confronted when planning outreach activities by hiring minority consultants and trainers to assist in building the capacity of local agencies to serve minorities (Washington Human Resource Development Task Force, 1981).

Some agencies have established satellite offices in neighborhoods or communities where many minorities live and hired minority staff members to provide services. The advantage of this approach is that services can be provided without having to overcome the barriers between Anglo staff and minority clients. The disadvantage is the tendency for that satellite to lose contact with the main office, lose status, and acquire fewer resources than other agency programs. In some communities, it is feasible to contract for mental health services with minority agencies, such as Indian tribal councils. The issues of confidentiality, acting with care and caution, knowing the culture, and personalizing the community contacts apply to service delivery with minority as well as Anglo rural populations.

Organization Maintenance

Small mental health organizations experience different administrative problems than large and complex organizations. Those problems are often exaggerated by state and national funding sources, which expect rural agencies to perform like miniversions of a large urban bureaucracy. Administrative problems are also complicated by the need to spread their services across large geographic areas and to perform many different functions.

One rural administrator, during a budget-cutting period, became fond of saying, "Ten percent of nothing is still nothing." Small budgets usually do not have flexibility. Staff turnover in a large agency provides the administrator with some reserve funds that can be used to cover deficits in other areas or for additional consultants, training sessions, or food for a client. Turnover may provide some budgetary relief in a small agency, too, but not without significant impact on staff work loads and client services. Small agencies must work even harder to budget for unexpected contingencies and special needs.

Most rural areas do not have the tax resources or philanthropic institutions that are available in industrialized metropolitan centers. Cities of 20,000 to 50,000 may have a United Way agency and may have a tradition of supporting some mental health services in private agencies, but this is not likely to be true in small towns. Most mental health services have been initiated within the past ten years as a result of federal intervention through the Community Mental Health Centers

Act of 1963 (PL 88–164). There is no tradition of local financial support for these services, and mental health administrators usually have few fund-raising skills. There is usually a potential reservoir of local financial support if administrators are able to develop good community relations. However, even with the maximum development of available resources, rural agency budgets will be small, and the administrative challenge is to maximize limited resources.

The most common method of working within small budgets has been to hire persons who have not completed professional degrees and pay them low salaries. With good in-service training and an intuitive ability to help others, many of these staff members perform excellent work, but few would advocate this approach. Other administrators stretch budgets with imaginative approaches to service delivery (Hagebak, 1980). For example, in one mining town, a mental health worker negotiated with the union and the mine owners to help support alcohol and family counseling programs. In other communities, outreach and prevention services have been developed by training local hairdressers, bartenders, and teachers to increase their ability to give emotional support to customers and to make appropriate referrals.

Budget Planning Process

Budget planning can be another headache, especially when the required forms were developed for use in a large organization that employs sufficient clerical and bookkeeping personnel to complete them. Small-agency directors and staff must take service delivery time to complete these forms and also must handle the criticism from funding sources when forms are not adequately prepared. Some of these problems can be averted by requesting technical assistance and on-site visitations from state and federal funding agency representatives. If the people who develop the forms become involved in helping small agencies comply with regulations, they might gain a better understanding of rural service delivery and translate new insights into more realistic reporting processes.

Agency boards need to be involved in the budget planning process, and administrators need to educate board members by identifying the purpose and rationale of financial reporting requirements. The following process for board involvement can be adapted to unique agency needs. It should begin with an explanation of the process and the role of board and staff in that process because board members may lack experience and have questions about the nature of their responsibilities.

	Staff	Board
Step 1: Assess Needs and Resources		
Evaluate achievements	X	X
Identify changes in community or client population	X	X
Review resources available	X	X
Step 2: Choose Goals and Priorities		
Input	X	X
Decision		X

	Staff	Board
Step 3: Prepare Budget		
Determine costs of goals and present to board	X	
Review, make any decisions, approve		X
Step 4: Budget Review		
Present reports of expenditure	X	X
Review financial report and budget and revise if necessary		X

When the planning process is understood, it can be initiated by staff members describing current programs to the board, including the extent to which last year's objectives have been accomplished. The agency administrator explains the financial picture, including grants and other funding sources, in order to identify budgetary flexibility, limitations, and the range of alternatives. The second step involves board and staff collaboration in developing program goals and/or altering previous goals. The third step is handled by the administrator in writing specific and measurable program objectives to achieve the goals, along with a proposed budget. The proposed budget and program plan is presented to the board for review and approval. The fourth and final step involves the board in budget review and monitoring throughout the year.

Participation in this planning process will help the board in a rural community identify with the decisions, interpret program and cost in the community, and prepare to give general support to the agency. Some administrators are reluctant to get the board too involved, fearing that they will not be able to interpret the complexity of the requirements or that they may lose some control of the budgeting process. Some agencies have used outside consultants to help build a productive executive-board relationship and thereby allay fear and confusion.

Formalizing Records

Formalization of records is an inevitable necessity in today's modern, complex society, even though it may not directly benefit small rural programs. State and federal agencies need certain types of information to aid them in decisions about fund distribution. Often when information is sent to state offices, it is like dropping it in a deep, dark hole. It is never heard of again; so local agencies do not benefit. From the state level, it seems impossible to get all the local agencies to collect data consistently. Consultation from state and federal administration is needed in order to comply with record management requirements. In addition, rural administrators need to request feedback on data they send to funding agencies.

In a similar fashion, administrators need to involve staff in a discussion of the type of information that could be useful to improving their practice or helping to distribute work assignments. They also might discuss what they would want to know about other programs, as well as from the record-keeping requirements of funding agencies. For example, the staff of a county mental health program was concerned with the difference in services provided to people living at great distances from the office. They decided to record travel distance and response time to emergency calls. They were then able to determine whether distance from the agency affected their decision to go out to see the client and how long it took before the client was seen. The fact that rural areas have been slow to formalize their records does not mean that they are "backward and illiterate," but only that such formalization was not a necessity until the local organization became a part of the larger, more complex mental health system.

Rural mental health administrators are frequently frustrated by the accountability requirements of state and federal agencies. The small populations in rural areas do not allow for the development of a wide range of services; yet federal guidelines for resource allocation all flow through rigid access channels that tend to deny the realities of rural life (President's Commission on Mental Health, 1978). An administrator in a rural area needs to find the balance needed to satisfy funding requirements and maintain a sense of independence and local control. This can be encouraged by gaining local financial commitment to programs that are mandated but are also relevant to local needs, engaging board and staff in consideration of local needs and advocating for them when they differ from funding guidelines, local fund raising for programs not included in state or federal guidelines, inviting representatives from state and national organizations to participate in dialogue of local needs, and participating with other small agencies to lobby for variations that will be relevant for rural programs.

Generalist Support Staff

Small organizations need not only generalist practitioners to provide client services, but also generalist support staff to maintain the organizations. The receptionist, intake worker, typist, and bookkeeper may all be the same person. Support staff must be able to meet and talk with clients, maintain records, type, answer the phone, and manage correspondence. They also often act as consultants on community culture, customs, and politics. The support staff is the backbone of agency operation; therefore, they need to be selected with special care. A new administrator might want to involve some board members who are longtime community residents on a recruitment and screening committee to select these generalists. Once they are selected, orientation to confidentiality and clients' needs should take place even before office procedures, appointments, and recordkeeping.

Support staff need support, too. Administrators and other professionals too often forget to include support staff in important meetings or decisions. Support staff should be part of the agency team, not simply to take notes and not speak. With everyone working together and providing mutual support, clients are able to experience warm, friendly, and helpful reception, with the support staff knowing what is going on and where to find people.

Visibility Issues

The agency is as visible and as vulnerable to public criticism as are the professionals who work there. Its reputation depends upon the relationships staff members have developed with the community, including the director, professional staff, and support staff. An effective rural mental health administrator is as likely to be found working on the Fourth of July celebration planning committee as at a professional association meeting. Active participation in community-wide activities is expected of anyone who cares about the community. People who cannot enjoy the typical local events, church socials, potlucks, and parades will probably not survive in rural areas.

Helping other community agencies can greatly enhance the public image of the mental health agency. For example, working agreements with law enforcement agencies to provide assistance with crises involving mental illness, alcohol situations, and family violence calls has led to the strong support of law enforcement for mental health programs. Mental health prevention services include community education programs, information booths at county fairs, and speaking engagements at local community club meetings. There is no way to hide in a small town. The only real alternative is to enjoy the visibility, building the agency reputation while enjoying community life.

Rural Cultures

There has not been sufficient time for rural communities to incorporate mental health services or professionals into their local culture. Mental health treatment is viewed as an urban phenomenon that has been transplanted into rural areas and is now adapting to that rural environment and culture. There is no local tradition for providing mental health services as there is, for example, for providing education. Most mental health programs were established by external forces with federal and state funds. Many are now beginning to look for local financial support as the federal funds diminish and new needs are identified.

Before a small community will assume any responsibility for support of mental health programs, they need to adopt them as their own. This can be difficult when the guidelines and the mandates are from national and state agencies. For example, in a county with three mental health professionals, there was an effort to comply with federal guidelines that require that twenty-four-hour emergency service be available in case of a need for hospitalization. The three professionals alternated being "on call," each taking a week at a time. Although there are few emergencies, a large proportion of their time "off work" was restricted by having to be available, and they objected to providing so much time without compensation. The director recognized the importance of the twenty-four-hour emergency services and took the problem to the board of directors, where someone suggested paying the workers fifty cents an hour during the time they are "on call," in recognition of the inconvenience. The problem in financing this plan was taken to the county supervisors, who were ultimately responsible for mental health programming in the county. It took some time for the board to be sure that they fully understood the problem, the guideline requirements, the need for that service in the county, and the need for the funds. They then met two times with the supervisors, eventually persuading them to approve the funds. With this small involvement, emergency services has become a county program rather than an imported urban program.

Rapid staff turnover can create serious problems for any program, but especially for small organizations. The ability of staff members to relate and identify with the local culture is a factor in their desire to stay in rural areas (Weber, 1976). Potential employees need a thorough orientation to the local culture, community expectations, and personal and professional life-styles before they decide whether they want to take the job. Rural agencies need to recruit people who like rural culture and rural people. It is often said that rural people are slow to accept newcomers, but it is also true that urban newcomers have difficulty accepting rural people and culture.

Professional Advancement

The rural setting offers some peculiar dilemmas for the professional development of the mental health administrators. There are rarely any opportunities for promotion within the same community. One cannot be a rural administrator for long and still follow the typical organizational career. One pattern is for the professional to seek a stable small town for self and family, assume an administrative position, and make that a life career. That is the typical pattern of small-town physicians and attorneys. Another pattern is to use small towns as learning opportunities and steppingstones to other larger cities and organizations with greater salaries and responsibilities. This tends to be a career pattern of public school administrators in rural areas.

Both patterns have advantages and disadvantages for individuals and for the programs they lead. The settled administrator provides stability to the agency and has time to develop strong and continuing relationships in the community. The person who moves from place to place must spend considerable time and energy developing relationships in each new position. Persons who stay in one place find it difficult to keep in touch with new developments. They are always in the position of the knowledgeable authority, giving information and consultation without the opportunity of exchange with other professionals of similar education and training. As is true of the small-town physician, they run a risk of becoming out of date and less effective than their urban colleagues. However, persons who move from one town to another are also limited. They can or will still be isolated from the professional environment of an urban area. There are only a limited number of positions available and few advancements within the rural environment.

It has been suggested that the federal government establish support for specialized research and program development focused on rural issues (President's

Commission, 1978). It has also been recommended that state mental health agencies employ rural specialists (Washington Human Resource Development Task Force, 1981). Should those recommendations be implemented, there would be a few opportunities for rural administrators to enter large bureaucracies based on their expertise in rural practice.

Rural mental health administrators also need to budget generously for professional advancement and continuing education travel to alleviate the effects of professional isolation. Both administrators and staff need opportunities to meet with other professionals and be informed of new developments in the field. Boards that resist travel allocations might be convinced if they can see that such travel helps provide them with improved service delivery. For example, an administrator learns from attending state conferences and reviewing professional literature that the state and federal priorities have shifted to improving services for chronically mentally ill. There may be a small number of chronic patients in the county. The administrator may introduce some ideas at the agency board and a local service club that relate to the priority, reminding them that "we have been wanting to see if we could fix up the Smith house for a group home, and maybe this is the time to do it." The rural mental health administrator has translated broad social policy into local needs by providing local leadership and thereby enhancing his or her professional image.

And finally, the professional advancement of rural administrators is likely to be limited if they are not sensitive to local cultures. There may be a personal conflict between the desire for promotion and advancement in bureaucratic structures and the rural orientation to persons rather than to institutions. Achievement or status for the rural administrator is based more on recognition of a job well done than on an upward promotion. Perhaps the recent revival of interest in rural mental health services will help to alleviate this dilemma.

Conclusion

Each rural community is different, but each will tend to operate on a personal rather than on an institutional basis. This means that the administrator and the staff need to carry out not mental health programs, but *community* mental health, in the fullest sense of the word "community." Rural life is clearly different from urban life. A small town is no place to go to get away from people; it is where you go if you want to get closer to people. In other respects, the administration and management functions of rural mental health are similar to those of urban mental health.

References

Burdge, R. J., and Rogers, E. M. *Social Change in Rural Societies.* (2nd ed.). Englewood Cliffs, N.J.: Prentice-Hall, 1972.

Cedar, T., and Salasin, J. *Research Directions for Rural Mental Health.* McLean, Va.: Mitre Corporation, 1979.

Conklin, C. "Rural Community Care-Givers." *Social Work,* 1980, *25,* 495-497.

Davenport, J., and Davenport, J. *Boomtowns and Human Services.* Laramie: Department of Social Work, University of Wyoming, 1979.

Dunbar, E. R. "Educating Social Workers for Rural Mental Health Settings." In *Symposium on Rural Mental Health.* Lincoln: University of Nebraska Press, in press.

Eisenhart, M., and Ruff, T. "Doing Mental Health Work in Rural versus Urban: Differences in the Organization and Meaning of Work." Paper presented at the Fifth National Institute on Social Work in Rural Areas, Southern Regional Education Board, 1980.

Fenby, B. L. "Social Work in a Rural Setting." *Social Work,* 1978, *23* (2), 162-164.

Flax, J. W., and others. *Mental Health and Rural America: An Overview and Annotated Bibliography.* Washington, D.C.: National Institute of Mental Health, 1979.

Hagebak, B. R. "Mental Health Services in Rural Areas: The Case for Interagency Coordination and Service Integration." Paper presented at the Third Annual Georgia Primary Health Care Conference, Atlanta, 1980.

Hargreaves, W. A., and Delay, E. A. "Program Evaluation in a Rural Community Mental Health Center." *Community Mental Health Journal,* 1979, *15* (2), 104-118.

Hartman, E. A., and Perlman, B. "Characteristics and Problems of Rural Mental Health Administrators." Paper presented at the Second National Assembly of State Mental Health Manpower Development Program, National Institute of Mental Health, Rockville, Md., July 1980.

Hassinger, E. W., and Whiting, L. R. *Rural Health Services: Organization, Delivery and Use.* Ames: Iowa State University Press, 1976.

Huessy, H. R. "Rural Models." In H. Barton and L. Bellak (Eds.), *Progress in Community Mental Health.* New York: Grune & Stratton, 1972.

Husaini, B. A., and Neff, J. A. *The Mental Health Needs of a Rural Middle Tennessee Community: A Preliminary Report.* Nashville: Tennessee State University, 1977.

Lamb, R. K. "Suggestions for a Study of Your Hometown." In F. M. Cox and others (Eds.), *Tactics and Techniques of Community Practice.* Itasca, Ill.: Peacock, 1977.

Luther, J. "Transactions Among Partners." Address to the Forum of the Partnership for Rural Improvement, Spokane, Washington, 1981.

Mazer, M. *People and Predicaments.* Cambridge, Mass.: Harvard University Press, 1976.

President's Commission on Mental Health. *Report to the President from the President's Commission on Mental Health.* Washington, D.C.: U.S. Government Printing Office, 1978.

Reynolds, R. C., Banks, S. A., and Murphee, A. H. *The Health of a Rural County: Perspectives and Problems.* Gainesville: University Presses of Florida, 1976.

Schott, M. "Casework: Rural." In W. H. Johnson (Ed.), *Rural Human Services, A Book of Readings.* Itasca, Ill.: Peacock, 1980.

Schwab, J., Warheit, G., and Holzer, C. *Mental Health: Rural-Urban Comparisons.* Proceedings of the Fourth International Congress of Social Psychiatry, 1972.

Srole, L. "Urbanization and Mental Health: Some Reformulations." *American Scientist,* 1972, *60* (5), 576–583.

U.S. Department of Health, Education, and Welfare. "A New Day in Rural Mental Health Services." In *New Dimensions in Mental Health.* Rockville, Md.: Alcohol, Drug, and Mental Health Administration, 1978.

Vidich, A. J., and Bensman, J. *Small Town in Mass Society: Class, Power, and Religion in a Rural Community.* Princeton, N.J.: Princeton University Press, 1956.

Warren, R. *Community in America.* Chicago: Rand McNally, 1978.

Washington Human Resource Development Task Force. *Rural Sub-Committee Report.* Olympia, Wash.: Division of Mental Health, 1981.

Weber, G. K. "Preparing Social Workers for Practice in Rural Social Systems." *Journal of Education for Social Work,* 1976, *12*(3), 108-115.

ॐ Name Index ॐ

⛦ Subject Index ⛦